A CLINICAL APPROACH TO NEURO-OPHTHALMIC DISORDERS

A CLINICAL APPROACH TO NEURO-OPHTHALMIC DISORDERS

Edited by

Vivek Lal MD (Medicine), DM (Neurology), FIAN, FRCP (Edin)

Professor and Head
Department of Neurology at PGIMER
Chandigarh, India

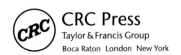

CRC Press
Taylor & Francis Group
Boca Raton London New York

CRC Press is an imprint of the
Taylor & Francis Group, an **informa** business

First edition published 2023
by CRC Press
6000 Broken Sound Parkway NW, Suite 300, Boca Raton, FL 33487-2742

and by CRC Press
4 Park Square, Milton Park, Abingdon, Oxon, OX14 4RN

CRC Press is an imprint of Taylor & Francis Group, LLC

© 2023 Taylor & Francis Group, LLC

Library of Congress Cataloging-in-Publication Data

Names: Lal, Vivek, editor.
Title: A clinical approach to neuro-ophthalmic disorders / edited by Vivek Lal.
Description: First edition. | Boca Raton, FL : CRC Press, 2022. | Includes
bibliographical references and index. | Summary: "Neuro-ophthalmology is
a merged subspecialty of neurology and ophthalmology dealing with
complex multisystem diseases presenting with visual manifestations. This
book helps the reader in recognizing, approaching, and managing such a
patient"-- Provided by publisher.
Identifiers: LCCN 2022002542 (print) | LCCN 2022002543 (ebook) | ISBN
9780367030513 (hardback) | ISBN 9781032251486 (paperback) | ISBN
9780429020278 (ebook)
Subjects: MESH: Vision Disorders | Nervous System Diseases
Classification: LCC RE951 (print) | LCC RE951 (ebook) | NLM WW 140 | DDC
617.7/5--dc23/eng/20220209
LC record available at https://lccn.loc.gov/2022002542
LC ebook record available at https://lccn.loc.gov/2022002543

ISBN: 978-0-367-03051-3 (hbk)
ISBN: 978-1-032-25148-6 (pbk)
ISBN: 978-0-429-02027-8 (ebk)

DOI: 10.1201/9780429020278

Typeset in Warnock Pro
by KnowledgeWorks Global Ltd.

Access the Support Material: www.routledge.com/9781032251486

To both my Patients and Residents—they are the joy of my world.

*To My Wife—Sadhna, My Children—Raghav, Parth & Gayatri
and my Retriever Biba—they are my world.*

*I wish my wife continuous good luck and my noble children all the
very best as they face the challenges life throws at them.*

CONTENTS

FOREWORD

When I was approached to write a Foreword for *A Clinical Approach to Neuro-Ophthalmic Disorders*, edited by my old friend Professor Vivek Lal, I was intrigued to see how this vastly experienced clinical neuro-ophthalmologist and educator would apply his experience to conceiving and executing such a manual, with a team of eminent Indian and international experts. Clinical neuro-ophthalmology, one of the sub-specialties in clinical medicine which spans major disciplines, in this case neurology and ophthalmology, is as a consequence often perceived as a difficult clinical subject. This is especially so since most practitioners with an interest migrate to the subject either from a purely neurological or ophthalmological training. To successfully achieve expertise in the subject requires considerable knowledge and practical skills in both, as well as a good knowledge of neuro-anatomy and neurophysiology. For example, the examination of the fundus, which is routinely achieved by the neurologist using a direct ophthalmoscope now needs to be supplemented by the ophthalmologist's direct ophthalmoscopy using a slit lamp and ocular coherence tomography to fully appreciate ongoing pathological processes affecting the fundus and optic nerve axons.

Upon reading through the chapters, it is apparent that this fusion of the relevant parts of these two specialties relevant to clinical neuro-ophthalmology has been extremely well addressed. The text is firmly based on the clinical approach to the patient with neuro-ophthalmological problems, but it also provides essential background knowledge that is fundamental to clinical practice. Of particular value to the trainee neuro-ophthalmologist is the first chapter of each section, providing a well-considered clinical approach to the patient presenting with specific neuro-ophthalmological symptoms, for example, visual loss, gaze disorder. There are also a couple of very useful chapters on clinical approaches to dealing with pediatric neuro-ophthalmological problems.

All in all, this textbook is very clearly written and is to be highly recommended for those who want to learn more about assessing and treating patients with clinical neuro-ophthalmological problems.

Christopher Kennard
Professor Emeritus in Clinical Neurology
University of Oxford

PREFACE

näsayämyätma-bhäva-stho jnäna-dépena bhäsvatä

10:11

Dispel—darkness born of ignorance by the illuminating lamp of knowledge.

Bhagavad Gita

Information is not knowledge. The only source of knowledge is Experience.

Albert Einstein

Neurology training involves apprenticeship with a disciplined clinical approach. Neurological illnesses are a perfect maze and require tying up of various loose ends diligently to reach a rational conclusion. Neuro-ophthalmological clues are vital to make a diagnosis but are often ignored and under narrated. Patients shuttle between Neurology, Medicine, Ophthalmology and Neurosurgery. The reason is simple – neither the ophthalmologists nor the neurologists are well versed with this interface branch of neuro-ophthalmology. Classical teaching focuses on core neurology, often missing out on subtle neuro-ophthalmic clues. On the periphery of neurology and ophthalmology is this subspeciality of neuro-ophthalmology that encompasses the symptoms related to vision, which have significant systemic bearings.

The eyes are undoubtedly the window to not just the brain but also the mirror of body. Silhouettes of many diseases are reflected in various forms, but as they say eyes don't see, what the mind doesn't know. Often, during medical meetings, I am asked about "ready to go to" and simplified references for common neuro-ophthalmic clinical syndromes. I conceptualized this book on table after I realized the lacunae in neuro-ophthalmology training of neurologists.

A mundane-looking optic disc edema may unfold an entire chronicle. Papilledema and papillitis are ominous ramifications of numerous diseases like idiopathic intracranial hypertension and various demyelinating disorders. Knowledge of these and many such neuro-ophthalmic manifestations is indispensable for an accurate diagnosis. Recognition of these abnormalities is the key and is of profound importance in daily practice.

As the title suggests, this book pivots around how to approach individual neuro-ophthalmic substrates. It focuses on clinical approach, which is the most priced armamentarium of a neuro-ophthalmologist.

This book is a humble attempt to amalgamate pearls of wisdom from masters of neuro-ophthalmology. It is broadly divided into sections – basics of neuro-ophthalmology, the afferent and the efferent systems for generating a structured thought process. Every chapter has been strategically textured keeping in mind the interest of young clinicians in training.

Normally, requesting authors of this stature is a herculean task. I am overwhelmed to put on record that every author sent their chapter well in time and supported me in every way. I cannot express my gratitude enough toward each author for their deep indulgence and extraordinary contributions to this academic venture.

I put together and consolidated the knowledge I have gathered from my teachers and the experience I have gained not just from my patients but also my students who are indeed a part of my extended family. I also acknowledge the immense contribution from my ophthalmology, radiology and pathology colleagues without whom this book wouldn't be seeing light of the day.

I am grateful to one person in particular Aastha Takkar Kapila. She has single-handedly midwifed the birth of this book. I am also grateful to my departmental research team and the publishing team consisting of Shivangi Pramanik and Himani Dwivedi from CRC Press/Taylor & Francis for their meticulous approach in planning the logistics.

I hope this academic endeavor benefits young neurologists, physicians and ophthalmologists in training.

This book has taken shape during the most painful and heart-rending pandemic that has taken an unprecedented toll globally. All the proceeds from this book, every single penny will go to the poor patients' fund of my institute.

ACKNOWLEDGMENTS

I gratefully acknowledge my parents DS Lt. Col H. G. Lal (AMC) and Amrit Lal – Their only passion in life was to educate their children.

I thank my younger brother Naveen and younger sister Namrata – they know why I thank them!

ABOUT THE EDITOR

Dr Vivek Lal [MD, DM-Neurology, FIAN, FRCP (Edin)] studied medicine and did his training in neurology at the prestigious Postgraduate Institute of Medical Education and Research (PGIMER), Chandigarh, India. He went on to become Professor, became the Chief of Department of Neurology and subsequently took the charge as Director of PGIMER, Chandigarh over his illustrious career spanning more than 30 years. He also served as the Dean of Baba Farid University of Health Sciences, Punjab, India and is a member of the editorial teams for journals on *Neuro-Ophthalmology, Annals of Indian Academy of Neurology* and the Indian edition of the *European Journal of Neurology*. He is a Fellow of Royal College of Physicians (Edin) (FRCP) and Indian Academy of Neurology (FIAN). He is also Chairman of the Neuro-Ophthalmology subsection of the Indian Academy of Neurology.

His major areas of interest are Headache and Neuro-Ophthalmology and he has done pioneering work in the identification and discovery of Ophthalmoplegic Migraine in India. He has the single largest series in world literature on Ophthalmoplegic Migraine and has several national and international publications, chapters in several books and awards to his credit. He runs a regular Neuro-Ophthalmology sub-specialty clinic catering to patients from all over India.

His presentations, especially 'The Grand Rounds' are extremely popular among his students, and he has been awarded 'Master Teacher' reward for his outstanding postgraduate neurology teaching. He has chaired/co-chaired and has been guest faculty for Neuro-Ophthalmology programs at XXIII—World Congress of Neurology (WCN), Kyoto, Japan in 2017; XXIV—WCN Dubai in 2019; and XXV—WCN in Rome 2021. He was guest faculty to the University of Oxford, UK, in March 2016 and was also a Teaching Faculty at Medical Ophthalmology Society (MOS), UK. He was an invited Neurologist in Rotary International Medical Mission to Ethiopia, Oct–Nov 2015. During this time, he was also the Visiting Neuro-Ophthalmologist, University of Addis Ababa, Ethiopia. He has been actively involved in medical public awareness programs and philanthropic works at regional and national levels. His concept of good research revolves around the adage "For the patients, By the patients and with the patients".

CONTRIBUTORS

Aniruddha Agarwal
Assistant Professor
Advanced Eye Center
Department of Ophthalmology
Post Graduate Institute of Medical
    Education and Research (PGIMER)
Chandigarh, India

Chirag Kamal Ahuja
Associate Professor
Department of Radiodiagnosis and
    Imaging (Division of Neuroradiology)
Post Graduate Institute of Medical
    Education and Research (PGIMER)
Chandigarh, India

**Mangayarkarasi Thandampallayam
    Ajjeya**
Resident Physician
Department of Neurology
University of Kentucky
Lexington, Kentucky

Muhammad Hassaan Ali
Senior Registrar and Consultant
    Ophthalmologist
Department of Ophthalmology
Allama Iqbal Medical College
Jinnah Hospital
Lahore, Pakistan

Fellow
Pediatric Ophthalmology and
    Strabismus
Stein Eye Institute
University of California
Los Angeles, California

Bayan Al-Othman
Clinical Assistant Professor
University of Rochester
Rochester, New York

Selvakumar Ambika
Director
Department of Neuro Ophthalmology
Medical Research Foundation
Sankara Nethralaya
Chennai, India

Giulia Amore
Doheny Eye Institute
UCLA Stein Eye Institute
Department of Ophthalmology
University of California
Los Angeles, California

IRCCS Istituto delle Scienze
    Neurologiche di Bologna
UOC Clinica Neurologica
Bologna, Italy

Samuel Asanad
Doheny Eye Institute
UCLA Stein Eye Institute
Department of Ophthalmology
University of California
Los Angeles, California

Jason J.S. Barton
Professor
Canada Research Chair
Marianne Koerner Chair in Brain
    Diseases
Departments of Medicine (Neurology),
    Ophthalmology and Visual Sciences,
    Psychology
University of British Columbia
Vancouver, Canada

Louis R. Caplan
Senior Neurologist
Beth Israel Deaconess Medical Center
Boston, Massachusetts

Professor Neurology
Harvard University
Cambridge, Massachusetts

Hui-Chen Cheng
Assistant Professor
School of Medicine
National Yang Ming Chiao Tung
    University
Taipei, Taiwan

Director
Neuro-Ophthalmology & Strabismus
    Section
Department of Ophthalmology
Taipei Veterans General Hospital
Taipei, Taiwan

Jared Ching
Cambridge Eye Unit
Addenbrooke's Hospital
Cambridge University Hospitals
Cambridge, United Kingdom

John Van Geest Centre for Brain
    Repair and MRC Mitochondrial
    Biology Unit
Department of Clinical Neurosciences
University of Cambridge
Cambridge, United Kingdom

Stacey Aquino Cohitmingao
Associate Professor
Department of Medicine
Cebu Institute of Medicine
Cebu City, Philippines

Fiona Costello
Professor
Departments of Clinical
    Neurosciences and Surgery
Cumming School of Medicine
University of Calgary
Calgary, Canada

Director, Roy and Joan Allen
    Chair in Vision and Visual Sciences
Hotchkiss Brain Institute
Calgary, Canada

Mangat R. Dogra
Professor (retired)
Advanced Eye Centre
Post Graduate Institute of Medical
    Education and Research (PGIMER)
Chandigarh, India

Mohit Dogra
Associate Professor
Advanced Eye Centre
Post Graduate Institute of Medical
    Education and Research (PGIMER)
Chandigarh, India

Mohamed Elkasaby
Cognitive Neurology Fellow
Daroff-Dell'Osso Ocular Motility
    Laboratory
Neurological Institute
University Hospitals

Department of Neurology
Case Western Reserve University

Neurology Service
Louis Stokes Cleveland VA Medical
    Center
Cleveland, Ohio

Zane Foster
Resident
Stanley H. Appel Department of
    Neurology
Houston Methodist Hospital
Houston, Texas

Neel Fotedar
Assistant Professor
Department of Neurology
Case Western Reserve University

Neurological Institute
University Hospitals Cleveland Medical
    Center

Neurology Service
Louis Stokes Cleveland VA Medical Center
Cleveland, Ohio

Ravindra Kumar Garg
Professor and Head
Department of Neurology
King George Medical University
Lucknow, India

Manoj K. Goyal
Additional Professor
Department of Neurology
Post Graduate Institute of Medical
    Education and Research (PGIMER)
Chandigarh, India

Amod Gupta
Emeritus Professor of Ophthalmology
Post Graduate Institute of Medical
    Education and Research (PGIMER)
Chandigarh, India

Vishali Gupta
Professor
Advanced Eye Center
Department of Ophthalmology
Post Graduate Institute of Medical
    Education and Research (PGIMER)
Chandigarh, India

Sabia Handa
Senior Resident
Advanced Eye Center
Department of Ophthalmology
Post Graduate Institute of Medical
    Education and Research (PGIMER)
Chandigarh, India

Simon J. Hickman
Consultant Neurologist
Royal Hallamshire Hospital
England, United Kingdom

Azad M. Irani
Consultant Neurologist
Jaslok Hospital & Research Centre
Mumbai, India

Mayank Jain
Fellow, Pediatric Ophthalmology,
    Adult Strabismus and
    Neuro-Ophthalmology
Child Sight Institute
Jasti V. Ramanamma Children's Eye
    Care Center
L V Prasad Eye Institute
Hyderabad, India

Sahil Jain
Senior Resident
Advanced Eye Centre
Post Graduate Institute of Medical
    Education and Research (PGIMER)
Chandigarh, India

Deeksha Katoch
Associate Professor
Advanced Eye Centre
Post Graduate Institute of Medical
    Education and Research (PGIMER)
Chandigarh, India

Sarosh M. Katrak
Neurologist
Sir JJ Group of Hospitals and GMC
    Hospital
Jaslok Hospital & Research Centre
Mumbai, India

Savleen Kaur
Assistant Professor
Advanced Eye Center
Department of Ophthalmology
Post Graduate Institute of Medical
    Education and Research (PGIMER)
Chandigarh, India

Ramesh Kekunnaya
Director
LVPEI Network, Child Sight Institute,
    Neuro Ophthalmology, Centre for
    Technology Innovation, Capacity
    Building
L V Prasad Eye Institute
Hyderabad, India

Ashwini Kini
Resident Physician
Department of Neurology
University of Kentucky
Lexington, Kentucky

Fellow
Department of Ophthalmology
Blanton Eye Institute
Houston Methodist Hospital
Houston, Texas

Gaurav Kumar
Department of Ophthalmology
King George Medical University
Lucknow, India

Neeraj Kumar
Department of Neurology
King George Medical University
Lucknow, India

Vivek Lal
Director
Post Graduate Institute of Medical
    Education and Research (PGIMER)
Chandigarh, India

Andrew G. Lee
Herb and Jean Lyman Centennial Chair
    of Ophthalmology

Adjunct Professor of Ophthalmology
Baylor College of Medicine

Department of Ophthalmology
Blanton Eye Institute
Houston Methodist Hospital
Houston, Texas

Departments of Ophthalmology,
    Neurology, and Neurosurgery
Weill Cornell Medicine
New York City, New York

Department of Ophthalmology
The University of Texas Medical Branch
    (UTMB)
Galveston, Texas

UT MD Anderson Cancer Center
Houston, Texas

Texas A and M College of Medicine
Houston, Texas

The University of Iowa Hospitals and
    Clinics
Iowa City, Iowa

The University of Buffalo
Buffalo, New York

M. Madhusudanan
Professor and Head of Neurology
Travancore Medical College and Hospital
Quilon, India

Adjunct Professor of Neurology
Manipal University
Manipal, India

Professor-Emeritus of Neurology
Medical College
PRS Hospital
Trivandrum, India

Senior Consultant Neurologist
PRS Hospital
Trivandrum, India

Hardeep Singh Malhotra
Department of Neurology
King George Medical University
Lucknow, India

Contributors

Kiran Preet Malhotra
Department of Pathology
Dr. RML Institute of Medical Sciences
Lucknow, India

Dan Milea
Singapore National Eye Centre

Visual Neuroscience Group
Singapore Eye Research Institute

Duke–NUS Medical School
Singapore

Usha K. Misra
Department of Neurology
Sanjay Gandhi Post Graduate Institute of
Medical Sciences (PGIMER)
Lucknow, India

Manish Modi
Professor
Department of Neurology
Post Graduate Institute of Medical
Education and Research (PGIMER)
Chandigarh, India

Bruttendu Moharana
Senior Resident
Assistant Professor, Ophthalmology
(Vitreo-Retina, Uveitis, ROP)
All India Institute of Medical Sciences
Bhubaneswar, India

Uchenna Francis Nwako
Doheny Eye Institute
UCLA Stein Eye Institute
Department of Ophthalmology
University of California
Los Angeles, California

Krishnakumar Padmalakshmi
Associate Consultant
Department of Neuro Ophthalmology
Sankara Nethralaya
Chennai, India

Stacy L. Pineles
Professor of Ophthalmology
Department of Ophthalmology
Stein Eye Institute
University of California
Los Angeles, California

Gordon Plant
Consultant Neurologist
National Hospital for Neurology and
Neurosurgery
Moorfields Eye Hospital
London, United Kingdom

Bishan Radotra
Professor of Neuropathology
Head, Department of
Histopathology
Post Graduate Institute of Medical
Education and Research (PGIMER)
Chandigarh, India

Imran Rizvi
Associate Professor
Department of Neurology
King George Medical University
Lucknow, India

Alfredo Sadun
Doheny Eye Institute
UCLA Stein Eye Institute
Department of Ophthalmology
University of California
Los Angeles, California

Aasef G. Shaikh
Associate Professor
Department of Neurology
Department of Biomedical
Engineering
Case Western Reserve University

Neurological Institute
University Hospitals Cleveland Medical
Center

Neurology Service
Louis Stokes Cleveland VA Medical
Center
Cleveland, Ohio

Paramjeet Singh
Professor
Department of Radiodiagnosis
and Imaging (Division of
Neuroradiology)
Post Graduate Institute of Medical
Education and Research (PGIMER)
Chandigarh, India

Ramandeep Singh
Professor
Advanced Eye Centre
Post Graduate Institute of Medical
Education and Research (PGIMER)
Chandigarh, India

Simar Rajan Singh
Assistant Professor
Advanced Eye Centre
Post Graduate Institute of Medical
Education and Research (PGIMER)
Chandigarh, India

Varun K. Singh
Assistant Professor
Department of Neurology
Institute of Medical Sciences
Banaras Hindu University
Varanasi, India

Monika Singla
Associate Professor
Department of Neurology
Dayanand Medical College and Hospital
Ludhiana, Punjab, India

Prem S. Subramanian
Professor of Ophthalmology, Neurology,
and Neurosurgery
Sue Anschutz-Rodgers Eye Center
University of Colorado School of
Medicine
Aurora, Colorado

Padmaja Sudhakar
Associate Professor
Department of Neurology
University of Kentucky
Lexington, Kentucky

Jaspreet Sukhija
Professor
Advanced Eye Center
Department of Ophthalmology
Post Graduate Institute of Medical
Education and Research (PGIMER)
Chandigarh, India

William Sultan
Doheny Eye Institute
UCLA Stein Eye Institute

Department of Ophthalmology
University of California
Los Angeles, California

Aastha Takkar Kapila
Associate Professor
Department of Neurology
Post Graduate Institute of Medical
Education and Research (PGIMER)
Chandigarh, India

Basavaraj Tigari
Assistant Professor
Advanced Eye Centre
Post Graduate Institute of Medical
Education and Research (PGIMER)
Chandigarh, India

An-Guor Wang
A/Professor
Department of Ophthalmology
Taipei Veterans General Hospital
Taipei, Taiwan

Department of Ophthalmology
School of Medicine
National Yang-Ming University
Taipei, Taiwan

P. Vinny Wilson
Professor
Armed Forces Medical College
Pune, India

Patrick Yu-Wai-Man
Professor of Ophthalmology
Cambridge Eye Unit
Addenbrooke's Hospital
Cambridge University Hospitals

John Van Geest Centre for Brain Repair
    and MRC Mitochondrial Biology Unit
Department of Clinical Neurosciences
University of Cambridge
Cambridge, United Kingdom

NIHR Biomedical Research Centre at
    Moorfields Eye Hospital
UCL Institute of Ophthalmology
London, United Kingdom

Part I
Basics of Neuro-Ophthalmology

1

CLINICAL EXAMINATION IN NEURO-OPHTHALMOLOGY

Selvakumar Ambika, Krishnakumar Padmalakshmi

Introduction

Neuro-ophthalmology disorders can be involving either afferent or efferent visual pathway, at times both. History taking is the key, along with proper clinical evaluation and interpretation would direct the practitioner in perfect topographic localization and management of the disease.

History taking

Careful history taking alone can help us to determine the etiology of these disorders. The first step is to identify the pathway involved. If the afferent pathway is involved, the most common symptom is visual loss. Inflammatory etiologies present with visual loss associated with pain, and visual loss without pain can be due to vascular or compressive etiology.

It is important to know whether loss of vision is unilateral or bilateral. Monocular vision loss would indicate a lesion anterior to optic chiasm and thus guide us to tailor the ancillary investigations. Figure 1.1 shows common causes of visual loss. Detailed history including onset, duration and progression will help us to plan appropriate investigations.

The most common complaint associated with efferent pathway defect is double vision or diplopia. Diplopia can be monocular or binocular double vision, monocular diplopia is commonly of non-neurological and often related to ocular causes. Uncorrected refractive errors that cause monocular diplopia will improve with pinhole. In case of binocular diplopia, it is important to note if the separation of images is horizontal, vertical or oblique. It is also important to find in which particular gaze the images have maximum separation, as it can guide us to localize the cranial nerve palsy.

Other common neuro-ophthalmic symptoms include drooping of the eyelids, proptosis, squint, transient vision loss, visual field deficits, headache and facial spasms. Figure 1.2 gives the list of tools needed for examination of neuro-ophthalmic disorders.

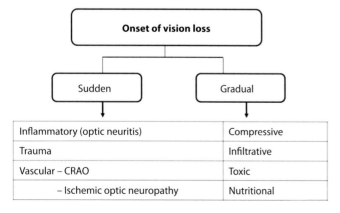

FIGURE 1.1 Causes of vision loss.

History of diurnal variation or symptoms worsening on exertion can be associated with ocular myasthenia gravis. Patients with generalized myasthenia gravis may give history of dysphagia, dysarthria, limb weakness, etc. if probed. Systemic history taking is important as diabetes, hypertension, dyslipidemia, etc. predispose to ischemic events. History of tuberculosis, any systemic malignancies, chronic medications like anti-tuberculous therapy, hydroxyquinolones, sildenafil, amiodarone, etc. need to be screened. Family history of vision loss secondary to any unexplained optic neuropathy should always be elicited. Personal history of smoking, alcohol, drug abuse, etc. has to be recorded to rule out toxic, drug-induced optic neuropathies. Table 1.1 shows the stepwise approach to clinical examination in neuro-ophthalmology.[1–3]

Visual acuity assessment

Visual acuity is a complex function of eye and is vital to monitor the progression of optic neuropathy. The distance and near visual acuity should be tested. The most widely used tool for measurement is the Snellen visual acuity chart.

The standard recording of visual acuity is by Snellen notation which is a fraction. The numerator denotes the testing distance (6 m or 20 feet) and the denominator is the distance at which a normal person is able to read the letter (Figure 1.3). Variations in the Snellen chart for patients who are unable to read include the "Landolt C" or the Illiterate E chart, which allows testing of acuity based on the orientation of the letters. Other visual acuity charts with better specifications include ETDRS, logMAR and Bailey-Lovie charts.

If the patient is unable to read visual acuity of 6/6, then it is necessary to look for improvement with pinhole, which will indicate a refractive error and complete refraction is mandatory in such cases. The best corrected visual acuity (BCVA) should always be established before proceeding further. Near visual acuity is tested at about 30 cm from the eye and the maximum smallest text the patient is able to read is recorded. Measurement of visual acuity in children requires expertise and patience. More time is to be spent with them in order to create a cordial atmosphere. The vision in children is tested by the response to light stimulus and whether child fixes and follows the light. The ability of a child to recognize faces, pick up an object and move freely in the examination room are additional clues to evaluate vision.

Optokinetic nystagmus drum is beneficial in assessing the vision in infants (Figure 1.4). It elicits jerk nystagmus with a slow phase following the target and a corrective jerk in the opposite direction. The degree of visual acuity can be assessed based on the size of target. The preferential looking test and visual-evoked potential (VEP) is also used to estimate visual acuity in infants. For older children, HOTV charts and Illiterate E test or pictorial charts can be used.[2,3]

Examination of pupils

Pupillary examination includes assessment of the size of the pupil in light/dark and also near stimulation with an accommodative target. The size of pupils is ascertained with the help of a

DOI: 10.1201/9780429020278-2

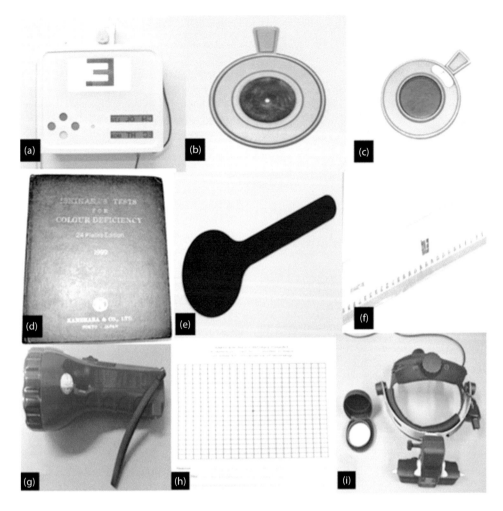

FIGURE 1.2 Basic requirements for examination—(a) Snellen visual acuity box, (b) pinhole, (c) red filter, (d) Ishihara chart, (e) occluder, (f) ruler, (g) torchlight, (h) Amsler grid, (i) indirect ophthalmoscope.

pupillary gauge (Figure 1.5). The shape and color of pupils should be documented.

The clues for pupillary examination are given in Table 1.2A.

The reaction of the pupil to light stimulus is usually tested in a dim lit room with the patient fixing at a distant target to eliminate accommodative response. Direct reflex to light is pupil constriction on exposure to light. The constriction of the pupil in the fellow eye (contralateral pupil) is called consensual response.

The best way to elicit a direct pupillary reflex is to have the patient fixate at a distance at least 3 m away and then shine the light approaching from slightly below. This would prevent the

TABLE 1.1: Stepwise Approach to Neuro-Ophthalmic Examination

Visual acuity assessment

Pupillary evaluation

External and anterior segment evaluation

Fundus examination

Assessment of ocular motility

Color vision

Contrast sensitivity

Visual field analysis

Electrophysiological tests

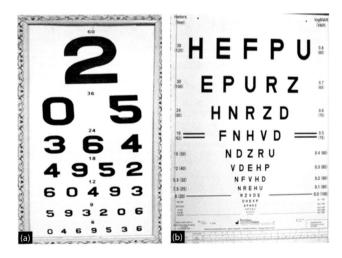

FIGURE 1.3 (a) Snellen Distant Visual Acuity chart, (b) Bailey-Love chart.

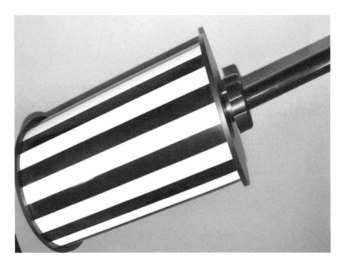

FIGURE 1.4   Optokinetic nystagmus drum.

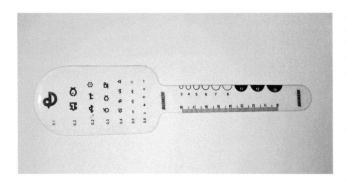

FIGURE 1.5   Pupillary gauge.

TABLE 1.2A: Prerequisites and Rules for Pupillary Examination

- Ensure presence of a dimly lit room before you start examination of pupils
- Hold the light for at least 3 seconds in the eye being examined for the direct light reflex
- While examining for indirect/consensual light reflex, ensure that the eyes are separated by patient's palm or a small cardboard held between the two eyes
- Record your observations under the headings below:
  1. Size of pupils
  2. Shape and color of the pupils
  3. Equality of size and shape
  4. Position of pupils in either eyes
  5. Direct and indirect light reflex
  6. Swinging light reflex—look out for RAPD
  7. Accommodation reflex
  8. Light near dissociation
  9. Tests for sympathetic/parasympathetic dysfunction if anisocoria is present

TABLE 1.2B: Grades of RAPD

Grade 1	Initial constriction followed by greater redilatation
Grade 2	Initial stall and greater redilatation
Grade 3	Immediate pupillary dilatation
Grade 4	Immediate pupillary dilatation following prolonged illumination of the good eye
Grade 5	Immediate dilatation with no secondary constriction

patient looking directly at the source of light and hence falsely generating an accommodation reflex (Figure 1.6).

The swinging flashlight test is used to test relative afferent pupillary defect (RAPD) and requires only one working pupil. In unilateral optic nerve diseases, RAPD is usually present. It may

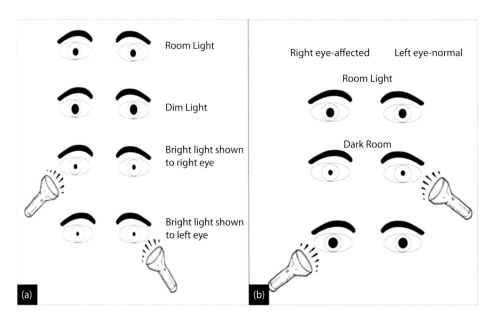

FIGURE 1.6   Normal pupillary light response. (a) Light projected into either elicit equal pupillary constriction. Swinging flash light test in a case of hypothetically affected right eye. (b) When light is shown into normal left eye, it elicits the same amount of pupillary constriction in both eyes; however, when light is shown to the abnormal right eye, it causes weaker pupillary constriction and both pupils dilate.

be present in bilateral cases if there is asymmetric involvement of optic nerves. Apart from optic neuropathy, RAPD can be present in severe vision loss like retinal detachment, dense amblyopia, ischemic retinal diseases, etc. Measurement of RAPD can be done using neutral density filters by 0.3 log units. Grades of RAPD are described in Table 1.2B.[3,4]

Absent reaction to light but brisk reaction to near target is called light-near dissociation (LND). It is seen in conditions like tonic pupil, Argyll Robertson pupil and Parinaud syndrome.

Usually, the pupil size is equal in both eyes. Anisocoria occurs due to efferent dysfunction of pupils and is referred to when the difference in the pupil size of either eye is 1.0 mm. About 20% of normal individuals may have physiological anisocoria.

It is important to look for associated ptosis and ocular motor restriction. Ptosis associated with pupil involving third nerve palsy is a surgical emergency and warrants immediate neuro-imaging. Partial pupil-sparing third nerve palsy also has to be watched closely as it can become pupil involving third nerve palsy at times. Usually, pupil-sparing complete third nerve palsy is of ischemic cause. Any patient with mild ptosis and miotic pupil should raise the suspicion of Horner's syndrome. Anisocoria more in bright light indicates that larger pupil has parasympathetic dysfunction, and anisocoria in dim illumination denotes that smaller pupil has sympathetic dysfunction.

Photostress test

Photostress test is used to differentiate vision loss due to macular pathology from optic nerve disease. When bright light is shown to the eye, the retinal pigments are bleached and the patient perceives a scotoma, and the time taken for patient to recover to the pre-test visual acuity is noted. The BCVA of the patient is documented and the patient is asked to fix at a bright light (light of indirect ophthalmoscope) for 10 seconds held 3 cm away. The photostress recovery time (PSRT) is the time taken for the patient to read the letters of the pre-test visual acuity line. The test is repeated with the other eye and then results are compared. In patients with macular pathology, PSRT will be longer compared to normal eye, while in patients with optic nerve pathology, there is usually no difference. Table 1.3 shows features to differentiate optic neuropathy from maculopathy.

External examination

Clinical assessment should start as soon as the patient enters the examination room, including gait, higher functions and external appearance. Abnormality of eyelid position such as ptosis or

TABLE 1.3: How to Differentiate Optic Neuropathy from Maculopathy

Optic Neuropathy	Maculopathy
RAPD present	Usually no RAPD
Decreased contrast	Metamorphopsia(Amsler test)
Normal photostress test	Abnormal photostress test

lid retraction needs to be noted. History of diurnal variation and fatiguability should be noted for any patient with lid droop to rule out ocular myasthenia. Simple clinical signs like improvement in ptosis after ice test and Cogan's lid twitch are more suggestive of myasthenia. Patients with third nerve palsy and certain myopathies as in chronic progressive external ophthalmoplegia and Miller Fisher syndrome also can present with ptosis, screening old photographs may help us to assess the onset of the findings. Ptosis should not be mistaken for conditions like blepharospasm or apraxia of lid opening. Measurement of palpebral fissure height, levator function and marginal reflex distance has to be done. Evaluation of proptosis is important as it may be associated with life-threatening intracranial and certain intraorbital tumors, carotid-cavernous fistulas, AV malformations, etc. Lid retraction can be a feature of thyroid eye disease or even dorsal midbrain syndrome.

Anterior segment

The anterior segment examination is done using slit lamp microscope, which helps in direct visualization of the cornea, lens, iris, anterior chamber and vitreous. Certain clinical conditions which can be picked up with clues on slit lamp examination (Figure 1.7) such as cork-screw vessels as seen in carotid-cavernous fistulas, exposure keratopathy changes in seventh cranial nerve palsy, vermiform movements in Adie's tonic pupil, Lisch nodules in neurofibromatosis 1, vitreous cells in papillitis.

Fundus evaluation

Posterior segment examination can be performed with direct ophthalmoscope or indirect ophthalmoscopy with a 20D, handheld lens and also by slit lamp biomicroscopy using 78- or 90D lens. On fundus examination, the optic nerve head size, shape, color and cup-disc ratio should be noted along with details of retinal vasculature, media clarity, retina appearance and particularly macular status (Figure 1.8).

Optic disc edema presents as blurred elevated disc with hyperemia. Optic disc swelling may occur due to various causes (Table 1.4) and it is necessary to differentiate between true edema

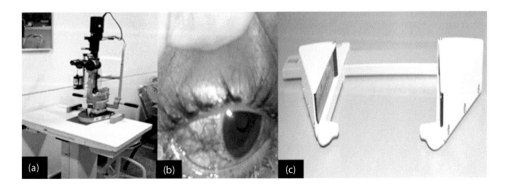

FIGURE 1.7 (a) Slit lamp, (b) cork-screw conjunctival vessels, (c) Hertel exophthalmometer.

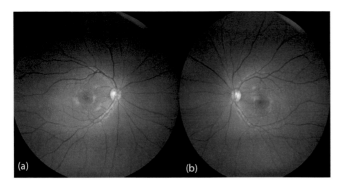

FIGURE 1.8 Normal fundus of right (a) and left eye (b).

TABLE 1.5: Optic Disc Features to Differentiate True and Pseudo Disc Edema

True Edema	Pseudo Disc Edema
Obscuration of surface vessels over disc	No vascular obscuration
Central cup present until late stage	Lack of physiological cup
Loss of spontaneous venous pulsations	SVP present
Disc hyperemia	Anomalous vascular branching
Dilatation of surface capillaries	Normal optic disc color/ hemorrhages, cotton wool spots rare

Abbreviation: SVP: Spontaneous Venous Pulsations

and pseudoedema (Table 1.5). Congenital optic disc anomalies like optic disc drusen can present as pseudoedema. Causes of pseudo disc edema are described in Table 1.6. Differentiating pseudoedema from true disc edema can avoid unnecessary investigations like neuroimaging brain and lumbar puncture. It is not necessary that all disc edemas are papilledema. It is important to differentiate an optic neuropathy from papilledema, as any disc edema with vision loss to begin with is an optic neuropathy. Papilledema patients will have normal optic nerve functions in early stages and worsen in later stages only.

Optic disc pallor can occur due to the various pathological processes. Disc pallor can be primary or secondary depending on the etiology causing the same (Table 1.7). It can be of any nature temporal, diffuse, segmental, bowties, etc. The presence of disc pallor indicated chronic nature of optic neuropathy and poor visual prognosis. Optic disc appearance should always be correlated with the optic nerve function as the vision and fields can improve after treatment in few instances like compressive optic neuropathy, optic neuritis. Figure 1.9 shows different types of abnormal optic discs.[5,6]

Extraocular movement abnormalities

Any patient with extraocular motility abnormality has to be watched for abnormal head posture. Both ductions and versions should be tested and limitation of movements recorded in all nine gazes (Figure 1.10). A subjective scale from +4 to −4 (+ indicates overaction and − indicates underaction) is used as it is helpful in the follow-up of patients with paralytic squint. Ocular misalignment can be horizontal or vertical. Horizontal can be eso- or exodeviations. Exodeviation (Exophoria/Exotropia) indicates outward deviation of the non-fixating eye and esodeviation (esophoria/esotropia) indicates an inward deviation of non-fixating eye. Tropia is a manifest squint, whereas phoria is latent and manifests when fusion is interrupted. Vertical misalignment can be hyper- or hypodeviation. In hypertropia, the non-fixating eye is higher, and in hypotropia, it is lower.

TABLE 1.4: Causes of Optic Disc Edema Based on Etiology

Inflammatory
Ischemic/vascular causes
Compressive
Infiltrative
Infective
Hereditary
Ocular hypotony
Post-trauma

If the ocular misalignment is constant in all directions, it is a concomitant strabismus but if the degree of misalignment varies depending on the direction of gaze, it is non-concomitant strabismus. Paralytic strabismus is usually non-concomitant.

Ductions are monocular eye movements. Medial movement of eye is termed as adduction, lateral is—abduction, upward—elevation/supraduction, downward-depression/infraduction. Vergences are binocular eye movements, which may be convergence or divergence. Convergence is tested by asking the patient to look at an accommodative target as it is brought closer to the nose and is associated with physiological constriction of pupils. Disorders of midbrain and Parkinson's disease can cause convergence insufficiency.

Saccades
These are rapid eye movements that quickly redirect the eye such that an image of an object is brought to the fovea. Peak velocity of saccades varies from 30 to 700 deg/second. Horizontal saccades are tested by asking the patient to look at the target (e.g., examiners index finger) straight ahead and then rapidly look at another object placed laterally at about 30 degrees. The patient is asked to look alternately between the central target and that placed laterally and the speed and accuracy are noted. In a similar manner, the vertical saccades are tested. Slowing of saccades is seen in cerebellar and supranuclear disorders.

Pursuits
Smooth pursuit stabilizes the image of an object on or near the fovea during slow movement of the object. To test smooth pursuit movement, the patient is asked to fixate at a target object which is moved across both in the horizontal and vertical directions. The target is moved at a speed of not more than 30 deg/second and not too laterally and the patient's eye movements are noted. Pursuits are affected in temporo-parieto-occipital cortex and ipsilateral deep parietal cortex lesions.

TABLE 1.6: Causes of Pseudo Disc Edema

Optic disc drusen
Crowded disc
Tilted disc
Myelinated nerve fibers
Megalopapilla
Morning glory disc

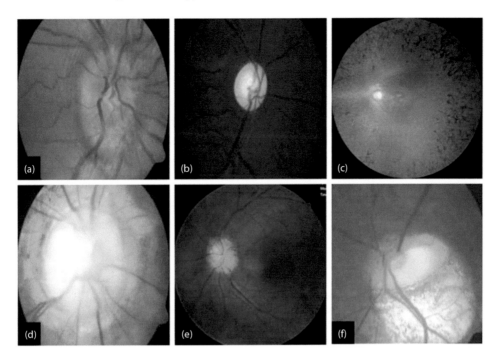

FIGURE 1.9   (a) Disc edema, (b) disc pallor, (c) retinitis pigmentosa, (d) disc coloboma, (e) optic disc drusen and (f) tilted disc.

TABLE 1.7: Classification of Optic Atrophy

Ophthalmoscopic	Pathological	Etiological
Primary	Ascending	Consecutive
Secondary	Descending	Circulatory
Consecutive	Hereditary	Pressure & traction
Cavernous		Post-inflammatory
Segmental or partial		Toxic
		Traumatic
		Metabolic
		Hereditary

Clinical tests to assess ocular misalignment

Cover-uncover test in patients with ocular misalignment along with prism bar cover test/Krimsky helps to characterize and quantify the deviation.

- *Prism bar cover test*—A prism is placed in front of deviating eye (apex of the prism toward the deviation). An alternate cover test is performed by alternately occluding one eye and observing the uncovered eye. The movement of eye behind the prism is watched as it takes up fixation. The prism strength is increased until there is no movement to take up fixation. Thus, the angle of deviation measured as the strength of the prism.

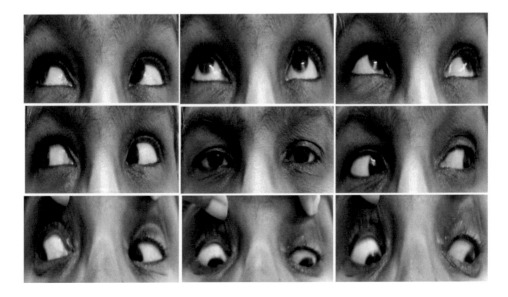

FIGURE 1.10   Composite of nine gaze photographs with normal extraocular movements.

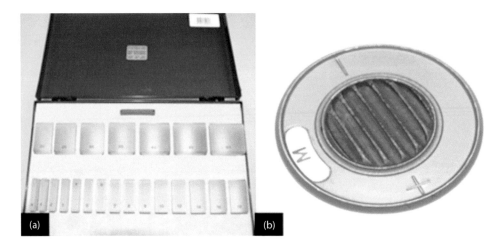

FIGURE 1.11   (a) Prism box, (b) Maddox rod.

- *Modified Krimsky test*—Prism bar is placed before the normal eye. Examiner observer the position of the corneal reflex as the patient fixates on a light source and prism strength is increased until the corneal reflex appears symmetrical, thus neutralizing the deviation.

Measurement is done for distance and near fixation with and without spectacle correction and abnormal head posture. In paralytic squint, deviation increases with gaze toward the direction of the action of the involved muscle. The primary deviation is referred to as the deviation of the normal eye when the prism is placed over the non-fixating paretic eye. The secondary deviation is the deviation of the sound eye when the paretic eye is fixing. According to Hering's law of equal innervations to yoke muscles, the secondary deviation is greater than the primary deviation. As an example, in case of sixth nerve palsy, esotropia will be greater when the normal eye fixates. This is due to strong stimulation of the paretic lateral rectus causing simultaneous equal innervations to the medial rectus in the non-paretic eye (secondary deviation).[1,3,6]

Maddox rod test

It is used to measure the amount of torsion. In a dim lit room, place the Maddox rods in front of each eye of the patient (Figure 1.11). Examiner stands in front of the patient and shines a light (direct ophthalmoscope) at the midline of the patient and asks how the lines are oriented with respect to each other. If the light streak seen by each eye is not parallel, the Maddox rods are rotated until they are parallel and horizontal, thus giving the torsional measurement.

Worth four-dot test

It is a test for red-green dissociation. The patient wears red-green goggles (red in front of the right eye, green in front of the left eye) and views a box of four dots as shown in Figure 1.12 (red on top, white at the bottom and two green placed horizontally).
  Interpretation:

- If all four dots are seen indicating:
  a. normal binocular response with no manifest deviation
  b. in the presence of manifest squint-harmonious anomalous retinal correspondence
- Only two red dots are seen—indicates left suppression
- If three green lights are seen—indicates right suppression
- If red and green dots alternate—alternate suppression
- If five dots are seen—diplopia is present

Forced duction test—FDT

This test is used to differentiate restrictive and paralytic pathology. After applying topical anesthetic with the patient is supine posture, lids are separated using a speculum. A forceps is held at the limbus and without pushing the globe posteriorly, the globe is rotated in the direction of action of the muscle being tested. If there is a free movement, FDT is negative, and if there is restriction, FDT is positive.

The forced generation test

Conjunctiva is grasped at the nasal limbus with the eye in adducted position after instilling topical anesthesia. The patient is instructed to abduct the eye. The examiner can feel a tug on the forceps if there is any residual lateral rectus function

Diplopia charting

Records the separation of images in nine different positions of gaze.

- *Requirement*—Dim lit room, Armstrong goggles or red-green filters (red in front of the right eye, green in front of the left eye), vertical streak of light (direct ophthalmoscope-streak).

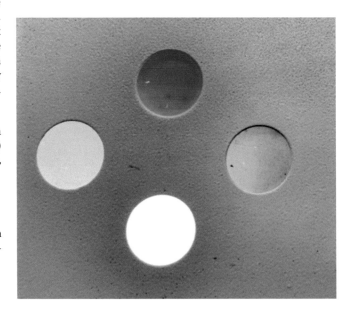

FIGURE 1.12   Worth four-dot test.

- The patient is seated 50 cm from the screen with the head still and erect wearing full refractive correction and able to appreciate the commands (either a superimposed image of red and green vertical streaks or separated red and green streaks at different gaze).

Separation is noted in both horizontal and vertical directions along with tilt if present. Separation increases in the direction of action of the paralyzed muscle. The distance between the streaks is measured in inches or centimeters. The chart is drawn from the patient's point of view.

Hess screen

The screen consists of a tangent pattern which is printed on a dark gray background. Red lights on the screen can be individually illuminated by a control panel, indicating the cardinal positions of gaze.

Method

The test is performed with each eye fixating in turn at the Hess screen placed at 50 cm from the patient. The patient wears red-green glasses to dissociate the two eyes. The red glasses are placed in front of the right eye first. The examiner should hold a red light projection pointer. The patient holds green light and superimposes green light over red light as shown by the examiner. Then the goggles are changed and the left eye has red goggles and the eye to be tested is the right eye (Figure 1.13).

Abducens nerve palsy

Here the patient complains of double vision more for distance and in the side of direction of the affected muscle. The images are usually uncrossed and are horizontally separated and the distance of the image increases in the direction of action of the affected muscle. There is a limitation of abduction in the affected eye with

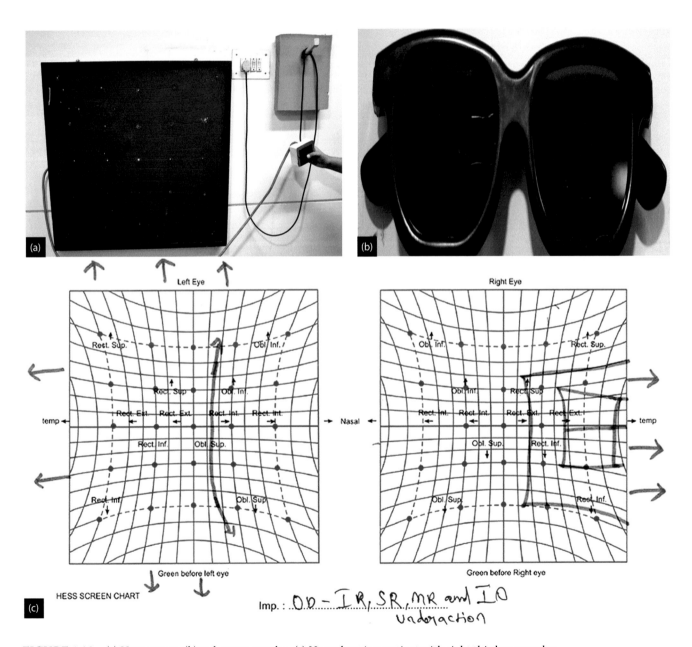

FIGURE 1.13 (a) Hess screen, (b) red-green goggles, (c) Hess chart in a patient with right third nerve palsy.

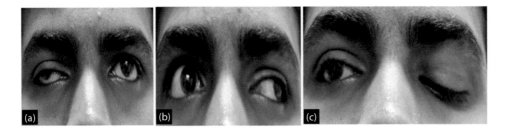

FIGURE 1.14   External photo of right third nerve palsy (a) with pseudo Duane's sign (b) and pseudo Van Graefe's sign (c).

esodeviation more for distance is seen. The sixth nerve can be affected due to neurogenic, myogenic or neuromuscular cause.

Oculomotor nerve palsy

Here the eye is usually down and out and the affected eye shows limitation of adduction, elevation and depression. Due to the involvement of levator muscle, ptosis may be present. The pupillary fibers are present in the superficial part of the third nerve and hence pupil may be dilated and fixed if involved as in compressive etiology. Contralateral elevation limitation and bilateral ptosis can be present in nuclear lesions. In ischemic causes as in diabetes or hypertension, the parasympathetic pupillomotor fibers are spared resulting in pupil-sparing third nerve palsy.

Aberrant regeneration of the third nerve is seen in long-standing third nerve palsy due to compressive or post-traumatic etiology (Figure 1.14).

*   Pseudo Duane's sign-widening of palpebral fissure on attempted adduction
*   Pseudo Argyll Robertson pupil—Constriction of the pupil on adduction
*   Pseudo Van Graefe's sign—Elevation of the eyelid on downgaze

Trochlear nerve palsy

Here the patient complains of double vision more in downgaze while getting downstairs or reading. Abnormal head posture may be present to overcome double vision. The patient may adopt a chin-up posture with an ipsilateral head turn and contralateral head tilt. The hypertropic eye can be recognized with the cover test. Bielschowsky-Parks three-step test is used to identify unilateral fourth nerve palsy.

Parks three-step test (for vertical diplopia)

Step 1 Which eye is hypertropic in primary gaze?
*   If the right eye is hypertropic, then there is weakness of depressors of the right eye (right inferior rectus/right superior oblique) or elevators of the left eye (left superior rectus/left inferior oblique)

Step 2 Hypertropia increases on right or left gaze?
*   Recti muscles have greater vertical action on abduction and oblique muscles have greater vertical action on adduction.
*   So if right hypertropia is worse on left gaze (right superior oblique/left superior rectus) is weak

Step 3 Hypertropia increase on right or left head tilt?
*   In the Bielschowsky head tilt test, the higher eye extorts, while the lower eye intorts.
*   If diplopia is worse on right head tilt, then the weak muscle in the lower (right) eye is the superior oblique and in the higher (left) eye is the inferior oblique.

Combining all three steps implies that the right superior oblique is weak.

In patients with the third, fourth or sixth cranial nerve involvement, basic cranial nerve examination is mandatory.[2,6]

Color vision

Color vision is the salient function of optic nerve and can be affected in diseases of the optic nerve and macula. Rarely, cerebral lesions may also affect color vision. In optic nerve disorders, even with mild visual drop, the degree of impairment of color perception may be severe; however, in macular pathology the degree of visual impairment is usually proportionate to dyschromatopsia.

Congenital color blindness is frequently present as red-green dyschromatopsia and is more common in males. Patients may not be aware of their condition and hence on testing with color vision charts, if the color perception is symmetrically affected, then congenital color blindness ought to be suspected.

Testing of color perception is done one eye at a time. Ishihara pseudo-isochromatic chart is commonly used to assess color vision in day-to-day practice. The test plate in the Ishihara chart is to determine whether or not the vision good because it cannot be read in patient with severe visual impairment. It is a simple screening tool as it can be performed rapidly. Hardy Rand Ritter is more accurate and is used to test both congenital and acquired color blindness. More detailed color vision testing is done using Farnsworth–Munsell 100 hue test and D15 test as they are more sensitive. The FM 100 needs placement of 85 caps in 4 rows and D15 requires arrangement of 15 color discs according to their hue and intensity (Figure 1.15).

Contrast sensitivity

Diseases of the optic nerve affect the contrast sensitivity and hence its measurement will help to access the visual dysfunction and quality of vision in such patients. During routine eye examination, the ability to recognize low contrast objects may be missed as Snellen acuity charts are of high contrast optotypes. Specially designed charts including Pelli-Robson chart consist of rows of optotypes of fixed size with decreasing contrast (Figure 1.16). The patient reads in a manner similar to visual acuity testing and the maximum contrast at which the letters can be detected is measured. Another method is using the Vistech chart, which has rows of circular targets with different special frequency and sinusoidal gratings.[2,6]

Visual field analysis

Visual field analysis is one of the fundamental tests to evaluate the afferent visual system. Various methods to access the visual fields were developed over the years. Visual field analysis helps in documentation and quantification of the field defect, localizing the lesion along the afferent visual pathways and also useful in follow up over time.

Patients with complaints of visual field defects, headache, neurological deficits and in unexplained vision loss, testing of visual fields will be helpful. Visual field examination is accomplished by two methods—static and kinetic. In static perimetry, the stimulus is held constant, while the intensity is varied to determine the threshold intensity values. Here, there is very little role for the operator.

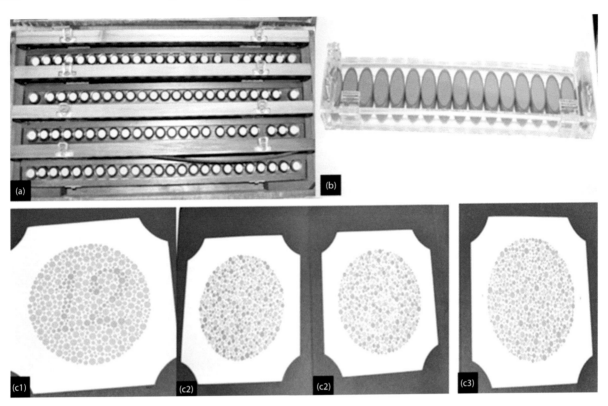

FIGURE 1.15 (a) Farnsworth–Munsell 100 hue test, (b) D15 test, (c1) Ishihara test plate, (c2) Ishihara color plates, (c3) tracing plate.

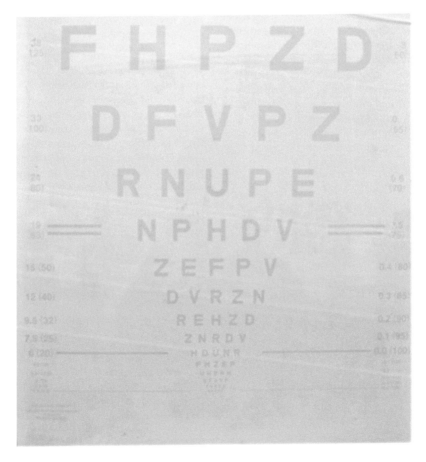

FIGURE 1.16 Contrast sensitivity chart.

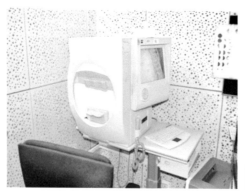
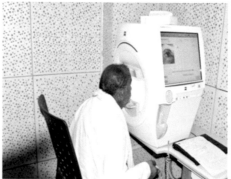

FIGURE 1.17   Testing of automated Humphrey visual field in a patient.

Examples include Humphrey, Octopus and Goldmann perimetry. In kinetic perimetry, the intensity and size of the stimulus remain constant and the stimulus is moved from the non-seeing area to the seeing area and depends on the experience of the operator. Examples include Goldmann perimetry and Tangent screen.

Nearly 80% of the visual cortex correlates to the central visual field and hence testing central 24 degrees or 30 degrees of the visual field is adequate for most visual defects. Goldmann perimetry can cover the largest isopter extending 90 degrees temporally and 60 degrees in other quadrants (full field) and is beneficial in children as there is constant supervision by perimetrist. The tangent screen is made of a black felt cloth mounted on a wall and the stimulus is mounted on a stick. It is useful within 30-degree fixation but can be extended. Radial meridian is marked at 30-degree interval and concentric circles are made at 10, 20, 30 for 1-m distance. Disadvantage includes strong dependence of results on the skill and technique of the perimetrist, difficulty in monitoring the patient's fixation while performing the examination and lack of standardization.

Automated perimetry is the most popular form of visual field testing. It is more sensitive, reproducible, standardized, less dependent on the technician and inter-technician variability less important; however, it is lengthy and tedious. Humphrey visual field 30-2 program tests 76 points in the central 30 degrees. The test locations are 6 degrees apart from each other (Figure 1.17).

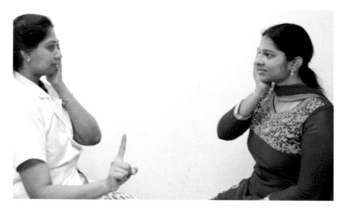

FIGURE 1.18   Confrontation method of visual field testing.

Confrontation method—Rapid, simple screening test performed easily at the bedside. Each eye is tested separately and the examiner compares the patient's visual field with his own. They are more sensitive when used properly but subtle defects cannot be detected by this method. The patient fixates on the examiner's nose and by this central scotoma can be identified if patients say a part of the face is missing. Finger mimicking or finger counting is performed in each quadrant. Hand comparison or color comparison is done by simultaneously presenting the target on either side of the vertical meridian to test the visual function simultaneously in both hemifields (Figure 1.18).

Amsler testing—It is a rapid screening test to access the central 20 degrees of visual field. Patient views a grid of vertical and horizontal lines at a reading distance (1/3 m) with spectacle correction and records response directly on the chart. One eye is tested at a time. Patient fixes on the central dot and is asked if the lines appear straight, wavy distorted or if any parts are missing. Maculopathies typically cause distortion of images or central scotoma, which can be easily detected using the Amsler chart.

BOX 1.1   CLINICAL PEARL 1

RELIABILITY INDICES

Fixation loss
- During the test itself, 5% of the stimulus will be presented to the blind spot. If the patient responds to this stimulus—it is due to the shift of fixation. Fixation loss > 20% is unreliable.

False positives
- Patient pushes the response button to the non-projected stimulus-trigger happy patients. False positives > 33% is unreliable.

False negatives
- Failure to respond to the brightest stimulus in an area previously determined to have some sensitivity and is due to inattention or tiredness. False negatives > 33% is unreliable.

BOX 1.2   CLINICAL PEARL 2

Homonymous defects—Are those present in both eyes with the same laterality (affect the same hemifield in both eyes)
Heteronymous defects—Different hemifield in the two eyes
Hemianopia—Refers to loss of half of the visual field, respecting the vertical (usually) meridian
Congruity—Refers to the symmetry of the field defect in both eyes

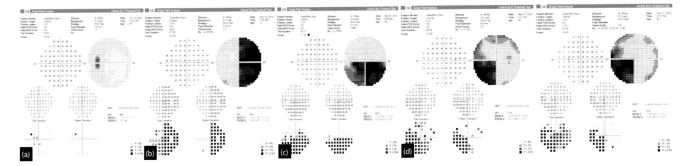

FIGURE 1.19 (a) Normal visual field, (b) right eye visual field with temporal hemianopia, (c) inferior altitudinal defect, (d) right inferior quadrantanopia.

Interpretation of visual fields should go hand in hand with clinical findings. Disease of the retina may produce focal defects or scotomas. Macular lesions produce central scotomas and branch retinal artery occlusion can cause focal field defects. Constricted visual fields not involving fixation are seen in retinitis pigmentosa. Central visual field defects in the absence of a macular lesion are typical, although not exclusively seen in optic nerve lesions. Altitudinal defects can be seen in optic neuritis and ischemic optic neuropathies. Toxic, nutritional and hereditary optic neuropathies produce central/paracentral defects. Lesions of chiasm cause bitemporal hemianopic defect due to the crossing over of nasal retinal fibers at the chiasm. Homonymous hemianopia is produced in retrochiasmal lesions (Figure 1.19). Thus, the vertical meridian separating the nasal and temporal hemifield has crucial importance in lesions of the chiasm, optic radiation and visual cortex. Table 1.8 describes visual field defects and its differential diagnosis.

Perimetry is an important tool in neuro-ophthalmology to know the extent and shape of visual field loss and provides diagnostic clues, which will aid in localizing the lesion on neuroimaging.[2,6]

Electrophysiological testing
Visual-evoked potential (VEP)

VEP is the electrophysiological recording of the occipital cortex and gives information regarding the integrity of optic nerve and the visual cortex. It is recorded by placing electrodes on the scalp in the occipital region and a stimulus is provided to evoke a potential. The stimulus here is visual which is either in the form of flash or pattern. The flash VEP is elicited by brief flash of light and is useful to access visual pathway in infants. The pattern VEP is the response to pattern stimulus (checkerboard—alternate black and white squares). It can be pattern onset-offset or pattern reversal. The pattern VEP has a component denoted as P100, which is the prominent positive wave at 100 ms. The P100 is preceded by a negative component at 75 ms which is N75 (Figure 1.20). In patients with optic neuritis, the pattern VEP shows a delay in P100 latency. It is characteristic of optic neuritis and is also useful in accessing subclinical visual pathway involvement. In compressive optic neuropathy, there is prolonged latency in early stage though not to the extent seen in optic neuritis. In ischemic optic neuropathies, there is reduced amplitude but latency is not significantly delayed. VEP is useful in functional vision loss as a normal pattern VEP to smaller checker size suggests intact visual pathway. Multifocal VEP (MFVEP) gives focal segmental defects just like the fields so useful in children/patients who are unable to do field tests.[6]

Electroretinogram—ERG

Electroretinogram is used to record the electrical activity of retina (Figure 1.20). Flash ERG is the mass response of retinal cells to full-field luminance stimulation and includes scotopic adaptation (scotopic rod response, maximal combined scotopic response and oscillatory potential) and photopic adaptation (photopic single flash cone response and 30-Hz flicker). Pattern ERG is the response of central retina to isoluminant stimulus (black- and white-checkerboard). It measures the central retinal

TABLE 1.8: Visual Field Defect—Differential Diagnosis

Visual Field Defect	Differential Diagnosis
Enlarged blind spot	Papilledema
	Optic disc coloboma
	Megallopapillae
	Staphyloma
	Acute idiopathic blind spot enlargement syndrome
	Acute Zonal Occult Outer Retinopathy with multiple evanescent white dot syndrome (AZOOR/MEWDS)
Arcuate/nasal step	Glaucoma
Altitudinal defect	Optic neuritis
	Ischemic optic neuropathy
	Other optic neuropathies like compressive etiologies
	Branch retinal artery occlusion
Central or cecocentral defects	Nutritional or toxic optic neuropathies
	Optic neuritis
	Macular pathology
Generalized depression in sensitivity	Cataract
	Corneal pathology and media opacities
Bitemporal hemianopia	More superiorly—pituitary adenoma
	More inferiorly—craniopharyngioma
Homonymous hemianopia	Retro chiasmal lesions
	Incongruous hemianopia—optic tract and anterior optic radiations
	Pie in sky defect—temporal lobe lesions
	Pie in floor defect—parietal lobe lesions
Congruous hemianopia	Posterior optic radiations
	Occipital cortex
Square visual field, spiraling, constricted or inconsistent patterns	Malingering

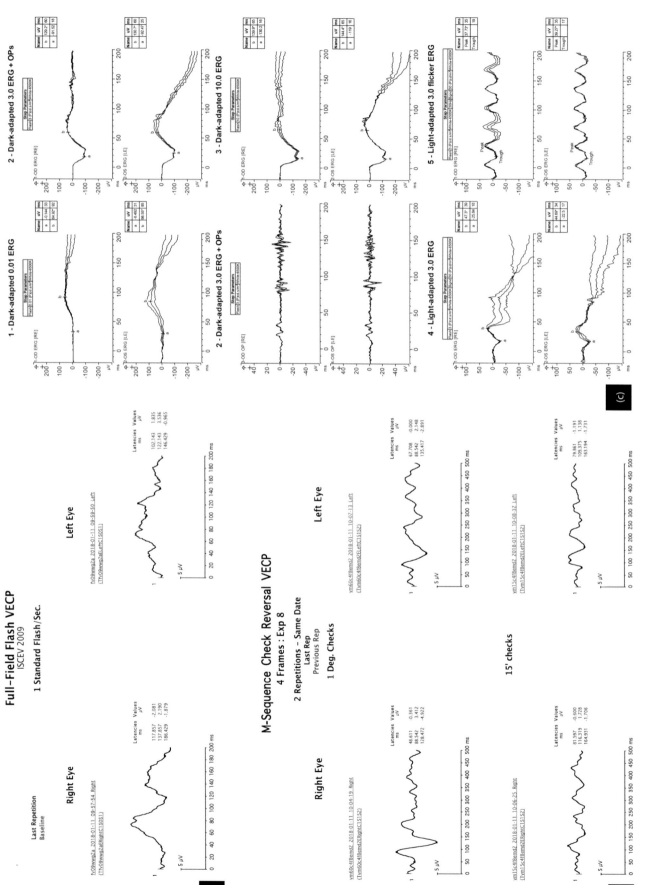

FIGURE 1.20 (a) Flash VEP, (b) Pattern VEP, (c) ERG.

function and uses in evaluation of retinal ganglion cells and thus helpful to differentiate between macular and optic nerve functions. It consists of two components—P50 (positive component at 50 ms) and N95 (large negative component at 95 ms). P50 reflects the macular photoreceptor function and N95 is related to retinal ganglion cell function. ERG is useful in diseases such as cancer-associated retinopathy, retinitis pigmentosa, cone dystrophy, congenital stationary night blindness and toxic retinopathies.[6,7]

Conclusion

The complexity in diagnosing neuro-ophthalmic disease can be simplified by basic skill and knowledge and proper interpretation of clinical findings. The essential element is proper history taking and clinical examination that will direct the clinician, and further evaluation including ancillary tests can be streamlined to guide in diagnosis and management of the disease.

CLINICAL CASES

CASE 1

A 28-year-old female presented with gradual painless progressive vision drop in both eyes since 1.5 months associated with transient visual obscurations. Visual acuity in right eye was 6/24 and left eye was 6/18 with defective color vision in both eyes. There was bilateral disc edema and visual fields were constricted. Her magnetic resonance imaging (MRI) brain and orbit showed large well-circumscribed extra-axial mass lesion in left frontal lobe with contrast enhancement causing mass effect on lateral ventricles, midline shift along with widened perioptic CSF space and empty sella. It is a case of papilledema secondary to intracranial space occupying lesion causing raised intracranial tension (Figure 1.21).

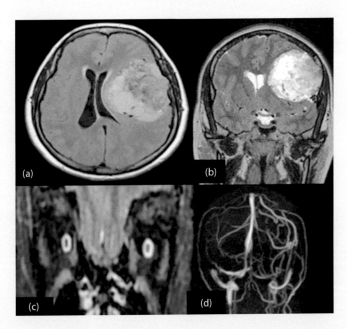

FIGURE 1.21 MRI brain and orbit showing well-circumscribed contrast-enhancing hyperintense with extra-axial lesion with areas of hypointensity within was seen in left frontal lobe meningioma (a, b) widened perioptic space (c) and bilateral narrowing of transverse sinuses in MR venogram (d).

CASE 2

A 45-year-old male came for routine eye checkup. His visual acuity was 6/6 in both eyes with normal color vision and visual fields. Disc swelling in both eyes had lumpy bumpy appearance without any vascular obscuration suggestive of pseudoedema. Ultrasound eye showed highly reflective clump echo in optic nerve head persisting in low gain suggestive of disc drusen. Optic disc drusen were also noted enhanced depth imaging-optical (EDI-OCT) coherence tomography. This is a case of pseudo disc edema and it does not require neuroimaging (Figure 1.22).

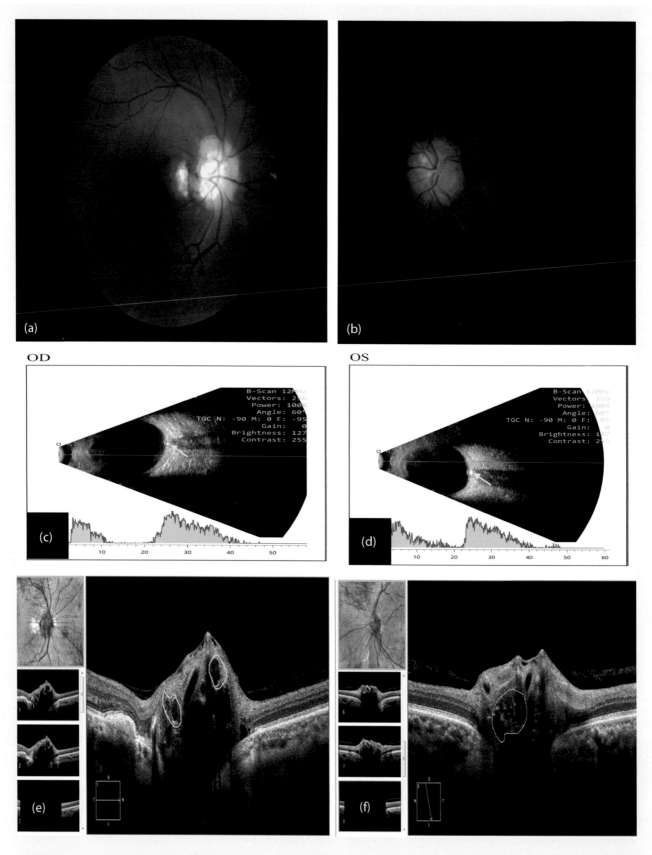

FIGURE 1.22 Optic disc drusen in both eyes on fundus examination (a, b). Ultrasound B scan suggestive of disc drusen (c, d) and drusen noted in EDI-OCT (e, f).

CASE 3

A 26-year-old female presented with headache since 6 months and nausea, tinnitus since 3 weeks. Visual acuity was 6/6 in both eyes with normal color vision and pupillary reaction. There was −4 abduction limitation in left eye. Fundus showed bilateral disc edema. Her blood pressure was 130/80 mm/Hg. Humphrey visual field analysis was suggestive of enlarged blind spot in both eyes. MRI brain and orbit showed widened perioptic CSF space and empty sella. MR Venography (MRV) brain was suggestive of hypoplastic left transverse sinus. She was referred to a neurologist for CSF opening pressure which was 30 cm of water and CSF analysis was normal. Patient was treated with antiedema drugs. This is a case of papilledema—secondary to idiopathic intracranial hypertension (Figure 1.23).

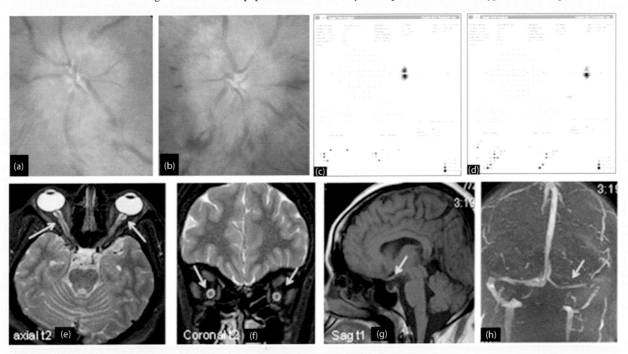

FIGURE 1.23 Bilateral disc edema (a, b) and enlargement of blind spot in visual fields (c, d). MRI brain and orbit showing widened perioptic CSF space (e, f) and empty sella (g) and MRV showing narrowing of left transverse sinus (h).

CASE 4

A 30-year-old female presented with sudden painful vision loss in left eye since 4 days. Vision acuity in right eye was 6/6 and 2/60 in left eye. There was relative afferent pupillary defect in left eye. Color vision by Ishihara plates was 21/21 in the right eye and 2/21 in the left eye. Visual fields were constricted in left eye and right eye had inferotemporal defect. MRI brain and orbit showed thickening and hyperintense signal in the left optic nerve up to the chiasm. Also there was subtle T2 hyperintense signal in right retro bulbar optic nerve along with right frontal T2 hyperintense signal, possibility of demyelination. This is a case of bilateral optic neuritis, where optic nerve functions are affected. Visual field helped to identify subclinical involvement of the fellow eye (Figure 1.24).

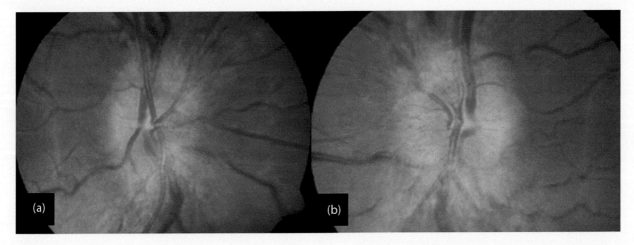

FIGURE 1.24 Bilateral disc edema (a, b) with visual field defect (c, d). MRI brain and orbit demonstrates signals in bilateral optic nerves in coronal T2 section (e) and hyperintense signal in frontal lobe suggestive of demyelination in sagittal flair image (f). *(Continued)*

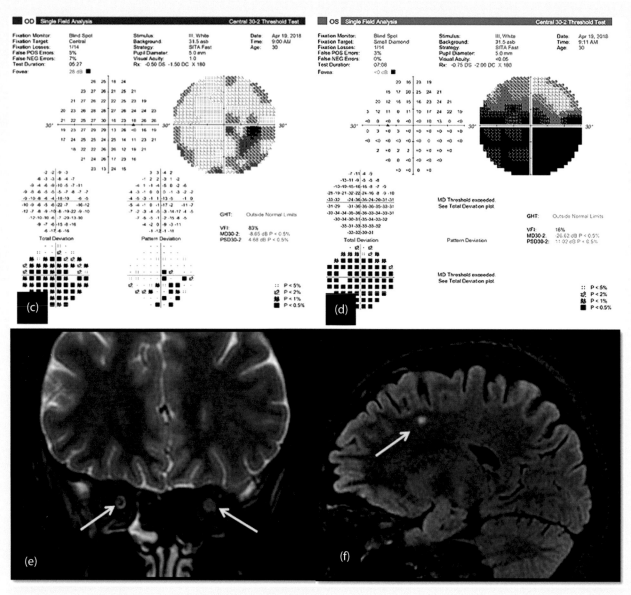

FIGURE 1.24 *(Continued)*

Multiple-Choice Questions

1. Optic nerve toxicity can happen with all these drugs, EXCEPT:
   a. Amiodarone
   b. Antitubercular
   c. Sildenafil
   d. Dexamethasone

   Answer:

   d. Dexamethasone

2. Tonic pupil
   a. Is caused by sympathetic pathway damage.
   b. Is caused by parasympathetic pathway damage.
   c. Is mostly bilateral.
   d. Patients are always asymptomatic.

   Answer:

   b. Is caused by parasympathetic pathway damage.

3. Basic optic nerve examination requirements include all of the following EXCEPT:
   a. Snellen chart
   b. Torch light
   c. Maddox rod
   d. Ishihara chart

   Answer:

   c. Maddox rod

4. A true optic disc edema
   a. Loss of SVP
   b. Filling of cup in late stages

c. Peripapillary hemorrhages
d. All of the above

Answer:

d. All of the above

References

1. Liu GT, Galetta SL. The neuro-ophthalmologic examination. Ophthalmol Clin North Am. 2001;14:23–39.
2. Miller NR, Walsh FB, Hoyt WF, editors. Walsh and Hoyt's clinical neuro-ophthalmology. Philadelphia: Lippincott Williams & Wilkins; 2006.
3. Rucker JC, Kennard C, Leigh RJ. The neuro-ophthalmological examination. Handb Clin Neurol. 2011;102:71–94.
4. Schiefer U, Wilhelm H, Hart W. Clinical neuro-ophthalmology: A practical guide. Berlin/Heidelberg/New York: Springer; 2007.
5. Bell RA, Waggoner PM, Boyd WM, Akers RE, Yee CE. Clinical grading of relative afferent pupillary defects. Arch Ophthalmol. 1993 July;111(7):938–942.
6. Heckmann JG, Vachalova I, Lang CJG, Pitz S. Neuro-ophthalmology at the bedside: a clinical guide. J Neurosci Rural Pract. 2018;9(4):561–573.
7. Lueck CJ, Gilmour DF, McIlwaine GG. Neuro-ophthalmology: examination and investigation. J Neurol Neurosurg Psychiatry. 2004;75(4):iv2–11.

2

VISUAL FIELDS IN NEURO-OPHTHALMOLOGY

Simon J. Hickman

Introduction

The field of vision is all that is visible at the same time during steady fixation of gaze. The normal visual field extends to approximately 90° temporally to central fixation, 50° superiorly and nasally, and 60° inferiorly.[1] The field of vision maps onto the retina. The electrical signals from the retina are transmitted via the anterior visual pathways to the visual cortex. From there the conscious visual percept is constructed by the brain. A lesion at any point in the anterior visual pathway can produce a visual field defect.[2,3]

This chapter will discuss the techniques available to map out the visual field and then the types of visual field defect that may be produced in non-organic (functional) illness and in neuro-ophthalmological disease. Figure 2.1 illustrates the usual visual field defects that can occur with damage to the different sites along the visual pathway. Absolute defects are not always seen. The depth of the defect depends on the degree of damage and the disease process involved.[2,3]

Examination of the visual field may be carried out by confrontation in the clinic or at the bedside. Alternatively, formal perimetry can be performed by a variety of techniques.[2] Before commencing any examination of the visual field, it is important to know the visual acuity in each eye. This will inform whether the target selected to map the visual field will be seen and will also allow the results to be put into context.[2]

Confrontation visual field examination

The confrontation visual field test is usually carried out with the subject seated opposite to the examiner so that the examiner can compare the subject's responses with their own visual field. Each eye is tested in turn and the subject is asked to fixate on the eye opposite to them. Testing can be carried out by a variety of techniques. The principal methods include: describing whether any part of the examiner's face is missing or distorted; finger counting in each of the four quadrants; comparison of simultaneously presented fingers in different quadrants of the visual field; comparison of simultaneously presented red targets in different quadrants of the visual field; detection of static wiggling finger in different portions of the visual field; detection of kinetic wiggling finger as it is brought in from the periphery in each quadrant; and detection of a kinetic red target as it is brought in from the periphery in each quadrant. When each of these techniques was compared with Humphrey automated perimetry, kinetic testing with a red target had the highest sensitivity (74.4%) and specificity (93.0%).[4] In practice, the test used needs to be tailored to the subject being tested and the clinical problem. It is usual to combine tests as well to understand the nature of the deficit more fully.

Perimetry

Perimetry is the technique of quantitatively assessing the field of vision.[3] It has advantages over confrontation visual field analysis in terms of accuracy but also in proving quantitative information so that change over time can be monitored.[2,3] It is important to understand the technique that has been used to be able to interpret the information provided and appreciate the limitations of the technique. When interpreting the output of perimetry, it is important to view the results from both eyes at the same time with the left eye visual field placed to the left and the right eye to the right. In this way, the plots are viewed from the perspective of the subject looking into the test bowl. By doing this both differences and similarities between the outputs from each eye can be interpreted, which may be very subtle. The identity of the patient having the test needs to be confirmed as well as the date on which it was performed.[5]

Suprathreshold static perimetry is often used by optometrists to screen for visual field defects.[6] In this testing, the machine projects a bright (suprathreshold) static stimulus target to each point being tested, typically within the central portion of the visual field, although driving assessments, which typically are performed with both eyes open (binocular), will test out into the peripheral visual field.[7] There are various methodologies employed. Each technique is fast to perform with easily interpretable results. All of the techniques tend to have high sensitivity with lower specificity.[6] It is important to emphasize that these techniques are designed to be screening tests and further examination is required if the patient has visual symptoms, even if the suprathreshold visual field result is normal.[8]

In Ophthalmology departments, two principal perimetric techniques are employed: static threshold perimetry, typically with the Humphrey visual field analyzer (HFA) (Humphrey Instruments Inc., San Leandro, California, USA) and kinetic perimetry, typically with the Goldmann perimeter and its newer stablemate the automated Octopus perimeter (Haag-Streit, Köniz, Switzerland).[5]

The HFA plots the luminance threshold at which static light stimuli are detected, while the subject fixates on a central target. Different test algorithms can be employed and the HFA is most commonly used to test the central 10°, 24° or 30° of the visual field. An example of a printout from a normal subject's HFA after testing the central 24° (termed 24-2) is shown in Figure 2.2. The reliability of the results need to be assessed to avoid over-interpretation of an apparent defect as this may just be due to poor performance with the test and not disease affecting the visual pathway. The automated perimetry machines will assess for fixation losses by retesting at the site of the blindspot. In addition, the machine will represent targets that have already been tested to assess for false-negative (failure to respond to a target at a threshold that had been previously detected) and false-positive (responding to a target at a threshold that had been previously undetected) responses. The visual field plot at the top of Figure 2.2 shows the visual sensitivity map in numbers and as a grayscale. This documents the threshold of detection in decibels at each point tested. The total deviation map charts the deviation of the subject's responses at each point compared with an age-matched control population. The pattern deviation map charts the deviation of the subject's responses from a normal pattern of responses where the peak of sensitivity is at the fovea. There are three additional outputs on the right

DOI: 10.1201/9780429020278-3

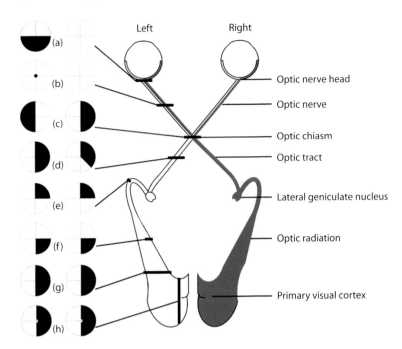

FIGURE 2.1 Diagrammatic view of the visual pathway with standard visual field defects illustrated: (a) altitudinal visual field defect due to a lesion at the optic nerve head; (b) central scotoma due to an optic nerve lesion; (c) bitemporal hemianopia due to a chiasmal lesion; (d) incongruous hemianopia due to an optic tract lesion; (e) superior homonymous quadrantanopia due to a lesion of the Flechsig-Meyer loop in the temporal lobe; (f) inferior homonymous quadrantanopia due to a lesion of the optic radiation in the parietal lobe; (g) homonymous hemianopia due to a complete optic radiation lesion; (h) homonymous hemianopia with macular sparing due to a lesion of the primary visual cortex. (Obtained from Hickman, 2011[3] with permission.)

of the plot, which provide an overall numerical indication of the degree of damage. The visual field index (VFI) gives an indication of overall percentage integrity. The mean deviation (MD) shows the overall difference against age-matched controls and the pattern standard deviation (PSD) shows the degree of localized visual field defects.[5]

Kinetic perimetry involves moving a light stimulus of different sizes and luminance from the periphery towards the center of the visual field with the subject fixating on a central target. In addition, scotomas and the blindspot may be plotted, both kinetically and statically. The output is a series of isopter lines that join points of equal visual sensitivity in the "hill of vision", akin to the contour lines on a map that join points of equal elevation.[5] In addition, single points of static testing can be plotted. An example of a Goldmann visual field plot from a normal subject is shown in Figure 2.3. The different sizes of target are denoted by the Roman numerals I–V from smallest to largest. The luminance of the target is denoted by the relative intensity ranging from 1a (the dimmest) to 4e (the brightest). The testing protocols for kinetic perimetry include tests for fixation losses (typically by retesting the site of the blindspot) and tests for consistency by re-testing at previously detected points in the visual field.[5]

Unreliable (functional) visual fields

An unreliable performance at visual field testing may be due to a poor understanding of how to perform the test, fatigue while doing the test, or due to non-organic (functional) illness.

What will result is an unreliable visual field due to poor reproducibility on re-testing and/or an output that is not consistent with an organic disease process. To confrontation a tubular rather than conical visual field may occur when re-testing at different distances. On Humphrey perimetry, a four-leaf clover pattern results when the response reliability tails off as the test progresses. The lowest threshold for detection is at the initial point tested in each quadrant (the apices of the four leaves of the clover) but then the threshold rises as the test progresses and reliability worsens (Figure 2.4). There will also be a high false-negative rate. On kinetic perimetry, there may be an inexplicably constricted visual field, spiraling and crossing of the isopter lines. The latter two are due to inconsistency and decreased apparent sensitivity over time (Figure 2.5). Physiologically, the isopter lines cannot cross just as contour lines on a map cannot cross.[5,9]

Another pattern that is occasionally seen in non-organic monocular visual impairment is an isolated monocular temporal hemianopic defect in the absence of retinal or optic nerve disease and with no detectable relative afferent pupillary defect. The non-organic nature of this may be elucidated by carrying out binocular testing. An organic monocular temporal visual field defect will become much smaller and more peripheral on binocular testing as the subject will be able to detect more points in the previously unseen portion of visual field as it overlaps with the contralateral nasal hemifield. Only the monocular temporal crescent of the affected eye will be abnormal. A non-organic monocular temporal visual field defect typically persists on binocular testing (Figure 2.6).[10]

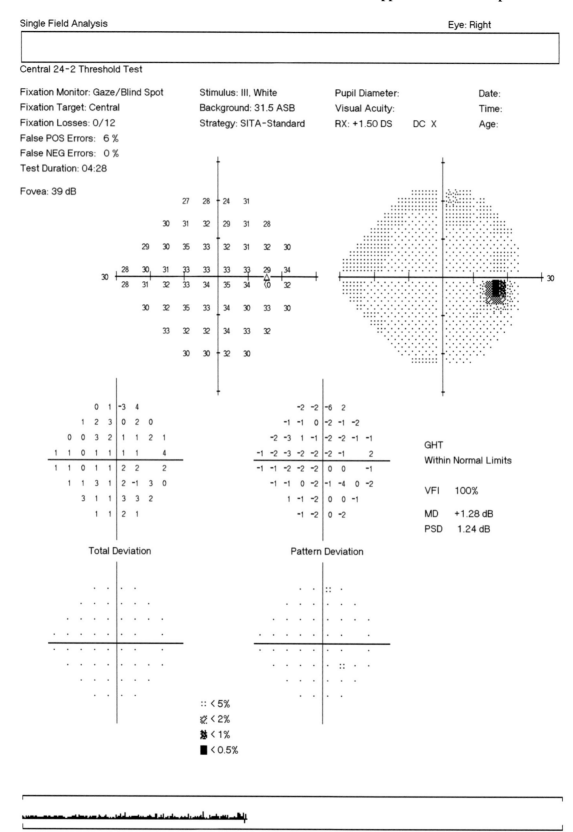

FIGURE 2.2   24-2 Humphrey perimetry output from a normal subject.

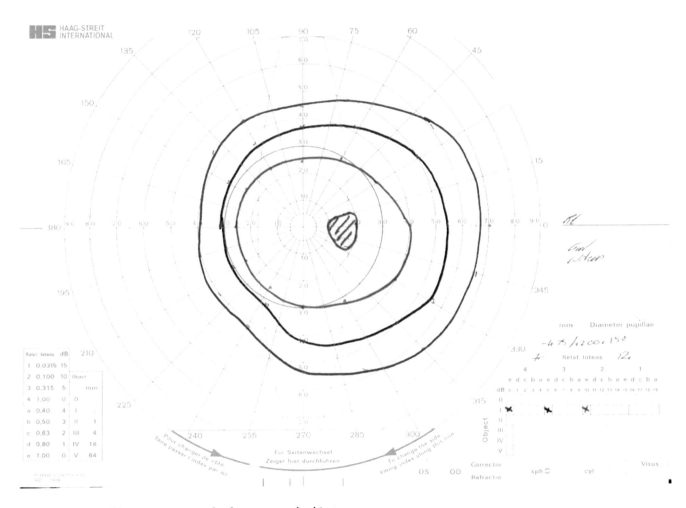

FIGURE 2.3   Goldmann perimetry plot from a normal subject.

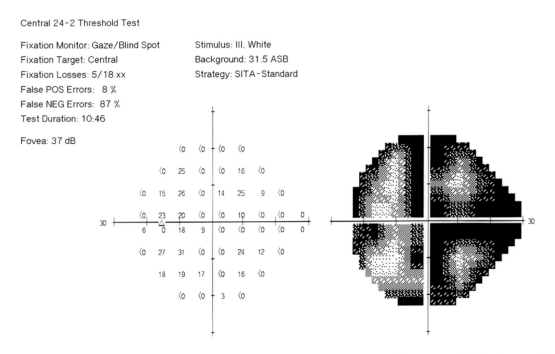

FIGURE 2.4   24-2 Humphrey perimetry numerical sensitivity plot and grayscale map from an unreliable witness with a very high false-negative rate and four-leaf clover pattern on the grayscale map.

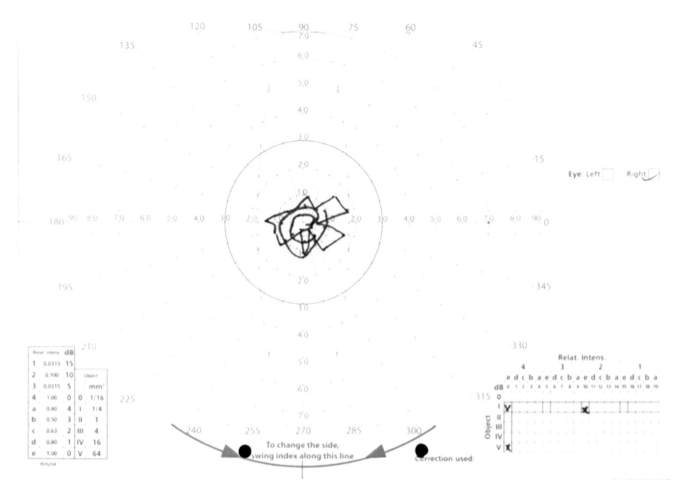

FIGURE 2.5 Goldmann perimetry plot from an unreliable witness demonstrating excessive constriction, spiraling and crossing of the isopter lines.

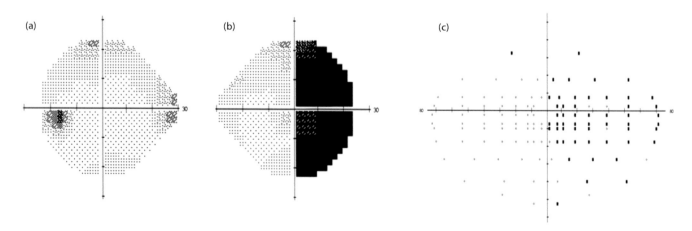

FIGURE 2.6 (a) Left and (b) right eye 24-2 Humphrey perimetry grayscale maps demonstrating a right monocular temporal hemianopia. (c) The temporal hemianopia is still present on binocular Esterman perimetry providing evidence that the defect is functional in origin.

(a)

(b)

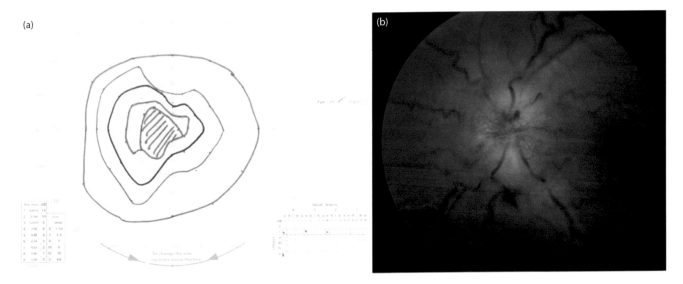

FIGURE 2.7   (a) Goldmann perimetry plot from a patient with papilledema, shown on (b) fundal photography. The visual field plot shows an enlarged blind spot and some depression of the inferonasal visual field.

Visual field defects resulting from lesions of specific structures

Optic nerve head

The commonest disease affecting the optic nerve head is glaucoma, which classically produces arcuate defects in the visual field.[11] The first visual field sign of papilledema is an enlarged blind spot due to optic nerve swelling. The optic nerve fibers most vulnerable to damage in papilledema are in the supero-temporal portion of the optic disc. Due to the inversion of the image by the lens the visual field defect that results is in the inferonasal visual field (Figure 2.7).[12] The optic nerve head is supplied by the short posterior ciliary arteries, with some separation of the supply to the superior and inferior halves. Infarction of the optic nerve head due to anterior ischemic optic neuropathy will usually affect one of these halves leading to an altitudinal visual field defect (Figure 2.8).[13]

Optic nerve

The papillomacular bundle, which projects from the macula into the optic nerve, contains more than 90% of all the retinal nerve fibers and principally contains small parvocellular axons, which are vulnerable to damage from toxins, nutritional deficiency, mitochondrial diseases such as Leber's hereditary optic neuropathy, and inflammation. Damage to these fibers will lead to a central or centrocecal (when the blindspot is affected as well) scotoma (Figure 2.9).[1,11] In acute optic neuritis, it has been shown that diffuse loss of the visual field is the commonest defect, although many other patterns are possible.[14] Compressional lesions of the optic nerve may also produce many types of visual field defect.[1,11]

Optic chiasm

The nasal optic nerve fibers, which subserve temporal vision, cross at the optic chiasm. The commonest visual field defect that occurs from damage to these crossing fibers across the center of the chiasm is a bitemporal hemianopia, typically by suprasellar extension of a pituitary adenoma. Initially, the inferior compression may cause an upper bitemporal quadrantanopia (Figure 2.10). The visual field defect may be asymmetrical or may involve the optic nerves or optic tracts, depending on the position of the optic chiasm in relation to the pituitary gland. Superior compression from a suprasellar mass, such as a craniopharyngioma, may result in an initial inferior bitemporal quadrantanopia.[1,11] Since the optic chiasm is relatively small, measured in one study to be a mean of 14 mm in width,[15] larger lesions, which involve both crossing and non-crossing fibers, can lead to complete blindness.[16]

Optic tract and lateral geniculate nucleus

For all retrochiasmal lesions, the principal causes are ischemic stroke, cerebral hemorrhage, trauma and tumors. Less common causes are iatrogenic following brain surgery, demyelination and neurodegenerative.[17]

Optic tract lesions will cause a hemianopic visual field defect contralateral to the lesion.[17–19] The classical visual field defect from an optic tract lesion is an incongruous (i.e., the defects in each eye do not exactly correspond to each other) hemianopic defect contralateral to the lesion, as fibers corresponding to the same part of the visual field from each eye have not yet completely joined together (Figure 2.11).[17,18] A complete homonymous (i.e., the visual field defect is the same in each eye) hemianopia is

(a)

(b)

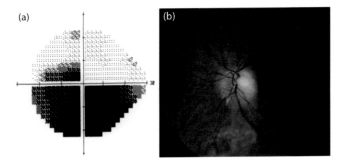

FIGURE 2.8   (a) 24-2 Humphrey grayscale map demonstrating an inferior altitudinal visual field defect consistent with anterior ischemic optic neuropathy, confirmed on fundal examination (b).

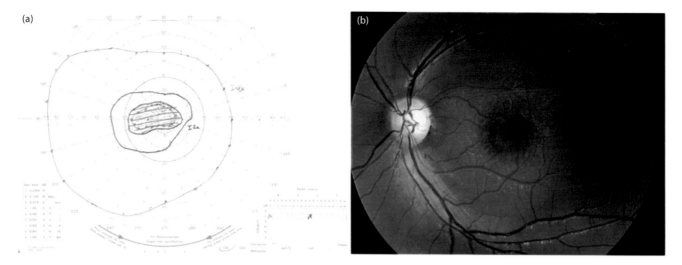

FIGURE 2.9   (a) Goldmann perimetry plot of a patient with Leber's hereditary optic neuropathy causing a centrocecal scotoma. (b) Fundus photograph of the resulting temporal pallor of the optic disc.

possible with an optic tract lesion; however, due to the small size of the tract.[19]

Clinical clues to the presence of an optic tract lesion include a relative afferent pupillary defect in the eye that has the temporal visual field involved (i.e., contralateral to the lesion) due to the larger visual field involved relative to the nasal field in the other eye[20] and bow-tie atrophy across the middle of the optic disc in the eye contralateral to the lesion.[18]

The synapse between the optic nerve and optic radiation fibers occurs at the lateral geniculate nucleus. A pure lesion here is quite rare but contralateral homonymous sectoral defects following infarcts have been reported.[21]

Optic radiation

The inferior portion of the optic radiation (that carries the visual field information from the contralateral superior visual quadrant)

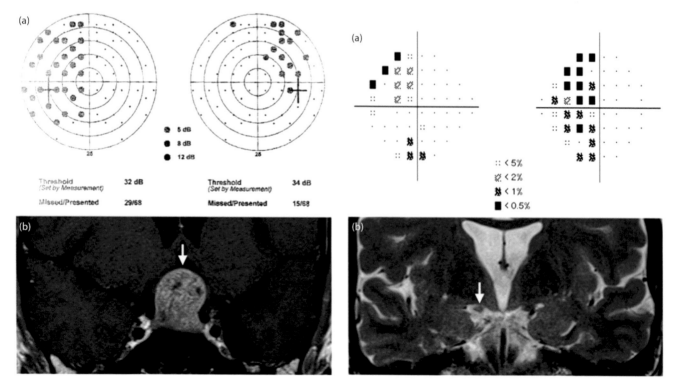

FIGURE 2.10   (a) Screening suprathreshold perimetry grayscale map of a superior bitemporal quadrantanopia, (b) confirmed to be due to optic chiasm compression and elevation by a pituitary macroadenoma (arrowed on coronal post-gadolinium T1-weighted magnetic resonance imaging).

FIGURE 2.11   (a) 24-2 Humphrey total deviation map showing a left incongruous hemianopia due to a traumatic lesion of the right optic tract. (b) Coronal T2-weighted magnetic resonance imaging demonstrating atrophy and high signal in the right optic tract (arrowed).

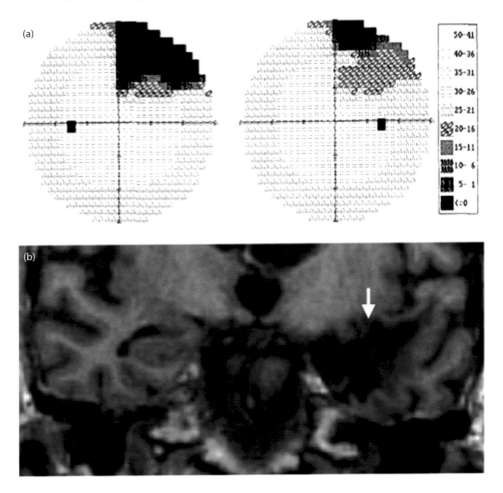

FIGURE 2.12   (a) Screening suprathreshold perimetry grayscale map demonstrating a right upper quadrantanopia in a patient following left amygdalo-hippocampectomy for intractable epilepsy. (b) Coronal T1-weighted magnetic resonance imaging showing the post-surgical changes in the left temporal lobe (arrowed).

takes it course round the temporal horn of the lateral ventricle (the Flechsig-Meyer loop) before continuing to the inferior part of the primary visual cortex. A lesion within the temporal lobe will produce a contralateral superior homonymous quadrantanopia (Figure 2.12).[22] The superior fibers of the optic radiation run within the parietal lobe before synapsing in the superior part of the primary visual cortex. A lesion here will lead to an inferior homonymous quadrantanopia (Figure 2.13).[22] Complete homonymous hemianopias are seen though in about 40% of optic radiation lesions.[18]

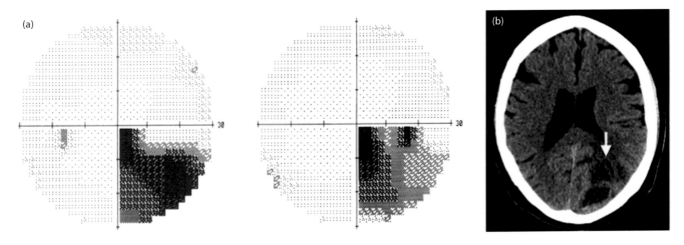

FIGURE 2.13   (a) 30-2 Humphrey perimetry grayscale map showing a right inferior homonymous quadrantanopia found to be due to left parietal lobe metastasis from bronchial small cell carcinoma, (b) shown on computed tomography scanning (arrowed).

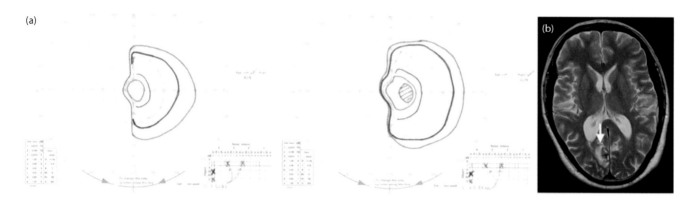

FIGURE 2.14 (a) Goldmann perimetry plot demonstrating a left homonymous hemianopia with macular sparing due to a right occipital infarct with sparing of the occipital pole, (b) as shown on axial T2-weighted magnetic resonance imaging (arrowed).

Occipital lobe

The primary visual cortex (or calcarine cortex, V1) lies within the medial occipital lobe and is divided into superior and inferior halves by the calcarine sulcus. A complete lesion of the calcarine cortex will produce a contralateral homonymous hemianopia. A complete lesion of the inferior cortex below the calcarine sulcus will cause a contralateral superior homonymous quadrantanopia and a complete lesion of the superior calcarine cortex will produce a contralateral inferior homonymous quadrantanopia.[1,11,18,22] For both superior and inferior homonymous quadrantanopias, the lesion responsible is most likely to be found in the occipital lobe than the temporal or parietal lobes, since ischemic stroke accounts for over 80% of the cases, which is most likely to occur in the occipital lobe.[22]

The majority of the arterial blood supply to the calcarine cortex is via the posterior cerebral artery, although there are variations between individuals and the occipital pole, which subserves macular vision, is often supplied by occipital branches from the middle cerebral artery.[23,24] Macular sparing therefore often results following posterior cerebral artery territory thrombo-embolic infarcts, in both hemianopias (Figure 2.14) and quadrantanopias.[1,3,11,18,25] Other patterns of sparing have also been reported, including along the horizontal and vertical meridia.[3,11]

Bilateral calcarine lesions are relatively common due to thrombo-embolism from the basilar artery into both posterior cerebral arteries causing simultaneous or sequential infarction. As with unilateral calcarine infarcts, partial sparing of vision can result, which may be asymmetrical.[1,3,11]

Lesions of the visual areas V2 and V3 may produce contralateral homonymous quadrantanopias, although pure lesions here are very rare.[26] Lesions in the ventromedial occipital cortex may produce hemi-achromatopsia (loss of color vision), which can occur with or without a visual field defect to white light.[27,28]

Driving

It is important to counsel patients with a visual field defect that this may have a bearing on whether they may be considered fit to drive. Each licensing authority has its own minimum requirements in terms of visual acuity and visual field restriction, although many will allow exceptions in individuals with long-standing stable defects who have also shown full adaptation.[29] The driving visual field assessment is usually by binocular suprathreshold perimetry.[7]

Conclusion

What will be apparent from the discussion is that the pattern of the presenting visual field defect, combined with other neurological signs, will provide a clue as to the most likely location of that lesion. This can then be combined with the history from the patient as to the speed of evolution of the visual symptoms to give the likely etiology. This will then inform the clinician as to what further investigations are required and the urgency of those investigations in case there may be a treatable cause. Once the cause has been found and appropriately treated, the patient will have to be assessed to determine whether there are any deficits in visual function that may be amenable to rehabilitation.[30]

Key points

- Any disease process along the visual pathway can lead to a visual field defect in one or both eyes.
- The pattern of defect will give a clue to the likely location of the lesion.
- Combining this with the history of onset will give a clue as to the likely etiology.

Multiple-Choice Questions

1. This visual field defect may be due to:

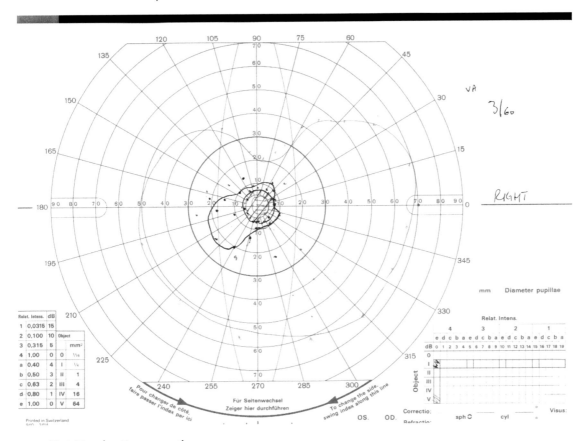

  a. Nutritional optic neuropathy
  b. Leber's hereditary optic neuropathy
  c. Optic neuritis
  d. All the above

Answer:

  d. This is a central scotoma due to involvement of optic nerve fibers in the papillomacular bundle. Hence, all of the above can cause preferential damage to these fibers and this visual field defect.

2. The most likely location of the lesion causing this visual field defect is:

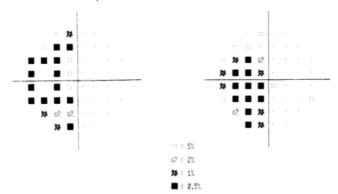

  a. Right occipital lobe
  b. Right optic tract
  c. Left optic tract
  d. Optic chiasm

Answer:

  b. This is a left incongruous hemianopia; therefore, the most likely location will be the right optic tract.

3. The most likely location of the lesion causing this visual field defect is:

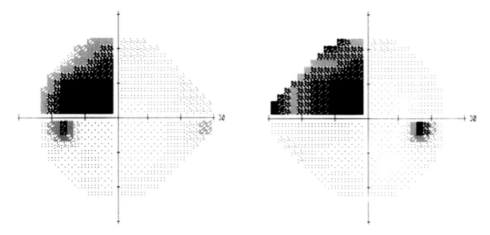

   a. Right optic tract
   b. Right temporal lobe
   c. Right parietal lobe
   d. Right occipital lobe

   Answer:

   d. This is a left superior homonymous quadrantanopia. As discussed in the text ischemic strokes are the most likely cause of this type of visual field defect and these predominantly affect the occipital lobes.

4. The most likely location of the lesion causing this visual field defect is:

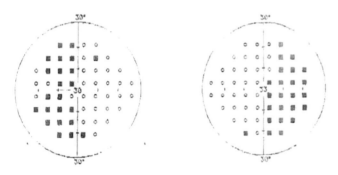

   a. Both optic radiations
   b. Both optic nerves
   c. Optic chiasm
   d. Both occipital lobes

   Answer:

   c. This is a bitemporal hemianopia so localizes the lesion to the optic chiasm due to interruption of the nasal crossing fibers that carry information from both temporal visual fields. The most likely cause is a pituitary macroadenoma.

References

1. Traquair HM. An introduction to clinical perimetry, 6th ed. London, UK: Henry Kimpton; 1949.
2. Cooper SA, Metcalfe RA. Assess and interpret the visual fields at the bedside. Pract Neurol. 2009;9:324–334.
3. Hickman SJ. Neurological visual field defects. Neuro-Ophthalmol. 2011;35:242–250.
4. Kerr NM, Chew SS, Eady EK, Gamble GD, Danesh-Meyer HV. Diagnostic accuracy of confrontation visual field tests. Neurology. 2010;74:1184–1190.
5. Wong SH, Plant GT. How to interpret visual fields. Pract Neurol. 2015;15:374–381.
6. Topouzis F, Coleman AL, Yu F, Mavroudis L, Anastasopoulos E, Koskosas A, Pappas T, Dimitrakos S, Wilson MR. Sensitivity and specificity of the 76-suprathreshold visual field test to detect eyes with visual field defect by Humphrey threshold testing in a population-based setting: the Thessaloniki eye study. Am J Ophthalmol. 2015;137:420–425.
7. Kotecha A, Spratt A, Viswanathan A. Visual function and fitness to drive. British Med Bull. 2008;87:163–174.
8. Petzold A, Plant GT. Failure to detect bitemporal field defects due to chiasmal compression on a screening perimetry protocol. Neuro-Ophthalmol. 2000;24:357–361.
9. Hickman SJ. Neuro-ophthalmology. Pract Neurol. 2011;11:191–200.
10. Acaroğlu G, Güven A, Ileri D, Zilelioğlu O. Monocular temporal hemianopia in a young patient. Turkish J Pediatr. 2004;46:98–100.
11. Harrington DO. The visual fields: A textbook and atlas of clinical perimetry. Saint Louis, MI: The C.V. Mosby Company; 1971.
12. Wall M, George D. Idiopathic intracranial hypertension: A prospective study of 50 patients. Brain. 1991;114:155–180.
13. Arnold AC. Ischemic optic neuropathies. In: Miller NR, Newman NJ, Biousse V and Kerrison, JB, editors. Walsh and Hoyt's clinical neuro-ophthalmology. 6th ed.; 2005. p. 349–384.
14. Keltner JL, Johnson CA, Spurr JO, Beck RW. Optic neuritis study group. Baseline visual field profile of optic neuritis: The experience of the optic neuritis treatment trial. Arch Ophthalmol. 1993;111:231–234.
15. Wagner AL, Murtagh FR, Hazlett KS, Arringhton JA. Measurement of the normal optic chiasm on coronal MR images. AJNR Am J Neuroradiol. 1997;18:723–726.

16. Agrawal D, Mahapatra AK. Visual outcome of blind eyes in pituitary apoplexy after transsphenoidal surgery: A series of 14 eyes. Surg Neurol. 2005; 63:42–46.

17. Zhang X, Kedar S, Lynn MJ, Newman NJ, Biousse V. Homonymous hemianopias: Clinical–anatomic correlations in 904 cases. Neurology. 2006;66:906–910.

18. Newman SA, Miller NR. Optic tract syndrome: Neuro-ophthalmologic considerations. Arch Ophthalmol. 1983;101:1241–1250.

19. Frisén L. The neurology of visual acuity. Brain. 1980;103:639–670.

20. Kardon R, Kawasaki A, Miller NR. Origin of the relative afferent pupillary defect in optic tract lesions. Ophthalmology. 2006;113:1345–1353.

21. Luco C, Hoppe A, Schweitzer M, Vicuña X, Fantin A. Visual field defects in vascular lesions of the lateral geniculate body. J Neurol Neurosurg Psychiatry. 1992;55:12–15.

22. Jacobson DM. The localizing value of a quadrantanopia. Arch Neurol. 1997;154:401–404.

23. Marinković SV, Milisavljević MM, Lolić-Draganić V, Kovačević MS. Distribution of the occipital branches of the posterior cerebral artery: Correlation with occipital lobe infarcts. Stroke. 1987;18:728–732.

24. Smith CG, Richardson WFG. The course and distribution of the arteries supplying the visual (striate) cortex. Am J Ophthalmol. 1966;61:1391–1396.

25. Wong AMF, Sharpe JA. Representation of the visual field in the human occipital cortex: A magnetic resonance imaging and perimetric correlation. Arch Ophthalmol. 1998;50:208–217.

26. Horton JC, Hoyt WF. Quadrantic visual field defects. A hallmark of lesions in extrastriate (V2/V3) cortex. Brain. 1991;114:1703–1718.

27. Short RA, Graff-Radford NR. Localization of hemiachromatopsia. Neurocase. 2001;7:331–337.

28. Kölmel HW. Pure homonymous hemiachromatopsia. Findings with neuro-ophthalmologic examination and imaging procedures. Eur Arch Psychiatr Neurological Sci. 1998;237:237–243.

29. Colenbrander A, De Laey JJ. *Vision requirements for driving safety with emphasis on individual assessment*. Sao Paulo, Brazil: Report prepared for the International Council of Ophthalmology at the 30th World Ophthalmology Congress, 2006.

30. Hickman SJ, Rhodes MJ. Management of neuro-ophthalmic disorders in neurorehabilitation. In: Nair KPS, González-Fernández M, Panischer JN, editors. Neurorehabilitation Therapy & Therapeutics; 2019. p. 166–177.

3A

OPTICAL COHERENCE TOMOGRAPHY (OCT) AND FUNDUS FLUORESCEIN ANGIOGRAPHY (FFA) IN NEURO-OPHTHALMOLOGY

Ramandeep Singh, Deeksha Katoch, Mohit Dogra, Basavaraj Tigari, Simar Rajan Singh, Sahil Jain, Bruttendu Moharana, Sabia Handa, Mangat R. Dogra

Optical coherence tomography in neuro-ophthalmology

Introduction

Optical coherence tomography (OCT) is now gaining popularity in the diagnosis and monitoring of several neuro-ophthalmological and neurological conditions. In neuro-ophthalmology, OCT can aid in the diagnosis, monitoring, and in some cases, provide prognostic information concerning diseases affecting the optic nerve. OCT is also emerging as an essential tool in the diagnosis and monitoring of neurodegenerative disorders such as Alzheimer's and Parkinson's disease.

OCT helps to pick the damage to the retinal ganglion cells (RGCs), especially macular retinal ganglion cells (mRGCs) and peripapillary retinal nerve fiber layer (pRNFL). RGCs are concentrated in the macula and loss of macular volume and thinning of the ganglion layer detectable by OCT, suggests damage to these first-order neurons in the visual afferent pathway. Unmyelinated axons of the RGC make up the retinal nerve fiber layer (RNFL) and reduction in the RNFL thickness can, therefore, be inferred due to axonal damage.

OCT can be useful to neuro-ophthalmologist in three ways:

1. Diagnostic tool
2. Monitoring tool
3. Prognostic tool

Diagnostic tool
Differentiating between optic neuropathy and retinopathy
Some rare retinopathies can mimic optic neuropathies. Acute zonal occult outer retinopathy (AZOOR) presents as subacute visual loss, relative afferent pupillary defect (RAPD) and near normal fundus. OCT can pick up the defect at the junction of outer and inner segments of photoreceptors or the cone outer segment tip line in the early stage of disease.[1]

Leber's hereditary optic neuropathy
Recent OCT literature[2–4] has shown that OCT is capable of detecting longitudinal changes in pRNFL and mRGC in different phases of Leber's hereditary optic neuropathy (LHON). In the presymptomatic stage, pRNFL thickness increases, whereas mRGC thickness decreases at an early stage as atrophy of the macular RGC is noticed.

True versus pseudo disc swelling
Conditions like crowded disc and optic disc drusen (ODD) can confuse and needs to be differentiated from true disc swelling. Spectral domain OCT has a sensitivity and specificity of 73% in distinguishing between pseudo-papilledema and true papilledema.[5] However, the earlier OCTs, that is, stratus (time-domain) and cirrus OCT, were not able to pick up this difference.[6,7]

For practical purposes, pRNFL would remain stable in the congenitally crowded disc, over repeated scans, whereas it might increase or decrease in true papilledema over repeated scans, provided some treatment was given or not.

ODD can be easily picked up by other non-invasive tools like fundus autofluorescence and ultrasonography. However, for knowledge purpose, OCT, especially enhanced depth imaging-OCT (EDI-OCT) can also pick up ODD as hyperreflective tumefactions with hyperreflective foci located anterior to lamina cribrosa.[8,9]

Functional visual loss
OCT is a useful test to exclude subtle macular diseases with macular scan and mRGC analysis in patients with long standing vision loss and normal clinical examination. Loss of mRGC in early stages of diseases like LHON is useful in differentiating between clinically normal LHON and functional vision loss patients.

Monitoring tool
Monitoring of any disease on OCT is highly dependent on test-retest variability. With the newer machines and technology, test-retest variability of pRNFL, mRGC and optic disc parameters has improved.

Compressive optic neuropathies
Surgical intervention in an otherwise asymptomatic non-secretory pituitary tumor may be dictated by evidence of visual dysfunction. OCT abnormalities (mRGC and pRNFL) in these patients are evident before symptomatic visual loss or abnormalities on perimetry. mRGC loss precedes the pRNFL damage.[10] Monitoring of vision with interval OCTs may be more cost-effective than serial MRIs and more relevant to planning surgical intervention.

Impaired ganglion cell layer (GCL) thickness in the nasal half of the retina in patients undergoing OCT as part of the routine ophthalmic evaluation or glaucoma assessment raises suspicion of chiasmal compression by a pituitary tumor[11] and warrants imaging.

Idiopathic intracranial hypertension
Papilledema is seen as thickened pRNFL. Sometimes OCT is unable to accurately pick up the condition in higher-grade papilledema due to OCT pRNFL algorithms failure. Serial monitoring of the pRNFL does not correlate exactly with the visual field damage due to onset of optic atrophy. The utility of OCT in the diagnosis and grading of papilledema has been described by Scott et al.[12]

ONH morphological assessment and peripapillary retinal thickness are better methods to monitor the disc edema than pRNFL monitoring.

Optic neuritis/multiple sclerosis
Optic neuritis (ON) is one of the manifestations of multiple sclerosis (MS) and is the presenting feature of MS in 25–50% of cases. OCT can detect subclinical axonal loss in eyes with normal visual

DOI: 10.1201/9780429020278-4

fields, and visual acuity in MS patients.[13] Peripapillary RNFL loss has been demonstrated even in the asymptomatic eye of MS patients with unilateral ON, although less than the affected eye. Since mRGC loss predicts axonal loss, mRGC measurement is a better investigative tool in all MS subtypes.[14] Longitudinal studies show mRGC thinning as an early phenomenon in MS and could occur independent of previous symptomatic episodes.[15] Macular RGC thickness analysis is more sensitive to detect damage and is reduced before detectable thinning of pRNFL in remitting-relapsing MS patients, even in the absence of a previous symptomatic event.[14]

Interestingly, OCT findings of inner retinal thinning, that is, inner plexiform layer correlates with brain atrophy and neurological disability in these patients suggesting that OCT may be used to monitor brain atrophy.[15] OCT has been now included in the most recent MS clinical trials, as it opens a window for quick and non-invasive monitoring of disease progression in MS. The rate of mGCA atrophy has been compared among different disease-modifying therapies in MS.[16]

Neuro-myelitis optica (NMO) spectrum disorder

Axonal loss in the optic nerve is more and visual prognosis poorer after an episode of ON in patients with NMO. Findings on OCT, although not conclusive in differentiating between MS and NMO, nevertheless reveal interesting differences between the two conditions. The RNFL thickness, macular volume and mRGC thickness are lower in NMO compared to MS. Patients with NMO have a reduction of 55−83 μm in pRNFL values as against a loss of around 20 μm in MS.[17] Unlike MS-associated ON which preferentially affects the temporal fields, it has also been shown that the superior and inferior quadrants are more intensely affected after NMO.[18]

Furthermore, unlike MS, unaffected eyes in patients with NMO do not have RNFL thinning. Microcystic macular edema (MMEO) on OCT is also encountered far more commonly in NMO than in MS or sporadic ON.[17]

Optic neuropathy due to other causes

In traumatic optic neuropathy, OCT shows pRNFL loss 2−4 weeks after the trauma, and it may be useful for monitoring and prognostication. In nutritional and toxic neuropathies, pRNFL may be normal or slightly increased on initial evaluation and become thinned, especially temporally on subsequent follow-up.[19]

Potential biomarker

mRGC thickness has been shown as a potential biomarker for diagnosis and progression of Alzheimer's disease and Parkinson's disease.[20] Disease severity of Huntington's has also been correlated with reduced macular volume and temporal pRNFL.[21]

Side effects of neurological treatment

Vigabatrin, an antiepileptic drug, causes visual field loss which is asymptomatic in early stages. Electrophysiological tests and perimetry are carried out regularly to pick up this visual loss. Problem is in children, where there is low reliability of these tests. Peripapillary RNFL examination on OCT has been shown to demonstrate characteristic nasal pRNFL thinning in patients exposed to vigabatrin[22] and these changes have been shown to correlate well with electrophysiological responses and visual field defects.[23]

Fingolimod, an oral agent for treating a relapsing form of MS, is known to cause Fingolimod-associated macular edema (FAME), which can be diagnosed with macular OCT.[24]

Prognostic information

Compressive optic neuropathy

Space-occupying lesions of the brain may cause visual dysfunction due to compression of the nerves in the visual pathways, especially in the vicinity of the chiasma. The most common among these are pituitary tumors which typically cause bitemporal hemianopia and progressive visual loss. OCT may help in the detection of presymptomatic pituitary tumors as well as aid in their management.

It has been shown that patients with normal preoperative pRNFL had significant visual or visual field improvement than those with pRNFL loss before surgery.[25] Among the four quadrants, temporal and inferior quadrants have a stronger correlation with visual recovery.[26] Furthermore, it has been shown that mRGC parameters correlate more with post-operative visual recovery than pRFNL.[26]

LHON

It has been demonstrated that LHON gene carriers have large optic nerve head (ONH) than LHON-affected eyes.[27] Similarly, LHON affected with the larger disc will have better visual outcome.[27]

Nonarteritic-anterior ischemic optic neuropathy

In the acute phase of nonarteritic-anterior ischemic neuropathy (NA-AION), the pRNFL loss cannot be predicted. However, it is known in primate eyes that degree of initial pRNFL swelling correlated with the severity of atrophy as well as functional impairment as seen on electrophysiological responses.[28] In early phase, mRGC thinning correlated more with visual field loss.[29] Further, it has been shown that macular ganglion cell inner plexiform layer (GCIPL) thinning is significant in AION eyes as compared to unaffected eye.[30]

Emerging advances in OCT technology

OCT-angiography (OCTA), extended depth imaging-OCT (EDI-OCT), and swept source-OCT (SS-OCT) are new advances in the field of OCT technology. OCTA has been shown to pick up telangiectatic vessels and dilated microvasculature over the temporal inner retinal layers in LHON eyes.[31] Peripapillary retinal and choroidal blood flow densities have been studied in the acute stage of AION, and its partial spontaneous recovery has also been shown.[32] EDI-OCT, due to its ability to pick deeper structures can detect etiologies related to ONH, lamina cribrosa, and choroid. Anterior displacement of lamina cribrosa has been shown in patients with IIH.[33]

Fundus fluorescein angiography in neuro-ophthalmology

Introduction

Fundus fluorescein angiography (FFA) allows a detailed assessment of retinal vasculature. In addition, it also helps to assess the blood supply of choroid and anterior part of the optic nerve, that is, optic nerve head. FFA has proved invaluable not only in the study of the blood supply of the optic disc in the health and disease, but it is also a method of clinical investigation in the diagnosis of many significant optic disc lesions, for example, optic disc edema, retrobulbar neuritis (RBN), pseudo-papilledema, drusen of the optic disc, optic atrophy, glial membrane covering the disc, optic disc pit, abnormal vessel on the disc, AION, optic disc vasculitis, glaucoma, normal tension glaucoma (NTG), and optic disc tumors, and in the better understanding of the disease.

For most of the above indications now, FFA is not carried out as better non-invasive tests such as ultrasonography, optical coherence tomography, and fundus autofluorescence are available. Serial fundus imaging alone is a great tool to monitor the response to treatment and explaining prognosis to the patient.

In the present era, FFA is indicated in various neuro-ophthalmological conditions mainly as a diagnostic tool.

Vascular disorders of the optic disc

Two important things about the blood supply of the optic disc are posterior ciliary artery (PCA) that supplies the optic disc and the choroid and this supply is sectoral. When the PCA supply to the optic disc is suddenly blocked as in temporal arteritis, arteriosclerosis, and a host of other systemic and vascular conditions, it produces anterior ischemic optic neuropathy. FFA in these cases shows filling defects in the optic disc, the peripapillary choroid, and sometimes, even in rest of the choroid. The involvement of the optic disc may be total or sectoral, depending upon the extent of vascular occlusion. FFA can pick up these lesions within the first few days of symptoms. Later the information is lost due to the collateral formation.[34]

Nonarteritic AION (NA-AION) is almost always due to transient non-perfusion or hypoperfusion of the nutrient vessels in the anterior part of the optic nerve.[35] On FFA, in NA-AION, during the very early stage, filling defects may be seen in the optic disc, peripapillary choroid, and choroidal watershed zone. Hence, these findings are very transient and recognized within the first days of disease. Rarely, NA-AION can occur due to embolic occlusion of the PCA. In nonarteritic AION, however, such massive choroidal non-filling is extremely rare.[36]

In arteritic AION (AION), by contrast, there is almost always evidence of PCA occlusion with the absence of choroidal and optic disc filling in its distribution.[36] Cilio-retinal artery occlusion, if associated with AION, is nearly always diagnostic of arteritic AION. With time after the onset of arteritic AION, there is collateral circulation in the choroid progressively results in filling of the involved choroid so that fluorescein angiography performed a week or more after the onset may not show any such massive filling defect. During the late phase of angiography, the disc stains with fluorescein, which is a non-specific finding for any optic disc edema.

Differentiating retinopathy from optic neuropathy

There are few uveitic conditions where optic disc edema is the initial sign of disease. Rest of the signs are so subtle that they can be missed in a casual examination. Intermediate uveitis, syphilis, Vogt-Koyanagi-Harada (VKH) syndrome,[37] and sympathetic ophthalmia are a few examples, where optic disc edema may be the first presenting feature of the disease. Other clinical signs may not have yet manifested. FFA can pick up early changes in the retina and choroid apart from the optic disc changes, thus can help in clinching the correct diagnosis.

Neuroretinitis is a morphological diagnosis, which can be funduscopically confused with papillitis or papilledema and occurs with hypertensive, renal failure, and infiltrative retinopathies, as well as with retinal vein occlusion or anterior ischemic optic neuropathy.[38] Here also, FFA helps to differentiate the retinal pathology from the optic nerve pathology.

Leber's hereditary optic neuropathy

In LHON, FFA shows telangiectatic vessels in the vicinity of the optic vessels and these vessels persist in the late phase but show no leakage.

Differentiating true disc edema from pseudedema

No abnormal changes or hyperfluorescence was seen in case of pseudo disc edema, whereas true disc edema will have the hyperfluorescent disc and blurred margins, as well as dilated capillaries and microaneurysms over the disc and the surrounding retina.

FFA is often normal in ON. It is reported that up to 25% of the patients demonstrate either dye leakage or perivenous sheathing.[39] These findings may identify patients at somewhat higher risk of developing multiple sclerosis. In RBN, FFA changes are sectoral, and staining of the disc may even appear before ophthalmoscopically visible optic disc edema.

REPRESENTATIVE CASES

CASE 1

LEBER'S HEREDITARY OPTIC NEUROPATHY

A 16-year-old male presented with the sudden, sequential, painless, progressive, bilateral decrease of vision since 24 days in the right eye followed by the left eye. Visual acuity was counting finger (CF) 1.5 m in the right eye (RE) and CF 3 m in the left eye (LE). RAPD was present in RE. On fundus examination, there was temporal pallor in RE (Figure 3A.1a) with nasal peripapillary edema. Rest of fundus was normal. LE showed hyperemic disc with surrounding nerve fiber layer edema along (Figure 3A.1b) with an increased number of capillaries in superotemporal as well as an inferonasal quadrant. Vascular tortuosity was also present in all quadrants.

Visual fields (Figure 3A.1c): RE showed generalized depression of visual fields, while LE showed cecocentral scotoma. Fundus fluorescein angiography: RE (Figure 3A.1d–f) showed few bulbous dilatations suggestive of telangiectatic capillaries (white arrows in Figure 3A.1e) in inferotemporal quadrant which persisted in the late phase but showed no leakage. Slight vascular tortuosity was noted in superotemporal vessels. LE (Figure 3A.1g–i) showed a marked increase in the number of telangiectatic vessels in superotemporal quadrant (white-dotted circle in Figure 3A.1h), which persisted in late phase along with vascular tortuosity in all four quadrants suggesting acute involvement. Late phase revealed disc staining (Figure 3A.1f) but no leakage. There was no arteriovenous delay or non-perfusion of the disc.

Optical coherence tomography (OCT): OCT RNFL of RE (Figure 3A.1l) revealed thinning of RNFL in inferior and temporal quadrant. OCT-RNFL showed thickening in superior and inferior quadrants due to thickening of the nerve fiber layer.

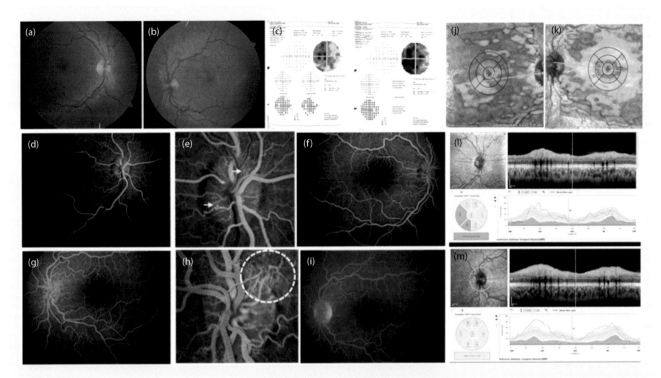

FIGURE 3A.1 Representative case of Leber's hereditary optic neuropathy. Fundus examination showed temporal pallor with nasal peripapillary retinal nerve fiber layer (RNFL) edema in the right eye (RE) (a). Hyperemic disc and peripapillary RNFL edema were noticed in the left eye (LE) (b). Visual fields showed generalized depression in RE and cecocentral scotoma in LE (c). Fundus fluorescein angiography (d–f) showed few bulbous dilatations suggestive of telangiectatic capillaries (e, white arrows) in the RE. Fluorescein angiography in LE (g–i) showed a marked increase in the number of telangiectatic vessels (h, white-dotted circle). Late phase revealed disc staining but no leakage (i). Macular ganglion cell analysis (GCA) showed a decrease in the ganglion cell volume in RE (j) as compared to LE (k), suggesting more damage to the ganglion cell layer in RE (darker colors depicts thinner areas). OCT RNFL of RE (l) showed RNFL thinning in the inferior and temporal quadrant. OCT-RNFL of LE (m) showed thickening in all quadrants due to nerve fiber layer edema.

OCT-RNFL of LE (Figure 3A.1m) showed thickening of all quadrants, especially supero- and infero-temporal due to nerve fiber layer edema. Ganglion cell analysis (GCA) of the macula (Figure 3A.1j and k) revealed a decrease in volume of RE as compared to LE, suggesting the loss of ganglion cell layer. (Darker colors depict more damage.) Recent studies suggest that ganglion cell layer thickness is a better predictor in comparison to the nerve fiber layer thickness as GCL decreases much earlier in comparison to the inner plexiform layer. OCT-angiography is also used to monitor LHON, which shows the spread of radial peripapillary capillary defects over some time in such patients.

CASE 2
TOXIC AND NUTRITIONAL OPTIC NEUROPATHY

A 22-year-old male presented with sudden, painless vision loss in both eyes. There was no previous history of similar episodes, trauma, or any ocular surgery. History was significant for chronic alcoholism in addition to the history of binge drinking just before visual loss. He was also a smoker and opioid user. His visual acuity was the light perception in both eyes, and the projection of rays was inaccurate. Pupils were mildly reacting with no RAPD or anisocoria.

On fundus examination, both discs showed pallor of the temporal neuroretinal rim (Figure 3A.2a and b). Fluorescein angiography showed no delay in perfusion of the disc or non-perfusion of disc in both eyes (Figure 3A.2c–f). OCT-RNFL showed severe bilateral loss of nerve fiber layer (Figure 3A.2g and h). He could not perform visual fields due to poor vision.

In toxic/nutritional optic neuropathy, RNFL thinning measured by OCT can help detect disease before fundus changes or optic disc pallor sets in. Thinning of the RNFL has been reported to begin in the inferotemporal quadrant of the papillomacular bundle and later involves all quadrants.

Retinal ganglion cell layer (RGL) analysis by spectral domain OCT (SD-OCT) has been shown to decrease both in thickness and volume. The most significant decrease in RGL thickness and volume has been reported in the inferonasal quadrants, supporting early papillomacular bundle impairment in its inferotemporal sector.

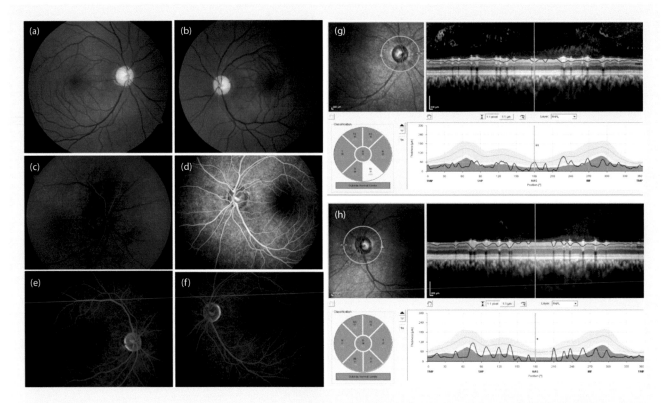

FIGURE 3A.2 Representative case of toxic and nutritional optic neuropathy. Temporal disc pallor was seen in both eyes (a, b). Fluorescein angiography was essentially normal in both eyes (c–f). OCT-RNFL showed severe bilateral loss of nerve fiber layer (g, h).

CASE 3

NMO SPECTRUM DISORDER

A 30-year-old female presents with the complaint of bilateral lower limb weakness, insidious in onset, gradually progressive for 2 months. She was diagnosed as a case of neuromyelitis optica-spectrum disorder (NMO-SD). She was positive for an anti-aquaporin-4 antibody test. She was referred for ophthalmological evaluation.

On examination, her visual acuity was 20/20 in both eyes. Anterior segment findings were normal. Fundus examinations (Figure 3A.3a and b) showed temporal pallor in bilateral optic discs without any other significant ocular findings. Fundus fluorescein angiography (Figure 3A.3c and d) was normal in both eyes. OCT pRNFL (peripapillary retinal nerve fiber layer) showed bilateral thinning of the temporal retinal nerve fiber layer. The patient was treated with intravenous methylprednisolone. She lost to follow up after that.

She presented after 3 years with sudden-onset progressive loss of vision in both eyes (R>L) for 1 week. She presented to the neurology department, and the diagnosis of relapse of NMOSD was made. On examination, her best-corrected visual acuity (BCVA) was counting finger 1 m in the right eye and 20/160 in the left eye. Fundus examination (Figure 3A.3e and f) showed bilateral temporal disc pallor (R>L) in both eyes. OCT macula (Figure 3A.3g and h) showed some changes in the inner nuclear layer (red arrowhead) in the right eye with the otherwise normal foveal contour in both the eyes. GCA analysis (Figure 3A.3i and j) revealed bilateral thinning. The ganglion cell loss was more evident in the right eye (Figure 3A.3i) (darker the color, thinner is the ganglion cell layer). OCT pRNFL in the right eye (Figure 3A.3k) showed thinning of retinal nerve fiber layer of around the entire optic disc. In the left eye (Figure 3A.3l), only temporal and inferior pRNFL was thinned out.

In NMO, optic disc pallor may be the only sign seen by the clinician. Fluorescein angiography is essentially normal. OCT shows substantial peripapillary retinal nerve fiber layer loss. Recent studies have demonstrated progressive retinal neuroaxonal damage in patients with NMOSD even without ON. The ganglion cell and inner plexiform (GCIP) layer thickness complements the pRNFL thickness as an imaging marker. The main targets of interest are the ganglion cell bodies associated with axons in the retinal fiber layers. It is mostly measured in the perifoveal area as the ganglion cells are concentrated over this area. Currently, pRNFL has a reasonably good standardization and is measured similarly across devices, whereas GCIP measurements lack it. After multiple attacks of ON, the pRNFL and GCIP layers are severely atrophic.

Further attacks don't lead to more thinning due to "flooring effect". There also have been reports of micro cystic macular edema in the inner nuclear layer (INL) in approximately 20% of patients of NMOSD. This is seen usually after an attack of ON. The presence of microcystic changes in INL could be used as a surrogate marker for the presence of inflammation.

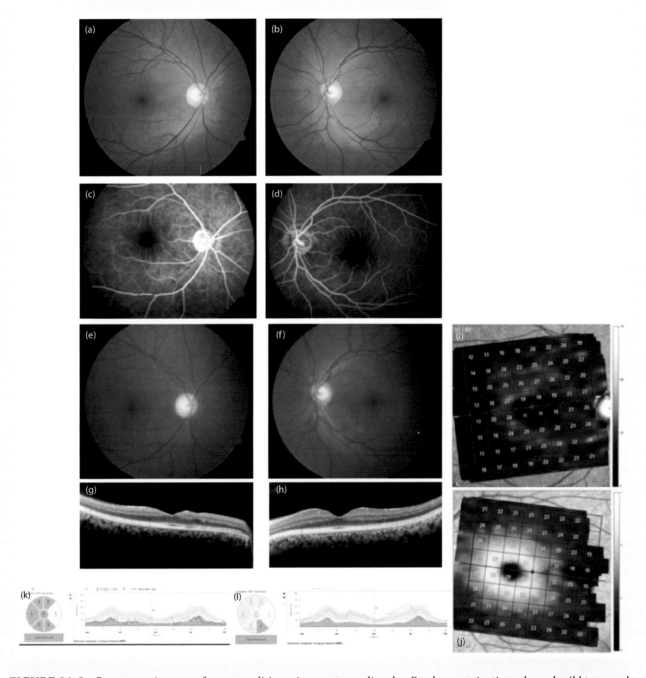

FIGURE 3A.3 Representative case of neuromyelitis optica spectrum disorder. Fundus examinations showed mild temporal pallor in bilateral optic discs (a, b). Fundus fluorescein angiography was normal in both eyes (c, d). Three years later, the patient presented with recurrence. Fundus examination showed bilateral temporal disc pallor (e, f). OCT macula (g, h) showed some changes in the inner nuclear layer (g, red arrowhead) in the right eye with the otherwise normal foveal contour in both eyes. GCA analysis (i, j) revealed bilateral ganglion cell layer thinning, which was more evident in RE (i, the darker the color, the thinner is the ganglion cell layer). OCT RNFL in RE (k) showed the retinal nerve fiber layer thinning in all quadrants. In the left eye (l), only temporal and inferior RNFL was thinned out.

CASE 4

OPTIC NEURITIS/MULTIPLE SCLEROSIS

A 35-year-old female who was well until 2 weeks before her clinic visit noticed the visual loss in her left eye. The visual loss was subacute in onset, progressive and accompanied by dull retro-orbital ache and pain on eye movements. She had no complaints of weakness, numbness, tingling, double vision, or headache. Her systemic history was uneventful for diabetes mellitus or hypertension.

On examination, her best-corrected visual acuity was 6/6 in the right eye and no perception of light in the left eye. Intraocular pressure was 10 and 12 mmHg in right and left eye, respectively. Extraocular movements were full and free in both eyes with pain on adduction and abduction in the left eye. Left eye pupil showed relative apparent pupillary defect (RAPD). Rest of the anterior segment examination was normal. Fundus examination revealed left eye hyperaemic disc edema. Right eye fundus examination was within normal limits (Figure 3A.4a and b). A clinical diagnosis of left eye ON was made, and the patient was scheduled for FFA. FFA revealed normal choroidal and optic disc perfusion with no perfusion delay. However, late disc staining was seen in the left eye (Figure 3A.4c and d). CSF analysis was normal. Laboratory investigations were negative for ANA, c-ANCA, p-ANCA, VDRL, and NMO antibodies. Serum angiotensin converting enzyme (ACE) levels were within normal limits. MRI brain and orbit with gadolinium contrast was within normal limits. The patient was administered intravenous methylprednisolone 1 g once a day for 3 days followed by oral steroids (starting with 1 mg/kg) and then in tapering doses.

On follow-up visit for 1 month, the best-corrected visual acuity improved to 6/18 in the left eye and there was temporal disc pallor in the left eye. GCA reveals decreased ganglion cell thickness in the left eye, as compared to left eye (Figure 3A.4e and f). OCT pRNFL showed thinning of the temporal retinal nerve fiber layer in the left eye as compared to the right eye (Figure 3A.4g and h).

After 3 months, the patient reported with visual loss in the right eye. It was associated with pain on eye movements. The best-corrected visual acuity was hand motions close to face in the right eye and 6/18 in the left eye. Right eye pupillary examination revealed RAPD. Fundus examination revealed right eye hyperaemic disc edema and left eye temporal disc pallor (Figure 3A.4i and j). A clinical diagnosis of right eye optic neuritis was made, and the patient was again started on intravenous methylprednisolone. FFA showed right eye normal choroidal perfusion with late staining of the disc suggestive of optic neuritis (Figure 3A.4k and l).

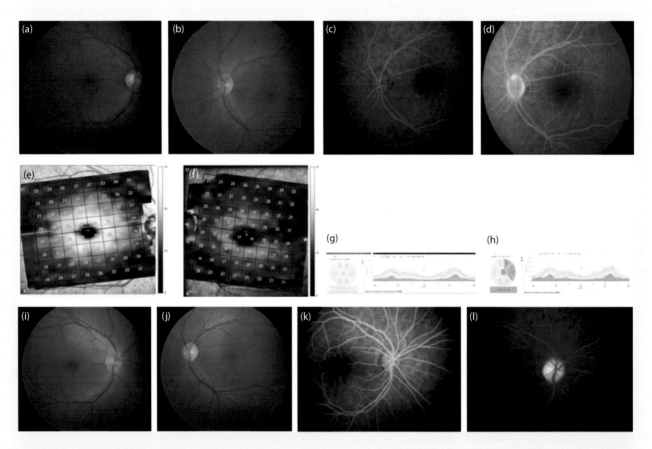

FIGURE 3A.4 Representative case of optic neuritis/multiple sclerosis (Case 1). Right eye fundus examination was within normal limits (a). The left eye showed disc edema (b). FFA revealed normal choroidal and optic disc perfusion with no perfusion delay (c, d). Late disc staining was seen in the left eye (d). Ganglion cell analysis showed a decrease in ganglion cell thickness in the left eye compared to the right eye (e, f). OCT RNFL showed thinning of the temporal retinal nerve fiber layer in the left eye compared to the right eye (g, h). The right eye was involved after three months. Fundus examination revealed right eye hyperemic disc edema and left eye temporal disc pallor (i, j). FFA showed normal choroidal perfusion with late staining of the disc in the right eye (k, l).

CASE 5

OPTIC NEURITIS/MULTIPLE SCLEROSIS

A 40-year-old female presented with complaint of diminution of vision in left eye for 2 days. The visual loss was subacute in onset and progressive in nature. It was accompanied by pain with eye movements and a dull retro-orbital ache. She did not have any other positive history. Her systemic history was not significant.

On examination, her best-corrected visual acuity (BCVA) was 6/6 in the right eye and counting fingers at 1 m in the left eye. Intraocular pressure was 10 and 12 mmHg with Goldmann applanation tonometry in right and left eye, respectively. Extraocular movements were full and free in both eyes with pain on adduction and abduction in the left eye. Left eye pupil showed relative apparent pupillary defect (RAPD). Rest of the anterior segment examination was within normal limits. Right eye fundus examination was within normal limits (Figure 3A.5a). Fundus examination revealed disc edema in the left eye (Figure 3A.5b). A clinical diagnosis of left eye optic neuritis was made. Fundus fluorescein angiography (FFA) findings were consistent with

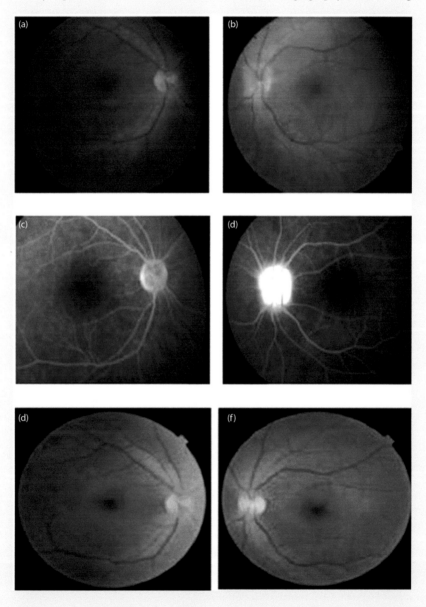

FIGURE 3A.5 Representative case of optic neuritis/multiple sclerosis (Case 2). Examination showed normal fundus in the right eye (a) and disc edema in the left eye (b). Fundus fluorescein angiography (FFA) findings were consistent with clinical diagnosis. The late phase of FFA showed normal findings in the right eye (c), whereas the left eye late phase of FFA showed disc leakage and staining (d). At 3-months follow-up, fundus examination of the right eye was normal (e), while the left eye showed temporal disc pallor (f). In all sectors, ganglion cell analysis (GCA) showed a decrease in macular ganglion cell volume in the left eye. GCA of the right eye was within normal limits (g). Peripapillary RNFL analysis revealed RNFL thinning in the temporal quadrant in the left eye and normal RNFL thickness in the right eye (h). *(Continued)*

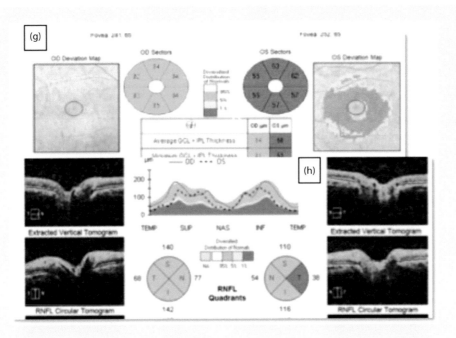

FIGURE 3A.5 *(Continued)*

clinical diagnosis. Late phase of FFA showed normal findings in the right eye, whereas left eye late phase of FFA showed disc leakage and staining (Figure 3A.5c and d).

She was seen by neurologist and her MRI was done. She was diagnosed as a case of multiple sclerosis presenting with optic neuritis in the left eye. The patient was given intravenous methylprednisolone 1 g OD for 5 days followed by oral steroids (starting with 1 mg/kg) and then in tapering doses. She was initiated on disease modifying therapy with teriflunomide (14 mg per day).

On follow-up visits, she did well with her BCVA improved to 6/6 and disc edema in left eye resolved. At 3 months follow-up, her BCVA was 6/6 in both eyes. Anterior segment examination was normal in both eyes. Fundus examination of the right eye was normal, while left eye revealed temporal pallor (Figure 3A.5e and f). GCA of macula revealed decrease in volume in the left eye in all sectors. GCA of the right eye was within normal limits (Figure 3A.5g). Peripapillary RNFL analysis revealed RNFL thinning in the temporal quadrant in the left eye and normal pRNFL thickness in the right eye (Figure 3A.5h).

CASE 6

ARTERITIC ISCHEMIC OPTIC NEUROPATHY

An 85-year-old male presented with complaint of sequential diminution in vision in 2 days. He noticed a decrease in vision, which was sudden in onset, painless, progressive, involving the right eye first and then the left eye within 48 hours. He was non-diabetic and non-hypertensive. He also had a history of bitemporal headache for 1 month and complained of difficulty and pain on opening his mouth which was suggestive of jaw claudication.

On ocular examination the patient could not perceive light from either eyes. There was no relative afferent pupillary defect. Right eye fundus view was hazy due to the presence of cataract. Fundus examination showed bilateral pale disc edema (Figure 3A.6a and b). On palpation, the bilateral temporal artery was palpable. Clinical diagnosis of Bilateral Arteritic Anterior Ischemic Optic Neuropathy was considered. The patient received intravenous methyl prednisone (1 gram per day for 5 days). Fundus fluorescein angiography was planned. FFA showed patchy and delayed choroidal filling (Figure 3A.6c) with disc perfusion defect in choroidal phase. Late phase (Figure 3A.6d) showed disc staining.

Temporal artery biopsy confirmed the diagnosis. No improvement in visual acuity was noted on follow up. The fundus photograph (Figure 3A.6e and f) at 3 months follow-up showed resolution of bilateral disc edema and development of disc pallor.

The degree of choroidal filling delay is directly proportional to the level of ischemia of the optic disc. This correlation disappears once the circulation is restored. As the choroidal circulation improves significantly within 1 week, the presence of ischemia might be missed if the clinician fails to get FFA within the first few days of onset of symptoms.

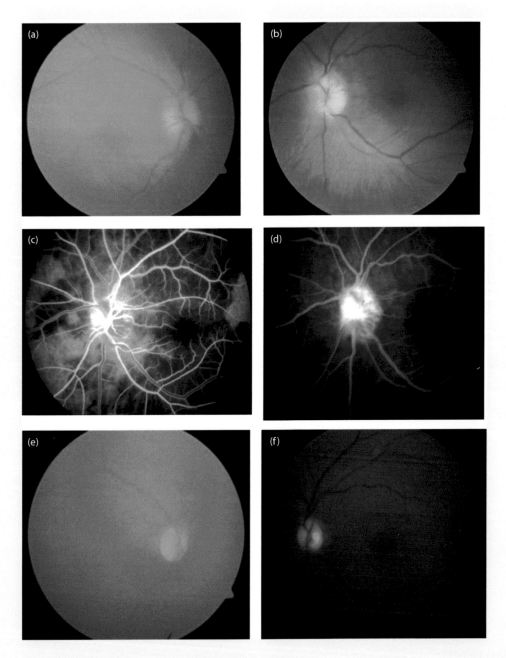

FIGURE 3A.6 Representative case of arteritic ischemic optic neuropathy. The right eye fundus view was hazy due to the presence of cataract. Fundus examination showed bilateral pale disc edema (a, b). FFA showed patchy and delayed choroidal filling (c) with disc perfusion defect in the choroidal phase (c). Late phase (d) showed disc staining. At the 3-months follow-up, the disc edema has resolved, and disc pallor has set in (e, f).

CASE 7

VKH SYNDROME PRESENTING AS PAPILLEDEMA TO NEUROLOGIST

A 45-year-old female presented with headache of one month duration. Gadolinium enhanced MRI suggested signs of increased intracranial pressure and she was diagnosed with Idiopathic Intracranial hypertension based upon high opening CSF pressure. All other blood and CSF investigations were normal. She was initiated on oral acetazolamide. On 2 weeks follow-up she complained of worsening visual function associated with redness of both eyes.

Her best-corrected visual acuity was 6/9P in both eyes. Anterior segment examination was normal in both eyes. Posterior segment examination showed 1+ vitreous cells along with disc edema with ILM folds in the peripapillary area due to fluid in both eyes (Figure 3A.7a and b).

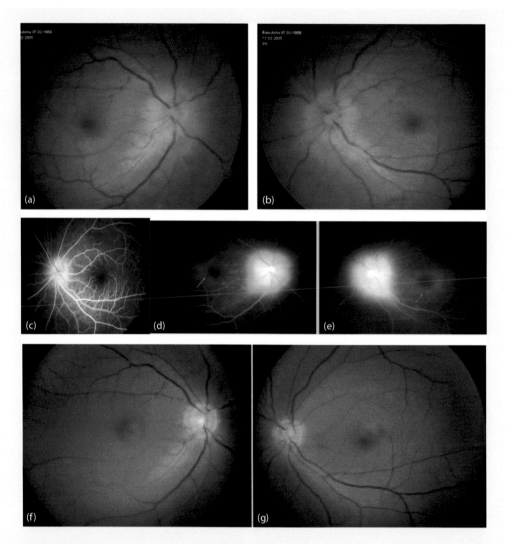

FIGURE 3A.7   Representative case of Vogt-Koyanagi-Harada (VKH) syndrome. Posterior segment examination showed bilateral disc edema with ILM folds in the peripapillary area (a, b). FFA showed disc leakage (c) and hyperfluorescent lesions in the choroidal circulation (c, red arrows). In the late phase, there was massive disc staining and pooling of dye in foveal areas (blue arrows) in both the eyes (d, e). On follow-up, papilledema has resolved (f, g).

In view of vitreous reaction and the disc edema, FFA was ordered. FFA showed hypolesion in the choroidal circulation along with leakage from disc in both eyes (Figure 3A.7c, red arrow). This became hyper in the late phase with massive disc staining due to peripapillary fluid with pooling of dye in foveal area (green arrow) in both the eyes (Figure 3A.7d and e).

Indocyanine green (ICG) angiography was also done, where more hypolesions were seen in the choroidal circulation. USG of both eyes revealed retinochoroidal thickening in the peripapillary area. These findings clinched the diagnosis of VKH syndrome. She was administered intravenous steroids followed by oral steroids. There was relief in her symptoms and signs. Her vision improved in 6/6 in both eyes with the resolution of inflammation and disc edema (Figure 3A.7f and g).

Conclusion

OCT is being used by neuro-ophthalmologists to precisely localize the damage, nail down the diagnosis, give a prognosis of visual recovery and to assess treatment. FFA is an invasive tool, with clear advantages of showing vascular blood supply of the anterior part of optic nerve and retina. Hence its use in understanding and diagnosing disorders of blood vasculature is irreplaceable. OCT-angiography (OCTA) (dyeless angiography) is becoming increasingly popular and may be able to replace FFA entirely in the future.

Multiple-Choice Questions

1. All of the following are true about FFA findings in AION EXCEPT:
    a. Optic nerve vasculature involvement is seen.
    b. Choroidal vasculature involvement is not seen.
    c. Early phase of FFA is of value.
    d. Angiography can provide useful information within first few days of AION.

Answer:

b. Choroidal vasculature involvement is not seen.

2. Which OCT is able to differentiate between true and pseudo disc swelling?
   a. Cirrus OCT
   b. Time-domain OCT
   c. Spectral domain OCT
   d. None of the above

Answer:

c. Spectral domain OCT

3. The following are the names of advances in OCT technology, EXCEPT:
   a. OCT-angiography (OCTA)
   b. Extended depth imaging-OCT (EDI-OCT)
   c. Swept source (SS-OCT)
   d. Time-domain OCT

Answer:

d. Time-domain OCT

4. Non-invasive tools to detect optic disc drusens, EXCEPT:
   a. FFA.
   b. OCT angiography
   c. Fundus autofluorescence (FAF)
   d. Ultrasonography

Answer:

a. FFA

References

1. Monson DM, Smith JR. Acute zonal occult outer retinopathy. Surv Ophthalmol. 2011;56:23–35.
2. Barboni P, Carbonelli M, Savini G, do VF Ramos C, Carta A, Berezovsky A, Salomao SR, Carelli V, Sadun AA. Natural history of Leber's hereditary optic neuropathy: Longitudinal analysis of the retinal nerve fiber layer by optical coherence tomography. Ophthalmology. 2010;117(3):623–627.
3. Mizoguchi A, Hashimoto Y, Shinmei Y, Nozaki M, Ishijima K, Tagawa Y, Ishida S. Macular thickness changes in a patient with Leber's hereditary optic neuropathy. BMC Ophthalmol. 2015;15(1):1–6.
4. Balducci N, Savini G, Cascavilla ML, La Morgia C, Triolo G, Giglio R, Carbonelli M, Parisi V, Sadun AA, Bandello F, Carelli V. Macular nerve fibre and ganglion cell layer changes in acute Leber's hereditary optic neuropathy. Br J Ophthalmol. 2016;100(9):1232–1237.
5. Fard MA, Fakhree S, Abdi P, Hassanpoor N, Subramanian PS. Quantification of peripapillary total retinal volume in pseudopapilledema and mild papilledema using spectral-domain optical coherence tomography. Am J Ophthalmol. 2014;158(1):136–143.
6. Karam EZ, Hedges TR. Optical coherence tomography of the retinal nerve fibre layer in mild papilledema and pseudo papilledema. Br J Ophthalmol. 2005;89:294–298.
7. Nguyen AM, Balmitgere T, Bernard M, Tilikete C, Vighetto A. Detection of mild papilloedema using spectral domain optical coherence tomography. Br J Ophthalmol. 2012;96(3):375–379.
8. Salo T, Mrejen S, Spaide RF. Multimodal imaging of the optic disc drusen. Am J Ophthalmol. 2013;156:275–282.
9. Park SC, De Moraes CG, Teng CC, Tello C, Liebmann JM, Ritch R. Enhanced depth imaging optical coherence tomography of deep optic nerve complex structures in glaucoma. Ophthalmology. 2012;119(1):3–9.
10. Zhang Y, Ye Z, Wang M, Qiao N. Ganglion cell complex loss precedes retinal nerve fiber layer thinning in patients with pituitary adenoma. J Clin Neurosci. 2017;43:274–277.
11. Yum HR, Park SH, Park HY, Shin SY. Macular ganglion cell analysis determined by cirrus HD optical coherence tomography for early detecting chiasmal compression. PLoS One. 2016;11(4):e0153064.
12. Scott CJ, Kardon RH, Lee AG, Frisén L, Wall M. Diagnosis and grading of papilledema in patients with raised intracranial pressure using optical coherence tomography vs clinical expert assessment using a clinical staging scale. Arch Ophthalmol. 2010;128(6):705–711.
13. Noval S, Contreras I, Rebolleda G, Muñoz-Negrete FJ. Optical coherence tomography versus automated perimetry for follow-up of optic neuritis. Acta Ophthalmol Scand. 2006;84(6):790–794.
14. Saidha S, Syc SB, Durbin MK, Eckstein C, Oakley JD, Meyer SA, Conger A, Frohman TC, Newsome S, Ratchford JN, Frohman EM. Visual dysfunction in multiple sclerosis correlates better with optical coherence tomography derived estimates of macular ganglion cell layer thickness than peripapillary retinal nerve fiber layer thickness. Mult Scler J. 2011;17(12):1449–1463.
15. Brandt AU, Martinez-Lapiscina EH, Nolan R, Saidha S. Monitoring the course of MS with optical coherence tomography. Curr Treat Options Neurol. 2017;19(4):15.
16. Button J, Al-Louzi O, Lang A, Bhargava P, Newsome SD, Frohman T, Balcer LJ, Frohman EM, Prince J, Calabresi PA, Saidha S. Disease-modifying therapies modulate retinal atrophy in multiple sclerosis: a retrospective study. Neurology. 2017;88(6):525–532.
17. Bennett JL, De Seze J, Lana-Peixoto M, Palace J, Waldman A, Schippling S, Tenembaum S, Banwell B, Greenberg B, Levy M, Fujihara K. Neuromyelitis optica and multiple sclerosis: Seeing differences through optical coherence tomography. Mult Scler J. 2015;21(6):678–688.
18. Monteiro ML, Fernandes DB, Apóstolos-Pereira SL, Callegaro D. Quantification of retinal neural loss in patients with neuromyelitis optica and multiple sclerosis with or without optic neuritis using Fourier-domain optical coherence tomography. Investig Ophthalmol Vis Sci. 2012;53(7):3959–3966.
19. Pasol J. Neuro-ophthalmic disease and optical coherence tomography: Glaucoma look alike. Curr Opin Ophthalmol. 2011;22:124–132.
20. Satue M, Obis J, Rodrigo MJ, Otin S, Fuertes MI, Vilades E, Gracia H, Ara JR, Alarcia R, Polo V, Larrosa JM. Optical coherence tomography as a biomarker for diagnosis, progression, and prognosis of neurodegenerative diseases. J Ophthalmol. 2016:8503859. doi: 10.1155/2016/8503859.
21. Kersten HM, Danesh-Meyer HV, Kilfoyle DH, Roxburgh RH. Optical coherence tomography findings in Huntington's disease: A potential biomarker of disease progression. J. Neurol. 2015;262(11):2457–2465.
22. Clayton LM, Devile M, Punte T, de Haan GJ, Sander JW, Acheson JF, Sisodiya SM. Patterns of peripapillary retinal nerve fiber layer thinning in vigabatrin-exposed individuals. Ophthalmology. 2012;119(10):2152–2160.
23. Kjellstrom U, Andreasson S, Ponjavic V. Attenuation of the retinal nerve fiber layer and reduced retinal function assessed by optical coherence tomography and full field electroretinography in patients exposed to Vigabatrin medication. Acta Ophthalmol. 2014;92:149-157.
24. Jain N, Bhatti MT. Fingolimod associated macular edema: Incidence, detection and management. Neurology. 2012;78:672–680.
25. Danesh-Meyer HV, Papchenko T, Savino PJ, Law A, Evans J, Gamble GD. In vivo retinal nerve fiber layer thickness measured by optical coherence tomography predicts visual recovery after surgery for parachiasmal tumors. Investig Ophthalmol Vis Sci. 2008;49(5):1879–1885.
26. Moon CH, Hwang SC, Kim BT, Ohn YH, Park TK. Visual prognostic value of optical coherence tomography and photopic negative response in chiasmal compression. Investig Ophthalmol Vis Sci. 2011;52(11):8527–8533.
27. Ramos CD, Bellusci C, Savini G, Carbonelli M, Berezovsky A, Tamaki C, Cinoto R, Sacai PY, Moraes-Filho MN, Miura HM, Valentino ML. Association of optic disc size with development and prognosis of Leber's hereditary optic neuropathy. Investig Ophthalmol Vis Sci. 2009;50(4):1666–1674.
28. Johnson MA, Miller NR, Nolan T, Bernstein SL. Peripapillary retinal nerve fiber layer swelling predicts peripapillary atrophy in a primate model of nonarteritic anterior ischemic optic neuropathy. Investig Ophthalmol Vis Scie. 2016;57(2):527–532.
29. Park SW, Ji YS, Heo H. Early macular ganglion cell-inner plexiform layer analysis in non arteritic anterior ischemic optic neuropathy. Grafes Arch Clin Exp Ophthalmol. 2016;254:983–989.
30. Dompablo ED, García-Montesinos J, Muñoz-Negrete FJ, Rebolleda G. Ganglion cell analysis at acute episode of nonarteritic anterior ischemic optic neuropathy to predict irreversible damage. A prospective study. Graefes Arch Clin Exp Ophthalmol. 2016;254(9):1793–1800.
31. Gaier ED, Gittinger JW, Cestari DM, Miller JB. Peripapillary capillary dilation in Leber hereditary optic neuropathy revealed by optical coherence tomographic angiography. JAMA Ophthalmol. 2016;134(11):1332–1334.
32. Sharma S, Ang M, Najjar RP, Sng C, Cheung CY, Rukmini AV, Schmetterer L, Milea D. Optical coherence tomography angiography in acute non-arteritic anterior ischaemic optic neuropathy. Br J Ophthalmol. 2017;101(8):1045–1051.
33. Villarruel JM, Li XQ, Bach-Holm D, Hamann S. Anterior lamina cribrosa surface position in idiopathic intracranial hypertension and glaucoma. Eur J Ophthalmol. 2017;27(1):55–61.
34. Hayreh SS. Anterior ischaemic optic neuropathy II. Fundus on ophthalmoscopy and fluorescein angiography. Br J Ophthal. 1974;58:964–980.
35. Hayreh SS. Anterior ischemic optic neuropathy. Arch Neurol. 1981;38:675–678.
36. Hayreh SS. Anterior ischaemic optic neuropathy differentiation of arteritic from non-arteritic type and its management. Eye. 1990;4(1):25–41.
37. Nakao K, Abematsu N, Mizushima Y, Sakamoto T. Optic disc swelling in Vogt-Koyanagi-Harada disease. Investig Ophthalmol Vis Sci. 2012;53(4):1917–1922.
38. Abdelhakim A, Rasool N. Neuroretinitis: A review. Curr Opin Ophthalmol. 2018; 29:514–519.
39. Lightman S, McDonald WI, Bird AC, Francis DA, Hoskins A, Batcholer JR, Halliday AM. Retinal venous sheathing in optic neuritis: its significance for the pathogenesis of multiple sclerosis. Brain. 1987;110(2):405–414.

3B

VISUAL-EVOKED POTENTIAL IN NEURO-OPHTHALMOLOGY

Usha K. Misra

Introduction

Visual-evoked potentials (VEPs) are the electrical potential differences recorded from scalp in response to visual stimuli. The role of VEP become important further in an uncooperative patient, fundus examination is not possible or when there is a question about localization of deficit within the visual pathways. However, VEP has poor localizing value as disturbances anywhere in the visual system can produce abnormality.

Anatomy

The optic nerves form connection between retina and the brain. Light impulses stimulate the photoreceptors (rods and cones) which further synapse with the inner nuclear or bipolar layers; bipolar cells synapse further with the ganglion cell layer. The axons of the ganglion cell form the optic nerve. The two optic nerves joined at optic chiasma. The optic tract starts from the optic chiasma and terminates in the lateral geniculate body. The optic tract contains ipsilateral temporal and contralateral nasal retinal fibers. The fibers carrying impulses from upper part of retina terminate in the ventromedial segment and those from lower part terminate in the ventrolateral segment of geniculate body. The ipsilateral temporal and contralateral nasal retinal fibers terminate alternatively in six layers in lateral geniculate body. Lateral geniculate body neurons form optic radiation, which pass posteriorly to terminate in the striate cortex (area 17). The macular fibers occupy the larger portion of occipital lobe at the occipital pole in a wedge-shaped area. The upper half and lower half of the retinal fibers relay superior and inferior to the calcarine fissure, respectively (Figure 3B.1).

The P100 waveform of VEP is generated in the striate and peristriate occipital cortex not only due to activation of primary cortex but also due to thalamocortical volleys. On stimulation, there is increased metabolism in primary visual area as well as in the visual association areas (area 18 and 19) [1].

VEP primarily reflects activity of central 3–6° of visual field, which is relayed to the surface of occipital lobe. The projections from the peripheral retina are directed to the regions deep within the calcarine fissure leading to attenuated or unrecordable VEP on peripheral retinal stimulation. In humans, the cortical representation of fovea is much greater than that of peripheral retina, which is known as *foveal magnification* [2].

Pre-test requirements

1. Patient should be explained about the test to get full cooperation
2. Avoid hair spray or oil application after the hair wash
3. The usual glasses if any should be put on during the test
4. The detailed ophthalmological examination such as visual acuity, pupillary diameter, and field charts should be reviewed
5. Avoid any miotic or mydriatic 12 h before the test
6. In patients with field defects, besides the midline electrode, lateral placement of electrode may be necessary

Methods: For VEP, standard disc electroencephalography (EEG) electrodes are commonly used. The preparation of skin is done by abrading and degreasing. The recording electrode is placed at Oz as per 10–20 international system of EEG electrode placement by using conducting jelly or electrode paste. The reference electrode site is Fpz or 12 cm above the nasion. Linked ear reference is also used as noncephalic reference. At Cz, ground electrode is placed. The electrode impedance is kept below 5 kΩ. An amplification ranging from 20,000 to 100,000 is used to record pattern shift visual-evoked potentials (PSVEPs). The low cut filters are set at 1–3 Hz and high cut at 100–300 Hz. Sweep time range between 250 ms and 500 ms. In common practice, usually 100 epochs are averaged. Averaging should be done twice and super imposed to check reproducibility of the wave form.

As per recommendation of International Federation of Clinical Neurophysiology (IFCN) Committee, montage consisting of two channels is sufficient for VEP recording [3]. The suggested montage for VEP is as follows:

- Channel 1: Oz–Fpz
- Channel 2: Oz–linked ear

Sometimes asymmetrical activation of visual cortex produced either by the changes in the shape of stimulus or lesions in the visual pathways results in lateral shift of P100 peak. Additional recording channels, therefore, are required as only midline recording may not be reliable (Figure 3B.2).

- Channel 1: Oz–Fpz
- Channel 2: Pz–Fpz
- Channel 3: L5–Fpz
- Channel 4: R5–Fpz

L5 and R5 denote sites 5 cm lateral to Oz on the left and right sides, respectively [4]. If required, the additional recording may be obtained from 10 cm right and left from Oz.

For PSVEP, alternating checks or alternating gratings are used for stimulation. The gratings can be either cine or square wave. The contrast should be between 50% and 80%, distance between subject's eye and screen should be 70 and 100 cm and fixation point for full field size greater than 8°. In routine clinical practice, black and white checks or gratings are employed. In multiple sclerosis patients, use of colored gratings will increase the yield of VEP abnormalities [5].

The size of pattern elements should be 14–16, 28–32, and 56–64 in. Smaller size is optimal for foveal stimulation and the larger for para foveal. However, foveal stimulation may be easily affected by visual acuity. Para foveal stimulation therefore may give normal results in patients with foveal dysfunction. The stimulation rate for transient PSVEP is 1 Hz and for steady-state PSVEP is 4–8 Hz. The mean luminance of the central field should be at least 50 cd/m² and the background luminance 20–40 cd/m². The difference of luminance between the center and periphery of field should not exceed 20%. The patient should fix his gaze at the center of the screen.

DOI: 10.1201/9780429020278-5

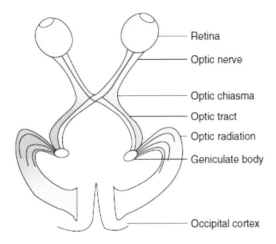

FIGURE 3B.1   A schematic diagram of visual pathway.

Normal PSVEP

The transient VEPs represent a series of waveform of opposite polarity. The negative waveform is represented as N and positive deflection as P, which is followed by the approximate latency in milliseconds. The commonly used wave forms are N70, P100, and N135, and the peak latency and peak-to-peak amplitudes of these waves are usually measured (Figure 3B.3). Normal values are given in Table 3B.1.

Steady-state VEP

Steady-state VEPs are the response to visual stimuli given at a rate of ≥3.5 Hz. These responses overlap one another and appear as somewhat sinusoidal oscillations, which persist during the period of stimulation. It can also be defined as repetitive evoked potentials (EPs), which constitute discrete frequency components and remain constant in amplitude and phase over an infinitely long period of time [6].

Variables influencing VEP

Age
Age has been found to affect the P100 latency at a rate of 2.5 ms/decade after the fifth decade [7, 8]. However, the amplitude is higher in the first decade and the mean amplitude is almost double that of the adult value.

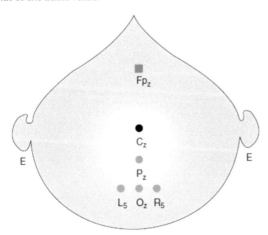

FIGURE 3B.2   Electrode placement in PSVEP (four channel). (●) Active, (■) reference and (●) ground electrode. L, Left; R, Right.

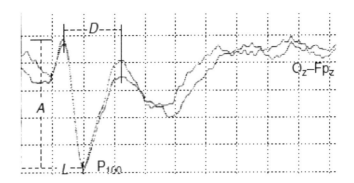

FIGURE 3B.3   A normal VEP with measurement of P100. *Abbreviations:* L, latency; D, duration; A, amplitude. Sweep speed 50 ms/division; sensitivity, 2 µV/division.

Gender
P100 latency is longer in adult males compared to that in females. Mean P100 amplitude is greater in females in comparison to males.

Eye dominance
Dominant eye stimulation produces VEP with P100 of shorter latency and higher amplitude.

Eye movement
Eye movement reduces the amplitude of P100, but its latency is not affected.

Visual acuity
The P100 latency is reported to be normal with visual acuity as low as 20/120; however, the amplitude reduces with further diminution of visual acuity.

Drugs
Miotics can increase P100 latency, due to the decreased area of retinal illumination. The mydriatics result in an opposite effect.

Other factors
* P100 latency increases with the decrease of luminance [9].
* P100 latency increases and amplitude decreases with the reduction of contrast between black and white squares [10].
* The pattern reversal frequency and not the direction of pattern shift affect P100 latency. Latency increases by 4.8 ms if frequency increased from 1 Hz to 4 Hz.

Clinical applications

Multiple sclerosis
In multiple sclerosis, focal demyelination in visual pathways leads to conduction abnormality, resulting in P100 latency prolongation with or without attenuation of amplitude (Figure 3B.4).The

TABLE 3B.1:   Normal Values of Visual-Evoked Potential, Mean (SD)

	Mean (SD)	
Parameters	Shahrokhi et al.	Misra and Kalita et al.
P100: latency (ms)	102.3 ± 5.1	96.9 ± 3.6
Amplitude (µV)	10.1 ± 4.2	7.8 ± 1.9
Duration	63.0 ± 8.7	55.9 ± 7.7

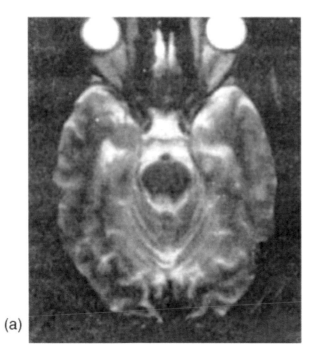

(a)

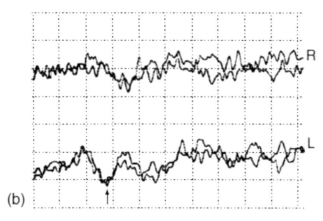

(b)

FIGURE 3B.4 Comparison of sensitivity of PSVEP with MRI in optic neuritis in a 22-year-old woman with multiple sclerosis. (a) MRI brain T2W axial image showing normal optic nerve, (b) PSVEP is unrecordable in right (R) eye and revealed prolonged P100 latency (134 ms) in left (L) eye. Sweep speed, 50 ms/division; gain, 10 μV/division; Oz-Fpz channel.

mean latency is prolonged by 10–30 ms in patients with definite MS [11]. The VEP abnormalities in MS have ranged between 50% and 96%. So diagnosis of MS depends on clinical evaluation and laboratory tests with exclusion of other differential diagnosis. PSVEP was found to be abnormal in 90–100% patients with history of optic neuritis [4, 9, 12]. VEP has been found to be more sensitive than MRI; MRI was positive in 84% symptomatic and 20% asymptomatic eyes [13].

In suspected MS patients, a clinically silent lesion detected by any EP study has 71% chance of clinical worsening and 48% developed definite MS. PSVEPs detected clinically silent lesion more frequently (22%) than BAEP (5%) and SEP (12%) [14].

The correlation between visual acuity and VEP improvement is not always present. Out of 39 eyes, visual acuity and VEP

improvement correlated in 61%, whereas in six eyes P$_{100}$ latency increased despite improvement in vision [15].

Therapeutic trial with methyl prednisolone did not show improvement in VEP [16]. A double-blind placebo-controlled study on azathioprine with or without corticosteroids revealed significant change in VEP after 1 year [17]. Interferon-β1a therapy for 1 year did not show significant VEP changes in RRMS [18].

To summarize, VEP is a valuable tool to detect visual pathway abnormalities in MS and is more sensitive than clinical and MRI examination of visual pathways.

Neuromyelitis optica

In a study of VEP in NMO patients, unrecordable P100 was present in 47.4%, reduced P100 amplitude with normal latency in 34.2%, prolonged latency with normal amplitude of P100 (similar to MS) in 5.3%, and normal VEP in 13.2% of patients [19]. So unrecordable P100 waveform and reduced amplitude of P100 have been reported to be characteristic unlike MS where prolonged P100 latency with normal P100 amplitude.

Optic neuritis

Some authorities believe optic neuritis to be at best form fruste of MS, and a majority of patients initially having optic neuritis turn out to have MS if followed up long enough. 11.5–85% patients with monosymptomatic optic neuritis developed MS [20]. Such patients are mostly females and with recurrent episodes and HLA BT101 [20, 21]. One hundred and forty-six patients of isolated optic neuritis were followed up for 6–7 years and 57% of these patients developed probable or definite MS [22].

VEPs from the involved eyes are often deformed and if recordable, these will be prolonged in nearly all the patients with optic neuropathy [23]. The VEPs help in detecting additional central nervous system (CNS) lesions, and evaluation in the fellow eye is important and helps in the diagnosis of MS. In a study on 33 patients evaluated by clinical examination, MRI, and VEP for 1 year, the factors associated with good recovery included short acute lesion on Gd-enhanced MRI, higher VEP amplitude, and early improvement in vision [24].

Ischemic optic neuropathy

Ischemic optic neuropathy refers to painless, irreversible, and non-progressive vision loss associated with nerve fiber bundle type of field defect, an afferent pupillary defect, and disc edema. The age range from 45 to 80 years. The affected blood supply is the ciliary circulation within the laminar portion of the optic disc [25]. Ischemic optic neuropathy is seen in hypertension, CNS vasculitis, connective tissue disorders, polyarteritis nodosa, and temporal arteritis. Disc edema is often segmental and accompanied by nerve fiber layer hemorrhage.

Ischemic optic neuropathy results in P100 amplitude reduction prior to latency prolongation. The VEP abnormality is related to area of retina involved [26, 27]. In 43 patients with ischemic optic neuropathy, VEP revealed reduction of P100 amplitude with normal latency in 65% patients and reduced amplitude with prolonged latency in 4.7% patients [28].

Nutritional and toxic optic neuropathy

Vitamin B12 is a common cause of myeloneuropathy and occasionally cognitive and behavioral change. B12 deficiency occurs in the patients who are unable to absorb it because of gastrointestinal disease, intrinsic factor deficiency, and widely variety of genetic and/acquired causes. Low vitamin B12 level is associated with megaloblastic anemia, involvement of posterior and lateral column of spinal cord and peripheral nerve resulting in subacute combined degeneration of the spinal cord (SACD). Vitamin B12 deficiencies usually manifest with sensory ataxia (distal paresthesia, joint position, and vibration sense impairment), spasticity and weakness, rarely optic neuropathy and may be the presenting sign of pernicious anemia [29]. Vitamin B12 deficiency results in bilateral prolongation of P100 latency, but the abnormality is generally asymptomatic. Visual acuity, field of vision, and color vision testing are normal. In a study on 17 patients with B12 deficiency neurologic syndrome, P100 latency was prolonged in 10 patients (17 eyes). There was no visual symptom and vision testing was also normal. After 6 months of treatment P100 latency improved in all except four eyes (Figure 3B.5). VEP changes were related to duration of illness [30].

In SACD, diffusion tensor imaging revealed fractional anisotropy ratio of optic nerve correlated well with P100 latency of VEP. Both of these parameter improved after B12 therapy [31].

A number of drugs and toxin like tobacco and ethanol result optic neuropathy. Tobacco amblyopia has been reported in pipe smokers and to a lesser extent in cigar smokers, tobacco chewers, and cigarette smokers. The patients with tobacco amblyopia have a lower level of thiocyanate in plasma and urine compared to unaffected smokers. Role of an inherent defect in detoxifying the cyanide in smokers has been postulated to be responsible for optic neuropathy [32, 33]. Occasionally, the patients may be addicted to both tobacco and alcohol and the term tobacco alcohol amblyopia has been used to describe these patients. VEP

abnormalities have been reported in 23 patients with tobacco–alcohol amblyopia [34]. Ethambutol produces dose-related optic neuropathy. In 59 patients treated with ethambutol, optic neuropathy detected in 18% at a dose of 35 mg/kg/day, which dropped to 2.25% at 25 mg/kg/day [35]. In recommended dose of ethambutol 15 mg/kg/day, visual acuity may be reduced, but central and para-central scotoma are a rule and fundus remains normal. On stopping ethambutol, recovery occurs within 2 months in majority of patients. VEP may be used to monitor visual toxicity of ethambutol. In 14 patients on ethambutol therapy, PSVEP was abnormal in 5 patients; but visual symptoms were present in 1 patient only [36].

Hereditary and degenerative diseases

Hereditary optic neuropathies are rare diseases and misdiagnosed as nutritional and toxic optic neuropathies. These are classified into recessive (rare) and dominant (common) types. The recessive optic atrophy is probably congenital and manifests as stable central visual loss with nystagmus. The dominant form manifesting between 4 and 8 years causes slowly progressing moderate visual impairment, moderate disc pallor and without nystagmus, centrocecal scotoma, and tritanopia color defect.

VEPs in the acute stage of LHON show reduction of amplitude without latency prolongation. P100 latency prolongation with normal amplitude has been reported in 65% patients with respiratory chain defect. Even 53% patients with normal vision have this abnormality [37]. Both VEP and electroretinography, therefore, may be recommended in the suspected mitochondrial disease evaluation as increased frequency of abnormalities present even in asymptomatic patients [38].

The abnormal VEPs have been reported in 2/3 patients with Friedreich's ataxia, but unrelated to severity or duration of illness [39]. Whereas in other hereditary disorders, such as late-onset autosomal dominant cerebellar ataxia, hereditary spastic paraplegia, and olivopontocerebellar atrophy, the VEPs remain unaffected [39–41].

In Parkinson's disease, the VEPs remain normal, although, few studies reported a significant group difference in P100 latency compared to controls [42, 43]. The plexiform layer of retina rich in dopaminergic cells proposed to be the likely site of conduction defect. Improvements with dopaminergic medication support the dopaminergic basis of VEP changes [44].

Malingering and hysteria

VEPs can remain normal with visual acuity as low as 20/120. Therefore, a normal VEP in a patient with visual loss may point toward hysterical blindness. Voluntary suppression of VEP can occur which can be reduced by using large fields, large checks, and binocular stimulation [45–47].

Conclusion

VEP is a simple non-invasive electrodiagnostic test, which has a great value in properly selected patients to evaluate an anterior visual pathway. In demyelinating diseases like multiple sclerosis, NMOSD, B12 deficiency, and ethambutol toxicity, it is very useful in supporting the diagnosis as well as in evaluating the therapeutic response. Due attention to normal values and correct technique are essential for proper interpretation.

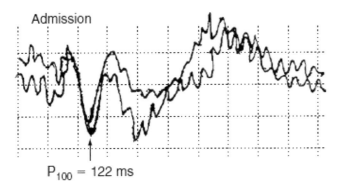

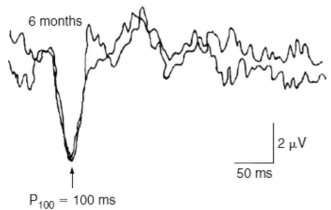

FIGURE 3B.5 Pattern reversal VEP of a patient with vitamin B12 deficiency suggestive of prolonged P100 latency at admission which normalizes at 6 months. Oz-Fpz recording.

Multiple-Choice Questions

1. Visual-evoked potential majorly reflects
   a. Central 15–20° of visual field.
   b. Primarily peripheral field of vision.
   c. Entire visual field.
   d. Central 3–6° of visual field.

   Answer:

   d. Central 3–6° of visual field.

2. Which statement is true about visual-evoked potentials?
   a. Mean P 100 amplitude is greater in males as compared to females.
   b. Mean P100 amplitude is higher in the first decade of life.
   c. Dominant eye produces VEP with P100 of longer latency.
   d. P100 amplitude is greater in moving eye.

   Answer:

   b. Mean P100 amplitude is higher in the first decade of life.

References

1. Phelps ME, Mazziotta JC, Kuhl DE, Nuwer M, Packwood J, Metter J, Engel J. Tomographic mapping of human cerebral metabolism: Visual stimulation and deprivation. Neurology. 1981;31(5):517–529.
2. Duke-Elder S, Scott GI. System of ophthalmology: The anatomy of the visual system. London: Henry Kimpton; 1971
3. Celesia GG, Bodis-Wollner I, Chatrian GE, Harding GF, Sokol S, Spekreijse H. Recommended standards for electroretinograms and visual evoked potentials. Report of an IFCN committee. Electroencephalograph Clin Neurophysiol. 1993;87(6):421–436.
4. Chiappa KH. Evoked potentials in clinical medicine. New York: Raven Press; 1990.
5. Hod Y, Pratt H, Schacham SE. Comparison of fiber optical and video monitor stimulators in normals and multiple sclerosis patients. Electroencephalogr Clin Neurophysiol. 1986;64(5):411–416.
6. Regan D. Some characteristics of average steady-state and transient responses evoked by modulated light. Electroencephalogr Clin Neurophysiol. 1966; 20(3):238–248.
7. Stockard JJ, Hughes JF, Sharbrough FW. Visually evoked potentials to electronic pattern reversal: latency variations with gender, age, and technical factors. Am J EEG Technol. 1979;19(4):171–204.
8. Celesia GG, Daly RF. Visual electroencephalographic computer analysis (VECA): A new electrophysiologic test for the diagnosis of optic nerve lesions. Neurology. 1977 Jul 1;27(7):637–641.
9. Halliday AM, McDonald WI, Mushin J. Visual evoked response in diagnosis of multiple sclerosis. Br Med J. 1973;4(5893):661–664.
10. Mackay DM, Jeffreys DA. Visually evoked potentials and visual perception in man. In: Jung R, editor. Handbook of sensory physiology. Vol. 8/3, Part B. New York: Springer; 1973. p. 647–678.
11. Cant BR, Hume AL, Shaw NA. Effects of luminance on the pattern visual evoked potential in multiple sclerosis. Electroencephalograph Clin Neurophysiol. 1978;45(4):496–504.
12. Matthews WB, Small DG, Small MA, Pountney E. Pattern reversal evoked visual potential in the diagnosis of multiple sclerosis. J Neurol Neurosurg Psychiatry. 1977;40(10):1009–1014.
13. Miller DH, Newton MR, Van der Poel JC, Du Boulay EP, Halliday AM, Kendall BE, Johnson G, MacManus DG, Moseley IF, McDonald WI. Magnetic resonance imaging of the optic nerve in optic neuritis. Neurology. 1988;38(2):175–179.
14. Hume AL, Waxman SG. Evoked potentials in suspected multiple sclerosis: Diagnostic value and prediction of clinical course. J Neurol Sci. 1988;83(2–3):191–210.
15. Matthews WB, Small DG. Serial recording of visual and somatosensory evoked potentials in multiple sclerosis. J Neurol Sci. 1979; 40(1):11–21.
16. Smith T, Zeeberg I, Sjö O. Evoked potentials in multiple sclerosis before and after high-dose methylprednisolone infusion. Eur Neurol. 1986;25(1):67–73.
17. Nuwer MR, Packwood JW, Myers LW, Ellison GW. Evoked potentials predict the clinical changes in a multiple sclerosis drug study. Neurology. 1987;37(11):1754–1761.
18. Lišèiæ RM, Brecelj J. Visual evoked potentials in multiple sclerosis patients treated with interferon beta-1a. Ophthalmology. 2004;45(3):323–327.
19. Neto SP, Alvarenga RM, Vasconcelos CC, Alvarenga MP, Pinto LC, Pinto VL. Evaluation of pattern-reversal visual evoked potential in patients with neuromyelitis optica. Mult Scler J. 2013;19(2):173–178.
20. Cohen MM, Lessell S, Wolf PA. A prospective study of the risk of developing multiple sclerosis in uncomplicated optic neuritis. Neurology. 1979;29(2):208–213.
21. Compston DA, Batchelor JR, Earl CJ, McDonald WI. Factors influencing the risk of multiple sclerosis developing in patients with optic neuritis. Brain: J Neurol. 1978;101(3):495–511.
22. Ebers GC. Optic neuritis and multiple sclerosis. Arch Neurol. 1985;42(7):702–704.
23. Halliday AM, Halliday E, Kriss A, McDonald WI, Mushin J. The pattern-evoked potential in compression of the anterior visual pathways. Brain: J Neurol. 1976;99(2):357–374.
24. Hickman SJ, Toosy AT, Miszkiel KA, Jones SJ, Altmann DR, MacManus DG, Plant GT, Thompson AJ, Miller DH. Visual recovery following acute optic neuritis. J Neurol. 2004;251(8):996–1005.
25. Knox DL, Duke JR. Slowly progressive ischemic optic neuropathy. Ophthalmology. 1971;75:1065–1068.
26. Asselman P, Chadwick DW, Marsden DC. Visual evoked responses in the diagnosis and management of patients suspected of multiple sclerosis. Brain: J Neurol. 1975;98(2):261–282.
27. Thompson PD, Mastaglia FL, Carroll WM. Anterior ischaemic optic neuropathy: A correlative clinical and visual evoked potential study of 18 patients. J Neurol Neurosurg Psychiatry. 1986;49(2):128–135.
28. Varga M. Visual evoked potentials and ultrasonography in ischemic optic neuropathy. Oftalmologia (Bucharest, Romania: 1990). 2002;53(2):41–45.
29. Lerman S, Feldmahn AL. Centrocecal scotomata as the presenting sign in pernicious anemia. Arch Ophthalmol. 1961;65(3):381–385.
30. Pandey S, Kalita J, Misra UK. A sequential study of visual evoked potential in patients with vitamin B12 deficiency neurological syndrome. Clin Neurophysiol. 2004;115(4):914–918.
31. Kalita J, Soni N, Dubey D, Kumar S, Misra UK. Evaluation of optic nerve functions in subacute combined degeneration using visual evoked potential and diffusion tensor imaging—A pilot study. Br J Radiol. 2018;91(1091):20180086.
32. Carr RE, Henkind P. Ocular manifestations of ethambutol: Toxic amblyopia after administration of an experimental antituberculous drug. Arch Ophthalmol. 1962;67(5):566–571.
33. Heaton JM, McCormick AJ, Freeman AG. Tobacco amblyopia: A clinical manifestation of vitamin-B12 deficiency. Lancet. 1958;2:286–290.
34. Kriss A, Carroll WM, Blumhardt LD, Halliday AM. Pattern- and flash-evoked potential changes in toxic (nutritional) optic neuropathy. Adv Neurol. 1982;32:11–19.
35. Leibold JE. The ocular toxicity of ethambutol and its relation to dose. Ann N Y Acad Sci. 1966;135(2):904–909.
36. Yiannikas C, Walsh JC. The variation of the pattern shift visual evoked response with the size of the stimulus field. Electroencephalogr Clin Neurophysiol. 1983;55(4):427–435.
37. Finsterer J. Visually evoked potentials in respiratory chain disorders. Acta Neurol Scand. 2001;104(1):31–35.
38. Scaioli V, Antozzi C, Villani F, Rimoldi M, Zeviani M, Panzica F, Avanzini G. Utility of multimodal evoked potential study and electroencephalography in mitochondrial encephalomyopathy. Ital J Neurol Sci. 1998;19(5):291–300.
39. Carroll WM, Kriss A, Baraitser M, Barrett G, Halliday AM. The incidence and nature of visual pathway involvement in Friedreich's ataxia. A clinical and visual evoked potential study of 22 patients. Brain: J Neurol. 1980;103(2):413–434.
40. Bird TD, Crill WE. Pattern-reversal visual evoked potentials in the hereditary ataxias and spinal degenerations. Ann Neurol: Off J Am Neurol Assoc Child Neurol Soc. 1981;9(3):243–250.
41. Livingstone IR, Mastaglia FL, Edis R, Howe JW. Visual involvement in Friedreich's ataxia and hereditary spastic ataxia: A clinical and visual evoked response study. Arch Neurol. 1981;38(2):75–79.
42. Bodis-Wollner I, Yahr MD, Mylin L, Thornton J. Dopaminergic deficiency and delayed visual evoked potentials in humans. Ann Neurol: Off J Am Neurol Assoc Child Neurol Soc. 1982;11(5):478–483.
43. Gawel MJ, Das P, Vincent S, Rose FC. Visual and auditory evoked responses in patients with Parkinson's disease. J Neurol Neurosurg Psychiatry. 1981;44(3):227–232.
44. Bodis-Wollner IV, Yahr MD. Measurements of visual evoked potentials in Parkinson's disease. Brain: J Neurol. 1978;101(4):661–671.
45. Tan CT, Murray NM, Sawyers D, Leonard TJ. Deliberate alteration of the visual evoked potential. J Neurol Neurosurg Psychiatry. 1984;47(5):518–523.
46. Lentz KE, Chiappa KH. Non-pathologic (voluntary) alteration of pattern-shift visual evoked-potentials. Electroencephalogr Clin Neurophysiol. 1985;61(2):30–30.
47. Chiappa KH, Yiannikas C. Voluntary alteration of evoked potentials? Ann Neurol. 1982;12(5):496–497.

Part II
Neuro-Ophthalmology
The Afferent Pathway

4

APPROACH TO "VISUAL LOSS"

Aastha Takkar Kapila, Monika Singla, Vivek Lal

Acute visual loss is a devastating symptom seen in clinical practice. The first step for the clinician is to anatomically localize the defect to anterior eye structures, retina, optic nerve, optic chiasma, the posterior visual pathways or the visual cortex. Initial approach to a patient with visual loss can be simplified into the following four steps.

Step 1. Is the visual loss unilateral (or monocular) or bilateral?
Step 2. Is the visual loss acute?
Step 3. If acute, is the visual loss transient or persistent?
Step 4. Is the visual loss progressive?

Step 1. Is the visual loss unilateral or bilateral?
Involvement of the pre-chiasmal axis leads to monocular visual loss, whereas chiasmal/post-chiasmal lesions cause binocular visual loss with or without visual field defects.

IN CASES OF ACUTE 'MONOCULAR' VISUAL LOSS

STEP 2. Is the Visual Loss Acute?
The differentials of acute monocular visual loss are varied depending upon the temporal profile of presentation, pattern of visual loss, triggers and associations. An important aspect to start interpreting a patient of acute monocular visual loss is to determine whether the visual loss is transient or persistent.

STEP 3. If Acute, Is the Visual Loss Transient, Persistent or Recurrent?
The various possible etiologies of transient visual loss are provided in Table 4.1.

Transient monocular visual loss

Transient monocular visual loss (TMVL) occurs when transmission across the optic nerve, disc or retina is interrupted transiently due to a reversible reduction in blood supply.

Interruption of vascular flow is the commonest cause of transient monocular blindness (amaurosis fugax). Determining the etiology of TMVL will guide the management. Vital information regarding onset, progression, duration, triggers, associated symptoms and field defects improves the yield of diagnosis. A simple approach to a patient with transient visual loss is given in Algorithm 4.1.

CLUES TO DIAGNOSIS IN PATIENTS WITH TRANSIENT VISUAL LOSS[1]

TEMPORAL PROFILE

Vascular and demyelinating disorders present acutely. Carotid stenosis is associated with TMVL lasting 1–10 minutes as against retinal migraine, which is usually of longer duration. Transient visual obscurations (TVOs) accompanying increased intracranial pressure (ICP) last for seconds and are usually binocular. In occipital epilepsy, duration may vary from less than a minute to days together.

TRIGGERS

TMVL related to demyelinating lesions is precipitated by high temperature. TVOs occur due to transient ischemia of optic nerve head on maneuvers, which increase intracranial pressure, like exercise, bending, coughing or on performing Valsalva. Retinal vasospasm can be precipitated by emotional stress, cold or exercise. Transient visual loss may occur on exposure to bright light due to impaired regeneration of photo pigments secondary to ocular ischemia in high-grade stenosis or occlusion of the internal carotid artery. In some retinal diseases (e.g., retinal dystrophies), patients may have evanescent visual loss in bright light too. This condition is often labeled as day blindness (or hemeralopia) and is usually binocular.

ASSOCIATIONS

Underlying atherosclerotic/embolic risk factors may be present in patients presenting with amaurosis fugax. Retinal claudication, transient focal neurological deficits and limb shaking transient ischemic attacks (TIAs) are the other accompaniments in a patient with carotid disease. Uhthoff's phenomenon is present in patients of optic neuritis, which may be related to an underlying demyelinating/inflammatory disorder. TVOs are seen in the setting of increased intracranial pressure. Ocular pain and unilateral headache should be differentiated from retinal claudication, while retinal claudication may occur in carotid stenosis, the presence of ocular pain necessitates the need to rule of local ocular causes (like glaucoma).

PATTERN OF VISUAL LOSS

Altitudinal field defects increase the odds of carotid disease. Optic nerve diseases are associated with early color desaturation and loss of contrast sensitivity. Patients with retinal migraine may have highly variable presentation. Visual loss is often described as black, gray, white or shaded areas of varying size that may appear instantaneously or gradually progress inward from the peripheral visual field. Retrochiasmal vascular or demyelinating disorders present with binocular visual field deficits respecting vertical meridian.

DOI: 10.1201/9780429020278-7

TABLE 4.1: Causes of Transient Visual Loss

Transient Visual Loss			
Amaurosis fugax	1–10 min	Monocular, altitudinal onset	Associated with vascular risk factors
Retinal migraine	10–30 min	Monocular blurring progressing inward from peripheral field	Migraine with or without aura
Uhthoff's phenomenon	Seconds–Minutes	Mono/binocular	History of optic neuritis/MS/other demyelinating disorders
Transient visual obscurations	Seconds	Binocular (rarely monocular). Vision may be preserved till last	Features of increased Intracranial pressure
Vertebro-basilar ischemia/posterior circulation transient ischemic attacks	1–10 min	Binocular, hemianopic field defects	Associated with vascular risk factors
Posterior reversible encephalopathy syndrome	Variable	Binocular vision loss, encephalopathy, seizures, focal neurological deficits	Associated with hypertensive emergencies, parenchymal renal disease, organ transplantation, sepsis, drugs
Occipital epilepsy	Seizure—minutes Postictal—minutes to hours	Binocular visual field loss, hallucinations, positive visual phenomenon	May be accompanied by positive visual phenomenon

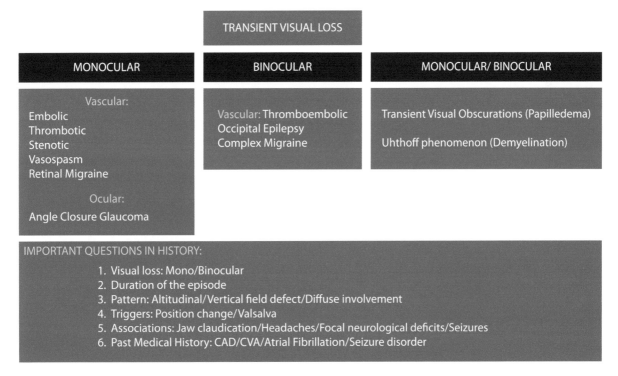

ALGORITHM 4.1 Approach to a patient with transient visual loss.

Amaurosis fugax (from the Greek *"Amaurosis"* meaning *darkening* and the Latin *"fugax"* meaning *fleeting*) is the commonest cause of transient visual loss. It is often caused by emboli from carotid vessels arising from atherosclerotic plaques causing stenosis of the carotid vessels at the ipsilateral carotid bifurcation leading to focal, repetitive, retinal ischemia. It is usually seen in elderly patients, with advanced atherosclerosis. The symptoms vary from partial field loss to complete loss of vision, curtain falling in front of the eye, shimmering blank spots, window shade or snow. This loss of vision may be present for a few seconds to several minutes, usually clears in the reverse pattern, and is often repetitive. They may rarely accompany contralateral motor or sensory loss as well. This is the hallmark of significant ipsilateral carotid vessel obstruction.[2]

CASE 1

A 63-year-old female with a known case of coronary artery disease, presented with a history of recurrent episodes of "blindness" of her right eye for 1 month. She complained that she has intermittent painless blurring of vision from the right eye, which begins from the upper half of her vision and progresses within seconds to complete loss of vision. The episode lasts for around 5–10 minutes and spontaneously resolves like clearing fog. During one of the recent episodes she had suffered a fall with transient loss of consciousness. General physical examination revealed prominent right carotid bruit. Rest of the systemic, ophthalmological and neurological examination was unremarkable. What is your diagnosis?

Repeated episodes of painless, transient monocular blindness in an elderly patient with coronary artery disease strongly suggest intermittent retinal ischemia or amaurosis fugax. The presence of normal ophthalmological examination and presence of carotid bruit further substantiates the diagnosis.

MRI-brain revealed mild microangiopathic changes (Figure 4.1a). MR angiogram of neck and cerebral vessels revealed advanced atherosclerotic changes along craniocervical arteries. Predominant soft plaque was seen at the right ICA origin causing near complete occlusion (Figure 4.1b and c).

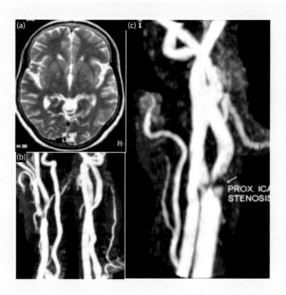

FIGURE 4.1 MRI brain T2-weighted axial image showing microangiopathic changes (a). MR angiogram of neck vessels (b, c) showing stenosis of proximal right internal carotid artery.

Retinal migraine

TMVL can also be caused by retinal artery vasospasm in patients of migraine and is called *retinal migraine.* Retinal migraine is the single commonest cause of transient monocular blindness in young adults less than 40 years.[3] Attacks of retinal migraine may mimic amaurosis fugax. While it is claimed by some researchers that "there are no distinguishing symptoms to separate retinal migraine from Amaurosis fugax due to retinal embolization"; others have noted that visual loss associated with retinal migraine is usually of longer duration and the evolution is slower. Moreover, the typical shade dropping over one visual field described by many patients who have amaurosis fugax has not been described in patients with retinal migraine.

CASE 2

A 23-year-old female presented with history of three episodes of transient loss of vision of right eye over the past 3 months. She was a known case of migraine for past 5 years and used to take non-steroidal anti-inflammatory agents for acute attacks. The episode of visual loss would begin as a shaded area in periphery and involves the whole visual field slowly. Complete blindness from the right eye was noted at the peak of headache. Each episode outlasted the headache and spontaneously resolved over 1–2 hours. In the first episode, the patient was noted to have retinal vasospasm in the right eye by an ophthalmologist.

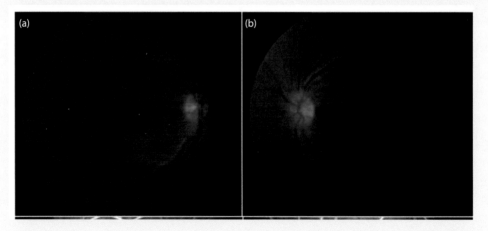

FIGURE 4.2 Images of normal optic discs on fundus examination (a, b). Fundus fluorescein angiography (FFA) (c, d) was normal. Delayed arm to retina time (right eye) was noted during the first episode of TMVL with headache suggesting transient retinal vasospasm. *(Continued)*

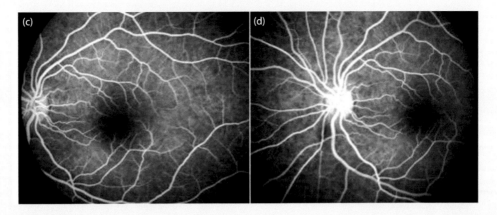

FIGURE 4.2   *(Continued)*

Subsequent ophthalmologic examinations were, however, unremarkable (Figure 4.2a and b). The patient was extensively worked up for her TMVL. Routine hemogram, biochemistry, electrocardiography, Echocardiography, Holter monitoring; fundus fluorescein angiography of both eyes; magnetic resonance imaging and angiography of neck and cerebral vessels were normal (Figure 4.2c and d). The screen for hypercoagulable conditions was also negative.

The diagnosis of retinal migraine was considered and the patient was initiated on migraine prophylaxis and aspirin. The symptoms of both headache and visual loss resolved remarkably on follow-up.

Uhthoff's phenomenon

Patients with demyelinating disorders may also present with TMVL when subjected to increased temperature (*Uhthoff's phenomenon*). It was described in 1890 by Wilhelm Uhthoff, who described the phenomenon of transitory visual disturbance in patients with multiple sclerosis occurring after physical exercise and an increase in body temperature, for example, after a hot bath. The phenomenon is thought to arise because of transient conduction block within the optic nerve.[4]

CASE 3

A 25-year-old female, known case of multiple sclerosis, presented with transient episodes of the visual loss of left eye during an intense sports performance in summers. The patient was diagnosed to have multiple sclerosis 3 years back when she had one episode of paraparesis. She had history of multiple attacks of optic neuritis (both right and left) over past 2 years. All episodes were managed with intravenous methyl prednisolone. The patient was not on any disease modifying agent. Ophthalmic examination suggested secondary optic atrophy of both eyes (Figure 4.3a and b). Visual fields were constricted bilaterally and bilateral retinal nerve fiber layer (RNFL) thickness was reduced on optical coherence tomography (OCT). Gadolinium enhanced MRI brain suggested typical T2 hyperintense lesions of multiple sclerosis (Figure 4.3c).

The transient episodes of visual loss in the above-described patient was due to Uhthoff's phenomenon. Transient fluctuation in neuronal conduction of the demyelinated axons is the cause of transient visual loss in these patients.

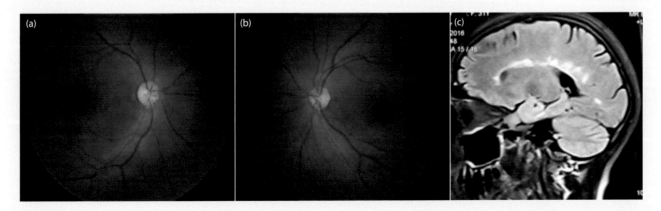

FIGURE 4.3   (a, b) Optic atrophy in both eyes, (c) MRI brain showing hyperintensities on T2-weighted images.

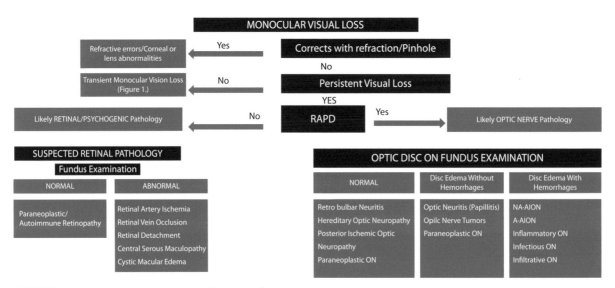

ALGORITHM 4.2   Approach to a patient with monocular visual loss.

Transient visual obscurations (TVOs) are episodes of transient blurring of vision (usually binocular), which usually last for less than 30 seconds and are followed by complete recovery. These are pathognomic of papilledema. Rarely, they can occur unilaterally too. The most likely underlying mechanism for TVOs is transient ischemia of the optic nerve head related to the increased tissue pressure. Though TVOs may provoke anxiety among the patients, they are usually not associated with poor visual outcomes.[5]

Local eye causes should always be borne in mind and ruled out. Hence, a thorough ophthalmologic examination is essential when suspected. While fading out of colors or a washed out appearance occurs in patients with optic nerve pathologies; monocular metamorphopsia (wavy, warped images) and positive phenomenon such as flashing or colored lights often indicate a retinal lesion.

Intermittent angle-closure glaucoma can present with transient episodes of pain, nausea, vomiting, blurry vision accompanied by other visual symptoms, such as halos around lights, during episodes. Rarely, these patients may also present with isolated painless TVL.[6]

Persistent monocular visual loss

Patients with monocular visual loss should be approached in a systematic way. Temporal profile of the visual loss, associations and vital information on examination may help in reaching a diagnosis. A simplified approach to a patient with persistent monocular visual loss is given in Algorithm 4.2.

CLUES TO DIAGNOSIS IN PATIENT WITH PERSISTENT VISUAL LOSS

TEMPORAL PROFILE

While both ischemic and inflammatory/demyelinating optic neuropathies can present acutely. Ischemic optic neuropathies (ION) (especially arteritic-anterior ischemic optic neuropathy (A-AION) are notorious to cause maximum deficit at the onset. Similarly, acute occlusions of central or branch retinal vessels can produce non-progressive vision loss. On the contrary visual loss in Optic Neuritis progresses over 1 week, remains static (if not treated) for around 2 weeks and spontaneously recovers over another 3 weeks. Traumatic optic neuropathies have a preceding history. Toxic and Hereditary optic neuropathies are usually binocular, but may present in one eye as well. These optic neuropathies usually present with painless progressive visual loss. Sequential involvement of eyes may be seen in ION (A-AION) and in patients of Leber's hereditary optic neuropathy.[7,8]

PATTERN OF VISUAL LOSS

Visual field defect in ischemic ON, specifically NA-AION, consists of altitudinal field defects (classically, inferior hemi-field defects), central or arcuate scotomas and quadrantic defects. In patients of posterior ischemic optic neuropathy (PION), central field defects are common.[8] Inflammatory ON usually presents with a central field defect; however, practically any part of the visual field may be involved depending upon the site of inflammation. Papilledema is usually associated with enlarged blind spot, peripheral field constriction and loss of nasal visual fields (especially inferonasal). The visual field loss in papilledema may resemble that of patients of glaucoma. Compressive optic neuropathies may present with hemianopia field defects depending upon the site of involvement (e.g., sellar lesions causing bitemporal field defects, junctional scotomas or unilateral temporal scotomas depending upon the exact site and the extent of the lesion). Toxic and hereditary optic neuropathies may cause variable field defects. Central field defects, centrocecal scotomas, peripheral field constriction, whole field loss and rarely even bitemporal field defects can be seen. Specific visual field patterns have also been described with drug-induced optic neuropathies (e.g., vigabatrin producing bi-nasal defects progressing to concentric bilateral field defects with preservation of central vision. Retrochiasmal lesions or disorders are associated with homonymous hemianopic defect.[8,9]

ASSOCIATIONS

Ocular pain is an important symptom. Pain on eye movements is typical of inflammatory optic neuropathy. Ocular trauma is associated with pain at the local site. Acute angle closure glaucoma is associated with red eye and severe periorbital pain and headache. Painful Horner syndrome with or without monocular vision loss should also prompt the investigations to rule out carotid artery dissection. Central retinal artery occlusion can also occur secondary to carotid dissection. Jaw claudication, scalp tenderness and polymyalgia are common associations of A-AION related to giant cell arteritis (GCAs). Pituitary apoplexy is associated with severe sudden headache and binocular visual loss. Patients of posterior circulation hypoperfusion/strokes may have associated focal neurological deficits. Similarly, patients with posterior reversible encephalopathy syndrome (PRES) may have altered mental status and seizures with visual loss[10–12] (Table 4.2). Elucidate causes and characteristics of pain are associated with visual loss.

TABLE 4.2: Causes and Characteristics of Painful Visual Loss

Etiology	Characteristics of Pain and Associations
MONOCULAR VISION LOSS	
Optic neuritis	Peri-orbital/Pain on eye movement
Vascular syndromes (AION, CRAO) associated with Carotid dissection	Neck Pain, Painful Horner Syndrome
Ocular Ischemic syndrome	Orbital pain, iris neovascularization, irido-cyclitis, narrowed retinal arteries, dilated retinal veins, retinal hemorrhages
A-AION (GCA)	Jaw claudication
Glaucoma(Acute angle closure)	Ocular Pain, Nausea, vomiting, conjunctival injection, increased IOP
Traumatic ON	History of trauma
Orbital apex syndrome	Periorbital pain with other cranial nerve involvement
BINOCULAR VISION LOSS	
Bilateral ON, Trauma	
Pituitary apoplexy	Sudden temporal headache/Periorbital pain associated with rapidly worsening visual field defect

Ischemic optic neuropathies (anterior/posterior) ischemic optic neuropathy can be anterior or posterior and often presents with sudden-onset visual deficit, often maximum at onset. Anterior ischemic optic neuropathy (AION) involves ischemic damage to the optic nerve head. It can be non-arteritic (non-arteritic anterior ischemic optic neuropathy [NAION]) or arteritic (A-AION), the latter being associated with giant cell arteritis. While NAION is the most common form of non-glaucomatous optic neuropathy in elderly individuals, arteritic AION is associated with vasculitis and is the most common ophthalmic manifestation of giant cell arteritis (GCA). It is a treatable neuro-ophthalmic emergency, which is exceedingly important to recognize and differentiate from more common NAION. The patients of AION usually have unilateral disc edema (pale disc edema with hemorrhages) and show a "classical" altitudinal horizontal field defect on visual field testing (because of the peculiar blood supply of the optic disc).[8,9]

CASE 4

An 67-year-old male presented with history of loss of vision in right eye since 1 day and of left eye since 7 days. He had noted sudden visual loss in the left eye when he woke up from sleep 2 days prior to presentation. The visual loss in the right eye was also noted suddenly the next day, while the patient was performing his routine activities of daily living. The visual loss was accompanied with severe throbbing bitemporal headache. Past history of jaw claudication and one episode of transient (lasting few seconds) right-sided visual loss were present 2 years prior to his current presentation. General physical examination revealed bilateral palpable temporal arteries and the left temporal artery was tender. The patient was having no perception of light at presentation and the fundus revealed bilateral disc edema (Figure 4.4a and b). Fundus fluorescein angiography suggested ischemic optic neuropathy in both the eyes (Figure 4.4c and d). The profile of the patient, rapid loss of vision and the intensity of visual involvement suggested an arteritic-anterior ischemic optic neuropathy and high dose pulse methylprednisone (1 g daily for 5 days) was initiated followed by oral steroids in tapering doses. Laboratory work-up was essentially normal except elevated ESR (104 mm/h) and CRP (60.5 mg/l). Temporal artery Doppler was showed the classical "halo sign" (concentric, hypoechogenic halo suggesting temporal artery inflammation) and the temporal artery biopsy was suggestive of giant cell arteritis. A-AION is notorious to cause severe, sequential and acute visual loss despite prompt therapy. It is often associated with systemic symptoms like headache, scalp tenderness and cord like palpable temporal arteries. The optic disc of the fellow eye is most often normal as opposed to NA-AION in which it is small in diameter (disc at risk).

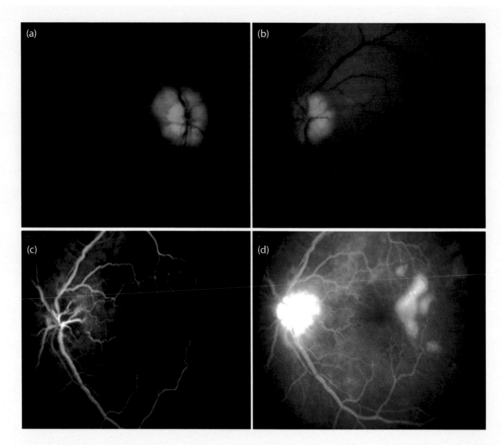

FIGURE 4.4 Fundus picture showing bilateral pale disc edema (a, b). FFA showing filing defect (hypofluorescence) in the choroid and the disc in the arterial phase (c). Late phase of FFA showing disc staining consistent with disc swelling (d).

CASE 5

A 57-year-old obese male with a 6-year history of uncontrolled diabetes and smoker (smoking index of 15 pack years) was referred to a tertiary care hospital with history of acute visual loss of right eye. The visual loss was sudden onset, painless and non-progressive. He noticed this visual loss on waking up from sleep 4 days prior to presentation. There was similar history of

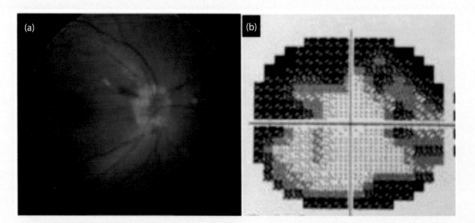

FIGURE 4.5 Fundus examination showing right optic disc edema with peri-papillary hemorrhages (a). Corresponding visual field (b) shows peripheral field constriction. Left eye shows optic disc pallor (more in the upper segment) (c). Corresponding visual field shows inferior altitudinal field defect (d). Fundus fluorescein angiography of the right eye showing leakage of dye from the optic disc with hypofluorescence corresponding to the hemorrhage (e–h). *(Continued)*

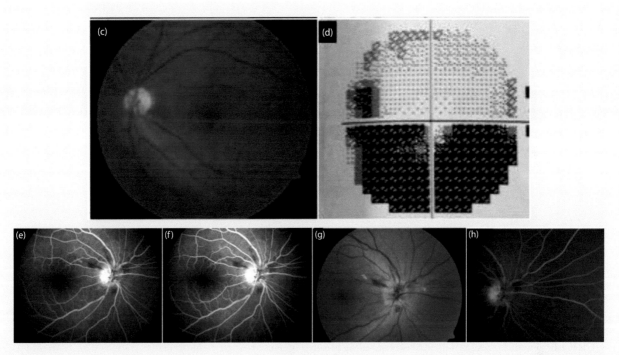

FIGURE 4.5   *(Continued)*

loss of vision of left eye 3 months back. At that time, the patient complained of his inability to see the lower half of his field of vision clearly from the left eye. He denied any history of painful eye movements, headache or any positive visual phenomenon. The diminution of vision is static since the onset. What is your diagnosis?

Painless unilateral visual loss in a diabetic/hypertensive, developing within hours is a signature presentation of anterior ischemic optic neuropathy (AION). The suddenness of the event defines its ischemic/vascular origin. Unilateral involvement, disc edema with hemorrhages and an altitudinal visual field of the corresponding eye strongly supports this diagnosis of AION in this diabetic/smoker of 57 years (Figure 4.5a–d). FFA disclosed minimal leakage of dye from the optic disc with hypofluorescence corresponding to the hemorrhage (Figure 4.5e–h). Rest of the retinal circulation was normal.

Optic neuritis (ON) is an acute to subacute illness due to inflammation/demyelination of optic nerve that leads to visual impairment causing loss of visual acuity, color vision and contrast sensitivity. When anterior part of optic nerve (optic nerve head, optic disc, optic papilla) is involved, it is termed as anterior optic neuritis/papillitis, and when posterior/rear part of the optic nerve is involved, it is termed as retro-bulbar optic neuritis. ON is defined with the triad of subacute unilateral loss of vision, periocular pain and impaired color vision. Typical visual field defect in optic neuritis has been central field defect; however, any area of visual field can be affected by ON. The presence of relative afferent pupillary defect (RAPD) is a rule, signifying the damage to the optic nerve. The examination of the optic disc reveals disc edema in papillitis. Normal healthy optic disc may be visible in patients with retro-bulbar ON. The absence of disc/peri-papillary hemorrhages is typical for an idiopathic ON or in ON associated with MS.

CASE 6

A 25-year-old female presented with headache and pain on movements of right eye for 7 days. She complained of blurring of vision and fading of colors for initial 5 days and noted progressive diminution of vision since then. There was a history of paraparesis around one and a half years back, when she was diagnosed and managed as "Idiopathic" Transverse myelitis. On ophthalmological examination, the patient could only count fingers close to face from the right eye. The visual field of the right eye was grossly depressed and optic disc on the right side was edematous (without hemorrhages) (Figure 4.6). RNFL on OCT was increased in the right eye. General and central nervous system examination was unremarkable expect generalized brisk deep tendon reflexes. What is the diagnosis?

The woman in question above had monocular painful vision loss progressive over 5–7 days duration. The right optic disc edema she had is suggestive of papillitis (Figure 4.6a–d). The findings are supportive of diagnosis of optic neuritis. Previous history of steroid responsive transverse myelitis further points out toward an inflammatory/demyelinating cause-likely optico-spinal multiple sclerosis or neuromyelitis optica. The patient was diagnosed as neuromyelitis optica based on MRI cervical spine, which was suggestive of longitudinally extensive transverse myelitis and presence of aquaporin-4 antibodies in serum.

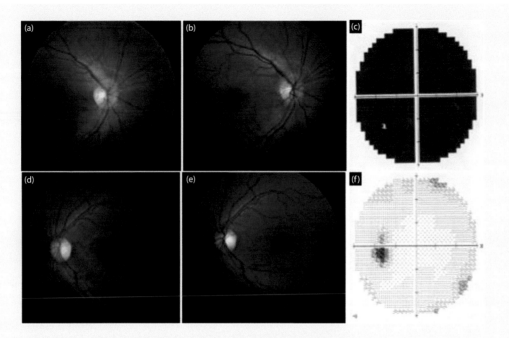

FIGURE 4.6 Fundus examination and corresponding red-free images showing right optic disc edema (a, b). Temporal pallor noted in the left optic disc (d, e) suggestive of previous insult). Corresponding visual fields showing grossly depressed field in the right eye and enlarged blind spot in the left eye (c, f).

Other primary ophthalmic causes of acute unilateral vision loss like *retinal artery/vein occlusion (central or branch)*, local eye *trauma; retinal detachment/vitreous hemorrhages* should always be ruled out in patients with monocular, persistent visual loss.

Central retinal vein occlusion (CRVO)

CRVO is a common sight-threatening retinal vascular disease. It is broadly classified into non-ischemic type or venous stasis retinopathy and ischemic type or hemorrhagic retinopathy. The presence of extensive retinal hemorrhages and cotton wool spots characterizes CRVO.[13]

CASE 7

A 26-year-old female presented with a history of headache and blurred vision of 20-day duration. Along with blurred vision she complained of intermittent flashes of light in her left eye which she described as transient bright light shining into her left eye. Ophthalmic examination revealed normal visual acuity and visual field in the right eye. Visual acuity in left eye was 6/9 and visual field examination was normal. Fundus examination was suggestive of optic disc edema in the left eye with tortuous vessels and splinter hemorrhages (Figure 4.7).

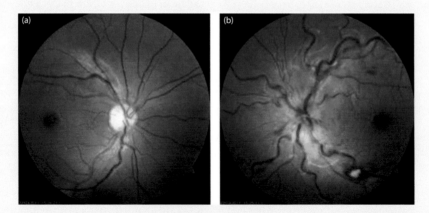

FIGURE 4.7 Fundus photographs showing normal right optic disc (a) and optic disc edema with multiple splinter hemorrhages and cotton wool spots in left eye. The retinal veins are prominently dilated and tortuous indicating slow vascular flow (b).

The presence of positive visual phenomenon, history suggests a retinal pathology in the given patient. The fundus findings were consistent with central retinal vein occlusion. FFA suggested the presence of non-ischemic central retinal vein occlusion (mild leakage of dye at disc with increased arm to retina time, slow arteriovenous phase and dilated tortuous veins). Patient's systemic workup revealed high positive titers for anticardiolipin antibodies.

Nonorganic (functional) visual loss can present with persistent monocular vision loss and is more common among younger age groups. Frequently reported non-organic visual complaints include a reduction of visual acuity with or without loss of field.[14] Vague history of onset, profound monocular visual loss with inconsistent or bizarre responses on vision testing, normal pupil function and ocular structures, known psychiatric or behavior disorders are often found in these patients. Clues to diagnose a patient of functional/non-organic visual loss are given in Table 4.3.

Recurrent monocular visual loss

Optic neuritis associated with MS, NMO or other systemic disorders may present with multiple recurrences. Sequential visual loss of one eye with the fellow eye following the involved eye after a few days is a key feature of arteritic ischemic optic neuropathy. Sequential vision loss may also occur in some form of hereditary optic neuropathies (LHON).

IN CASES OF ACUTE "BINOCULAR" VISUAL LOSS

STEP 3. If Acute, Is the Visual Loss Transient, Persistent or Recurrent

Transient binocular visual loss (TBVL)

TBVL is far less common than TMVL. The approach to TBVL is similar to that of TMVL (Figure 4.1). Common causes are *migrainous aura, posterior circulation transient ischemic attacks, occipital lobe seizures, posterior reversible encephalopathy (PRES) and transient visual obscurations.*[5]

Migrainous aura
Visual prodrome of migraine or migrainous aura may present with scotomas in visual field surrounded by shimmering zig-zag lines, which gradually enlarge and then break up over a period of 15–30 minutes. Complete binocular loss of vision or loss of vision in either visual fields may be seen. The aura is characteristically followed by a hemi-cranial throbbing headache on the side opposite to the involved hemi-field. Visual disturbances of migraine generally last less than an hour, most commonly 10–30 minutes.[15]

Transient ischemic attacks
TBVL may be seen in transient ischemic attacks involving the posterior circulation. These symptoms usually accompany vertebrobasilar insufficiency and are warning signs of impending stroke. Depending upon the site of hypoperfusion patient may present with homonymous hemianopia or complete blindness. Unlike migrainous auras, these are not associated with positive visual symptoms and do not evolve over time.[2] Outcome is grim because of their strategic vascular character.

Posterior reversible encephalopathy syndrome (PRES)
PRES is a reversible and treatable cause of acute encephalopathy with blindness and has been commonly seen in hypertensive emergencies secondary to the inability of posterior circulation to autoregulate in response to acute changes in blood pressure. The encephalopathy develops due to reversible cerebral edema. Other accompanying symptoms include headache, seizures and focal neurological deficits. Apart from malignant hypertension, eclampsia, renal parenchymal disease, organ transplantation and some chemotherapeutic agents have been implicated as the cause.[16]

Occipital lobe seizures
TBVL may be seen in occipital lobe seizures as an ictal as well as postictal phenomenon. They often manifest with elementary visual hallucinations, headache and vomiting with blindness. If the occipito-temporal cortex is involved, the hallucinations can be more vivid, colorful and complex. Duration can be variable lasting from minutes to days.[17]

TABLE 4.3: Clues to Diagnose a Patient with Non-Organic/Functional Visual Loss

Clues to Non-Organic/Functional Visual Loss
• Absence of RAPD
• Visual Field Defect- "Tunnel Vision"
• Positive Menace reflex
• Preserved Spasm of the Near Triad/Convergence reflex (purposeful convergence with associated pupillary miosis) may also be witnessed
• Impaired tests of stereopsis (In monocular Visual Loss)
• Impaired tests of proprioception (In binocular Visual Loss)

CASE 8

A 24-year-old female presented with history of intermittent episodes of binocular visual loss of 1-month duration. These episodes were preceded by flashes of light lasting a few seconds, after which the patient complained of complete loss of vision lasting less than a minute. The episodes spontaneously aborted and there was no history of headache, pain on eye movements or any other focal neurological deficits. There was a past history of right focal seizures with secondary generalization around 12 years back when the patient was started on anti-epileptics (Carbamazepine). General physical, systemic, ophthalmic and neurological examination was unremarkable.

Occipital lobe epilepsy was considered in view of very short lasting episodes and previous history of seizure disorder. EEG suggested occipital lobe discharges during the episode and gadolinium enhanced magnetic resonance imaging (MRI) of the brain revealed band hypertropia (Figure 4.8).

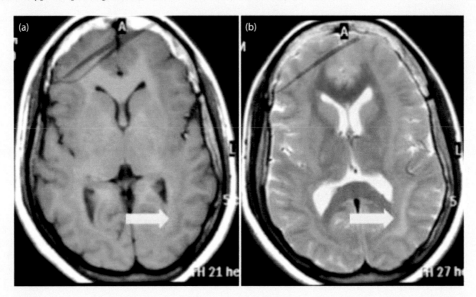

FIGURE 4.8   MRI brain axial images showing thick band of T1 hypointense (a) and T2 hyperintense (b) signal intensity deep to the cerebral cortex associated with diminished gyral sulcations. Altered hyperintense T2W signal seen in bilateral parieto-occipital regions.

Ophthalmic examination is normal in the causes mentioned above. TBVL associated with bilateral papilledema suggests transient visual obscurations.

Transient Visual Obscurations (TVOs) are triggered by maneuvers that increase ICP as described above and are frequently binocular.[5]

CASE 9

A 34-year-old obese woman (BMI = 30 kg/m^2) presented with history of headache of 3 months duration and episodes of transient loss of vision for 15 days. Headache was holo-cranial, associated with nausea, vomiting and photophobia. The headache was worse early morning and would wake the patient up from her sleep. Episodes of transient visual loss were recent and were triggered when the patient got up after prolonged sittings, upon bending and during coughing.

Ophthalmic examination revealed normal visual acuity and color vision, but visual fields were constricted peripherally in the left eye (Figure 4.9c, d). Fundus examination revealed bilateral disc edema (Grade 5: Modified Frisen grading) (Figure 4.9a, b).

The history is suggestive of the presence of transient visual obscurations, which are accompanying the increased intracranial type of headache in the above-described patient. The presence of constricted visual fields and disc edema further substantiate the diagnosis. Retinal nerve fiber layer thickness was increased in both eyes on optical coherence tomography (Figure 4.9e).

MRI-brain suggested normal brain parenchyma, optic nerve tortuosity and scleral indentation of the globe and empty sella (Figure 4.9f). Bilateral transverse sinuses were stenosed on MR venography. CSF pressure on lumbar puncture was noted to be high (300 mm of CSF) and the CSF composition was normal. Patient was diagnosed to be a case of idiopathic intracranial hypertension and was initiated on acetazolamide and topiramate.

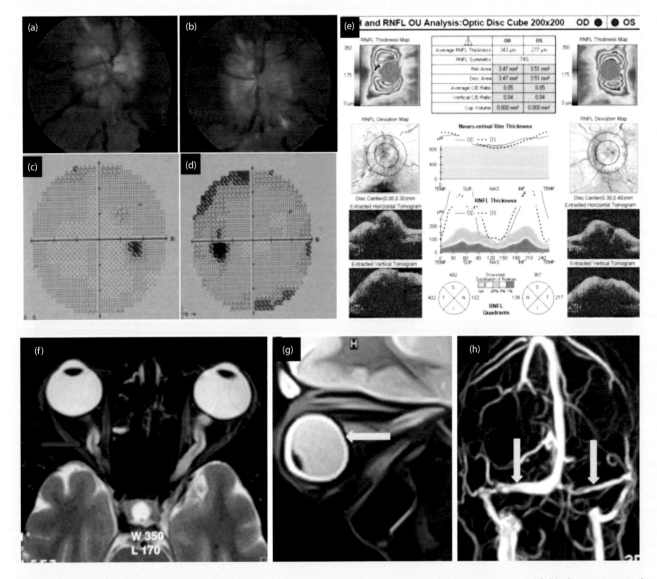

FIGURE 4.9 Bilateral papilledema on fundus examination (a, b). (c, d) A visual field examination and (e) shows increased RNFL thickness on OCT. MRI brain showing optic nerve tortuosity (f) and scleral flattening (g). MR venography suggests bilateral transverse sinus stenosis (h).

Persistent binocular visual loss

Binocular visual loss can be caused by bilateral anterior optic pathway involvement or involvement of uni/bilateral posterior optic pathway. Bilateral asymmetric optic neuropathies are also associated with RAPD (symmetric optic neuropathies do not present with RAPD). Chiasmal and retrochiasmal disorders are associated with visual field defects respecting a vertical meridian. Other details regarding clues to diagnosing persistent visual loss are given above. Algorithm 4.3 gives the systematic approach to a patient with binocular visual loss.

Ischemic/vascular brain lesion should always be kept as an important differential. Strokes involving retrochiasmal regions cause homonymous visual field defects. Bilateral occipital lobe infarcts can cause tubular visual field defects or complete blindness (cortical blindness). Cortical blindness may be associated with denial of visual loss (Anton's syndrome). Tiny islands of vision may persist,

and the patient may report fluctuating vision in the preserved portions. *Occipital lobe strokes* may be associated with other features of posterior circulation ischemia like dizziness, vertigo, ataxia and blindness with normal retinal/ocular examination.[2]

Posterior ischemic optic neuropathy (PION) often causes bilateral involvement. Postoperative vision loss (POVL) after major non-ocular surgery is a very rare but devastating complication since it has the potential to cause bilateral, severe and permanent loss of vision. The common major procedures resulting in POVL are cardiac and spinal procedures. While posterior ischemic optic neuropathies have widely been reported in the literature to be associated with prolonged systemic surgical procedures, occurrence of even bilateral anterior ischemic optic neuropathies is known. PION is more common with spinal surgeries or radical neck dissections, whereas AION is more common with cardiac surgeries. Arteritis is another important cause of PION.[8–10]

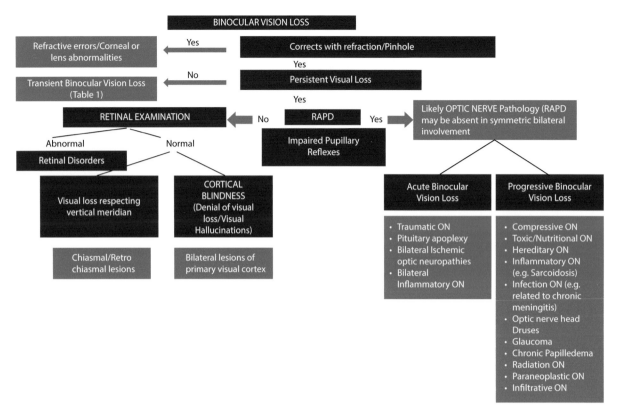

ALGORITHM 4.3   Approach to binocular visual loss.

CASE 10

A 32-year-old male presented to emergency department with a history sudden-onset, severe and constant epigastric pain of 2 days duration and two episodes of massive hematemesis followed by altered sensorium since morning of the day of admission. The patient had a similar history around 9 months back when he was diagnosed as a case of peptic ulcer disease. On presentation, patient was in altered sensorium, not oriented to surroundings and unresponsive to commands. Presenting systolic blood pressure was 64 mmHg, pulse rate of 132/min and respiratory rate of 38/min. The patient was identified to be in hypovolemic shock, was shifted to the intensive care unit and all measures to resuscitate him. Initial laboratory evaluation of this patient revealed the hemoglobin of 4.7 g/dL and he received 4 units of blood transfusion. Upper GI endoscopy revealed bleeding peptic ulcer and endoscopic hemostasis was achieved.

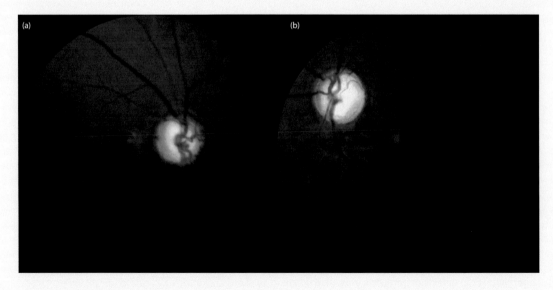

FIGURE 4.10   Fundus showing optic atrophy following posterior ischemic optic neuropathy.

The patient regained sensorium after 72 hours of his admission and was noted to have loss of vision of both eyes. The patient could only perceive light from both eyes and bilateral pupillary reflexes were sluggish. Fundus examination done on Day 5 after admission showed primary optic atrophy of both eyes (Figure 4.10). Contrast MRI brain and orbits were within normal limits.

The patient was diagnosed to be having posterior ischemic optic neuropathy because of massive blood loss and persistent hypotension. He did not improve on follow up.

Pituitary apoplexy (apoplexy meaning to be struck down) is a potentially life-threatening disorder due to acute ischemic infarction or hemorrhage of the pituitary gland. The rich, peculiar and complex vascular supply of the pituitary gland makes it susceptible to apoplexy. Headache, the most frequent presentation, is often sudden, severe, retro-orbital and may precede other symptoms. Loss of visual acuity occurs in 45–90% of the afflicted patients. Patients may present with altered visual fields depending upon the site of affliction. Cranial nerve involvement (III, IV, V and VI) is also common, cavernous sinus being the vulnerable site.

Other associated symptoms may include altered mental status, neck stiffness, nausea, vomiting, focal neurological deficits and frontal lobe syndrome.[11]

CASE 11

A 50-year-old male known case of hypertension presented to emergency room with history of severe headache associated with bilateral loss of vision of 2 days duration. On examination, the patient was febrile, confused and restless. On ophthalmic examination, patient had absent perception of light in the right eye and could only count fingers at 3 m from the left eye. Neurological examination revealed right third and fourth nerve palsy.

An emergency CT scan without contrast revealed a hyperdense lesion (with an air-fluid level) in the pituitary gland and optic chiasm suggesting pituitary apoplexy (Figure 4.11). A follow-up MRI was obtained and confirmed the existence of a pituitary macroadenoma with acute hemorrhage. Because of the patient's acute visual loss, emergency transsphenoidal resection was planned.

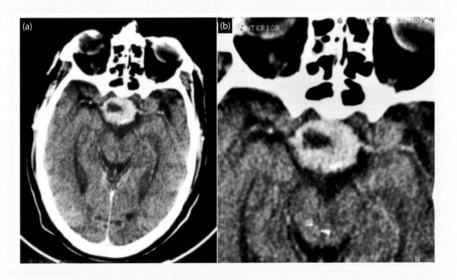

FIGURE 4.11 Non-contrast CT head showing hyperdense lesion (suggestive of bleed) in the sellar region with central hypodensity (suggestive of air-fluid level).

Toxic/nutritional/hereditary optic neuropathies

Vision loss in hereditary and toxic/nutritional optic neuropathies is usually chronic and progressive over months to year. Centrocecal scotoma is considered as a hallmark.[21] Though usually chronic, these can also present with acute vision loss. Earliest ophthalmological findings of toxic optic neuropathies (e.g., ethambutol induced) are color vision loss or central scotomas. Some drugs like ethambutol also have an affinity for the optic chiasm and may cause bitemporal visual field defects manifesting with their toxicity.[21]

In specific, Leber's hereditary optic neuropathy often has a rapid-onset painless loss of vision of one eye followed by the similar loss of vision in the fellow eye within days to months. The visual loss from one eye may often get unnoticed and many times patients notice loss of vision from both eyes together. Bilateral simultaneous involvement is also known to occur. In acute-subacute phase of LHON, circumpapillary telangiectatic microangiopathy and elevation of the RNFL around the disc (pseudo edema) is noted. There is no true disc edema, as is demonstrated by the absence of disc leakage on fluorescein angiography. Tortuosity of the retinal vasculature has also been described.

In up to 50% of acute LHON cases, the optic disc may appear normal. In the chronic phase, extensive axonal loss occurs in the papillomacular bundle. At this stage, primary optic atrophy is noted on fundus examination.[18]

CASE 12

A 32-year-old male presented with painless progressive loss of vision in the right eye of 15 days duration. There was a similar history of loss of vision of the left eye around 4 months back. On ophthalmic examination, the patient could count fingers at 6 m from the right eye and had only perception of light from the left eye. The visual fields were grossly depressed bilaterally. Fundus examination revealed increased tortuosity of the retinal vessels, and elevation of the disc margins (Figure 4.12a). FFA revealed circumpapillary telangiectatic microangiopathy with elevation of nerve fiber layer without leakage of the dye (Figure 4.12b). Fundus examination of the left eye showed primary optic atrophy. Routine hemogram and biochemistry, gadolinium enhanced MRI brain, MR venography and CSF analysis were all within normal range. The patient had already received five grams of methylprednisolone over 5 days but to no benefit. Genomic workup of patient's serum showed wild status for G3460A, T14484C and mutant status for G11778A mutation, which is commonly associated with LHON syndrome. The patient was started on coenzyme Q and Idebenone. On 6 months follow-up, both eyes revealed primary optic atrophy.

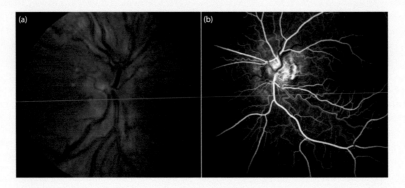

FIGURE 4.12 Fundus photograph (a) and fundus fluorescein angiography (b) of right eye showing features consistent with acute-subacute phase of LHON.

Massive head trauma causing chiasmal or retrochiasmal injuries, intra-parenchymal hemorrhage and diffuse axonal injury are other causes of binocular vision loss.

Recurrent binocular visual loss

Vascular episodes involving posterior circulation may be recurrent. Bilateral optic neuritis also has recurrences, especially in patients of neuromyelitis optica.

STEP 4: Is the visual loss progressive?

The common causes of progressive vision loss with their salient features have been described in Table 4.4. Local eye causes *like optic nerve head drusen, glaucoma* and even *chronic papilledema* should always be ruled out in such patients as these have a potential to cause vision loss over time. All these optic neuropathies have been covered in detail elsewhere in this book.

TABLE 4.4: Causes of Progressive Vision Loss

Etiology	Onset	Mono/Binocular	Pain	Vision Loss	Visual Prognosis
Demyelinating/ Inflammatory[19]	Acute-subacute	Usually monocular	Periorbital/with eye movements	Progressive over 7–10 days. Disc edema (without hemorrhages) in papillitis; normal disc in retrobulbar neuritis Central visual field defects	Good
Compressive[20]	Chronic	Monocular for orbital/optic nerve compressive lesions Binocular for chiasmal/ retrochiasmal lesions	Absent	Chronic progressive vision loss with variable visual field defects depending upon the site of lesion	Variable, usually poor
Toxic/nutritional[21]	Chronic	Binocular, usually symmetric	Absent	Usually central/centrocecal field defects. Disc may be normal, edematous or atrophied	Variable, usually poor
Hereditary[18]	Chronic May be acute-subacute in some patients of LHON	Binocular Sequential in LHON	Absent	Central/centrocecal field defects. Optic disc is usually atrophied; (fundus examination in LHON may show telangiectatic capillaries and pseudo edema of the optic disc with surrounding swelling of the RNFL	Poor

(Continued)

TABLE 4.4: **Causes of Progressive Vision Loss** *(Continued)*

Etiology	Onset	Mono/Binocular	Pain	Vision Loss	Visual Prognosis
Papilledema[5]	Visual acuity usually preserved	Binocular	Associated with increased ICP headache	Enlarged blind spot and peripheral constriction of the fields is common. Fundus examination reveals disc edema with peripapillary hemorrhages	Good
Optic nerve drusen[22]	Chronic	Mono/binocular	Painless	May have peripheral field defects. Fundus shows lumpy bumpy appearance confined to the disc, absence of venous congestion, hemorrhages or exudates and preservation of spontaneous venous pulsations	Usually good
Infiltrative[23]	Subacute to chronic	Mono/binocular	May be associated with increased ICP headache	Fundus may be normal or may reveal an infiltrated optic disc/disc edema	Variable, usually poor
Radiation[24]	Rapid deterioration over a period of days to weeks	Mono/binocular (simultaneous/sequential)	Absent	Peak incidence at 1–1.5 years after radiation (range 3 months to 8 years (or longer) Fundus may be normal, pale or edematous	Poor

CASE 13

A 50-year-old female presented with 6 months history of painless progressive diminution of vision of both eyes. On examination, visual acuity was 6/18 in the right eye and 6/12 in the left eye. Visual fields showed peripheral field defects (Figure 4.13c, d). Fundus examination revealed unevenly elevated disc margins (with lumpy-bumpy appearance) (Figure 4.13a, b). Gadolinium enhanced MRI brain, MR venography and CSF analysis were all within normal range. The disc elevation was thought to be optic nerve drusen and their presence was confirmed on B-scan ultrasound which revealed hyper-reflective echoes at optic nerve head with acoustic shadow persisting at low gain (Figure 4.13e, f). On fluorescein angiography, these lesions demonstrated auto-fluorescence on optic disc in the pre-injection phase.

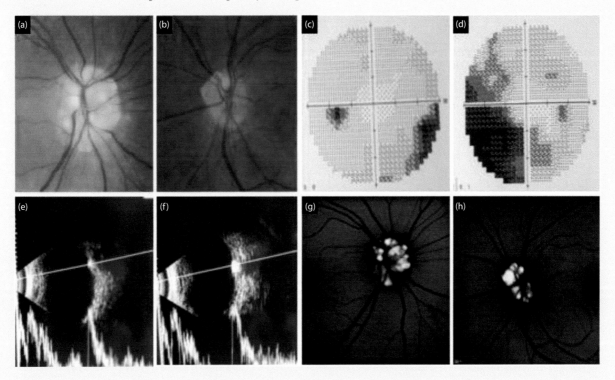

FIGURE 4.13 Fundus photographs of right and left optic discs (a, b) showing unevenly elevated and indistinct disc margins with lumpy bumpy appearance of the optic discs. Visual fields of right and left eyes (c, d) show peripheral field defects corresponding to the sites of optic nerve drusen, sparing the central fields. B-scan ultrasonography reveals hyper-reflective echoes at the optic head with acoustic shadows persisting at low gain (e, f). Fluorescein angiography shows auto-fluorescence on optic discs in the pre-injection phase (g, h).

Conclusion

The visual pathway is often a target of many systemic as well as neurological disorders. Early diagnosis and prompt treatment of patients with visual loss is often challenging. Visual loss can arise from disturbances in local ocular structures, optic nerves and the visual cortex. Recognition of the anatomical target and the ongoing pathology are the first steps to management of these patients. The temporal profile, triggers, associations and pattern of visual loss are vital clues to diagnosis. While monocular visual loss often arises from the anterior visual pathway, binocular loss is common in posterior visual pathway involvement. Systematic examination of visual acuity, visual fields and fundus solves most mysteries. A careful clinical examination and a step-wise approach are rewarding. While vasculitis is a devastating cause of visual loss, it often causes involvement of the peripheral nervous system before causing visual damage. This chapter is only an introduction to a horde of disorders with the potential to cause significant visual morbidity. The other causes described in this chapter will be covered in detail subsequently.

Multiple-Choice Questions

1. Following are the causes of painful loss of vision, EXCEPT:
   a. Optic neuritis
   b. Posterior ischemic optic neuropathy
   c. Ocular ischemic syndrome
   d. Acute angle closure glaucoma

   Answer:

   b. Posterior ischemic optic neuropathy

2. Following are false for ischemic optic neuropathies, EXCEPT:
   a. Diabetes is a risk factor for NA-AION.
   b. Usually presents with visual field defects respecting vertical meridian.
   c. Complete visual recovery is a rule.
   d. Does not occur in patients with vasculitis.

   Answer:

   a. Diabetes is a risk factor for NA-AION.

3. Uhthoff's phenomenon
   a. Implies loss of stereopsis in high temperature.
   b. Occurs due to transient hypoperfusion of retinal vasculature.
   c. May be associated any inflammatory optic neuropathy.
   d. Associated with periorbital pain.

   Answer:

   c. May be associated any inflammatory optic neuropathy.

4. Posterior reversible encephalopathy syndrome is associated will all of the following, EXCEPT:
   a. Eclampsia
   b. High-grade carotid artery stenosis
   c. Hypertensive crisis
   d. Chemotherapeutic agents like cyclosporine

   Answer:

   b. High-grade carotid artery stenosis

References

1. Pula JH, Kwan K, Yuen CA, Kattah JC. Update on the evaluation of transient vision loss. Clin Ophthalmol. 2016;10:297–303.
2. Newman N, Biousse V. Diagnostic approach to vision loss. Continuum (Minneap Minn). 2014;20(4):785–815.
3. Pradhan S, Chung SM. Retinal, ophthalmic, or ocular migraine. Curr Neurol Neurosci Rep. 2004 Sep;4(5):391–397.
4. Frohman TC, Davis SL, Beh S, Greenberg BM, Remington G, Frohman EM. Uhthoff's phenomena in MS—clinical features and pathophysiology. Nat Rev Neurol. 2013;9: 535–540. doi:10.1038/nrneurol.2013.98
5. Wall M. Idiopathic intracranial hypertension. Neurol Clin. 2010;28(3):593–617.
6. Amerasinghe N, Aung T. Angle-closure: Risk factors, diagnosis and treatment. Prog Brain Res. 2008;173:31–45.
7. Newman-Toker DE, Horton J, Lessell S. Clinicopathologic reports, case reports, and small case series–recurrent visual loss in Leber hereditary optic neuropathy. Arch Ophthalmol. 2003;121(2):288–291.
8. Hayreh SS. Ischemic optic neuropathy. Prog Retin Eye Res. 2009;28(1):34–62.
9. Purvin V. Ischemic optic neuropathy. Seminars in cerebrovascular diseases and stroke. 2004;4(1):18–38. doi: 10.1053/j.scds.2004.07.002
10. Francis CE. Giant cell arteritis. J Neuro Ophthalmol. 2016; 36:e2–e4.
11. Boellis A, di Napoli A, Romano A, Bozzao A. Pituitary apoplexy: An update on clinical and imaging features. Insights Imaging. 2014; 5:753–762. doi:10.1007/s13244-014-0362-0
12. Bi WL, Dunn IF, Laws ER Jr. Pituitary apoplexy. Endocrine. 2015;48(1):69–75.
13. McIntosh RL, Rogers SL, Lim L, Cheung N, Wang JJ, Mitchell P, Kowalski JW, Nguyen HP, Wong TY. Natural history of central retinal vein occlusion: An evidence-based systematic review. Ophthalmology. 2010;117(6):1113–1123.e15. doi: 10.1016/j.ophtha.2010.01.060
14. Bruce BB, Newman NJ. Functional visual loss. Neurol Clin. 2010;28(3):789–802. doi:10.1016/j.ncl.2010.03.012
15. Agostoni E, Aliprandi A. The complications of migraine with aura. Neurol Sci. 2000;27:S91–S95. doi: 10.1007/s10072-006-0578-y
16. Faske SK. Posterior reversible encephalopathy syndrome: A review. Semin Neurol. 2011;31:202–215. doi: http://dx.doi.org/10.1055/s-0031-1277990
17. Taylor I, Scheffer IE, Berkovic SF. Occipital epilepsies: Identification of specific and newly recognized syndromes. Brain. 2003;126:753–769.
18. Yen MY, Wang AG, Wei YH. Leber's hereditary optic neuropathy: A multifactorial disease. Prog Retin Eye Res. 2006;25(4):381–396.
19. Voss E, Raab P, Trebst C, Stangel M. Clinical approach to optic neuritis: Pitfalls, red flags and differential diagnosis. Ther Adv Neurol Disord. 2011 Mar;4(2):123–134. doi: 10.1177/1756285611398702
20. Behbehani R. Clinical approach to optic neuropathies. Clin Ophthalmol. 2007;1(3): 233–246.
21. Sharma P, Sharma R. Toxic optic neuropathy. Indian J Ophthalmol. 2011 Mar–Apr;59(2):137–141. doi: 10.4103/0301-4738.77035.
22. Davis PL, Jay WM. Optic nerve head drusen. Semin Ophthalmol. 2003; 18(4): 222–242.
23. Takkar A, Naheed D, Dogra M, Goyal MK, Singh R, Gupta N, Gupta K, Mittal BR, Lal V. Infiltrative optic neuropathies: Opening doors to sinister pathologies. Neuro-Ophthalmol. 2017; Published online: 08 May 2017. doi:10.1080/01658107.2017.130851
24. Danesh Meyer HV. Radiation-induced optic neuropathy. J Clin Neurosci. 2008;15(2): 95–100.

5

OPTIC NEUROPATHIES ASSOCIATED WITH MULTIPLE SCLEROSIS (MS) AND NEUROMYELITIS OPTICA SPECTRUM DISORDERS (NMO-SD)

Gordon Plant, Vivek Lal

CASE STUDY

A 35-year-old woman presented with sudden-onset right eye visual loss associated with painful eye movements for 5 days. On examination, visual acuity of the right eye was 6/36 with normal visual acuity in the left eye. Visual field examination from the right eye suggested central field defect. Fundus examination was normal. MRI brain demonstrated multiple T2 hyperintense lesions involving juxta-cortical and subcortical white matter. What are the differentials and likely diagnosis in this patient?

Introduction—Optic nerve in demyelinating disorders

Multiple sclerosis (MS) and neuromyelitis optica (NMO) are chronic, relapsing, inflammatory demyelinating conditions of the central nervous system (CNS). These two entities are phenotypically similar and may pose a diagnostic dilemma, particularly at first presentation. NMO was in the past considered a monophasic disorder (better known as Devic disease). It has also been confused with a subtype of MS, the Opticospinal form, commonly diagnosed in East Asia. It was the groundbreaking discovery of Aquaporin-4 (AQP-4 IgG) antibodies by Lennon et al. in 2004 that enabled a serological diagnosis of NMO to be made, and the disorder has subsequently become clearly distinct from MS (1). The term NMO spectrum disorder (NMO-SD) was subsequently introduced to describe cases where a serological diagnosis is made, but the phenotype is missing one or both of the classical manifestations in the optic nerve or spinal cord. While MS is primarily considered to be a demyelinating disease, with axonal loss being responsible for chronic deficits, NMO-SD is recognized as an astrocytopathy with demyelination. In MS demyelinating plaques with relative preservation of axons are a frequent manifestation, whereas in NMO severe damage is noted in both myelin and the axons, which may even lead to necrotic cavitation (2).

The immunological and pathological differences between these two entities explain the difference in their response to some specific treatment modalities like interferons. Interferon Beta, which is widely used in MS, is known to exacerbate NMO-SD (3). Figure 5.1 shows the differences in the immunological differences involved in MS and NMO. The long-term prognosis also differs between these two distinct diseases.

Wrongly classified in classical anatomy with the cranial nerves, the optic nerves (which together with the optic chiasm and optic tracts form the anterior visual pathway) should be considered white matter tracts of the CNS analogous to the white matter columns and tracts of the spinal cord. Anterior visual pathway involvement is a common presenting feature of immune-mediated disorders of the CNS including MS and NMO.

Optic neuritis (ON) is one of the common initial manifestations of MS, NMO-SD and allied disorders underscoring the importance of recognizing the differences in its presentation.

In this chapter, we will discuss how to approach a patient presenting with ON. We shall specifically be elaborating about similarities and differences in ON related to MS and NMO-SD.

Optic neuritis

Optic neuritis is inflammation of one or both optic nerves characterized by the triad of subacute vision loss, dyschromatopsia and, often, periocular pain. ON has varied etiologies, demyelinating being the most common. Other differential diagnoses of ON include infectious, and post-infectious autoimmune conditions and for subacute visual loss neoplastic, toxic and other causes must be considered. The incidence of optic neuritis varies across the geographical territories and range from 1.03 to 6.4/100,000 per year (4, 5). Optic neuritis can be subdivided into four categories depending upon the site of involvement (Figure 5.2) as follows (4):

1. *Anterior optic neuritis (ON) (sometimes referred to as papillitis although in most cases there is involvement of the retrobulbar optic nerve):* On fundus examination, swelling at the optic disc is visible, signifying involvement of the anterior optic nerve.
2. *Retro-bulbar neuritis (RBN):* Inflammation of the posterior (retro-bulbar portion) of the optic nerve, sparing the optic disc. Normal disc appearance on fundus examination. The optic nerve involvement may be intracranial in which case the patient is unlikely to experience pain. Anterior and retro-bulbar optic neuritis are the most common forms seen in MS.
3. *Optic perineuritis:* Inflammation of the optic nerve sheath within the orbit with secondary involvement of the optic nerve. This form does not occur in MS.
4. *Neuro-retinitis:* In this form of optic neuritis, there is optic disc swelling acutely accompanied by the generation of subretinal fluid leading to the development of a macular star in the recovery phase. Whether this indicates involvement of the neural retina is uncertain as this may result from primary involvement of the prelaminar optic nerve alone. This form does not occur in MS (6).

Anterior ON and RBN are the two most common forms, in which a neuro-ophthalmologist encounters in relation to MS and NMO-SD. Neuro-retinitis is more commonly associated with post-infectious or other autoimmune conditions and optic

DOI: 10.1201/9780429020278-8

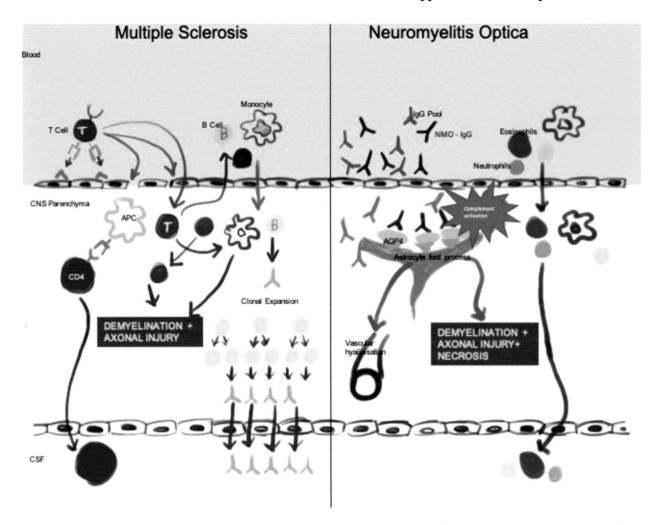

FIGURE 5.1 Immunological mechanisms involved in multiple sclerosis (MS) and neuromyelitis optica spectrum disorder (NMO-SD). The former is mediated by entry of activated lymphocytes to the CNS compartment, whereas the latter is mediated by a systemic IgG antibody against Aquaporin-4 (AQP-4) channels found on astrocytes.

perineuritis (OPN) may be part of a more generalized orbital inflammatory syndromes or a durally based granulomatous disorder such as sarcoidosis or IgG4 spectrum disease.

Based upon the etiology, some authors have classified ON into typical ON – ON related to MS and atypical ON – ON due to any other cause (7). Unfortunately, this designation is inappropriate in the global context and reflects the domination of the literature concerning ON by work carried out in populations of white

European descent living in temperate latitudes. It is certainly recommended that MS-associated optic neuritis (MSON) be clearly distinguished as this occurs worldwide and management differs considerably from other forms of ON. Other conditions can usefully be grouped together as non-MSON as management is very different in the acute situation in this group of disorders, some of which are seen more commonly than MSON in some parts of the world. Optic neuropathies related to causes like infectious, autoimmune, vasculitis, malignancies, etc. are included in this group. Recognizing red flags is important in wake of long-term implications. Table 5.1 shows the primary distinguishing features between MSON and non-MSON.

In this chapter, we shall be concentrating on MS-related ON (MSON) and ON related to NMO-SD (NMO-ON).

Optic Neuropathy in MS (MSON)

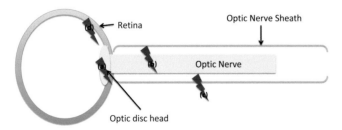

FIGURE 5.2 Types of optic neuritis depending upon the site of involvement. (a) anterior optic neuritis (papillitis, AON); (b) retro-bulbar neuritis (RBN); (c) optic perineuritis (OPN); (d) neuro-retinitis.

ON has been seen as a harbinger of MS. In an epidemiological study, 13–15% patients of MS presented with ON and 27–37% MS patients showed evidence of ON during the disease course (8). In the ONTT, the cumulative probability of developing MS within 15 years of developing ON was 50% (25% in patients with no baseline lesions and 72% in patients with one or more lesions) (9).

TABLE 5.1: Differences between MSON and Non-MSON

	MSON	Non-MSON
Onset	Acute or subacute	May be sudden, acute, subacute or chronic
Progression	Progresses to peak in 1 week, remains stable over 2 weeks, recovers over 3 weeks spontaneously with variable residual deficit.	No specific pattern, may peak to nadir rapidly within hours to a few days or may progress beyond 2 weeks
Age group	Usually young adult 15–45 years	Variable
Gender	Female > Male	Either
Periocular pain	90%, increase on eye movements. Spontaneous resolution within days.	May be absent (particularly if intracranial optic nerve involved) or may progress > 2 weeks from onset
Laterality	Usually unilateral – variable severity	May be bilateral simultaneous or sequential
Visual acuity	Variable, usually mild to moderate at nadir; better than 6/36 or 20/125	Severe visual loss at nadir – light perception or no light perception
Optic nerve head	Swollen in 35% (anterior ON) Normal in 65% (retrobulbar ON) Rarely hemorrhages	Markedly swollen with hemorrhages and Macular star in neuroretinitis cases
Visual field deficit	Variable, usually central	Variable, may be hemianopic, altitudinal, etc.
Ocular/retinal/ vitreous changes	None or minimal, mild venous sheathing (if present) scant vitreous cells	Marked anterior and/or posterior segment inflammation; marked periphlebitis
Improvement	Spontaneous in >90% over 4 weeks regardless of treatment	Lack of Improvement within 4 weeks or continuous deterioration
Steroid Response	Responsive, no relapse on discontinuing treatment, even short 3-day high dose regimen.	May or may not be responsive. If responds, usually steroid dependent (may relapse when treatment discontinued).
Optic disc pallor	Develops 4–6 weeks after the acute episode	Early optic disc pallor (within 4 weeks)

Optic neuritis associated with MS is one of the most common causes of acute/subacute unilateral visual loss in young individuals in temperate latitudes, where MS has the highest prevalence. The loss of color vision and contrast sensitivity may be early and out of proportion to the loss of visual acuity. MS-ON occurs more commonly in women as compared to men, usually in the age group of 15–45 years.

Classical clinical presentation is a triad of

1. *Subacute unilateral visual loss:* While a wide range of visual acuity loss has been observed, visual field losses are universal, seen in 97.5% cases.
2. Peri-ocular pain is present in 92% patients.
3. Impaired color vision is seen in 93.8%.

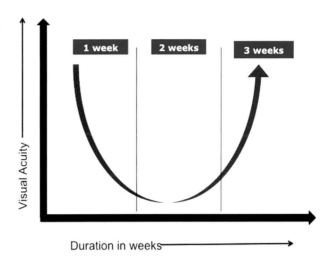

FIGURE 5.3   Typical course of MSON.

Natural course of MS-ON. The rule of 1-2-3 should always be borne into mind. Initially, the symptoms (severity of visual loss) worsen over a period of 1 week, remain stable for next (second) week and then spontaneously improve by the end of the third week (Figure 5.3). As a rule in typical optic neuritis, recovery of vision (to variable extent) should occur within 30 days of onset. The improvement is noted regardless of the administration of steroids or any other treatment, although corticosteroids will hasten the recovery.

Most data about MSON have been derived from the ONTT, a prospective multicenter, randomized trial that enrolled patients between 1988 and 1991. Fifteen-year follow-up data from this trial are available. The majority of cases are unilateral, although there are exceptions. The visual loss is usually mild to moderate and presenting visual acuity is usually above Snellen 6/36 (20/125).

The loss of vision is associated with pain in around 92% of patients, of which in 40%, pain precedes the visual loss. Orbital pain on eye movements is frequently reported (10, 11).

Color desaturation is often the earliest manifestation with patients reporting that colored objects appear darker, dirty or pale. Earliest desaturation develops for red color and object which may appear washed out, faded or pinkish in patient's terminology.

History suggestive of Uhthoff's phenomenon may be present. Transient visual deterioration occurs when body temperature rises, due to physical activity, hot bath, eating, etc. Recovery occurs as core temperature returns to normal. In a study of 125 patients of ON, Uhthoff's phenomenon was seen to occur in 32.8% patients (12, 13). Uhthoff's phenomenon was, however, not related to poor prognosis (13).

Another phenomenon experienced by patients of ON is Pulfrich phenomenon, which is the abnormal perception of movement in depth (14). The Pulfrich effect is due to a delay in neural conduction along the optic nerve and can be simulated in normal vision by placing a neutral density filter (dark glass) in front of one eye.

On assessment of visual function, as mentioned above, visual loss is usually mild to moderate. In ONTT, 89.5% patients presented with abnormalities of visual acuity, 35.3% suffered mild visual loss (better than 20/40 (6/12)), 28.8% had visual acuity of 20/50 to 20/190 (6/24–6/36)) and 35.9% population had a visual acuity worse than 20/200(6/60). Only 7% of the cohort had a visual acuity of light perception or no perception of light. Even when visual acuity was good, abnormalities were noted in other visual symptoms. Relative afferent pupillary defect is present in patients with unilateral or asymmetric involvement.

On fundus examination, optic disc swelling is seen in 39.5% patients of ON according to the ONTT. Patients with RBN are more likely to develop MS on follow up. The finding of a markedly swollen optic disc, retinal exudates and excessive retinal hemorrhages should raise alarm toward an alternative diagnosis. The asymptomatic eye may show optic disc pallor in a few patients suggesting a previous subclinical ON (Table 5.1).

Abnormal contrast sensitivity has been found in up to 98.2% involved eyes and color vision has been noted to be abnormal in 88.2%. In the ONTT 97.5%, patients had visual field deficits with 44.8% having diffuse field loss and 55.2% presenting with various types of focal deficit (11). Central field defects are most common in patients with MSON.

In the ONTT, it was also noted that the asymptomatic fellow eye also showed abnormalities on examination in a considerable number of patients. While the visual acuity was affected in 13.8% cases, other abnormalities included visual field deficits (48%), color vision deficits (20%) and abnormal contrast sensitivity (15.4%).

MRI is considered the gold standard in the diagnosis of MS (refer to Annexure 5.1. – for Diagnostic Criteria of MS), but diagnostic confusion may occur in certain clinical scenarios (15). Newer neuro-ophthalmic tools like spectral domain optical coherence tomography (OCT) to measure the retinal nerve fiber layer (RNFL), ganglion cell inner plexiform layer (GCIP) may have a role as potential novel biomarkers of MS. Greater neuro-retinal loss may be a marker of greater disease activity (16). OCT is rather a novel biomarker to study the disease activity and progression of MS (17). Objective markers have the potential to explore such manifestations as subclinical involvement of the asymptomatic fellow eye. Structural changes in retinal layers other than the optic nerve fiber and ganglion cell layers have been observed. Variously known as "microcystic maculopathy" or "retrograde maculopathy," there is controversy as to whether inner nuclear layer pathology represents a primary pathological process or the result of retrograde trans-synaptic changes. However, this change certainly reflects more advanced disease (17, 18).

Where available, neuroimaging is mandatory in all cases of ON at first presentation unless the patient is already known to have MS, and the clinical picture is of MSON. T2-weighted and gadolinium enhanced T1-weighted MRI of the brain should be carried out. Where ON presents as a clinically isolated syndrome, the morphology and distribution of the lesions seen on T2-weighted imaging of the brain can give a diagnosis of MS with a high degree of certainty. The addition of T1 gadolinium enhanced imaging can give an indication of disease activity by identifying active lesions in addition to the ON. The 10-year risk assessment of developing MS in patients of ON was done in ONTT. While 56% patients with one or more MRI white matter lesions developed MS; 22% patients without any specific MRI lesions also went on to develop MS. MRI techniques developed since this study was carried out have considerably increased the sensitivity and specificity. At the time of writing, dissemination of lesions is needed in time as well as space (two of the four areas – periventricular, juxta cortical, infratentorial and spinal cord) to fulfill the diagnostic criteria for MS (Annexure 5.1), but these criteria are constantly being reviewed and refined.

Orbital imaging is useful particularly where the diagnosis may not be MSON. T2-weighted or STIR imaging can identify the location of the inflammation in the anterior visual pathway. T1-weighted gadolinium enhanced imaging can confirm the changes seen on T2 as being acute and identify inflammation outside the optic nerve such as in OPN.

In acute stage, up to 90% patients may show ON hyper-intensity on dedicated MRI (19). Focal and anterior involvement of the optic nerve is commonly seen in MS. Posterior, long segment optic nerve involvement or involvement of the intracranial optic nerve or optic chiasma favor NMO-SD and important in the differential diagnosis of ON.

Cerebrospinal fluid (CSF) is usually acellular but may reveal mild mononuclear pleocytosis. Proteins may be normal or mildly increased. Pleocytosis of >100 cells/mm^3 or proteins of >100 mg/dl should alarm a clinician toward an alternative diagnosis. CSF total IgG levels and 24 hour intrathecal production of IgG are increased resulting in oligoclonal bands in 85% of MS patients (20, 21). As per the 2017 Mc Donald criteria (Annexure 5.1), the presence of CSF-specific OCBS can substitute for requirement of DIT in a patient with clinical evidence of a single attack.

Treatment

Corticosteroids are the chief line of management for patients presenting with acute ON. Intravenous methyl-prednisone should be used. Medical comorbidities, caregiving status, status of vision of the unaffected eye should be kept in consideration before initiating the therapy. While various dose regimens are available, most widely used is the administration 500–1000 mg intravenously or orally daily for 3–5 days. Low dose oral prednisone is not advised as a stand-alone therapy because of limited efficacy and higher recurrence rates of ON demonstrated in the ONTT.

Patients fulfilling the diagnostic criteria of MS should be offered disease modifying therapy (DMT). Glatiramer acetate, interferon beta, dimethylfumarate, teriflunomide and fingolimod are commonly used first-line agents. Natalizumab and mitoxantrone may be needed for an aggressive disease. Rituximab and stem cell therapy are the latest additions to the treatment armamentarium. The decision is usually taken after noting the patient's clinical status, expanded disease status scale and neuroimaging.

CASE 1

A 35-year-old woman presented with sudden-onset right eye visual loss of 5 days duration. On examination, visual acuity of the right eye was 6/36 and fundus examination was normal (Figure 5.4a, b). Color vision was impaired and visual field examination suggested central field. On OCT, the average RNFL thickness was 95 μm in both eyes (Figure 5.4c). T2W coronal imaging of orbit with fat suppression showed increased signal in the right optic nerve (Figure 5.5a, yellow arrow). Axial gadolinium enhanced MRI of the orbit with fat suppression shows involvement of the entire extent of the orbital portion of the optic nerve in this case of RBN (Figure 5.5b, blue arrow). MRI brain demonstrated multiple T2 hyperintense lesions involving juxta-cortical and subcortical white matter (Figure 5.5c, red arrow) confirming the diagnosis of MS. CSF analysis was acellular, with protein of 64 mg/dl, glucose of 45 mg/dl and oligo-clonal bands were noted further supporting the diagnosis of MS.

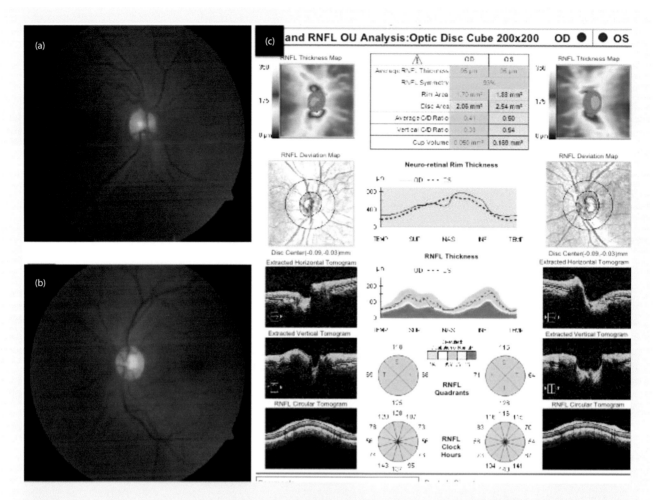

FIGURE 5.4 Fundus examination showing Normal Fundus Examination (a, b) with Normal OCT/RNFL thickness (c) of Case 1.

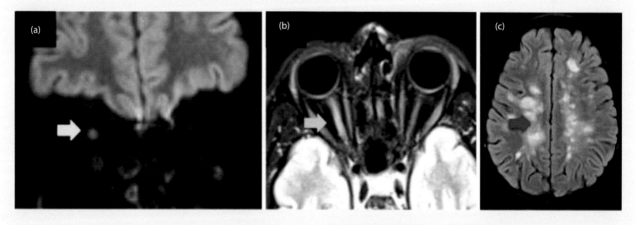

FIGURE 5.5 Findings on MRI brain and optic nerves of Case 1 showing Hypertintense Right Optic Nerve on Coronal T2-weighted (a) and Axial T2-weighted (b) orbital images, (c) MRI Brain images showing T2W Hyperintensities.

Optic neuropathy related to NMO-SD and related disorders

In the past, NMO-SD, as mentioned above, has been confused with MS. Devic disease was the term given to the optico spinal syndrome, which occurred more in the Asian subgroups, hence naming these as Asian variant MS. As compared to MS, NMO has an even stronger predilection towards affecting women (M:F = 1:8), especially in young age groups (22). Though age of presentation has a wide range, it usually afflicts patients in their mid-thirties. In contrast to MS, the pediatric and elderly populations are certainly affected, as evidenced by many published series (23, 24). The relapsing nature of the disease is well accepted, though monophasic forms are also known, and indeed were previously considered the archetypal disorder.

Prevalence rates of 0.3−4.4 per 100,000 people have been seen in population-based studies on NMO, major variations in prevalence have been seen depending upon the geographic and ethnic factors (25).

ON is a core criterion to diagnose patients with NMO, and the term NMO-SD was introduced to classify cases with either only one or neither of the classic features: optic nerve and spinal cord involvement (Annexure 5.1). Optic neuritis is a presenting feature in at least half of NMO patients. Twenty percent of these present with bilateral involvement, which is rare in MS, where inflammation occurring in both optic nerves simultaneously, occurs as a coincidence. In NMO, however, due to the presence of a systemic antibody, this occurs particularly in the post-infectious situation. In the past, some cases diagnosed as bilateral simultaneous retrobulbar, optic neuritis may have been a single lesion in the chiasm (chiasmitis). This is common in NMO but also occasionally seen in MS. Lag period between was initial ON and disease defining myelitis can vary from days to years. Recurrent attacks may occur before, along or after the myelitis attacks (26).

Differences between MSON and ON related to NMO-SD (referred to as typical and atypical ON, respectively, in some series) are important to appreciate owing to the vast differences in response to treatment and prognosis. Notably, even in ONTT, the presence of atypical features had low likelihood of developing MS on follow up (9).

Patients with ON related to NMO-SD usually present with severe visual loss. It has been noted that up to 80% of patients have presenting visual acuity of 20/200 (6/60) or worse (25). Around 30% of patients have no perception of light at presentation. The

visual loss does not meet the classical 1-2-3 rule of typical ON. Rather rapidly progressive visual loss may commonly occur. While patients may reach their nadir vision in 1–2 days, progressive visual loss over weeks may also occur. As stated earlier, bilateral ON is another harbinger of NMO-SD, as against MS and indeed this was an exclusion criterion for the ONTT. This exclusion contributed to the bias of the study toward MSON. In another series of ON in MS, it was noted that only 0.4% patients had bilateral ON as their presenting neurological manifestation (27). These episodes may or may not be associated with pain and indeed are less likely to be painful because of the frequent involvement of the intracranial optic nerve. Various series have reported pain as presenting feature in 27– 67% patients (26, 28). Recurrent ON is common. NMO has a predilection toward the posterior part and involves the intracranial portion of the optic nerve, optic chiasma, optic tracts. Hence, various corresponding field defects have been noted like altitudinal field defect, bitemporal hemianopia, homonymous hemianopia, etc. depending upon the location of the lesion. Associated specific syndromes like longitudinally extensive transverse myelitis (LETM), acute brainstem syndrome, acute area postrema syndrome, symptomatic narcolepsy or acute diencephalic syndrome should further raise suspicion of NMO-SD (Annexure 5.1). In common with other conditions associated with a systemic autoantibody and in contrast to MS, NMO-SD has been noted to be associated with autoimmune conditions like rheumatological disorders (Sjögrens syndrome, SLE, RA, etc.) or other autoimmune disorders like myasthenia gravis, autoimmune thyroiditis, etc.

CASE 2

A 59-year-old woman presented with history of sudden-onset bilateral visual loss of 2 days duration. She also had a past history of sudden-onset paraplegia 9 months prior to the current episode. On examination, vision of 6/60 in the right eye and absent perception of light in the left eye were noted. Fundus examination revealed bilateral severe optic disc edema (Figure 5.6a, b). Visual field examination revealed diffuse field loss in both eyes (Figure 5.6c, d). Average pRNFL on optical coherence tomography was 81 μm in the right eye and 27 μm in the left eye (Figure 5.6e, f). T1-weighted gadolinium enhanced MRI suggested thickened and enhancing optic nerve (involving middle and posterior segment) and optic chiasma (Figure 5.7a, b). CSF examination showed pleocytosis with 550 cell/dl, protein of 94 mg/dl and glucose of 55 mg/dl. OCBs were not found in CSF. AQP-4 antibodies tested positive in serum, confirming the diagnosis of NMO. Previous MRI spine demonstrated a LETM further supporting the diagnosis.

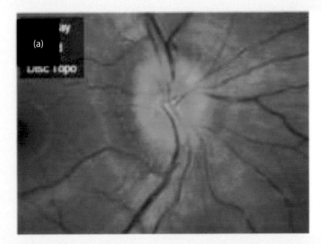 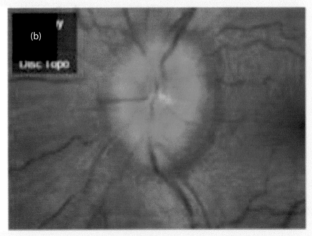

FIGURE 5.6 Fundus findings (a, b); visual field (c, d) and optical coherance tomography/retinal nerve fiber layer thickness (e, f) of Case 2. *(Continued)*

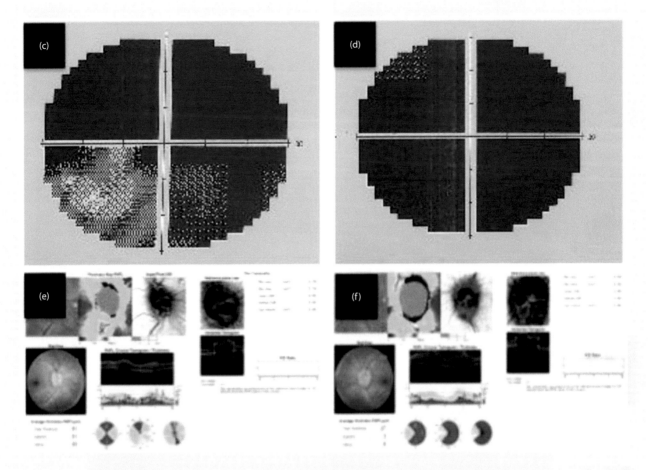

FIGURE 5.6   *(Continued)*

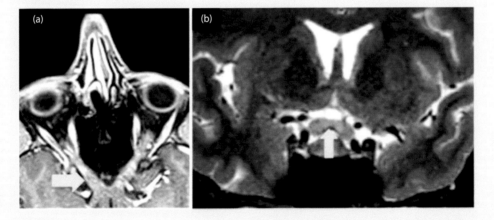

FIGURE 5.7   T1-weighted gadolinium enhanced MRI suggesting thickened and enhancing optic nerve (involving middle and posterior segment) and optic chiasma (a, b).

Diagnostic confusion usually arises on the first episode of ON. Examination should be focused on finding subtle signs, which can lead on to a definite conclusion. Compared to MSON, in NMO, bilateral involvement and severe visual loss are more common. The likelihood of NMO is higher if the presenting visual acuity is LP or NLP. If best vision after recovery is 20/50 or worse, suspicion is again of NMO-SD. Specific field defects like bitemporal hemianopia or homonymous hemianopia again point toward NMO, although both of these can occur in MS due to chiasmitis,

a plaque in the optic tract or a tumefactive lesion involving the optic radiation.

Optic neuropathy associated with anti-MOG syndrome

NMO-SD as discussed is most frequently associated with anti-AQP4-IgG antibodies. Damage to myelin oligodendrocyte glycoprotein (MOG), which is expressed on the surfaces of oligodendrocytes and myelin sheath causes anti-MOG syndromes. The presence of anti-MOG IgG antibodies may cause clinical syndrome similar to NMO-SD. Of special interest is the ON related to MOG IgG antibodies, which is the most common presentation of anti-MOG syndromes and is present in about 60% of cases. Forty percent of AQP-4 sero-negative optico spinal syndromes have been found to have MOG IgG antibody disease (29). Myelitis is the next most frequent presentation and cerebral changes, and rarely may manifest as ADEM -like syndrome or encephalitis or epilepsy. Like AqP4 antibody disease, MOG IgG associated ON is a female predominant disease and occurs more frequently in individuals older in age as compared to MSON (average age of onset approximately 40 years) and is a female predominant disease. Around 40% patients have bilateral disease and most present with prominent optic disc edema. About 80–93%

have recurrent disease and this was considered to the most common antibody found in cases of chronic relapsing inflammatory optic neuropathy (CRION) (30). MOG IgG ON extensively involves the optic nerve along its whole length but less frequently extend up to optic chiasm. Involvement is predominantly anterior with comparative sparing of the intracranial optic nerve, optic chiasm and optic tract and the retro chiasmatic segment. Involvement of the optic nerve sheath and surrounding orbital fat may be present. This radiological picture with features of OPN may be seen more frequently than with AQP-4 antibody ON. The majority of patients with MOG IgG ON have a normal MRI of the brain. MOG antibody disease is less frequently associated with other autoimmune disease when compared with AQP-4 IgG ON. While vision loss is severe at presentation, recovery and overall prognosis tends to be better (7).

CASE 3

A 45-year-old woman presented with sudden-onset bilateral vision loss of 4 days duration. On examination, she had absent perception of light in both eyes and fundus examination suggested severe optic disc edema (Figure 5.8a, b). Visual field analysis was not possible owing to severe vision loss. T1-weighted gadolinium enhanced MRI of the brain and CSF examination showed no abnormality. Serum AQP-4 antibodies were negative. A closer look at the MRI of the orbits suggested an extensive bilateral optic neuritis involving the whole optic nerve along with involvement of the perineural sheath (OPN) on contrast enhanced images (Figure 5.9a, b). Serum anti-MOG-antibodies were positive, confirming the diagnosis of anti-MOG antibody-mediated ON.

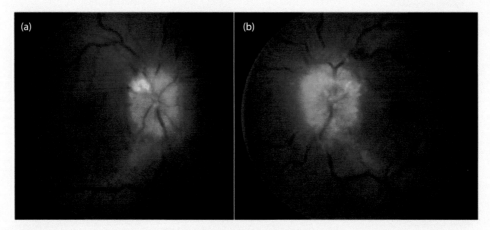

FIGURE 5.8   Fundus examination showing severe optic disc edema (a, b).

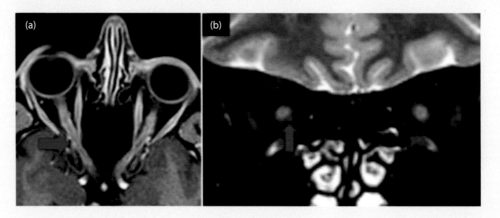

FIGURE 5.9   MRI of the orbits suggesting an extensive bilateral optic neuritis involving the whole optic nerve along with involvement of the perineural sheath (OPN) on contrast enhanced images (a, b).

Neuroimaging clues

Conventional neuroimaging shows changes of acute ON. Gadolinium enhanced fat-suppressed images of the orbits are ideal. MRI Changes include optic nerve swelling, increase signal intensity on T2 weighted with fat suppression or STIR images and nerve enhancement on T1 weighted gadolinium enhanced images with fat suppression. All the changes are more extensive when compared to MS. Importantly the site of involvement gives a major clue toward the etiology. While MS usually involves anterior part of ON, NMO involves the posterior segment (31). Storoni et al. noted the extent and location of inflammation in the anterior visual pathway and found that intracranial and long segment involvement of the anterior visual pathway favors NMO-SD over MS (31). Long involvement of optic nerve (usually > ½ the length of optic nerve) is seen. Bilateral involvement, involvement of optic chiasma and optic tract favor NMO. Optic chiasm may be thickened – symmetrically or asymmetrically. Extensive, bilateral involvement sparing the optic chiasm or optic tract favors anti-MOG syndrome.

Involvement of optic nerve sheath and intraorbital fat is more common in anti-MOG syndrome, optic perineuritis (OPN) may be noted in a few patients of NMO-SD. OPN is an inflammatory disorder that involves the sheath of the optic nerve as discussed above (Figure 5.2). Figure 5.10 schematically shows the sites of involvement of optic nerve in ION, MS-ON and NMO-SD-ON (31).

A typical MRI spine lesion of NMO-SD is a longitudinally extensive intramedullary lesion extending ≥3 contiguous vertebral segments. The cervical cord is more commonly involved in AQP-4 positive syndromes and caudal cord (conus) is involved more in MOG antibody disease (32, 33). Patchy heterogenous involvement of the cord with blurred margins (cloud like enhancement) may be seen along with nodular meningeal enhancement in MOG antibody disease (34).

On axial images, NMO-SD and anti-MOG syndromes frequently involve the central cord area around the canal as against MS lesion, which are typically peripheral extending to the subpial surface.

Though MRI brain can be normal, it may show non-specific white mater changes or occasionally have MRI changes overlapping with MS. NMO-SD typical patterns include lesions of dorsal medulla, area postrema, peri-ependymal regions of brainstem, diencephalic structures, cortico-spinal tracts and long lesions spanning the corpus callosum. Large confluent cerebral lesions and tumefactive (space-occupying) lesions can occur both in NMO-SD and atypical MS. Lesions of NMO-SD are subcortical and are not traversed by a central venule as seen in MS, both in pathological studies and high resolution MRI. It should be remembered that the typical Dawson fingers (perpendicular orientation of periventricular plaques) occurring in MS, also following the venular architecture and periventricular lesions located in inferior temporal lobe and cortical lesions, are only rarely seen in NMO-SD (32, 33). In anti-MOG syndromes, nonspecific supratentorial or infratentorial changes may be seen. ADEM-like lesions may be seen with diffuse signal changes in cortical/deep gray matter or subcortical/deep white matter. Poorly delineated, patchy enhancement in anti-MOG syndrome may give rise to cloud like enhancing lesions. Leptomeningeal enhancement may also be seen in some patients (34).

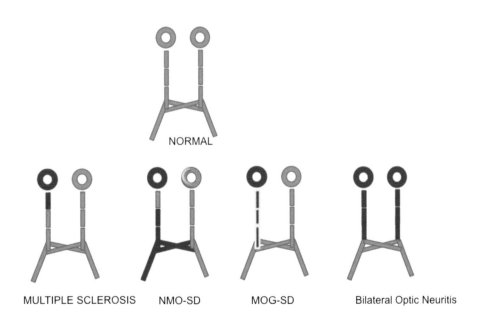

NORMAL

MULTIPLE SCLEROSIS   NMO-SD   MOG-SD   Bilateral Optic Neuritis

FIGURE 5.10   Sites of involvement of optic nerve in ION, MS-ON, NMO-SD-ON, MOG-SD and bilateral ON.

▌ – Normal optic nerve   ▌ – Affected ON

◎ – Clinically normal eye   ◉ –Clinically affected eye

▯ – Normal Optic Nerve Sheath   ▯ –Affected Optic Nerve Sheath

◉ – Variable Visual Field Involvement (depending upon the extent of optic chiasma and optic tract involvement

Other neuro-ophthalmic biomarkers

Optical coherence tomography measures of retinal nerve fiber layer thickness could also be used to differentiate between MS and NMO. Mean OCT-pRNFL values <70 μm measured 3 or more months after an attack favor NMO to idiopathic ON or MS related ON (25, 35). A cross-sectional study on retinal features of ON between MS and NMO patients concluded that the presence of vascular changes (focal arteriolar narrowing and attenuation of peripapillary vascular tree) and lower pRNFL are seen in NMO-SD when compared to MS (36). VEP may be absent or delayed in both NMO and MS patients.

Serological clues

Serological testing is diagnostic. Due to the recent advances in serological testing, diagnostic sensitivity and specificity of these assays have markedly improved. Cell-based serum assays are advisable. (Mean sensitivity in a pooled analysis – 76.7%.) (37). Serum MOG-IgG antibodies form another serological group in patients who are seronegative for AQP-4 IgG antibodies (25, 32).

Other diagnostic clues

CSF examination often shows prominent pleocytosis (> 50×10^6 leucocytes/l), lymphocytes predominate but polymorphonuclear cells and monocytes are more likely to be seen than in MS.

CSF-restricted oligoclonal IgG bands, which are hallmark of MS, are rarely seen (15–30%) (21, 32, 38). Total CSF proteins and albumin CSF/serum ratios correlate with disease activity, especially with the length of the spinal cord lesions in patients with acute myelitis (38).

Rheumatological diseases may coexist with NMO-SD, specifically Sjögrens syndrome, autoimmune thyroiditis, Rheumatoid arthritis. This association is less common in anti-MOG syndromes and further less frequent with MS.

Treatment

Acute treatment of ON
Steroids are the chief line of management for patients presenting with acute ON. Intravenous methyl prednisone should be used where possible. Medical comorbidities, caregiving status, status of vision of the unaffected eye should be kept in consideration before initiating the therapy. While various dose regimens are available, most widely used is the administration 1000 mg daily intravenous for 3–5 days. Low dose oral prednisone is not advised as a stand-alone therapy because of limited efficacy and higher recurrence rates of optic neuritis reported in the ONTT, although this has not been confirmed in later studies. Many studies have shown that in MSON treatment with corticosteroids hastens the recovery but does not influence the eventual outcome in terms of visual function. However, it is essential to understand that this is not the case for non-MSON.

Hyperacute treatment
In patients who have experienced pain preceding visual loss in an acute episode, it is advisable to ask them to report if there is a recurrence of pain. MRI at this point may confirm recurrent optic neuritis prior to visual loss and treatment with corticosteroids prior to visual loss may be beneficial.

In patients of NMO-SD-ON/anti-MOG syndrome also intravenous methyl prednisolone is the first choice. In patients who do not or partially respond to the steroid treatment, therapeutic plasma exchange (PLEX) should be planned. A retrospective analysis also suggests use of combine steroid+PLEX for patients of NMO-SD to improve disability outcomes (39). Limited data on any role of IVIG in acute stages of isolated ON are available.

Chronic relapsing inflammatory optic neuropathy (CRION)
CRION was introduced to describe a clinically defined syndrome, where the optic neuritis is recurrent and corticosteroid dependent as well as being corticosteroid responsive. That is to say when the acute treatment is withdrawn, the patient relapses. It is indeed remarkable that in MSON, it is possible to give 3 days of high dose corticosteroids and to discontinue this abruptly without fear of relapse. Although often a short tapering dose of oral treatment is given, it is not required to prevent early relapse. This certainly would not be recommended in NMO-SD, but a particular group of patients with a tendency to long-term corticosteroid dependence have been identified. Where the diagnosis is not certainly MSON, then a longer course of oral treatment is recommended with a gradual taper instructing the patient to report immediately if there is a return of symptoms. The clinically defined entity of CRION is most likely to be associated with anti-MOG antibodies or to be seronegative.

Long-term management

Long-term immune-suppression/Disease modifying therapy (DMT) is advocated in all cases of CRION and NMO-SD in order to avoid future relapses and associated cumulative disability. First-line agents used are azathioprine, rituximab and mycophenolate mofetil (MMF was used as a second-line drug by the neuromyelitis optica study group). Drugs like methotrexate and mitoxantrone are considered second-line agents. Drugs for which clinical trials are underway are tocilizumab, inebilizumab, eculizumab, aquapuromab (40). A general approach to treatment is given in Figure 5.11.

Special populations

Pediatric optic neuropathy (23)
ON is a common symptom occurring in acquired syndromes of demyelination. Based on one Canadian study, the annual incidence is lower as compared to adults (0.2%).

ON is the initial event in 25% children with acquired demyelinating disorders. ON is a presenting feature in 10–22% of children with MS and in 50–75% of children with NMO-SD.

Increased age at presentation is an independent risk factor for the development of MS. As per a meta-analysis with every 1 year increase in age, the odds of developing MS increase by 32% (41). Recurrent or sequential optic neuritis, typical MRI changes and the presence of CSF OCBs are the other risk factors.

Children show high heterogeneity in their presentation. Monophasic illness is common, although recurrent isolated ON or recurrent ON in relation to other inflammatory illnesses is known. As with adults, ON can be idiopathic, associated with demyelinating diseases like acute disseminated encephalomyelitis (ADEM), MS or NMO-SD. The clinical features are similar to the ones occurring in adults, but children less than 10 years of age are more likely to present with bilateral simultaneous ON, which as stated above is more likely to be a post-infectious disorder. Even

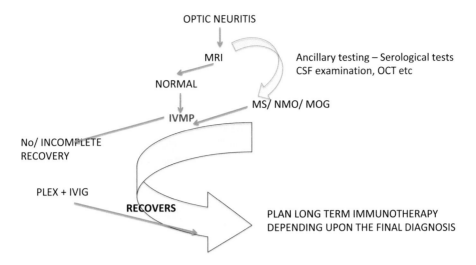

FIGURE 5.11 Approach to treatment of optic neuritis.

the ON episodes that present unilaterally rapidly involve the other eye and become bilateral. Around 72% children older than 10 years had bilateral involvement in a meta-analysis (41). Around 33–77% children report pain on eye movements. Sixty percent children report to have a severe visual loss (20/200 or worse) and only 20% had visual acuity better than 20/40. Optic disc swelling on fundus examination is seen in 46–69% (as compared to 30% in adults). MRI changes and other investigations are described above.

Speculations of relation of MOG antibodies with ON related to ADEM have been made though definite role and significance of these antibodies in ADEM-ON is unknown (23, 24).

As children frequently have severe visual loss and bilateral optic disc swelling, it is imperative to rule out infectious and neoplastic causes. Investigations focused on ruling out tuberculosis, Lyme disease, cat scratch disease, syphilis, sarcoidosis, etc. should be considered. Management strategy is as followed for adults: methyl prednisolone at a dose of 30 mg/kg/day (maximum of 1 g) daily for 3–5 days. PLEX and IVIG therapy may be considered in refractory cases. DMT is decided based upon the underlying diagnosis. Excellent visual recovery, often despite optic atrophy, is the rule.

Visual outcome of children of NMO with AQP-4 IgG antibodies may not favorable, and many are left with permanent severe visual loss (23).

Optic neuritis in pregnancy

Pregnancy is considered to be an immune privileged state; hence, there is a relative decline in incidence of ON during pregnancy and of MS relapses in general. The incidence may increase after pregnancy. It is important to rule out other causes of visual loss during pregnancy.

Pregnancy itself can bring changes in refraction due to progesterone-related shifts in corneal morphology. Similarly, one should rule out ophthalmic manifestations of pre-eclampsia and eclampsia such as optic disc edema, hypertensive retinopathy, choroidal infarction, serous retinal detachment, posterior circulation stroke and posterior reversible encephalopathy. Cerebral venous sinus thrombosis and idiopathic intracranial hypertension are the other common disorders that can cause visual loss with headache during pregnancy.

Other diagnostic considerations in pregnancy is safety of neuroimaging. CT scan should be avoided as far as possible. MRI is comparatively safe but gadolinium administration should be avoided, as it is a Food and Drug Administration (FDA) class C agent.

MS and pregnancy

Corticosteroids can be safely used in second and third trimesters during pregnancy. For a patient with MS who is pregnant or breast feeding preferred option is not to use any DMT. Selected pregnant patients may continue glatiramer or interferon beta. These DMTs are also compatible with breast feeding.

Given its teratogenic and lethal effects on the embryo, it is advisable not to use Teriflunomide during pregnancy. Other DMTs including fingolimod and dimethyl fumarate have been associated with high teratogenicity (42).

NMO-SD and pregnancy

First symptoms of NMO-SD may initially occur in 20–47% women during pregnancy. Relapses remain more or less unchanged in pregnancy, but some authors have noted that relapses may be increased in the first trimester of pregnancy, probably owing to the increased synthesis of B-cell activating factor by estrogens. NMO-SD carries a higher risk of miscarriages and pre-eclampsia. Antenatal use of high dose steroids is recommended (class C). PLEX and IVIG have been used at various stages of gestation.

Rituximab is the only class C drug in pregnancy, which can be used in NMO-SD. Azathioprine, mycophenolate mofetil and cyclophosphamide are all class D agents. Oral corticosteroids may be continued at low dose in selected patients, but risk of systemic adverse effects due to prolonged steroid usage should always be considered (43).

Approach to a patient presenting with optic neuropathy related to MS/NMO-SD

As noted above, there is an overlap of symptoms and signs in a patient presenting with an acute ON. A systematic approach becomes important while evaluation. History taking should include important points like onset, progression, laterality, nature of visual loss, vision at nadir and time taken to reach the vision at nadir. Associated symptoms defining specific syndromes like area postrema syndrome, LETM, conus syndrome, etc. should be specifically looked for. Specific neuro-ophthalmic examination like OCT, VEP and dedicated neuroimaging can provide major clues. Ancillary investigations like CSF analysis and serological tests should be looked into in wake of the above. Table 5.2 is a general guide, which can provide diagnostic clues.

TABLE 5.2: General Guide and Diagnostic Clues for Diagnosis of Optic Neuritis

Feature	Nature		Likely Diagnosis
Laterality	Unilateral		MS > NMO-SD > MOG-SD
	Bilateral		MOG-SD > NMO-SD > MS
Nature Of ON	Typical (Rule of I-2-3)		MS
	Atypical		NMO-SD/MOG-SD
Visual loss	Mild-moderate		MS > NMO-SD > MOG-SD
	Severe		MOG-SD/ NMO-SD
Involvement of peri-optic nerve sheath/ other orbital structures/fat/EOM	Yes		MOG-SD> NMO-SD
Response to steroid	Responsive		MS (NMO and MOG-SD are also responsive)
	Dependent		NMO-SD > MOG-SD
Improvement	Spontaneous and complete		MS
	None or incomplete		NMO-SD
Optic disc pallor	Early		NMOSD > MOG-SD
	Late		MS
Neuroimaging	Optic nerve	Anterior	MS/MOG-SD
		Posterior	NMO-SD
		> 1/2 of the length	NMO-SD
		extensive involvement	MOG-SD/NMO-SD
		Involvement of optic nerve sheath/ orbital fat	MOG-SD
	Spine	Short segment	MS
		LETM	NMO-SD
		Central	NMO-SD/ MOG -SD
		Eccentric	MS
		Cervical region	NMO-SD
		Conus	MOG-SD
	Brain	Dawson's fingers	MS
		Brainstem/area postrema diencephalon	NMO-SD/ MOG-SD
		ADEM like lesions	MOG-SD
		Leptomeningeal involvement	MOG-SD
CSF analysis	Pleocytosis> $> 50 \times 10^6$ leucocytes/l		NMO-SD
	OCBs		MS> NMO-SD
Average RNFL on OCT	< 70 μm		NMO-SD

Abbreviations: MS: Multiple sclerosis; NMO-SD: Neuromyelitis optica spectrum disorders; MOG: Myelin oligodendrocyte; ON: Optic neuritis; LETM: Longitudinally extensive transverse myelitis; ADEM: Acute disseminated encephalomyelitis; OCB: Oligoclonal bands.

Annexure 5.1

1. 2017 McDonald Criteria for Diagnosis of Multiple Sclerosis (MS) (44)

No. of Clinical Attacks Needed	Number of Lesions with an Objective Clinical Evidence	Additional Data Required
≥2	≥2	None
≥2	1 with a definite previous attack with a lesion in a distinct anatomical location	None
≥2	1	DIS
1	≥2	DIT
1	1	DIS or DIT

DIS: Demonstrated by either an additional clinical attack in a distinct anatomical location or by neuroimaging (MRI)

DIT: Demonstrated by either an additional clinical attack or by MRI OR CSF-specific oligo-clonal bands (OCBs)

Neuroimaging/MRI criteria DIS and DIT

- DIS: One or more T2-hyperintense MS lesions in two or more of four areas—periventricular, cortical or juxta-cortical, and infra-tentorial brain regions, and the spinal cord
- DIT:
  a. Simultaneous presence of gadolinium-enhancing and non-enhancing lesions at any time
  b. New T2-hyperintense or contrast-enhancing lesion on follow-up

DIS: Dissemination in Space
DIT: Dissemination in Time

2. International Consensus Diagnostic Criteria for Neuromyelitis Optica Spectrum Disorder (NMO-SD) (32)

NMO-SD with AQP4-IgG	1. At least 1 core clinical characteristic
	2. Positive test for AQP4-IgG (preferably using cell-based assay)
	3. Exclusion of alternative diagnoses

Diagnostic criteria for NMO-SD without AQP4-IgG or NMO-SD with unknown AQP4-IgG status	1. At least 2 core clinical characteristic, as a result of one or more clinical attacks
	  a. Plus all of the following—At least 1 core clinical characteristic must be optic neuritis, acute myelitis with LETM, OR area postrema syndrome
	  b. DIS (2 or more different core clinical characteristics)
	  c. Fulfillment of additional MRI requirements
	2. Unavailable testing or negative tests for AQP4-IgG using best available detection method
	3. Exclusion of alternative diagnoses

Core clinical characteristics

1. Optic neuritis
2. Acute myelitis
3. Area postrema syndrome

4. Acute brainstem syndrome
5. Symptomatic narcolepsy or acute diencephalic clinical syndrome with NMO-SD-typical diencephalic MRI lesions
6. Symptomatic cerebral syndrome with NMO-SD-typical brain lesions

Additional MRI requirements for NMO-SD without AQP4-IgG and NMO-SD with unknown AQP4-IgG status

1. Acute optic neuritis—Brain MRI with either
   a. Normal findings or only nonspecific white matter lesions
   b. Optic nerve MRI with T2-hyperintense lesion or T1 contrast enhancing lesion extending more than 1/2 optic nerve length or optic chiasm involvement
2. Acute myelitis: Lesion extending 3 or more than 3 contiguous segments (LETM)
3. Area postrema syndrome: Lesions in dorsal medulla/area postrema
4. Acute brainstem syndrome: Lesions in periependymal brainstem

Conclusion

As ON can be a presenting manifestation of common autoimmune demyelinating or inflammatory conditions, care should be taken while analyzing it. Subtle differences in presentation can provide major clues. While ancillary testing is an important part of diagnosis, the importance of detailed history taking with regard to onset, progression and associated symptoms and a thorough neuro-ophthalmic examination cannot be understated.

Multiple-Choice Questions

1. Which statement is true for a patient with optic neuritis associated with multiple sclerosis?
   a. Around 65% cases have retrobulbar involvement.
   b. CSF pleocytosis is common association, usually more than 250 cells/mm³ are seen.
   c. Periphlebitis is a common fundus finding.
   d. More than 2/3 of optic nerve is involved in MRI.

   Answer:
   a. Around 65% cases have retrobulbar involvement.

2. Pulfrich phenomenon is
   a. Worsening of vision on increased body temperature.
   b. Early color desaturation associated with optic neuritis.
   c. Can be simulated in normal vision by placing a neutral density filter (dark glass) in front of one eye.
   d. Related to poor visual prognosis.

   Answer:
   c. Can be simulated in normal vision by placing a neutral density filter (dark glass) in front of one eye.

3. Pediatric optic neuritis
   a. Is presenting feature in more than half of patients with MS.
   b. Younger age is an independent risk factor for the development of MS.

   c. Is mostly unilateral.
   d. Presence of CSF OCBs in pediatric patients with ON increases the odds of diagnosis of MS.

   Answer:
   d. Presence of CSF OCBs in pediatric patients with ON increases the odds of diagnosis of MS.

4. Which of the following statements is INCORRECT?
   a. Patients with MOG antibody associated optic neuritis are more likely to have associated orbital inflammation as compared to aquaporin-4 antibody positive NMO-SD are more likely.
   b. Extensive optic nerve involvement can occur in MOG antibody associated ON.
   c. Average RNFL of below 70 μm on OCT points toward NMO-SD as the etiology.
   d. Patients of ON associated with multiple sclerosis usually reach the nadir of their vision by the third week.

   Answer:
   d. Patients of ON associated with multiple sclerosis usually reach the nadir of their vision by the third week.

References

1. Lennon VA, Wingerchuk DM, Kryzer TJ, Pittock SJ, Lucchinetti CF, Fujihara K, et al. A serum autoantibody marker of neuromyelitis optica: Distinction from multiple sclerosis. Lancet Lond Engl. 2004;364(9451):2106–2112.
2. Masaki K, Suzuki SO, Matsushita T, Matsuoka T, Imamura S, Yamasaki R, et al. Connexin 43 astrocytopathy linked to rapidly progressive multiple sclerosis and neuromyelitis optica. PLoS ONE [Internet]. 2013;8(8).
3. Kim S-H, Kim W, Li XF, Jung I-J, Kim HJ. Does interferon beta treatment exacerbate neuromyelitis optica spectrum disorder? Mult Scler Houndmills Basingstoke Engl. 2012;18(10):1480–1483.
4. Pau D, Al Zubidi N, Yalamanchili S, Plant GT, Lee AG. Optic neuritis. Eye. 2011; 25(7):833–842.
5. Ishikawa H, Kezuka T, Shikishima K, Yamagami A, Hiraoka M, Chuman H, et al. Epidemiologic and clinical characteristics of optic neuritis in Japan. Ophthalmology. 2019;126(10):1385–1398.
6. Purvin V, Sundaram S, Kawasaki A. Neuroretinitis: Review of the literature and new observations. J Neuro-Ophthalmol Off J North Am Neuro-Ophthalmol Soc. 2011;31(1):58–68.
7. Abel A, McClelland C, Lee MS. Critical review: Typical and atypical optic neuritis. Surv Ophthalmol. 2019;64(6):770–779.

8. Percy AK, Nobrega FT, Kurland LT. Optic neuritis and multiple sclerosis: An epidemiologic study. Arch Ophthalmol. 1972;87(2):135–139.

9. Optic Neuritis Study Group. Multiple sclerosis risk after optic neuritis: Final optic neuritis treatment trial follow-up. Arch Neurol. 2008;65(6):727–732. doi: 10.1001/archneur.65.6.727.

10. Voss E, Raab P, Trebst C, Stangel M. Clinical approach to optic neuritis: pitfalls, red flags and differential diagnosis. Ther Adv Neurol Disord. 2011;4(2):123–134.

11. The clinical profile of optic neuritis. Experience of the optic neuritis treatment trial. Optic neuritis study group. Arch Ophthalmol Chic Ill 1960. 1991;109(12):1673–1678.

12. Perkin GD, Rose FC. Uhthoff's syndrome. Br J Ophthalmol. 1976;60(1):60–3.

13. Fraser CL, Davagnanam I, Radon M, Plant GT. The time course and phenotype of Uhthoff phenomenon following optic neuritis. Mult Scler Houndmills Basingstoke Engl. 2012;18(7):1042–1044.

14. Farr J, McGarva E, Nij Bijvank J, van Vliet H, Jellema HM, Crossland MD, et al. The Pulfrich Phenomenon: Practical implications of the assessment of cases and effectiveness of treatment. Neuro-Ophthalmol. 2018;42(6):349–355.

15. Barkhof F. The clinico-radiological paradox in multiple sclerosis revisited. Curr Opin Neurol. 2002;15(3):239–245.

16. Pisa M, Guerrieri S, Di Maggio G, Medaglini S, Moiola L, Martinelli V, et al. No evidence of disease activity is associated with reduced rate of axonal retinal atrophy in MS. Neurology. 2017;89(24):2469–2475.

17. Costello FE, Burton JM. Multiple Sclerosis: Eyes on the Future. J Neuro-Ophthalmol Off J North Am Neuro-Ophthalmol Soc. 2018;38(1):81–84.

18. Gelfand JM, Nolan R, Schwartz DM, Graves J, Green AJ. Microcystic macular oedema in multiple sclerosis is associated with disease severity. Brain. 2012;135(6):1786–1793.

19. Rizzo JF, Andreoli CM, Rabinov JD. Use of magnetic resonance imaging to differentiate optic neuritis and nonarteritic anterior ischemic optic neuropathy. Ophthalmology. 2002;109(9):1679–1684.

20. Rammohan KW. Cerebrospinal fluid in multiple sclerosis. Ann Indian Acad Neurol. 2009;12(4):246–253.

21. Wingerchuk DM, Lennon VA, Lucchinetti CF, Pittock SJ, Weinshenker BG. The spectrum of neuromyelitis optica. Lancet Neurol. 2007;6(9):805–815.

22. Borisow N, Kleiter I, Gahlen A, Fischer K, Wernecke K-D, Pache F, et al. Influence of female sex and fertile age on neuromyelitis optica spectrum disorders. Mult Scler Houndmills Basingstoke Engl. 2017;23(8):1092–1103.

23. Yeh EA, Graves JS, Benson LA, Wassmer E, Waldman A. Pediatric optic neuritis. Neurology. 2016;87(9):S53-S58.

24. Chang MY, Pineles SL. Pediatric Optic Neuritis. Semin Pediatr Neurol. 2017;24(2):122–128.

25. Morrow MJ, Wingerchuk D. Neuromyelitis optica. J Neuro-Ophthalmol Off J North Am Neuro-Ophthalmol Soc. 2012;32(2):154–166.

26. Burman J, Raininko R, Fagius J. Bilateral and recurrent optic neuritis in multiple sclerosis. Acta Neurol Scand. 2011;123(3):207–210.

27. Fardet L, Généreau T, Mikaeloff Y, Fontaine B, Seilhean D, Cabane J. Devic's neuromyelitis optica: Study of nine cases. Acta Neurol Scand. 2003;108(3):193–200.

28. Papais-Alvarenga RM, Carellos SC, Alvarenga MP, Holander C, Bichara RP, Thuler LCS. Clinical course of optic neuritis in patients with relapsing neuromyelitis optica. Arch Ophthalmol Chic Ill 1960. 2008;126(1):12–16.

29. Narayan R, Simpson A, Fritsche K, Salama S, Pardo S, Mealy M, et al. MOG antibody disease: A review of MOG antibody seropositive neuromyelitis optica spectrum disorder. Mult Scler Relat Disord. 2018;25:66–72.

30. Lee H-J, Kim B, Waters P, Woodhall M, Irani S, Ahn S, et al. Chronic relapsing inflammatory optic neuropathy (CRION): a manifestation of myelin oligodendrocyte glycoprotein antibodies. J Neuroinflammation. 2018;15(1):302.

31. Storoni M, Davagnanam I, Radon M, Siddiqui A, Plant GT. Distinguishing optic neuritis in neuromyelitis optica spectrum disease from multiple sclerosis: A novel magnetic resonance imaging scoring system. J Neuroophthalmol. 2013;33(2):123–127.

32. Wingerchuk DM, Banwell B, Bennett JL, Cabre P, Carroll W, Chitnis T, De Seze J, Fujihara K, Greenberg B, Jacob A, Jarius S. International consensus diagnostic criteria for neuromyelitis optica spectrum disorders. Neurology. 2015;85(2):177–189.

33. Kim HJ, Paul F, Lana-Peixoto MA, Tenembaum S, Asgari N, Palace J, Klawiter EC, Sato DK, de Seze J, Wuerfel J, Banwell BL. MRI characteristics of neuromyelitis optica spectrum disorder: An international update. Neurology. 2015;84(11):1165–1173.

34. Denève M, Biotti D, Patsoura S, Ferrier M, Meluchova Z, Mahieu L, et al. MRI features of demyelinating disease associated with anti-MOG antibodies in adults. J Neuroradiol. 2019;46(5):312–318.

35. Ratchford JN, Quigg ME, Conger A, Frohman T, Frohman E, Balcer LJ, et al. Optical coherence tomography helps differentiate neuromyelitis optica and MS optic neuropathies. Neurology. 2009;73(4):302–308.

36. Green AJ, Cree BAC. Distinctive retinal nerve fibre layer and vascular changes in neuromyelitis optica following optic neuritis. J Neurol Neurosurg Psychiatry. 2009;80(9):1002–1005.

37. Ruiz-Gaviria R, Baracaldo I, Castañeda C, Ruiz-Patiño A, Acosta-Hernandez A, Rosselli D. Specificity and sensitivity of aquaporin 4 antibody detection tests in patients with neuromyelitis optica: A meta-analysis. Mult Scler Relat Disord. 2015;4(4):345–349.

38. Jarius S, Paul F, Franciotta D, Ruprecht K, Ringelstein M, Bergamaschi R, et al. Cerebrospinal fluid findings in aquaporin-4 antibody positive neuromyelitis optica: Results from 211 lumbar punctures. J Neurol Sci. 2011;306(1–2):82–90.

39. Abboud H, Petrak A, Mealy M, Sasidharan S, Siddique L, Levy M. Treatment of acute relapses in neuromyelitis optica: Steroids alone versus steroids plus plasma exchange. Mult Scler J. 2016;22(2):185–192.

40. Trebst C, Jarius S, Berthele A, Paul F, Schippling S, Wildemann B, et al. Update on the diagnosis and treatment of neuromyelitis optica: Recommendations of the Neuromyelitis Optica Study Group (NEMOS). J Neurol. 2014;261(1):1–16.

41. Waldman AT, Stull LB, Galetta SL, Balcer LJ, Liu GT. Pediatric optic neuritis and risk of multiple sclerosis: meta-analysis of observational studies. J AAPOS Off Publ Am Assoc Pediatr Ophthalmol Strabismus. 2011;15(5):441–446.

42. Coyle PK. Management of women with multiple sclerosis through pregnancy and after childbirth. Ther Adv Neurol Disord. 2016;9(3):198–210.

43. Shosha E, Pittock SJ, Flanagan E, Weinshenker BG. Neuromyelitis optica spectrum disorders and pregnancy: Interactions and management. Mult Scler Houndmills Basingstoke Engl. 2017;23(14):1808–1817.

44. Thompson AJ, Banwell BL, Barkhof F, Carroll WM, Coetzee T, Comi G, et al. Diagnosis of multiple sclerosis: 2017 revisions of the McDonald criteria. Lancet Neurol. 2018;17(2):162–173.

6

PAPILLEDEMA
Diagnosis and Management

Prem S. Subramanian

CASE STUDY

A 34-year-old obese female presented with history of headache of 3 months duration and episodes of transient loss of vision for 15 days. The headache was worse during early morning and would wake the patient up from her sleep. Episodes of transient visual loss were recent and were triggered when the patient got up after prolonged sitting, upon bending and during coughing.

Ophthalmic examination revealed normal visual acuity and color vision, but visual fields were constricted peripherally in both eyes. Fundus examination revealed bilateral disc edema. What is the likely diagnosis?

Introduction

Although the term "papilledema" may be used commonly to describe any type of optic disc swelling, it is preferable to confine its application to conditions in which the optic nerve swells secondary to elevated intracranial pressure (ICP). This definition is specific to the English language, as there is no similar means of separating different types of optic disc swelling by nomenclature alone in other languages. Other types of optic disc swelling from inflammation, infection, demyelinating disease, and other processes have a separate means of pathogenesis; in fact, it is this distinctive causation of papilledema that allows the clinician to differentiate it from other types of disc swelling. Except in unusual circumstances or in cases in which there is optic atrophy as well as optic disc swelling, the objective severity of the optic disc swelling in papilledema is usually much greater than the degree of vision loss (swelling out of proportion to vision loss). A similar degree of swelling from inflammation or infection will, in contrast, result in severe loss of both visual acuity and visual field. Indeed, true papilledema with severe vision loss should be considered a very ominous sign of advanced disease that may portend a poor visual prognosis (Figure 6.1).

Thus, in this chapter, the diagnosis of papilledema and its differentiation from conditions such as pseudopapilledema and optic disc drusen will be considered, as will the common causes of papilledema and their medical and surgical management.

Pathogenesis

Experiments in non-human primates have demonstrated the relationship between ICP elevation and optic disc swelling, establishing that cerebrospinal fluid (CSF) pressure is transmitted along the optic nerve sheath and propagated to the back of the globe. Using an intraventricular balloon, Hayreh and colleagues tracked the development of optic disc swelling as ICP was raised and also observed the subsequent loss of axons and optic atrophy that results from sustained ICP elevation [1]. These studies led to the theory that axonal compression and stasis of axoplasmic transport, rather than ischemia from neurovascular compression, is the primary mechanism by which papilledema occurs [2]. In extremely severe papilledema, optic disc infarction may occur (Figure 6.2), and permanent vision loss often ensues. In most cases, restoration of normal ICP restores axoplasmic flow, and visual dysfunction, if present, often remits. However, prolonged axoplasmic stasis will lead to apoptosis and axonal/ganglion cell loss, and the goal of therapy is to intervene before this irreversible process starts.

A more recent discovery is that free flow of CSF along the optic nerve sheath may not occur in some patients, with restriction of flow coming at the level of the optic canal and/or from trabeculations within the arachnoid layers [3–5]. In this scenario of CSF compartmentation, fluid enters the optic nerve sheath under pressure and then cannot flow back into the basilar cisterns because of the restriction. Continued pulsation of CSF into the sheath may lead to pressurization that is not relieved even if ICP returns to normal. Such instances are fortunately uncommon but should be considered in unusual cases of optic disc swelling.

Signs and symptoms of papilledema

Since vision loss is a late finding in patients with papilledema, other signs and symptoms must be used to raise suspicion for the disease. Visual symptoms include transient visual obscurations (TVOs), which often occur with positional changes (lying to standing, sitting to standing, bending over and then returning upright). Vision may become gray or black in the periphery of one or both eyes; complete loss of vision also may occur. Symptoms may last for several seconds before vision returns to baseline. The occurrence and severity of TVO is proportional to the degree of papilledema, and increasing or decreasing symptoms may be used as evidence for change in the underlying disease severity. True TVOs are highly characteristic of papilledema and are much briefer than other types of transient vision loss from embolic or vasospastic disease. They are thought to be caused by transiently decreased optic nerve head perfusion in the setting of swelling; vision returns as perfusion is rebalanced and restored, and the transient symptoms do not result in permanent visual deficits [6].

More advanced papilledema, in which axonal dysfunction starts to occur on a constant basis, may cause peripheral vision loss that is relatively asymptomatic, perhaps in part because, as in glaucoma, it starts in the inferonasal quadrant which overlaps entirely with the corresponding temporal field of the fellow eye. If the optic disc swelling extends toward the macula and foveal center, then decreased visual acuity and/or visual distortion may be noticed by the patient. This loss of central visual acuity must be differentiated from central visual loss or scotoma from optic

DOI: 10.1201/9780429020278-9

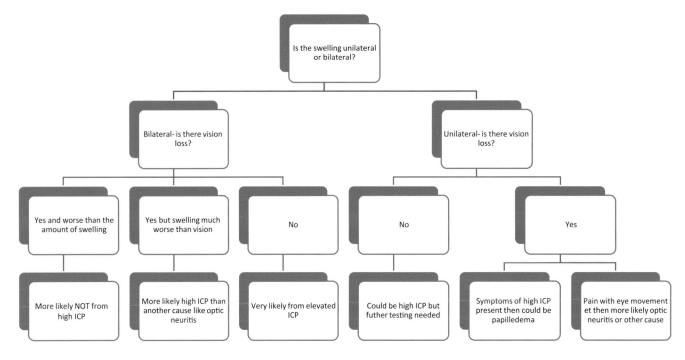

FIGURE 6.1   Schema for differentiating papilledema from other causes of optic disc swelling.

nerve dysfunction itself, which is a late finding in papilledema and may indicate that vision loss is both severe and irreversible (unlike vision loss from macular edema, which often improves markedly as the swelling remits) (Table 6.1). Non-visual symptoms of papilledema will be considered with the specific etiologies of this condition.

Causes of papilledema

The most common cause of elevated ICP in the Western world is idiopathic intracranial hypertension (IIH), in which ICP elevation occurs with disproportionate frequency in young women (ages 15–40) who are obese or overweight and often recently gained weight [7]. Diagnostic criteria for IIH have been defined (Annexure 6.1), most recently modified in 2013, with patients required to have (i) signs and symptoms of elevated ICP (e.g., papilledema), (ii) an absence of focal neurological deficits other

than sixth cranial nerve palsy, (iii) neuroimaging with no lesions directly causing CSF outflow obstruction (i.e., tumor, cerebral venous sinus thrombosis [CVST]), and (iv) elevated CSF pressure (defined as an opening pressure [OP] on lumbar puncture [LP] >25 cm H_2O in adults and >28 cm H_2O in children). Patients who do not satisfy all of these criteria may be considered to have a probable pseudotumor cerebri syndrome, although alternative diagnoses other than disorders of ICP must be considered as well [8]. A minority of patients with ICP elevation may satisfy the diagnostic criteria for IIH (including the presence of MRI findings such as empty sella turcica, venous sinus stenosis and vertical optic nerve tortuosity that support chronic ICP elevation) but lack papilledema. This condition, termed IIH without

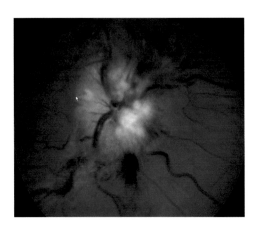

FIGURE 6.2   Color photo of right optic disc in a patient with severe papilledema and vision loss. The white area on the nasal aspect of the disc represents retinal nerve fiber layer infarction.

TABLE 6.1: Signs of Early and Late Papilledema

Optic Disc Sign	Cause	Visual Implication
Hyperemic disc swelling	Venous congestion and/or obstruction of axoplasmic flow	Usually no permanent change acutely but can lead to late atrophy
Peripapillary hemorrhages	Increased capillary pressure and rupture (hypothesized)	Does not predict visual function or outcome
Cotton wool spots	Retinal nerve fiber layer infarction	May cause permanent micro- or macroscotoma because of loss of nerve fiber architecture
Peripapillary choroidal folds (Paton lines)	Longstanding swelling with alteration of choroidal architecture	None permanently
Disc pallor with swelling	Axonal loss over time with chronicity of papilledema	Slow vision loss, either peripheral or central, may occur

TABLE 6.2: Etiology of Elevated Intracranial Pressure

Source of High ICP	Rate of Onset	Treatment
CSF outflow obstruction	Often acute on chronic	Removal of obstruction and/or CSF diversion
Cerebral venous sinus thrombosis	Acute, often with severe symptoms	Anticoagulation, rarely direct neuroradiology intervention
Decreased CSF compliance	Depends upon causative process, i.e., rapid with scarring from meningitis, slow onset if idiopathic	Medical reduction of CSF production or surgical increase of CSF outflow
Idiopathic	Slow or rapid- unknown factors influence rate	Weight loss (in most patients), medical reduction of CSF production or surgical increase of CSF outflow

papilledema (IIHWOP), does not appear to cause vision loss and also seems to respond better to migraine therapeutic strategies than to ICP lowering in terms of symptomatic headache relief. Patients with IIHWOP with visual impairment are often considered to have non-physiological visual field losses, though posterior nerve compression has also been conceived as one of the causes in the available literature [9, 10].

Since CSF production rates appear to be normal in IIH, the working hypothesis for the cause of the ICP rise is decreased CSF absorption (Table 6.2). There is increasing evidence for impaired cerebral venous sinus outflow as a cause of ICP rise in many IIH patients [11] (see Treatment), and decreased compliance within the spinal canal also may contribute to ICP elevation in a subset of individuals. As there appears to be a rather strong relationship between obesity and the incidence of IIH, this disease has been historically less common in Asia and other parts of the world; however, the rise of wealth in these regions has had the untoward effect of increased obesity rates and thus a greater incidence of IIH as well. It does appear that the degree of obesity in such regions may not be as great before ICP elevation occurs; in the IIH Treatment Trial, conducted in North America (see below), the average body mass index (BMI) was 40 [7, 12], whereas a BMI of 26–28 may be sufficient to contribute to IIH occurrence in patients of Indian or Chinese ethnicity.

CVST, distinct from the obstruction of venous outflow mentioned above, is an infrequent but potentially severe cause of ICP elevation [11, 13]. It may occur after trauma, with dehydration, clotting disorders or spontaneously with no identifiable cause. The papilledema that occurs with CVST may be particularly acute because of the rapid ICP rise and can be associated with extensive peripapillary and intraretinal hemorrhages, cotton wool spots and retinal venous tortuosity and/or dilation. Prompt diagnosis and treatment are needed to optimize the visual outcome (see below).

Elevated ICP also may occur at any age due to obstructive hydrocephalus, in which a mass lesion obstructs normal CSF outflow from the ventricular system. Either communicating or non-communicating hydrocephalus may cause papilledema, and the rapidity of onset of the obstruction and the subsequent ICP rise may be evident in the severity of hemorrhage and/or cotton wool spots appearing on or immediately adjacent to the swollen optic nerve. Because obstructive hydrocephalus may decompensate and progress to cerebral herniation and permanent neurologic compromise and even death, all patients with newly diagnosed papilledema should be evaluated immediately for a potential space-occupying lesion as the cause.

Finally, medications such as vitamin A or its derivatives, tetracycline and similar antibiotics, exogenously administered growth hormone, excess lithium and a host of other agents may lead to a secondary ICP elevation that may be mistaken for IIH if a full medication and diet history is not obtained. ICP elevation and papilledema usually remit within weeks upon cessation of the offending substance. Other less common causes of ICP elevation include androgen excess, anemia, and right heart failure with cerebral venous pressure elevation. A secondary or non-idiopathic cause of ICP elevation as noted here should be considered in all patients but particularly in atypical presentations (i.e., males, patients older than age 45, non-obese individuals).

Diagnostic evaluation

It is uncommon that patients are found to have papilledema in the setting of a known condition that could explain their ocular findings and symptoms (if any). Rather, the discovery of optic disc swelling on ophthalmic examination usually prompts the workup for an etiology of the condition. Patients with papilledema may have no symptoms at all, or they may have non-specific concerns such as blurred vision or "tired eyes" after extensive computer or mobile device use (which is probably unrelated to the papilledema). Headache is a common condition in the population demographic that gets elevated ICP from IIH (the most common cause of ICP elevation), and its presence or absence is not a reliable predictor of papilledema being present in a given patient. However, headache may prompt a visit to a neurologist or ophthalmologist, who will then find papilledema on examination.

Once papilledema is found on exam, and another cause for the optic disc swelling (inflammation, infection, etc.) is not evident, then urgent neuroimaging of the head is required. Obstructive hydrocephalus (Figure 6.3) may present with precisely the same symptoms as other, more common causes of high ICP and must be diagnosed immediately to allow for appropriate interventions that can prevent cerebral herniation, a neurological and neurosurgical emergency.

What imaging study or studies should be ordered? The preferred imaging modality is magnetic resonance imaging (MRI) and magnetic resonance venography (MRV) of the head, both with contrast. These two studies should identify any mass lesion causing obstructive hydrocephalus (if present), venous sinus anomalies (including venous sinus thrombosis) and also reveal other processes such as meningeal inflammation that can increase ICP and cause papilledema as well. Although not needed to make the diagnosis of papilledema, the presence of signs such as empty sella turcica, vertical optic nerve tortuosity within the orbits, and dilated optic nerve sheaths can support the presence of elevated ICP. An important note, these changes on MRI may not reverse or resolve with normalization of the ICP, and their persistence can lead to diagnostic confusion at a later date if the patient has a repeat MRI brain for other reasons.

If MRI and MRV cannot be obtained, then CT head with CT venography with contrast can be substituted, although the information derived from the CT head is not equivalent in terms of alternative diagnoses (it will not show inflammation, for example). In fact, CT venography may be more specific in the detection of venous sinus abnormalities seen in many patients with IIH, but that does not suggest it should be used routinely in lieu of MRV.

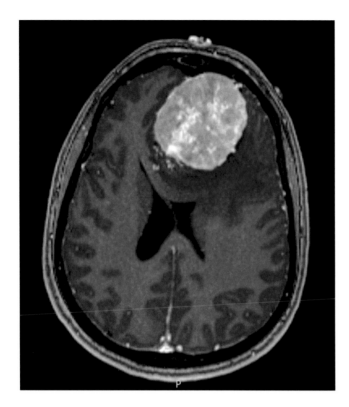

FIGURE 6.3 MRI brain with contrast demonstrates a large left-sided meningioma causing lateral ventricular obstruction left greater than right. This patient had moderate papilledema in both eyes.

Once neuroimaging has been performed and a mass lesion excluded, Lumbar Puncture (LP) both for measurement of Opening pressure (OP) and CSF analysis should be done. Contraindications to LP in patients with suspected IIH may include Arnold-Chiari type I malformation with moderate to severe tonsillar descent. Less common reasons to defer LP include unusual spinal anatomy and/or prior lumbar surgery or trauma. The LP should be performed with the patient in the left lateral decubitus position; this can be challenging, especially in obese patients in whom anatomic landmarks are more difficult to identify. LP under fluoroscopy in the prone position can be done; the patient can then be moved to the lateral decubitus position before OP measurement. Some studies suggest that OP in the prone position is equivalent to the lateral decubitus, but that assertion remains controversial. Ideally, the OP should be measured in the lateral decubitus position with the legs extended, head supported by a pillow and with normal respiration and a lack of sedation. Valsalva maneuver, leg flexion, breath holding and discomfort all may cause a false elevation of the OP and mislead the physician diagnostically. Routine CSF studies (protein, glucose, cell count) are adequate in patients with typical IIH, while in atypical cases, CSF cytology and infectious investigations should be considered, based on the overall clinical scenario.

Papilledema and pseudopapilledema

It is rarely, if ever, a challenge to distinguish a completely normal optic nerve from one with moderate to severe swelling (Figure 6.4). Reliable discrimination of a mildly swollen optic disc from one that is only elevated presents an important clinical challenge to ophthalmologists, neurologists and others who provide eye care to large populations of patients who may or may not have symptoms that would raise concern for elevated ICP. In a typical clinical scenario, a patient presents for a routine optometric or ophthalmologic examination and is found to have abnormal appearing optic nerve heads in the absence of any visual or neurological symptoms. Similarly, a patient may experience headache and/or blurred vision, and when a fundus examination is performed, the optic disc appearance is judged to be abnormal. It is important to recognize the role that cognitive bias may play in such situations. A patient may have small or anomalous optic nerve heads that are elevated but not swollen. This patient may have had prior eye exams in which the optic nerve appearance raised no concern with the optometrist or ophthalmologist. However, if the same patient presents with a concern about headache, and if in addition he or she is obese, then a concern for true papilledema and elevated ICP may be raised, even though the fundus appearance is more consistent with elevation alone and may even be unchanged from prior exams. Studies of diagnostic error regarding IIH (the most common cause of papilledema) indicate at least 40% of patients given this

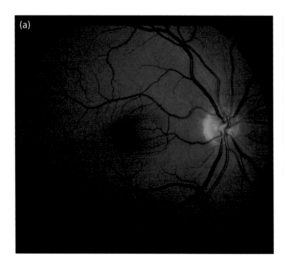
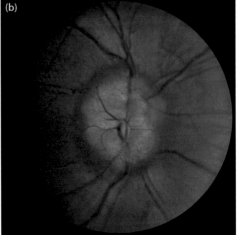

FIGURE 6.4 (a) Normal optic nerve with clearly visible central cup, disc margins and retinal vessels. (b) Moderately swollen optic nerve with loss of sharp disc margins and obscurations of vessels.

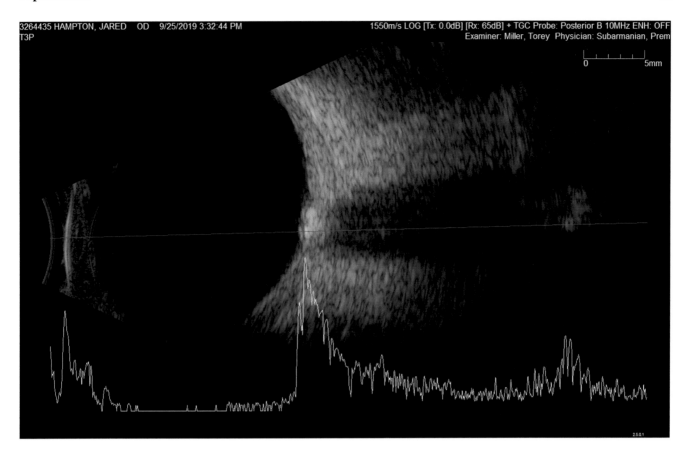

3264435 HAMPTON, JARED   OD   9/25/2019 3:32:44 PM   1550m/s LOG [Tx: 0.0dB] [Rx: 65dB] + TGC Probe: Posterior B 10MHz ENH: OFF
T3P   Examiner: Miller, Torey Physician: Subarmanian, Prem

                                                                      0   5mm

FIGURE 6.5   B-scan echography with overlaid A-scan demonstrating highly reflective optic disc drusen of the right eye.

diagnosis receive it in error [14]. Since a diagnosis of papilledema will require expensive and potentially invasive testing and potential treatment with medication or eye surgery, it is important to differentiate papilledema from pseudopapilledema at the earliest juncture.

Aside from ophthalmoscopy, ancillary testing in the ophthalmology clinic may be used to distinguish these two conditions. Fluorescein angiography may discriminate true papilledema from disc elevation because of the presence of late (and possibly early) disc leakage, in contrast to the late staining (or normal result) seen with disc drusen or other anomalies [15, 16]. Oral fluorescein administration in children may be used in lieu of intravenous injection, since early phase images are not necessary. B-scan echography will show hyperreflectivity within the optic disc in many cases of optic disc drusen (Figure 6.5), but obtaining adequate images may be challenging for an untrained examiner. Autofluorescence images may reveal optic disc drusen but only if they are relatively superficial (Figure 6.6). Optical coherence tomography (OCT) also may be used to identify optic disc abnormalities that are characteristic of pseudopapilledema, including optic disc drusen. A protocol has been published in which enhanced-depth imaging (EDI)-OCT is used to visualize buried drusen with high sensitivity and specificity [17] (Figure 6.7). If drusen are not present, then other OCT measures, such as peripapillary total retinal volume, may differentiate the two conditions [18]. OCT-angiography (OCT-A) shows promise in separating the two entities as well, with alterations of peripapillary and macular capillary density being associated with true disc swelling [19–21].

Ultimately, clinical judgment along with examination must be used to make the final determination of whether or not true disc swelling is present. Serial examinations with photographic comparison may be necessary to convince the clinician that there is no change in optic disc appearance over time, as papilledema should evolve (increasing or decreasing). On the other hand, both pseudopapilledema and true disc swelling may coexist in the

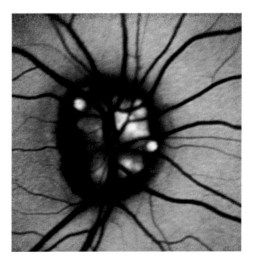

FIGURE 6.6   Autofluorescence photo of the same individual in Figure 6.5, demonstrating superficial optic disc drusen (areas of brightness).

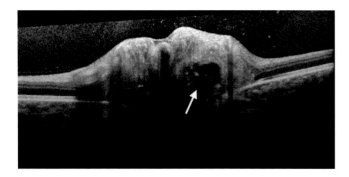

FIGURE 6.7   OCT cross-sectional imaging through the optic disc showing lesions with a hyporeflective core and hyperreflective edge (arrow), indicating drusen.

same patient, and in the setting of a prior diagnosis of disc drusen but new symptoms and signs that suggest elevated ICP, the same diagnostic evaluation listed above should be performed.

Management

This chapter is not intended to be a specific guide to the care of the individual patient, as each doctor must formulate an appropriate plan of care based on current evidence, individual patient factors and local resources, among other considerations. Rather, it reflects the author's experience and the existing literature at the time of writing. In this context, most patients with papilledema from elevated ICP can be managed in the outpatient setting. Exceptions include those who have an underlying condition such as CVST or intracranial mass, in which case neurosurgical intervention should be undertaken. The rapidity with which treatment should be instituted for papilledema often depends upon the degree of vision loss that is measured. As noted above, central visual acuity is affected late, and interventions should be considered before this occurs. If the patient presents with severe vision loss, then urgent surgical intervention often is undertaken (see below). A small number of patients with IIH will have a rapidly progressive, fulminant condition that may lead to severe and permanent vision loss if not recognized and treated quickly; this variant of IIH should not be overlooked, as delay in treatment is not only detrimental to the patient's long-term visual outcome but also may expose the physician to medicolegal risk [22, 23].

In most cases of IIH, however, regular outpatient visits present the opportunity to assess symptoms and to reinforce treatment strategies (below). Papilledema can lead insidiously to permanent vision loss, and thus visual field testing with automated perimetry, in addition to checking visual acuity and color vision, should be a routine part of the management of patients with papilledema, as it will both guide the clinician in terms of severity of disease and also allow tracking of the effect of the treatment rendered. If the treating physician/neurologist does not have access to automated perimetry in their own office or clinic, then collaboration with an ophthalmologist is crucial to help with management. Other tests to be considered at each visit include optic disc photography and OCT, both of which will document changes over time in severity of the optic disc swelling.

Medical treatment of IIH

In most patients, the goal of treatment is to reduce headache burden and to prevent permanent vision loss. The main "medical" therapy for IIH, supported by a number of studies, is directed

weight loss [24–26]. It is insufficient for the treating doctor simply to tell the patient that they must lose weight to put their disease into remission and prevent complications of disease such as vision loss. A weight loss plan must be developed, either by the treating doctor or other professionals, including the patient's primary care physician and/or a nutritionist or dietitian, that provides specific guidance and goals for the patient to follow. Many towns and cities have medically directed weight loss clinics whose services may be used by patients with IIH. Results of the IIH Treatment Trial (IIHTT, discussed further below) showed that patients with IIH are able to lose weight with success rates comparable to individuals without IIH when provided with a structured program to follow. Even if not managing the patient's weight loss directly, the treating neurologist should chart the patient's progress and reinforce their successes or guide them to new strategies if unsuccessful.

Patients with mild or no vision loss and/or headache may benefit from medical treatment with drugs to lower ICP as well as migraine headache therapy [27, 28]. Randomized clinical trial evidence from the IIHTT supports the use of acetazolamide as an adjunct to weight loss in patients with mild vision loss, defined as a mean deviation (MD) on Humphrey visual field (HVF) testing between −2 dB and −7 dB [26]. This study demonstrated that acetazolamide use resulted in a greater improvement (+0.71 dB) of HVF MD as compared with placebo. More rapid resolution of papilledema, especially from higher grades, also was reported as a secondary outcome. OP on LP also was significantly lower in acetazolamide-treated subjects than placebo after 6 months of treatment.

In the IIHTT, patients were given up to 4 g of acetazolamide daily (divided in twice daily dosing) with a median dose of 2500 mg daily; each treating physician must determine the appropriate starting dose and escalation plan for a given patient. Common side effects of acetazolamide include paresthesias of the fingers, toes, lips and tongue as well as dysgeusia, particularly for carbonated beverages. In the IIHTT, subjects on acetazolamide developed neither serum metabolic abnormalities nor hematopoietic problems at higher rates than subjects using placebo. Despite the greater lowering of ICP in subjects taking the actual drug, headache status was no different between the two groups [29], suggesting that sustained ICP elevation may trigger a pressure-independent headache that does not respond to ICP-lowering medication. For this reason, it is often necessary to offer the patient other methods for headache relief. Migraine prophylactic medications such as topiramate or tricyclic antidepressants may be useful in obtaining headache control. While topiramate has a weak carbonic anhydrase inhibitory action, its efficacy is more likely due to headache relief and appetite suppression (thus enhancing weight loss). Other diuretic agents, such as furosemide, are used occasionally in patients who are intolerant of acetazolamide or who are worsening despite maximal dosing of the drug. The physician must consider any possible interactions between these medications and acetazolamide, if using it (i.e., hypokalemia with concomitant furosemide use), and also anticipate potentially undesirable weight gain with tricyclic antidepressants.

Surgical treatments

Invasive procedures should be considered for patients whose disease is refractory to medical management. The most common reason for proceeding to surgery is progressive vision loss. Severe, pressure-related headache also may be improved by appropriate surgical intervention, although the patient must be cautioned that a pressure-independent headache often persists and requires ongoing medical treatment. The most commonly used surgical procedures include optic nerve sheath fenestration (ONSF), CSF diversion and venous sinus stenting. No direct prospective, randomized evidence has been generated at the time of this writing to support the use of one technique over another, and factors such as local expertise and patient preference often weigh heavily in the surgical decision-making process. Furthermore, existing retrospective studies are subject to significant patient selection bias, making it difficult to rely upon them to guide individual treatment decisions. Indeed, a prospective, randomized trial (designated SIGHT—the Surgical IIH Treatment Trial) in which patients were to be randomized to maximal medical therapy, ONSF or CSF diversion by ventriculoperitoneal (VP) shunting was recently closed to enrollment of new patients after failing to meet recruiting goals; only a handful of patients were enrolled, and thus no conclusion will be forthcoming.

ONSF relieves papilledema by the creation of a dural window in the retrobulbar optic nerve sheath. A variety of surgical approaches may be used to reach the optic nerve sheath with no proven superiority of a particular method, and this procedure may be performed under local anesthesia if general anesthesia is contraindicated. The procedure itself carries a 1–2% risk of vision loss; in addition, long-term patency of the fenestration may be difficult to achieve [30–32]. Other potential complications include diplopia, ptosis and pupillary abnormalities (depending upon the surgical approach). Advantages of ONSF include absence of an implanted device and ease of performance relative to CSF diversion in extremely obese or pregnant patients. It has been reported that unilateral surgery frequently results in bilateral papilledema improvement [33]. However, CSF compartmentation or sequestration may occur as noted previously [5]. In such cases, unilateral surgery may be ineffective for the fellow eye, and the patient must have close follow-up after unilateral surgery to ensure that the anticipated improvement is occurring in both eyes, as second eye surgery still may be required. ONSF usually results in rapid papilledema resolution with concomitant improvement in visual acuity and visual fields. Headache also may improve after ONSF, although the mechanism by which this occurs is not known, as there is no evidence that enough CSF drainage occurs through the orbit(s) to lower ICP globally.

CSF diversion, either by ventriculoperitoneal (VP) or lumbo-peritoneal (LP) shunting, will relieve CSF shunting throughout the cerebrospinal system and is expected to reduce papilledema as well [34, 35]. There is no clear evidence that one procedure is superior to the other, and each has its own surgical advantages and challenges that are beyond the scope of this chapter. In both procedures, plastic tubing is implanted into the CSF space and tunneled subcutaneously to the peritoneal cavity. A valve (fixed-pressure or adjustable) may be used to regulate CSF drainage and reduce the risk of intracranial hypotension. Challenges to VP shunting include finding the normal or small ventricles in IIH patients, although modern radiographic and endoscopic techniques have largely obviated these concerns. Similarly, some studies suggest a higher failure rate of LP than VP shunting, but more modern data do not support this contention [34]. In retrospective analyses, CSF diversion appeared as effective as ONSF in reducing papilledema and improving HVF MD [36]. Potential complications of the procedure include shunt infections, shunt failure, and neurological morbidity or mortality from damage to intracranial contents.

Venous sinus stenting aims to reverse venous outflow obstruction at the distal transverse sinus that may contribute to IIH pathogenesis. Focal narrowing of the distal transverse sinus has been observed in >90% of IIH patients compared to 18% of obese controls [37], and a significant venous pressure gradient often is present across the stenosis. A number of retrospective studies indicated that stenting these stenoses (usually unilaterally) using interventional neuroradiologic techniques results in IIH resolution, as measured by visual function, papilledema improvement, and headache relief [38–41]. A prospective, nonrandomized study of 13 patients demonstrated similar outcomes [42], with a meta-analysis supporting the use of the procedure as well [43]. Patients must be treated with antiplatelet agents after the procedure, and hemorrhage is thus a potential complication as is intraoperative damage to the cerebral venous structures. As with ONSF and CSF diversion, long-term failure can occur; typically, this results from a restenosis proximal to the treated segment. Factors that may contribute to restenosis are being studied and may include stent size as well as patient BMI [39].

A final surgical treatment to consider in IIH patients is bariatric surgery. Small retrospective studies show that surgical weight loss often is dramatic (in excess of 44 kg) and leads to IIH remission [44, 45]. Bariatric surgery carries a number of short- and long-term surgical and medical risks that must be considered carefully by the patient and the surgeon, and evaluation by an experienced surgical team may be appropriate in selected patients who meet the medical indications for surgical treatment.

Long-term prognosis

The goal of treatment is disease remission, as indicated by papilledema and headache remission. OP on LP should not be used as a measure of disease activity or resolution, as patients with clinical remission of these symptoms and signs of IIH may have persistently elevated OPs on LP. Although the medical and surgical treatments discussed here have good short-term success rates, they should be considered as temporizing and not curative treatments that will protect vision while the patient continues to pursue weight loss for long-term disease remission. Patients may remain on acetazolamide for months if necessary, but most patients are eager to stop its use when possible. Since the majority of IIH patients are women of childbearing age, they may be interested in becoming pregnant, and the safety of acetazolamide use in pregnancy has not been studied prospectively [46]. As noted, weight loss remains the most effective means of achieving a long-term and durable remission of IIH. Recurrence or worsening of papilledema often occurs when acetazolamide is stopped in the absence of weight loss, and late surgical failures also may be more likely in patients who are unable to lose weight. Similarly, the most important predictor of IIH recurrence in successfully treated patients is weight gain [47], and patients must be counseled that maintenance of weight loss is usually required for long-term IIH control. Ongoing neurologic and ophthalmologic surveillance of treated IIH patients may detect recurrent symptoms or signs and should be considered in patients at risk for recurrent IIH.

Conclusion

Optic disc swelling from increased ICP most commonly results from IIH but can occur from any process that obstructs CSF outflow or reduces outflow facility. Pseudopapilledema must be differentiated from true papilledema to avoid unnecessary treatment of patients with ICP-lowering methods, and a number of modern diagnostic tools are available to assist the clinician in this task. When true papilledema is present, an appropriate evaluation for causative lesions must be pursued, although the majority of cases are idiopathic. When a secondary cause is present, papilledema remission should occur upon treatment of the responsible lesion. In IIH, medical and/or surgical treatments may be used as adjuncts to weight loss to help the patient achieve long-term disease control. Although up to 25% of patients may suffer from long-term vision loss from IIH, timely diagnosis and intervention will minimize the likelihood of long-term damage to the optic nerve and help the patient with headache management as well.

Annexure 6.1

Diagnosis of IIH

a. **Diagnostic criteria for pseudotumor cerebri syndrome (PTCS) [8]**

1. Diagnosis of pseudotumor cerebri syndrome (PTCS) (Definite if criteria A–E are fulfilled; probable if criteria A–D are met but the opening CSF pressure is lower than described for making a definite diagnosis)

    A. Presence of papilledema
    B. Neurological examination is normal (except abnormal cranial nerve examination)
    C. Neuroimaging is normal with normal brain parenchyma (without hydrocephalus, space-occupying lesion, meningeal enhancement) for typical patients
    D. CSF composition is normal.
    E. Opening CSF pressure is elevated (>250 mm CSF in adults; >280 mm CSF in children [250 mm CSF in a non-sedated, non-obese child])

2. Diagnosis of pseudotumor cerebri syndrome without papilledema

    If papilledema is absent, diagnosis of pseudotumor cerebri syndrome should be considered if B–E from above are satisfied, and the patient has abducens nerve palsy (unilateral or bilateral) in addition.
    If both papilledema and abducens nerve palsy are absent, a diagnosis of pseudotumor cerebri syndrome can only be suggested, if in addition to presence of criteria B–E from above at least three of the following neuroimaging criteria are present:

    i.   Presence of an empty sella
    ii.   Posterior globe flattening or indentation
    iii. Perioptic nerve sheath prominence or distention with or without presence of tortuous optic nerves
    iv.   Stenosis of transverse venous sinus

b. **Diagnostic criteria for IIH ICHD3 [48]**

A. New headache, or a significant worsening of a pre-existing headache, fulfilling criterion C

B. Both of the following:
    1. Idiopathic intracranial hypertension (IIH) has been diagnosed
    2. CSF pressure exceeds 250 mm CSF (or 280 mm CSF in obese children)

C. Either or both of the following:
    1. Headache has developed or significantly worsened in temporal relation to the IIH, or led to its discovery
    2. Headache is accompanied by either or both of the following:
        a. Pulsatile tinnitus
        b. Papilloedema

D. Not better accounted

Multiple-Choice Questions

1. Which of the following MRI findings is not associated with elevated intracranial pressure in idiopathic intracranial hypertension?
   a. Posterior globe flattening
   b. Transverse sinus stenosis
   c. White matter edema
   d. Optic nerve tortuosity

   Answer:

   c. White matter edema

2. Which of the following is the most characteristic visual symptom of papilledema?
   a. Transient visual obscuration
   b. Scintillating scotoma
   c. Metamorphopsia
   d. Monocular diplopia

   Answer:

   a. Transient visual obscuration

3. Which of the following medications may lead to ICP elevation?
   a. Azathioprine
   b. Cabergoline
   c. Dalfamprine
   d. Minocycline

   Answer:

   d. Minocycline

4. Which of the following is the most effective long-term therapeutic intervention for patients with typical IIH?
   a. Acetazolamide
   b. CSF diversion
   c. Observation
   d. Weight loss

Answer:

d. Weight loss

References

1. Tso M, Hayreh S. Optic disc edema in raised intracranial pressure. III. A pathologic study of experimental papilledema. Arch Ophthalmol. 1977; 95:1448–1457.
2. Tso M, Hayreh S. Optic disc edema in raised intracranial pressure. IV. Axoplasmic transport in experimental papilledema. Arch Ophthalmol. 1977; 95:1458–1462.
3. Killer H, Jaggi G, Miller NR, Huber AR, Landolt H, Mironov A, Meyer P, Remonda L. Cerebrospinal fluid dynamics between the basal cisterns and the subarachnoid space of the optic nerve in patients with papilloedema. Brit J Ophthalmol. 2011; 95:822–827.
4. Jaggi GP, Harlev M, Ziegler U, Dotan S, Miller NR, Killer HE. Cerebrospinal fluid segregation optic neuropathy: An experimental model and a hypothesis. Brit J Ophthalmol. 2010;94:1088–1093.
5. Killer HE, Subramanian P. Compartmentalized cerebrospinal fluid. Int Ophthalmol Clin. 2014;54:95.
6. Hayreh S. Optic disc edema in raised intracranial pressure. VI. Associated visual disturbances and their pathogenesis. Arch Ophthalmol. 1977;95:1566–1579.
7. Wall M, Kupersmith MJ, Kieburtz KD, Corbett JJ, Feldon SE, Friedman DI, Katz DM, Keltner JL, Schron EB, rmott MP. The Idiopathic Intracranial Hypertension Treatment Trial: Clinical profile at baseline. JAMA Neurol. 2014;71:693–701.
8. Friedman DI, Liu GT, Digre KB. Revised diagnostic criteria for the pseudotumor cerebri syndrome in adults and children. Neurology. 2013;81:1159–1165.
9. Salgarello T, Tamburrelli C, Falsini B, et al. Optic nerve diameters and perimetric thresholds in idiopathic intracranial hypertension. Br J Ophthalmol. 1996;80:509–514.
10. Digre KB, Nakamoto BK, Warner JEA, et al. A comparison of idiopathic intracranial hypertension with and without papilledema. Headache. 2009 February;49(2):185–193. doi:10.1111/j.1526-4610.2008.01324.x.
11. Subramanian PS, Haq A. Cerebral venous sinus thrombosis and stenosis in pseudotumor cerebri syndrome. Int Ophthalmol Clin. 2014;54:61.
12. Friedman DI, McDermott MP, Kieburtz K, et al. The Idiopathic Intracranial Hypertension Treatment Trial: Design considerations and methods. J Neuroophthalmol. 2014;34:107.
13. Brodsky MC, Biousse V. A bloody mess! Surv Ophthalmol. 2018;63:268–274.
14. Fisayo A, Bruce BB, Newman NJ, Biousse V. Overdiagnosis of idiopathic intracranial hypertension. Neurology. 2016;86:341–350.
15. Chang MY, Velez FG, Demer JL, Bonelli L, Quiros PA, Arnold AC, Sadun AA, Pineles SL. Accuracy of diagnostic imaging modalities for classifying pediatric eyes as papilledema versus pseudopapilledema. Ophthalmology. 2017;124:1839–1848.
16. Pineles SL, Arnold AC. Fluorescein angiographic identification of optic disc drusen with and without optic disc edema. J Neuroophthalmol. 2012;32:17.
17. Malmqvist L, Bursztyn L, Costello F. The optic disc drusen studies consortium recommendations for diagnosis of optic disc drusen using optical coherence tomography. J Neuroophthalmol. 2018;38:299.
18. Fard M, Fakhree S, Abdi P, Hassanpoor N, Subramanian PS. Quantification of peripapillary total retinal volume in pseudopapilledema and mild papilledema using spectral-domain optical coherence tomography. Am J Ophthalmol.2014;158:136–143.
19. Fard M, Sahraiyan A, Jalili J, Hejazi M, Suwan Y, Ritch R, Subramanian PS. Optical coherence tomography angiography in papilledema compared with pseudopapilledema. Invest Ophth Vis Sci. 2019;60:168–175.
20. Fard M, Okhravi S, Moghimi S, Subramanian PS. Optic nerve head and macular optical coherence tomography measurements in papilledema compared with pseudopapilledema. J Neuroophthalmol Publish Ahead of Print. 2018;28–34.
21. Fard M, Jalili J, Sahraiyan A, Khojasteh H, Hejazi M, Ritch R, Subramanian PS. Optical coherence tomography angiography in optic disc swelling. Am J Ophthalmol. 2018;191:116–123.
22. Elder BD, Goodwin RC, Kosztowski TA, Radvany MG, Gailloud P, Moghekar A, Subramanian PS, Miller NR, Rigamonti D. Venous sinus stenting is a valuable treatment for fulminant idiopathic intracranial hypertension. J Clin Neurosci. 2015;22:685–689.
23. Thambisetty M, Lavin PJ, Newman NJ, Biousse V. Fulminant idiopathic intracranial hypertension. Neurology. 2007;68:229–232.
24. Sinclair AJ, Burdon MA, Nightingale PG. Low energy diet and intracranial pressure in women with idiopathic intracranial hypertension: Prospective cohort study. Br Med J. 2010;341:c2701.
25. Ball AK, Howman A, Wheatley K. A randomised controlled trial of treatment for idiopathic intracranial hypertension. J Neurol. 2011;258:874–881.
26. Wall M, McDermott MP, Kieburtz KD, Corbett JJ, Feldon SE, Friedman DI, Katz DM, Keltner JL, Schron EB, Kupersmith MJ. Effect of acetazolamide on visual function in patients with idiopathic intracranial hypertension and mild visual loss: The Idiopathic Intracranial Hypertension Treatment Trial. JAMA. 2014;311:1641–1651.
27. Mollan SP, Davies B, Silver NC. Idiopathic intracranial hypertension: Consensus guidelines on management. J Neurol Neurosurg Psychiatry. 2018;89:1088–1100.
28. Kanagalingam S, Subramanian PS. Update on idiopathic intracranial hypertension. Curr Treat Options Neurol. 2018;20:24.
29. Friedman DI, Quiros PA, Subramanian PS, Mejico LJ, Gao S, rmott M, Wall M, and the NORDIC IIHTT Study Group. Headache in idiopathic intracranial hypertension: Findings from the Idiopathic Intracranial Hypertension Treatment Trial. Headache. 2017;57:1195–1205.
30. Obi EE, Lakhani BK, Burns J, Sampath R. Optic nerve sheath fenestration for intracranial hypertension: A seven year review of visual outcomes in a tertiary centre. Clin Neurol Neurosurg. 2015;137:94–101.
31. Pineles SL, Volpe NJ. Long-term results of optic nerve sheath fenestration for idiopathic intracranial hypertension: Earlier intervention favours improved outcomes. Neuroophthalmology. 2013;37:12–19.
32. Feldon SE. Visual outcomes comparing surgical techniques for management of severe idiopathic intracranial hypertension. Neurosurg Focus. 2007;23:E6.
33. Alsuhaibani AH, Carter KD, Nerad JA, Lee AG. Effect of optic nerve sheath fenestration on papilledema of the operated and the contralateral nonoperated eyes in idiopathic intracranial hypertension. Ophthalmology. 2011;118:412–414.
34. Sinclair AJ, Kuruvath S, Sen D, Nightingale PG, Burdon MA, Flint G. Is cerebrospinal fluid shunting in idiopathic intracranial hypertension worthwhile? A 10-year review. Cephalalgia. 2011;31:1627–1633.
35. Tarnaris A, Toma AK, Watkins LD, Kitchen ND. Is there a difference in outcomes of patients with idiopathic intracranial hypertension with the choice of cerebrospinal fluid diversion site: A single centre experience. Clin Neurol Neurosurg. 2011;113:477–479.
36. Fonseca PL, Rigamonti D, Miller NR, Subramanian PS. Visual outcomes of surgical intervention for pseudotumour cerebri: Optic nerve sheath fenestration versus cerebrospinal fluid diversion. Br J Ophthalmol. 2014;98:1360–1363.
37. Farb R, Vanek I, Scott JN, Mikulis DJ, Willinsky RA, Tomlinson G, terBrugge KG. Idiopathic intracranial hypertension: The prevalence and morphology of sinovenous stenosis. Neurology. 2003;60:1418–1424.
38. Radvany MG, Solomon D, Nijjar S, Subramanian PS, Miller NR, Rigamonti D, Blitz A, Gailloud P, Moghekar A. Visual and neurological outcomes following endovascular stenting for pseudotumor cerebri associated with transverse sinus stenosis. J Neuroophthalmol. 2013;33:117.
39. Kumpe DA, Seinfeld J, Huang X, Mei Q, Case DE, Roark CD, Subramanian PS, Lind KE, Pelak VS, Bennett JL. Dural sinus stenting for idiopathic intracranial hypertension: Factors associated with hemodynamic failure and management with extended stenting. J Neurointerv Surg. 2017;9:867–874.
40. Kumpe DA, Bennett JL, Seinfeld J, Pelak VS, Chawla A, Tierney M. Dural sinus stent placement for idiopathic intracranial hypertension. J Neurosurg. 2012;116:538–548.
41. Smith KA, Peterson JC, Arnold PM, Camarata PJ, Whittaker TJ, Abraham MG. A case series of dural venous sinus stenting in idiopathic intracranial hypertension: Association of outcomes with optical coherence tomography. Int J Neurosci. 2017;127:145–153.
42. Dinkin MJ, Patsalides A. Venous Sinus Stenting in Idiopathic Intracranial Hypertension: Results of a Prospective Trial. J Neuroophthalmol. 2017; 37:113.
43. Nicholson P, Brinjikji W, Radovanovic I, Hilditch C, Tsang A, Krings T, Pereira V, Lenck S. Venous sinus stenting for idiopathic intracranial hypertension: A systematic review and meta-analysis. J Neurointerv Surg. 2019;11:380–385.
44. Fridley J, Foroozan R, Sherman V, Brandt ML, Yoshor D. Bariatric surgery for the treatment of idiopathic intracranial hypertension. J Neurosurg. 2011;114:34–39.
45. Sugerman H, Felton W, Sismanis A, Kellum J, DeMaria E, Sugerman E. Gastric surgery for pseudotumor cerebri associated with severe obesity. Ann Surg. 1999;229:634–640.
46. Falardeau J, Lobb BM, Golden S, Maxfield SD, Tanne E. The use of acetazolamide during pregnancy in intracranial hypertension patients. J Neuroophthalmol. 2013;33:9
47. Ko M, Chang S, Ridha M. Weight gain and recurrence in idiopathic intracranial hypertension: A case-control study. Neurology. 2011;76:1564–1567.
48. Headache Classification Committee of the International Headache Society (IHS). The international classification of headache disorders. 3rd ed. Cephalalgia. 2018;38:1–211.

7

OPTIC NEUROPATHIES ASSOCIATED WITH SYSTEMIC DISORDERS AND RADIATION-INDUCED OPTIC NEUROPATHY

Fiona Costello

CASE STUDY

A 38-year-old woman presented with progressive painless vision loss affecting the left eye for 2 months duration. She also noted diplopia for approximately 15 days. Neuro-ophthalmological examination revealed left periorbital swelling, proptosis and a left lateral rectus palsy. Media of the left eye was hazy and optic disc examination of the left eye suggested papillitis. Gadolinium-enhanced magnetic resonance imaging (MRI) of the brain and orbits suggested thickening and hyperintense signal change affecting the left optic nerve along with enlargement of both lacrimal glands. What are the probable causes of such presentation? What are the investigations which will aid in rendering the final diagnosis?

Introduction

The optic "nerve" is a functionally eloquent tract of the central nervous system (CNS) that may be injured by a variety of different pathological mechanisms. Symptoms of an inflammatory optic nerve injury include variable pain, dyschromatopsia (decreased color perception), and vision loss (1). The neuro-ophthalmic examination in affected individuals may reveal evidence of decreased central visual acuity, visual field loss that follows the topography of the retinal nerve fiber layer, a relative afferent pupil defect in the ipsilateral eye (or in the case of bilateral optic nerve involvement, the more severely affected eye); and, with chronicity, optic atrophy (1). During the acute phase of injury, the optic nerve may appear swollen (papillitis), or be otherwise normal in appearance. Optic neuritis, either sporadic in type, or associated with multiple sclerosis (MS), represents the most common inflammatory optic neuropathy (1). Yet, there are several "red flags" that should raise concern for an underlying systemic inflammatory disorder, mimicking the clinical presentation of typical optic neuritis (Table 7.1). Identifying non-demyelinating, inflammatory optic neuropathies associated with systemic disorders is important, because these conditions may be both vision- and life-threatening. In this section, the approach to diagnosing inflammatory optic neuropathies will be reviewed, with emphasis on clinical features that should prompt early recognition of an underlying systemic disease. This, in turn, will facilitate effective management and optimize patient outcomes (Figure 7.1).

Sarcoidosis

Overview

Sarcoidosis is an immune-mediated disease, which causes tissue injury through inflammation, granuloma formation and consequent fibrosis (1, 2). While this disorder can affect any part of the body, the lungs, skin, liver and joints are most frequent anatomical sites involved (1, 2). Sarcoidosis typically affects women more than men, and disease manifestations can be more severe among African Americans (2). Optic nerve involvement may be unilateral or bilateral, and arise from a myriad of pathological mechanisms, including: inflammation of the nerve (optic neuritis), parachiasmal structures, or the optic nerve sheath (perineuritis); compression or infiltration by an inflammatory mass adjacent to the anterior visual pathway (orbital apex, or pituitary gland); or, as a consequence raised intracranial pressure (dural venous sinus thrombosis, aseptic meningitis, or hydrocephalus) (1, 2).

Key clinical features

Optic neuropathy is infrequently associated with sarcoidosis, affecting only 5–10% of patients (1). Yet, ocular involvement can occur in up to 10–50% of sarcoid cases (1, 2). Associated features include anterior uveitis with mutton fat keratic precipitates, iris nodules, vitritis (with a so-called "string of pearls"), periphlebitis, candle wax drippings and choroidal involvement (1, 2). Lacrimal gland enlargement is another common association of orbital sarcoidosis. The optic nerve head appearance in sarcoid-related optic neuropathy may mimic other causes of optic neuritis. Notably, direct granulomatous infiltration of the optic nerve head is a distinctive feature of this condition (Figure 7.2) (3). These granulomas may present as small, discrete lesions at the optic disc margins, or large lesions that protrude into the vitreous (3). Sarcoidosis may also manifest as an orbital inflammatory syndrome characterized by pain, proptosis and ocular motility deficits (1). In this scenario, the optic nerve may be damaged due to contiguous inflammation. In a recent prospective observational cohort study, Kidd and colleagues characterized the clinical features of 52 cases of sarcoid-related optic neuropathy (2). All affected individuals demonstrated decreased central visual acuity, dyschromatopsia and visual field defects. In some cases, optic nerve dysfunction evolved over days, whereas other patients manifested a more slowly progressive optic neuropathy. Ocular inflammation was associated with optic neuropathy in approximately one-third of cases (36%). Pain was a less common feature than is seen in demyelinating optic neuritis (affecting only 27% of sarcoid cases, relative to 92% if "typical" optic neuritis cases), a feature which may help distinguish optic neuritis associated with MS, from sarcoid-related optic neuropathy (1, 2).

Approach to diagnosis

In some cases of neurosarcoidosis, the patient may not have pulmonary features, therefore establishing the diagnosis can be challenging (1–5). Cranial MRI may show meningeal enhancement, particularly at the base of the skull, in close proximity to the chiasm (1, 5). Orbital MRI often discloses T2-weighted and fluid-attenuated inversion recovery (FLAIR) hyperintense signal changes in the optic nerve, with variable

DOI: 10.1201/9780429020278-10

TABLE 7.1: **Atypical Clinical Features of Optic Neuritis Suggesting an Underlying Systemic Inflammatory Disorder**

History

Younger (<20 years) or older age (>50 years)

Absence of pain

Bilateral optic nerve involvement

Hyper acute visual loss

Severe visual loss

Symptoms progressing beyond 2–3 weeks

Absence of visual recovery

Frequent relapses

Examination

Optic disc pallor at presentation

Severe optic disc edema, with hemorrhage and/or vitreous inflammation

Visual field showing altitudinal field defects

Associated uveitis and/or retinal vasculitis

Associated systemic symptoms or signs (lymphadenopathy, rash, fever, weight loss, myalgias, arthropathy, end-organ involvement)

Neuroendocrine dysfunction

Evidence of orbitopathy

degrees of optic nerve sheath thickening and enhancement (5). Notably, sarcoidosis, tuberculosis, syphilis, IgG4-related disease and Lyme disease represent a heterogeneous group of disorders that may also cause hypertrophic pachymeningitis. This finding can help localize the diagnosis of neurosarcoidosis in the appropriate clinical context (5). Cerebrospinal fluid (CSF) analysis may reveal a lymphocytic pleocytosis and an elevated protein level in cases of sarcoid-related optic neuropathy (1). Moreover, chest imaging may disclose evidence of hilar lymphadenopathy, or other features of pulmonary sarcoidosis (1). A *definite* diagnosis of neurosarcoidosis is achieved in a relative minority of patients because this requires histologic confirmation of non-caseating granulomas in affected CNS tissue (4). A *probable* diagnosis may be determined from ancillary evidence of CNS inflammation with MRI or CSF in combination with proof of systemic disease (with histological confirmation and/or at least two indirect indicators consisting of fluorodeoxyglucose positron emission tomography [FDG-PET], gallium scan, chest imaging and serum angiotensin-converting enzyme). Finally, *possible* neurosarcoidosis is defined if there is appropriate clinical suspicion, exclusion of other diagnoses, and if the criteria for definite and presumed sarcoidosis are not fulfilled (4).

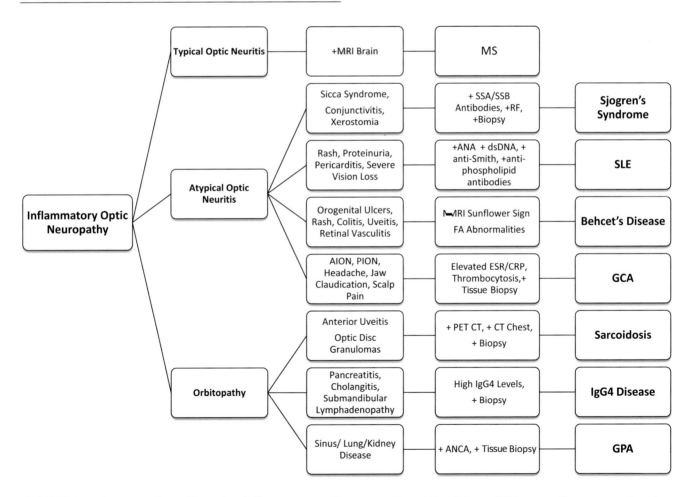

FIGURE 7.1 An approach to diagnosing inflammatory optic neuropathies. *Abbreviations*: MRI, magnetic resonance imaging; AION, anterior ischemic optic neuropathy; PION, posterior ischemic optic neuropathy; MS, multiple sclerosis; SSA/B, Sjogren's specific antibody A/B; RF, rheumatoid factor; ANA, anti-nuclear antibody; FA, fluorescein angiography; TAB, temporal artery biopsy; ESR, erythrocyte sedimentation rate; CRP, c-reactive protein; PET CT, positron emission tomography computed tomography; ANCA, anti-nuclear cytoplasmic antibodies; SLE, systemic lupus erythematosus; GPA, granulomatosis with polyangiitis.

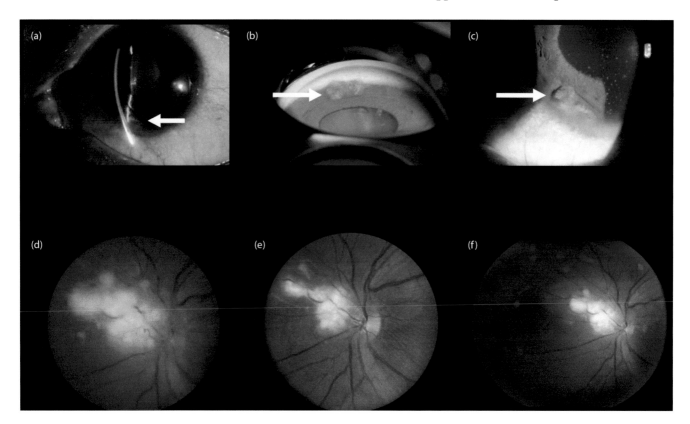

FIGURE 7.2 A biopsy-proven case of sarcoidosis (conjunctival biopsy) with a conjunctival lesion (a–c) (arrows), and extensive granulomatous changes on the left optic disc (d–f). The patient's optic nerve appearance (e, f) and visual field function improved with corticosteroids. (Images provided courtesy of Dr. Randy Kardon, University of Iowa.)

Treatment and prognosis

In cases of proven, presumed or suspected sarcoidosis presenting with optic nerve involvement, it is recommended that patients receive high-dose corticosteroids, with a slow taper (2). Relapses should be managed with the addition of an immunosuppressive agent. Patients who experience an inflammatory version of sarcoid optic neuropathy often respond to treatment, whereas those with infiltrative or progressive optic nerve involvement may recover less robustly (2). Methotrexate, azathioprine, hydroxychloroquine, mycophenolate mofetil and cyclosporine A represent second-line therapy considerations (4, 6). Third-line therapies include cyclophosphamide and tumor necrosis factor (TNF)-alpha antagonists (4, 6). Treatment responses include total remission (27%), incomplete remission (32%), stable disease (24%) and deterioration (6%) (4).

IgG4-related disease

Overview

IgG4-related disease is a multi-organ, fibro-inflammatory condition, which has recently been recognized as the cause of several systemic and neurological inflammatory syndromes previously regarded as idiopathic in nature (7, 8). This disorder has a predilection for involving anatomical structures in the head and neck, including the orbits, meninges, pituitary gland and peripheral nerves (7, 8). Less frequently, IgG4-related disease affects the brain parenchyma and vasculature (7, 8). Autoimmune pancreatitis, sclerosing cholangitis, chronic sclerosing sialadenitis (especially of the submandibular glands), dacryoadenitis and retroperitoneal

fibrosis are common systemic features (7, 8). IgG4-related disease is most commonly reported among middle-aged to elderly men. Yet, when disease manifestations involve the head and neck, both sexes may be equally affected. Ocular involvement is relatively common among pediatric patients (7, 8). Since disease manifestations may wax and wane over time, the diagnosis of IgG4-related disease is often delayed. Yet, early identification of this condition is important, because treatment response is often favorable.

Key clinical features

Patients with IgG4-related disease manifest an orbital syndrome in a quarter of cases, characterized by periorbital swelling, proptosis, ptosis and lacrimal gland enlargement. These features arise from inflammation involving the extraocular muscles, orbital fat and connective tissue (7, 8). Evaluation of anatomical structures in the neck often demonstrates lymphadenopathy and enlargement of the major salivary and thyroid glands. Submandibular gland involvement is characteristic (7, 8). Unlike thyroid eye disease, which favors the inferior and medial recti, the lateral rectus is the most commonly involved muscle in IgG4-related disease (7, 8). Optic neuropathy, secondary to IgG4-related diseases, may be caused by a variety of mechanisms (Table 7.2), including hypophysitis as shown in Figure 7.3.

Approach to diagnosis

Identifying IgG4-related disease requires consideration of clinical, radiographic, serological, and pathological sources of evidence. High IgG4 serum concentrations in isolation are not sensitive or specific enough to render the diagnosis (8). Approximately 30% of patients

TABLE 7.2: Mechanisms of Optic Neuropathy Caused by IgG4-Related Disease (7, 8)

Syndrome	Clinical Features	Imaging Findings	Mechanisms of Optic Nerve Injury	Alternative Diagnoses
Orbitopathy	Periorbital swelling, enlargement of the infraorbital nerve	Enlargement of the lacrimal, salivary and parotid glands. MRI shows lesions to be isointense on T1W and iso/hypointense with T2W and FLAIR sequences. Involvement of the trigeminal nerve is characteristic. A key distinguishing feature of IgG4-related orbital disease is the involvement of the infraorbital nerve.	Compressive, inflammatory, orbital apex lesions	Idiopathic orbital inflammation, lymphoma, metastatic disease, infection, sarcoidosis, GPA, thyroid eye disease, Erdheim–Chester disease
Hypertrophic pachy-meningitis	Headache, cranial nerve palsies, motor deficits, sensory loss, gait instability, vision loss, seizures, cognitive deficits	Contrast-enhanced MRI shows pachymeningeal thickening and enhancement. CT shows IgG4-related pachymeningitis as isodense lesions. MRI reveals hypointense or isointense relative to the brain parenchyma on T1W and T2W imaging.	Infiltrative, compressive, and raised intracranial pressure	Tuberculosis, lymphoma (and other malignancies) sarcoidosis, rheumatoid arthritis, Behçet's, GPA, GCA
Hypophysitis	Involves the pituitary gland and stalk; vision loss and neuro-endocrine dysfunction	MRI shows a symmetrically enlarged pituitary gland with thickening of the stalk. MRI shows hypointense T2W characteristics that enhance homogeneously with gadolinium.	Compression or chiasmal infiltration	Pituitary tumors, sarcoidosis, meningioma, GPA, Langerhans cell histiocytosis, syphilis, TB, lymphocytic hypophysitis

Abbreviations: MRI = magnetic resonance imaging; T1W = T1-weighted; T2W = T2-weighted; FLAIR = fluid-attenuated inversion recovery; GPA = granulomatosis with polyangiitis; CT = computed tomography; GCA = giant cell arteritis; TB = tuberculosis.

with histopathological proof of diagnosis have normal serum IgG4 concentrations. Additionally, among patients with increased serum IgG4 concentrations, the range of values is extremely variable. IgG4 concentrations correlate imprecisely with disease activity and do not predict the need for additional treatment (8). Since corticosteroid therapy lowers IgG4 concentrations, these levels should be measured before initiating treatment (7, 8). Patients with IgG4-related disease may have associated eosinophilia, elevated IgE levels and hypocomplementemia of C3 and C4 (8). Erythrocyte sedimentation rate (ESR) spikes may be associated with hypergammaglobulinemia (8). In contrast, C-reactive protein concentrations are uncommonly elevated and usually disproportionately low compared with the serum ESR (8). Head and neck imaging shows enlargement of the lacrimal, salivary and/or pituitary gland and/or localized nodules or masses. With MRI, lesions appear isointense on T1-weighted imaging, isointense or hypointense on T2/FLAIR imaging and demonstrate homogeneous enhancement (7, 8). The orbital myositis associated with IgG4-related disease causes smooth swelling of the muscles and tendons, unlike thyroid eye disease, which primarily affects the muscle bellies of the extraocular muscles (5, 7, 8). A characteristic feature of IgG4-related disease is radiologic involvement of branches of the trigeminal nerve. In particular, enlargement of the infraorbital nerve (with expansion of its canal) is relatively specific for IgG4-related disease. Notably, the diagnosis should be suspected when the coronal section of the infraorbital nerve is larger than that of the optic nerve (7, 8). As mentioned, tissue biopsy is critical to confirming the diagnosis, and also serves a role in excluding clinic mimics. Major histopathological features to look for include lymphoplasmacytic infiltration (sometimes associated with eosinophilia), "storiform" fibrosis and obliterative phlebitis (8). Immunohistochemistry typically shows a large percentage of IgG4-positive cells (8).

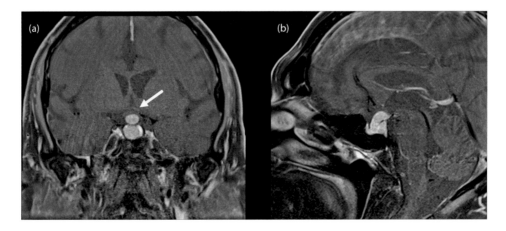

FIGURE 7.3 Coronal (a) and sagittal (b) T1-weighted gadolinium-enhanced MRI sequences showing thickening, enhancement and hyperintense signal changes of the pituitary gland and stalk in a 72-year-old man with biopsy-proven IgG4-related disease. Despite chiasmal compression (arrow) caused by IgG4-related hypophysitis, the patient had normal afferent visual pathway function.

Treatment and prognosis

An international consensus statement from more than 40 investigators from Europe, North America and Asia has recommended monotherapy with glucocorticoids as first-line treatment for systemic IgG4-related disease (7). In patients with therapeutic failure on first-line treatment, alternative immune-suppressive agents have also proven useful. B-cell depletion with rituximab has also shown efficacy, and radiotherapy may be used in refractory cases (7, 8). The manifestations of this condition generally respond well to treatment, but chronic or recurrent courses of corticosteroid therapy may be required (7, 8).

Granulomatosis with polyangiitis (GPA)

Overview

GPA is a systemic necrotizing vasculitis. As such, it is linked with polyarteritis nodosa (PAN) and other anti-neutrophil cytoplasm antibody (ANCA)-associated vasculitides, namely microscopic polyangiitis (MPA) and eosinophilic granulomatosis with polyangiitis (EGPA) (9). The clinical features of these conditions are protean and can be both life- and organ-threatening (9). For the purpose of this review we will focus on GPA, because it is the most common systemic necrotizing vasculitis subtype associated with optic neuropathy (9). GPA typically targets vessels in the upper and lower respiratory tracts, paranasal sinuses, kidneys and lungs (1, 9, 10). Unlike some of the other systemic inflammatory conditions described, GPA affects both sexes equally, with 40–55 years representing the typical age range of diagnosis (1, 9, 10). Caucasians are the most commonly affected ethnic group, whereas African Americans represent only 2–8% of this patient population, in most studies (1, 9, 10).

Key clinical features

Ocular involvement is seen in approximately 50–60% of GPA patients and 8% of affected individuals experience disease-related vision loss (10). Any part of eye may be affected, albeit the condition most often manifests as orbital disease, followed by scleral, episcleral, corneal and nasolacrimal abnormalities (10). Early recognition of the ocular features can be pivotal to identifying active disease, and preventing vision loss. Optic nerve involvement may develop from contiguous inflammation in the setting of orbital inflammation, or local compression (1). When orbital disease occurs, it can extend from its origin in the maxillary or ethmoid sinuses, and spread to involve the extraocular muscles, nerves or blood vessels (1, 10). Alternatively, inflammation can arise in the orbit, and spread throughout the retrobulbar space (1, 10). Patients may present with proptosis, ocular motility deficits and pain (1). In some cases, affected individuals develop exposure keratopathy and corneal ulceration, which in turn, leads to permanent vision loss.

Approach to diagnosis

Serum ANCA levels are positive in approximately 80–90% of GPA patients (10). Yet, when GPA disease manifestations are confined to the sinuses and orbits, ANCA may be negative in 50% of cases (1). In this clinical setting, biopsy of affected tissue may be required to support the diagnosis (1, 10). In ANCA-positive cases, the antibody targets cytoplasmic proteinase-3 80% of the time, whereas in 20% of cases the antibody targets cytoplasmic myeloperoxidase (10). Other serological findings noted in GPA are relatively non-specific, and include anemia, thrombocytosis,

leukocytosis and elevated acute phase reactants (ESR and CRP) (10). Computed tomography imaging of the orbits may demonstrate sinus opacification and osseous invasion (5). Specifically, orbital lesions appear as slightly hyperdense relative to nasal mucosa, with contrast-enhanced CT scans. Moreover, GPA infiltrates appear hypointense compared to orbital fat in both T1-weighted and T2-weighted MRI sequences, and typically enhance with gadolinium (5, 10). Histologic changes noted in GPA cases include granulomatous inflammation within the wall of an artery, and/or the presence of necrotizing vasculitis (10).

Treatment and prognosis

The combination of glucocorticoids and either cyclophosphamide, methotrexate or azathioprine can lead to disease remission and prolonged survival (1, 10). Unfortunately, treatment-related morbidity remains a challenge in GPA. This has led to exploration of numerous alternative therapies, including rituximab, mycophenolate mofetil, leflunomide and plasmapheresis, with variable results reported (9, 10). The choice of systemic therapies depends on the extent of disease, the organs involved, rate of progression, response to therapy, and side effects.

Despite several case reports and a strong therapeutic rational suggesting a role for TNF-alpha inhibition, a randomized, double-masked, placebo-controlled trial failed to demonstrate efficacy of the TNF-alpha inhibitor (etanercept) in GPA (10). This trial also demonstrated an increased risk of solid organ malignancy among patients who received concurrent therapy with both etanercept and cyclophosphamide, for severe disease (10). Treatment of ocular manifestations of GPA is most successful when a multidisciplinary approach is employed. Surgical intervention is indicated in the setting of locally destructive disease, or to obtain tissue diagnosis (10).

Giant cell arteritis (GCA)

Overview

GCA is a systemic vasculitis affecting large to medium-sized arteries. This disease shows preferential involvement of the ophthalmic artery and its branches, including the posterior ciliary arteries and the central retinal artery. Pathologically, GCA is characterized by granulomatous inflammation and narrowing (or occlusion) of extradural arteries with an internal elastic lamina (11–13). Giant cell arteritis is diagnosed predominantly in elderly adults, with cases under the age of 50 years being rare, and the incidence increasing with advancing age (13). The diagnosis is more common in females, with a threefold relative risk in women compared to men (13). Of note, GCA is more likely to affect Caucasians relative to other ethnic groups (13).

Key clinical features

The most common causes of visual loss in GCA patients include arteritic anterior ischemic optic neuropathy (A-AION), central retinal artery occlusion and posterior ischemic optic neuropathy (12, 13). Less commonly, GCA patients can present with an orbital inflammatory syndrome, perineural sheath enhancement and chiasmal enhancement (14). While many GCA patients report symptoms such as myalgias, weight loss, fever headache, scalp tenderness, jaw claudication and transient vision loss, A-AION may represent the only clinical manifestation of otherwise clinically silent GCA (13). In fact, 21% of GCA patients with visual loss secondary to A-AION do not have any other cranial or systemic manifestations at disease onset (13). At presentation, A-AION patients present with optic disc edema. Over time, pallor of the nerve head becomes evident as the edema resolves and loss of the retinal ganglion cell axons comprising the optic nerve fully manifests (11). For some GCA patients, late cupping of the optic nerve head evolves; this feature can help distinguish cases of A-AION from non-arteritic AION (11). For this reason, a patient presenting with AION in one eye and a relatively large optic nerve head cup in the fellow eye should prompt suspicion for GCA (11). In less frequently observed cases of arteritic posterior ischemic optic neuropathy, there is no evidence of optic disc edema or pallor acutely. Yet, over weeks, optic nerve pallor becomes evident (11).

Approach to diagnosis

GCA is typically diagnosed based on clinical grounds, and supported by the observation of elevated serum ESR, CRP and platelet count. Despite the utility of other diagnostic modalities (Table 7.3), temporal artery biopsy remains the gold standard for GCA diagnosis. A positive temporal artery biopsy confirms the disease, yet a negative biopsy does not exclude it, given the potential for inflammatory lesions to "skip" some artery segments.

Treatment and prognosis

When GCA patients present with vision loss, high dose intravenous or oral corticosteroid therapy is recommended for 3–5 days, prior to initiating an oral taper (11, 13, 15–18). Treatment is offered with the intention of salvaging the patient's remaining vision, since the potential for reversing the effects of A-AION is generally low. Aspirin is sometimes given to offer anti-thrombotic and anti-inflammatory benefits to GCA patients presenting with vision loss, albeit there are no randomized controlled trials validating the role of aspirin for the prevention of ischemic complications from this condition (18, 19). A recent landmark study has shown the beneficial, steroid sparing effects of tocilizumab

administered weekly or every other week, combined with a prednisone taper, in the treatment of GCA (20).

Behçet's disease

Overview

Behçet's syndrome is an autoimmune, inflammatory condition of uncertain etiology characterized by recurrent orogenital ulceration, skin lesions, arthropathy and colitis (21–23). The incidence and prevalence of Behçet's syndrome are highest in the Middle East and Asia (22). There is no evidence of a gender predilection with respect to the neurological manifestations of this disease (22). The ocular features of Behçet's include uveitis and vaso-occlusive retinal vasculitis (21). Optic nerve injury may arise from primary inflammatory infiltration of the optic nerve, spread of inflammation into the nerve from an adjacent meningitis, compression of the nerve by an inflammatory mass, raised intracranial pressure, uveitic glaucoma, or contiguous spread from adjacent retinal vasculitis (21–23).

Key clinical features

Common ophthalmic complications of Behçet's include uveitis (70% of cases), which is classically anterior in type (21). In addition, 30% of these patients can develop a sight-threatening retinal vasculitis, leading to retinal and macular edema, perivascular sheathing and an occlusive arterial vasculopathy (21). Less commonly, patients may develop a subacute painless optic neuropathy, similar to the clinical presentation seen with demyelinating or other inflammatory optic nerve injuries (21–23). Optic disc edema (papillitis) is common. The presence of peripapillary hemorrhages can help distinguish Behçet's optic neuropathy from demyelinating optic neuritis (21, 22).

Approach to diagnosis

Behçet's optic neuropathy may be characterized by MRI evidence of perineural enhancement around the orbital optic nerve (21, 22). This finding is significantly more common than increased signal in the optic nerve itself and is referred to as the "sunflower-like sign" on coronal MRI views (21, 22). The observation of perineural enhancement suggests that optic nerve inflammation in Behçet's originates in the adjacent optic nerve sheath, akin to the mechanism of meningoencephalitis (21). Hyper-fluorescence of the optic disk may be observed in Behçet's optic neuropathy, whereby leakage of dye is seen mostly in papillary or peripapillary capillaries (22). In contrast to patients with uveitis (in which 98% of eyes may show dye leakage from retinal capillaries), retinal vessels are rarely affected (22). In some cases of Behçet's optic neuropathy, patients may have evidence of CSF leukocytosis and/or raised protein (21, 22).

Treatment and prognosis

The first-line treatment of optic neuropathy in Behçet's syndrome is corticosteroids, with adjunctive immunosuppression required if there is evidence that the systemic condition is particularly severe, there is concurrent CNS inflammation, or the condition relapses (21, 23). Short-term recurrence of primary optic neuropathy in Behçet's syndrome is very rare (21, 23), and the prognosis for visual recovery tends to be favorable (23). This observation regarding the clinical course helps differentiate primary optic neuropathy in Behçet's syndrome from myelin oligodendrocyte glycoprotein IgG antibody associated neuropathy, which frequently relapses (22). The diagnosis of optic neuropathy with Behçet's should dissuade use of cyclosporine, since this agent can promote the development of neurologic involvement in this disease (23).

TABLE 7.3: **Imaging Modalities Used to Diagnosis Giant Cell Arteritis (5, 12, 17)**

Imaging Modality	Findings in GCA
Fluorescein angiography	Choroidal filling defects have been reported in patients with arteritic AION, and filling times may normalize after therapy
Ultrasound	A hypoechoic halo around a perfused lumen of affected temporal arteries has been reported, and may normalize after therapy
MRI	High resolution MRI using contrast-enhanced, fat saturated, T1W spin-echo sequences have shown luminal stenosis and enhancement of the superficial temporal and superficial occipital arteries
MRA	Detects vasculitis of the extracranial vessels, with the most common vessels involved being the axillary and subclavian arteries
CTA	This imaging study has shown evidence of arteritis in the aorta, the brachiocephalic trunks, the carotids and the subclavian arteries
PET-CT	PET and PET-CT have shown significant tracer uptake of the walls of the ascending aorta, aortic arch and subclavian arteries

Abbreviations: MRI = magnetic resonance imaging; T1W = T1-weighted; MRA = magnetic resonance angiography; CTA = computed tomography angiography; PET-CT = positron emission tomography CT.

Sjogren's syndrome

Overview
Sjogren's syndrome is a systemic autoimmune disease characterized by keratoconjunctivitis and xerostomia (dry mouth) (1). Primary Sjogren's tends to be limited to the oral and lacrimal glands, causing sicca syndrome. When the condition is associated with rheumatoid arthritis, systemic lupus erythematosus (SLE), vasculitis, scleroderma, polymyositis, primary biliary cirrhosis or chronic active hepatitis, patients are deemed to have secondary Sjogren's syndrome (1). Middle-aged adults are most commonly affected, with a female-to-male sex ratio of 9:1 (1).

Key clinical features
CNS involvement occurs in the minority (2–25%) Sjogren's cases and is much less common than peripheral nerve involvement in this condition (24, 26). The optic neuropathy may be related to immune-mediated small vessel vasculitis or demyelinating disease (24). Sjogren's related optic neuropathy may be more likely to recur than optic neuritis associated with MS (25).

Approach to diagnosis
The diagnosis of Sjogren's syndrome can be determined by testing for rheumatoid factor (50% of patients), and antibodies against antigens known as Ro (SSA), and La (SSB) (1). Studies have demonstrated that the presence of anti-SSA and anti-SSB antibodies associate with an earlier disease onset and the presence of extra-glandular manifestations. Ultrasonic testing and lip biopsy may also be used to confirm the diagnosis of primary Sjogren's syndrome.

Treatment and prognosis
Treatment of Sjogren's commonly involves corticosteroids and immunosuppressive therapies (1).

Systemic lupus erythematosus

Overview
Systemic lupus erythematosus (SLE) is an immune-mediated connective tissue disorder. While the condition is more common in individuals of Asian and African extraction, thrombotic events may be more common in Caucasians. Notably, SLE is nine times more common in women relative to their male counterparts. Ocular manifestations may affect one in three SLE patients. (1, 27).

Key clinical features
Optic nerve involvement in SLE may manifest as optic neuritis or ischemic optic neuropathy (1, 27). The onset of vision loss is usually painless, and subacute in nature. Moreover, the course tends to be both progressive and severe (1). Visual acuity in SLE-associated optic nerve injury is usually worse than 20/200 acutely, with only 50% of patients recovering better than 20/25 visual acuity (1, 27). The more dire outcomes are attributed to the fact that SLE optic neuropathy is believed to arise from ischemic injury as opposed to a primary demyelinating insult to the optic nerve (1, 27).

Approach to diagnosis
In cases of SLE optic neuropathy, the serum anti-nuclear antibody (ANA) level is typically abnormal, with a speckled pattern (1). Anti-double-stranded DNA and anti-Smith antibodies can help confirm the diagnosis (1). Anti-phospholipid antibodies are also seen with increased frequency particularly in association with ophthalmic and neurological features of SLE (1). Notably, patients with Sjogrens Syndrome (SS) and SLE may develop optic neuritis as a manifestation of co-existing neuromyelitis optic spectrum disorders (NMOSD). It is therefore important to check serum Aquaporin 4 IgG status in SS and SLE patients presenting with neurological deficits.

Treatment and prognosis
The inflammatory optic neuropathy associated with SLE may respond to corticosteroid therapy. Early treatment is associated with better visual outcomes. A standard regimen includes high-dose corticosteroids followed by an extended oral taper. Therapeutic benefits have been reported with numerous immunosuppressive agents including: methotrexate, cyclosporin, cyclophosphamide, and azathioprine (1, 27).

Radiation-induced optic neuropathy

Introduction
Radiation therapy is a frequently employed treatment modality for tumors of the skull base, nasopharynx cancers, choroid, retina and cranial fossa. Generally, this treatment is well tolerated by patients, and provides therapeutic benefits by ameliorating tumor growth or recurrence. Yet, on rare occasions, radiation-induced injury to the anterior visual pathway can occur. Unfortunately, when radiation-induced optic neuropathy (RION) manifests, it can have devastating effects on visual function. Recognition of this clinical syndrome is important, because any opportunity to ameliorate the effects of optic nerve injury may be augmented with early intervention.

Overview
The pathophysiology of RION is believed to be a chronic progressive vasculopathy (radionecrosis) that predominantly affects white matter (28–30). In animal studies, a time-dependent and dose-sensitive pathologic reaction in endothelial cells has been demonstrated to cause blood–brain barrier disruption in the setting of radiation-induced tissue injury (28–30). Aside from depleting vascular endothelial cells, radiation exposure is believed to cause somatic mutations in glial cells, leading to demyelination and neuronal degeneration (28–30). Pathological studies have shown ischemic demyelination, reactive astrocytosis, endothelial hyperplasia, obliterative endarteritis and fibrinoid necrosis as features associated with RION (28).

There are several risk factors that have been reported to potentiate the risk for RION including female gender, diabetes, older age, hyperlipidemia and chemotherapy (28–33). Yet, in a recent small, retrospective case-controlled study, Ferguson and colleagues (32) did not find any association between vascular risk factors, adjuvant chemotherapy, age or gender and a higher odds ratio for RION. In fact, the most significant risk factor for this condition has consistently been shown to be the total dose of radiation received, with the risk of RION increasing from 0% when the total dose of radiation is less than 50 gray units (Gy), and increasing to 16% for doses exceeding 70 Gy (32, 33). Radiosurgery in doses of greater than 8 Gy has also been associated with this condition. Moreover, cases of RION have been reported with lower radiation doses (34), particularly in patients treated for pituitary tumors (42–50 Gy), possibly due to the concomitant deleterious effect of chiasmal compression.

Key clinical features
Vision loss in cases of RION is generally severe. Patients may manifest monocular symptoms, or develop simultaneous (or sequential) involvement of both eyes (28–30). Bilateral optic nerve involvement can be as high as 75% of cases, when the field

of radiation involves the optic chiasm, or both optic nerves. Patients affected by RION typically develop vision loss months to years (mean time of onset is 18 months) after radiation treatment (29, 34). Vision loss is unaccompanied by pain (29). The onset of symptoms may be abrupt, and is often progressive. For cases caused by radiation focused on the eye or orbit, the optic nerve head can be directly affected (radiation papillopathy). In this context, the optic nerve may appear edematous, with surrounding subretinal fluid, peripapillary hard exudates and cotton–wool spots (29). Fluorescein angiography in cases of radiation papillopathy shows nonperfusion of the superficial disc vasculature. The optic disc generally remains swollen for weeks to months and then eventually atrophies (29). Retrobulbar RION is associated with a normal optic disc appearance at onset of vision loss, but atrophy ultimately develops over time (29, 30).

Approach to diagnosis

The diagnosis of RION depends on a thorough knowledge of the patient's potential risk for this condition, and early recognition of the cardinal clinical findings. In the appropriate clinical setting, MRI can be extremely helpful in localizing the diagnosis of RION by demonstrating enhancement of the optic nerve on T1-weighted images (30, 34). In a small series of 12 cases, Archer et al. (34) reported a pre-chiasmatic imaging abnormality in 87% (13 of 15 affected eyes) of RION eyes, which was most readily apparent on axial imaging. This study demonstrated evidence of segmental expansion and abnormal T2 signal within the optic nerves (34). These imaging abnormalities were felt to be pathognomonic for the diagnosis of RION, because discrete areas of enhancement (accompanied by expansion or T2-high signal) are not seen with neoplastic infiltrative optic neuropathies (34). In some cases, pre-chiasmatic enhancement was apparent on MRI scans performed 3–6 weeks before the onset of vision loss, indicating a potential predictive role for this imaging modality in the diagnosis of RION (34). In the study by Archer et al. (34), the duration of enhancement among eyes affected by RION was at least 2 months (averaging 6 months) and in one case extending to 17 months, in keeping with published reports indicating persistent optic nerve enhancement ranging from 3 to 13 months after vision loss (34).

Optical coherence tomography angiography has been recently used to establish a putative grading system for RION, by characterizing effects on the radial peripherally capillary plexus (35). Findings may range from no detectable radial peripapillary capillary plexus abnormality to complete radial peripapillary capillary plexus dropout (35). Notably, more severe grades of peripapillary capillary injury correlate with worse visual acuity in affected eyes (35).

Treatment and prognosis

Unfortunately, treatment of RION can be quite disappointing, with systemic corticosteroids and anticoagulation showing little benefit (36). Hyperbaric oxygen might offer some positive therapeutic effects if treatment is initiated within 72 hours of visual loss (28). Recently, bevacizumab, a recombinant human monoclonal antibody that blocks angiogenesis by inhibiting vascular endothelial growth factor A has shown promise in the treatment of radiation necrosis affecting the CNS and RION (37–39). Gonzalez et al. (39) demonstrated the benefit of using bevacizumab as monotherapy or bevacizumab with a chemotherapeutic agent (carboplatin, irinotecan, temozolomide) in 15 patients diagnosed with CNS radiation necrosis. Affected patients demonstrated improvement in both FLAIR and post-contrast

T1-weighted MRI abnormalities. Torcuator et al. (40) described improvement in both FLAIR and contrast-enhanced T1 images in patients with biopsy-proven cerebral radiation necrosis. Levin et al. (41) enrolled 14 patients into a placebo-controlled, randomized, double-blind study to evaluate the effect of bevacizumab in treating CNS radiation necrosis. The MRI findings from this study showed that bevacizumab-treated patients demonstrated regression of necrotic lesions. Hence, there may be promise for the treatment of RION, which requires additional study. Given the devastating natural history of this condition, it may be reasonable to initiate therapy with bevacizumab, ideally at earliest point possible after diagnosis.

Conclusion

Optic neuropathies caused by underlying inflammatory systemic disorders and radiation treatment present with distinct clinical features, radiological findings and/or serological markers. In recent years, there have been novel developments in the diagnostic evaluation and treatment options for these conditions. Early recognition of these optic nerve syndromes is paramount to optimizing visual recovery, and in some cases, reducing morbidity and mortality for patients.

Multiple-Choice Questions

1. The mean time of onset of radiation-induced optic neuropathy (RION) after treatment is:
   a. 3 months
   b. 6 months
   c. 18 months
   d. 3 years

   Answer:
   c. 18 months

2. Patients with IgG4-related disease manifest an orbital syndrome in what percentage of cases?
   a. 10%
   b. 25%
   c. 75%
   d. 100%

   Answer:
   b. 25%

3. Which of the following steroid-sparing agents has recently been approved for the treatment of GCA?
   a. Tocilizumab
   b. Natalizumab
   c. Rituximab
   d. Bevacizumab

   Answer:
   a. Tocilizumab

4. Which of the following statements is false?
   a. Sarcoid optic neuropathy may be unilateral or bilateral.
   b. Sarcoid optic neuropathy is more likely to be heralded by pain than optic neuritis associated with multiple sclerosis.

c. Sarcoidosis can cause optic nerve injury from orbital apex syndrome.

d. Sarcoidosis may be associated with a hypertropic pachymeningitis.

Answer:

b. Sarcoid optic neuropathy is more likely to be heralded by pain than optic neuritis associated with multiple sclerosis.

References

1. Costello F. Inflammatory optic neuropathies. Continuum. 2014;20(4):816−837
2. Kidd DP, Burton BJ, Graham EM, Plant GT. Optic neuropathy associated with systemic sarcoidosis. Neurol Neuroimmunol Neuroinflamm. 2016;3:e270.
3. O'Neil EC, Danesh-Meyer HV, Connel PP, et al. The optic nerve head in acquired optic neuropathies. Nat Rev Neurol. 2010;6:221−236.
4. Fritz D, van de Beek D, Brouwer MC. Clinical features, treatment and outcome in neurosarcoidosis: Systematic review and meta-analysis. BMC Neurol. 2016;16(1):220.
5. Costello F, Scott JN. Imaging in neuro-ophthalmology. Continuum. 2019;25(5):1438−1490.
6. Radwan W, Lucke-Wold B, Robadi IA, Gyure K, Roberts T, Bhatia S. Neurosarcoidosis: Unusual presentations and considerations for diagnosis and management. Postgrad Med J. 2017;93:401−405.
7. AbdelRazek MA, Venna N, Stone JH. IgG4-related disease of the central and peripheral nervous systems. Lancet Neurol. 2018; 17:183−192.
8. Chwalisz BK, Stone JH. Neuro-ophthalmic complications of IgG4-related disease. Curr Opin Ophthalmol. 2018;29(6):485−494.
9. Rothschild PR, Pagnoux C, Seror R, et al. Ophthalmologic manifestations of systemic necrotizing vasculitides at diagnosis: A retrospective study of 1286 patients and review of the literature. Semin Arthritis Rheum. 2013;42:507−514.
10. Tarabishy AB, Schulte M, Papaliodis GN, Hoffman GS. Wegener's granulomatosis: Clinical manifestations, differential diagnosis, and management of ocular and systemic disease. Surv Ophthalmol. 2010;55(5):429−444.
11. Vodopivec I, Rizzo JF. Ophthalmic manifestations of giant cell arteritis. Rheumatology. 2018;57:ii63−ii72.
12. Frohman L, Wong AB, Matheos K, Leon-Alvarado LG, Danesh-Meyer HV. New developments in giant cell arteritis. Surv Ophthalmol. 2016;61(4):400−421.
13. Patil P, Karia N, Jain S, Dasgupta B. Giant cell arteritis: A review. Eye Brain. 2013;5:23−33.
14. Souza NM, Morgan ML, Almarzouqi S, Lee AG. Magnetic resonance imaging findings in giant cell arteritis. Eye. 2016;30:758−762
15. Dasgupta B. Concise guidance: Diagnosis and management of giant cell arteritis. Clin Med (Lond). 2010;10(4):381−386.
16. Roberts J, Clifford A. Update on the management of giant cell arteritis. Ther Adv Chronic Dis. 2017;8(4−5):69−80.
17. Sammel AM, Fraser CL. Update on giant cell arteritis. Curr Opin Ophthalmol. 2018;29(6):520−527.
18. Palkovacs EM, Costello F, Golnik KC. Giant cell arteritis. Neuroophthalmology. 2019;41−51.
19. Mollan SP, Sharrack N, Burdon MA, Denniston AK. Aspirin as adjunctive treatment for giant cell arteritis. Cochrane Database Syst Rev. 2014;8.
20. Stone JH, Tuckwell K, Dimonaco S, et al. Trial of tocilizumab in giant-cell arteritis. N Engl J Med. 2017; 77:317−328.
21. Kidd DP. Optic neuropathy in Behçet's syndrome. J Neurol. 2013;260:3065−3070.
22. Yang Q, Sun L, Wang Q, et al. Primary optic neuropathy in Behçet's syndrome. Mult Scler. 2019;25(8):1132−1140.
23. Akdal G, Toydemir HE, Saatci AO, et al. Characteristics of optic neuropathy in Behçet disease. Neurol Neuroimmunol Neuroinflamm. 2018;5:e490.
24. Tang WQ, Wei SH. Primary Sjogren's syndrome related optic neuritis. Int J Ophthalmol. 2013;6(6):888−891.
25. Li H, Zhang Y, Yi Z, Huang D, Wei S. Frequency of autoantibodies and connective tissue diseases in Chinese patients with optic neuritis. PLoS ONE. 2014;9(6):e99323.
26. Colaci M, Cassone G, Manfredi A, et al. Neurologic complications associated with Sjögren's disease: Case reports and modern pathogenic dilemma. Case Rep Neurol Med. 2014;590292.
27. Palejwala NV, Walia HS, Yeh S. Ocular manifestations of systemic lupus erythematosus: A review of the literature. Autoimmune Dis. 2012;290898.
28. Malik A, Golnik K. Hyperbaric oxygen therapy in the treatment of radiation optic neuropathy. J Neuroophthalmol. 2012;32:128−131.
29. Lessell S. Friendly fire: Neurogenic visual loss from radiation therapy. J Neuroophthalmol. 2004;24:243−250.
30. Danesh-Meyer HV. Radiation-induced optic neuropathy. J Clin Neurosci. 2008; 15:95−100.
31. Wang W, Yang H, Guo L, Hongyu Su, Wei S, Zhang X. Radiation-induced optic neuropathy following external beam radiation therapy for nasopharyngeal carcinoma: A retrospective case-control study. Mol Clin Oncol. 2016;4:868−872.
32. Ferguson I, Huecker J, Huang J, McClelland C, Van Stavern G. Risk factors for radiation-induced optic neuropathy: A case−control study. Clin Exp Ophthalmol. 2017;45:592−597.
33. Peeler CE, Cestari DM. Radiation optic neuropathy and retinopathy with low dose (20 Gy) radiation treatment. Am J Ophthalmol Case Rep. 2016;3:50−53.
34. Archer EL, Liao EA, Trobe JD. Radiation-induced optic neuropathy: Clinical and imaging profile of twelve patients. J Neuroophthalmol. 2019;39:170−180.
35. Parrozzani R, Frizziero L, Londei D, et al. Peripapillary vascular changes in radiation optic neuropathy: An optical coherence tomography angiography grading. Br J Ophthalmol. 2018;102:1238−1243.
36. Lee SM, Borruat FX. Should patients with radiation-induced optic neuropathy receive any treatment? J Neuroophthalmol. 2011;31:83−88.
37. Farooq O, Lincoff NS, Saikali N, et al. Novel treatment for radiation optic neuropathy with intravenous bevacizumab. J Neuroophthalmol. 2012;32(4):321−324.
38. Dutta P, Dhandapani S, Kumar N, Ahuja C, Mukerjee KK. Bevacizumab for radiation induced optic neuritis among aggressive residual/ecurrent suprasellar tumors: More than a mere antineoplastic effect. World Neurosurg. 2017;107:1044.e5-1044.e10.
39. Gonzalez J, Kumar A, Conrad CA, Levin VA. Effect of bevacizumab on radiation necrosis of the brain. Int J Radiat Oncol Biol Phys. 2007;67(2):323−326.
40. Torcuator R, Zuniga R, Mohan YS, et al. Initial experience with bevacizumab treatment for biopsy confirmed cerebral radiation necrosis. J Neurooncol. 2009;94(1):63−68.
41. Levin VA, Bidaut L, Hou P, et al. Randomized double-blind placebo-controlled trial of bevacizumab therapy for radiation necrosis of the central nervous system. Int J Radiat Oncol Biol Phys. 2011;79(5):1487−1495.

8

INFECTIOUS OPTIC NEUROPATHIES

Imran Rizvi, Ravindra Kumar Garg

CASE STUDY

A 22-year-old male presented with history of fever and headache for 2 months and bilateral visual loss for 15 days duration. Bilateral pupils were dilated, and the patient could only perceive light in both eyes. Fundus examination revealed bilateral optic atrophy. Gadolinium-enhanced MRI brain suggested thick exudates in the optochiasmatic region. What is your diagnosis?

Introduction

Neurologists as well as ophthalmologists frequently encounter patients with optic neuropathies. The usual presenting complaint these patients have is vision loss. Optic nerve examination, in addition to diminished visual acuity, reveals dyschromatopsia, a relative afferent pupillary defect (RAPD), and other ophthalmoscopic abnormalities.[1] A variety of conditions like demyelinating disorders, inflammatory and autoimmune diseases, vascular disorders, toxic, nutritional, neoplastic diseases and infections cause unilateral or bilateral optic nerve involvement. Infections are leading cause of optic neuropathies, especially in South East Asia. In infectious optic neuropathies, there can be involvement of optic nerve or adjacent structures like meninges, sinuses and orbital wall. A variety of viruses, bacteria, fungi, parasites and rickettsia are known to cause optic neuropathies[2] (Table 8.1). In this chapter, we will focus on salient features of various infectious optic neuropathies.

Approach to infectious optic neuropathies

The optic neuritis is the commonest type of optic nerve involvement in neurological practice. Optic neuritis is a demyelinating condition of the optic nerve commonly observed in multiple sclerosis and neuromyelitis optica. In large number of patients, optic neuritis is idiopathic in nature.[1] The clinical features and the course of a patient with idiopathic optic neuritis are different from that in secondary optic neuritis. The features that are suggestive of a secondary optic neuritis are involvement of both the eyes, inflammation involving several eye structures with optic nerve involvement, unusual clinical course along with systemic manifestations.[2] An atypical optic neuritis/neuropathy can be caused by a number of infections and non-infectious causes like inflammatory and autoimmune diseases, vascular disorders, toxic, nutritional and neoplastic diseases[1,2] (Table 8.2). A recent infectious illness, diabetes mellitus, human immunodeficiency virus infection, organ transplant, diseases of orbits, paranasal sinuses and meninges, bilateral optic nerve involvement suggest the possibility of an infectious optic neuropathy.[1] Drug-induced, especially antimicrobial-induced, optic neuropathy is a close differential diagnosis. A variety of antimicrobial agents

can produce optic neuritis[2] (Figure 8.1 and Table 8.3). Table 8.4 shows the investigations in a suspected patient with Infectious Optic Neuropathy.

Viral

Herpes simplex virus

Optic nerve can be affected in patients with herpes simplex encephalitis. Vision loss in herpes simplex encephalitis can also occur because of retinal involvement (acute retinal necrosis syndrome).[2] The common presenting symptoms are blurred vision, floaters and ocular discomfort. There are patchy retinal necrosis, vitritis and inflammation of anterior chamber.[3] About 11–57% of acute retinal necrosis syndrome patients can have an optic nerve involvement.[4,5] The presenting clinical features are acute severe vision loss. Eye examination reveals papillitis, neuroretinitis or optic atrophy. Optic perineuritis (enhancement of optic nerve sheath) can be demonstrated on MRI of optic nerves. The prognosis of untreated patients is very poor. Acyclovir is often efficacious. Corticosteroids should be added 48 hours after starting antiviral treatment.[2]

Varicella zoster virus

Varicella zoster infection can present as chicken-pox in children, as herpes zoster in elderly or in an immunocompromised host. Optic nerve involvement can occur in both these settings.

Optic neuropathy commonly occurs 2–6 weeks after onset of the rash.[6] The patient can present with unilateral or bilateral vision loss. On eye examination, papillitis can be demonstrated. The role of corticosteroids is not clear although they are advocated to accelerate recovery. Usually majority patients recover vision. Optic neuropathy can be part herpes zoster ophthalmicus, either at time of rash or later in post-herpetic phase.[7] Patient can report unilateral or bilateral vision. Optic disc is either normal or infrequently oedematous. Acyclovir and steroids are used for the treatment. The visual prognosis is generally good. Varicella zoster infection can also cause retinal necrosis in immunocompromised patient. In patients with retinal necrosis, optic nerve can also be affected. The visual prognosis in patients with retinal necrosis is generally poor.[8]

Cytomegalovirus

Cytomegalovirus is a common viral cause producing vision loss in HIV-infected patients. Cytomegalovirus infection characteristically produces hemorrhagic retinitis. Optic nerve involvement is seen in 14–73% patients.[9] Cytomegalovirus-associated optic neuropathy can occur even without retinitis. Ganciclovir or foscarnet can be used for treatment. Prognosis remains grim.[10]

Epstein-Barr virus

The Epstein-Barr virus is associated with many non-malignant and malignant conditions, like infectious mononucleosis, Burkitt's lymphoma, nasopharyngeal malignancy and central nervous system lymphoma. Epstein-Barr virus can also cause optic neuropathy. The involvement of optic nerve in such

DOI: 10.1201/9780429020278-11

TABLE 8.1: Common Causes of Infectious Optic Neuropathies

Viruses

Herpes simplex virus 1 and 2
Varicella zoster virus
Cytomegalovirus
Epstein-Barr virus
Human immunodeficiency virus
West Nile virus
Chikungunya
Dengue
Measles
Mumps
Rubella

Bacteria

Mycobacterium tuberculosis
Bartonella henselae
Treponema pallidum
Borrelia burgdorferi
Bacillus anthracis
Tropheryma whipplei

Fungi

Aspergillus
Candida
Coccidioides
Cryptococcus
Mucor

Parasites

Toxocara
Toxoplasma

TABLE 8.2: Clinical Features Suggestive of Infectious Optic Neuropathy (1)

History of a recent infectious illness
Diabetes
Immunocompromised states (HIV/AIDS, medications that can suppress immunity)
Residents of developing countries/travel to endemic zones
Bilateral involvement
Presence of neuroretinitis
Involvement of other parts of nervous system (cerebillitis/meningio encephalitis)
Diseases of the paranasal sinuses, orbits or meninges

cases is usually bilateral. Papillitis, neuroretinitis, retrobulbar neuritis and involvement of optic chiasm all have been described.[11–13] Corticosteroids are often helpful in restoring the vision.[14]

Measles

Measles virus is an important cause of optic nerve and retinal involvement. Optic nerves are likely to be involved during acute measles infection as well in patients with subacute sclerosing panencephalitis (SSPE). The optic nerve can be involved approximately 1 week after febrile illness. Optic neuropathy is usually part of acute disseminated encephalomyelitis.[15] The optic neuropathy manifests either with papillitis or retrobulbar neuritis. Methyl prednisolone is treatment of choice. Majority of patients recover vision after treatment.

SSPE is a progressive brain disorder that is caused by a persistent mutated measles virus infection. SSPE is characterized by rapid cognitive decline, periodic myoclonic jerks and

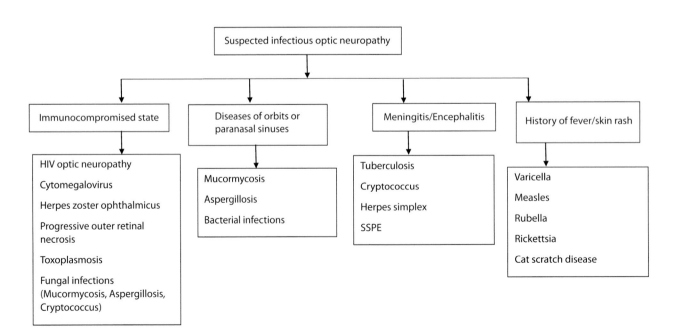

FIGURE 8.1 Approach to a case of infectious optic neuropathy.

TABLE 8.3: **Common Antibiotics Which Can Cause Optic Neuropathy**

Category	Drugs
Anti-bacterial agents	Linezolid, sulfonamides, chloramphenicol
Anti-tuberculosis drugs	Ethambutol, isoniazid
Anti-malarial drugs	Quinine, chloroquine

TABLE 8.4: **Investigations in Suspected Infectious Optic Neuropathy**

Complete blood count

Blood sugar

Serological testing of HIV/Syphilis

C-reactive protein, ESR

Blood culture

Chest X-ray

Examination of cerebrospinal fluid for protein, sugar, total and differential cell count.

Cerebrospinal fluid culture, GeneXpert for tuberculosis, India ink staining, fungal culture.

Cerebrospinal fluid for detection of antibodies against specific viruses.

Antibodies/PCR of aqueous or vitreous.

MRI brain with contrast including orbital cuts

raised antimeasles antibody titer in cerebrospinal fluid.[16] Up to 50% of the SSPE patients have ocular complications.[17] In some visual manifestations precedes neurological manifestations. Visual manifestations in SSPE are either because of the optic nerve, retina or the visual cortex involvement.[17–19] Necrotizing retinitis is the most common ocular manifestation in SSPE. The optic nerve involvement can manifest as papilledema, papillitis and optic atrophy.[17,18,20,21] Retinal changes may dominantly be present in macular region.[22] The involvement of cortex manifest with cortical blindness (Box 8.1).

CASE 1   OCULAR INVOLVEMENT IN SSPE

A 12-year-old boy presented with history of cognitive decline from last 5 months and recurrent falls from last 3 months. Parents also gave history that he has difficulty in seeing objects from his right eye. There was history suggestive of measles in early childhood.

On examination, periodic myoclonus was seen. Vision in the right eye was 6/36 and in the left eye was 6/6. Both the pupils were of normal size and showed normal reaction to light. Fundus examination was suggestive of slightly hyperaemic optic disc on the right side, there was a pale diffuse lesion temporal to the disc (retinitis) and a healed choroiditic patch inferonasally (Figure 8.2). Left fundus was normal. His EEG was suggestive of periodic discharges and cerebrospinal fluid and serum were positive for anti-measles antibodies. This case is an example of SSPE with ocular involvement.

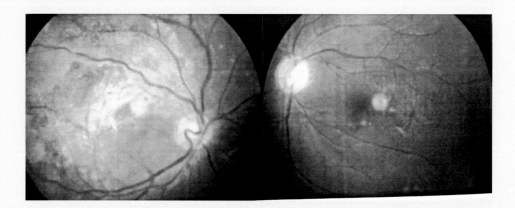

FIGURE 8.2   Fundus photograph of subacute sclerosing panencephalitis patient shows retinitis (a pale diffuse lesion) and a healed choroiditis. The left fundus is normal.

Human immunodeficiency virus

Vision involvement in HIV-infected patients can occur because of opportunistic infections. Human immunodeficiency virus can itself cause optic nerve damage. HIV-associated optic neuropathy can be unilateral or bilateral. It can manifest as papillitis, retro bulbar optic neuritis or optic atrophy.[23,24] HIV DNA had been demonstrated in the optic nerve.[25] HIV-associated optic neuropathy can be treated with anti-retroviral drugs.[24]

Dengue

Dengue virus is a flavivirus. *Aedes* mosquitos are responsible for its transmission in humans. The clinical spectrum of dengue fever ranges from mild self-limiting febrile disorder to severe life-threatening clinical syndromes, like dengue hemorrhagic fever and dengue shock syndrome. Ophthalmological complications, in dengue fever, occur in the form of subconjunctival hemorrhage, anterior uveitis, vitritis, retinal hemorrhages, retinochoroiditis, choroidal effusion, panophthalmitis and optic neuropathies.[26] The reported incidence of optic neuropathy in dengue is up to 1.5%.[27] Optic nerve involvement manifests with optic neuritis, optic disc swelling or neuroretinitis. Vision loss is often self-limiting.

Chikungunya

Chikungunya is also transmitted by bite of infected *Aedes* mosquitos. Clinical features of chikungunya infection are fever, headache, joint pain, myalgia, rash or sometimes multi-organ dysfunction. Ocular involvement is described in the form of uveitis, sclerites, retinitis, vitritis, retinal detachment and optic neuropathy. Optic neuropathy in chikungunya can occur at the time of acute infection. A direct viral infection or an immune-mediated damage of optic nerve are possible etiopatho genetic mechanisms. Corticosteroids are often used. The visual prognosis is generally good.[28]

Bacterial

Tuberculosis

Vision loss is a common complication of tuberculosis in South East Asia. Vision loss is seen both in pulmonary as well as in extrapulmonary tuberculosis. Tuberculous meningitis is the most frequent extrapulmonary tuberculosis that leads to vision impairment. Vision impairment occurs in approximately 25% tuberculous meningitis patients.[29] In tuberculous meningitis, a variety of causes are responsible for vision loss. Causes include tuberculous optic neuropathy, optico-chiasmatic arachnoiditis, compression by enlarging third ventricle, optic nerve tuberculoma and ethambutol toxicity. Tuberculous optic neuritis can occur as a result of direct *Mycobacterium tuberculosis* infection, Bacillus Calmette-Guerin vaccination or hypersensitivity reaction.[30] Tuberculous optic neuritis often presents with unilateral painless vision loss. Eye examination demonstrates papillitis along with neuroretinitis, optic nerve tubercle and papilledema.[31]

Tuberculous optochiasmatic arachnoiditis is a common complication of tuberculous meningitis that presents with profound vision loss. In optochiasmatic arachnoiditis, there is dominant affection of optic nerve and optic chiasm secondary to marked basal exudates and associated cranial arachnoiditis. Exudates are dominantly present in interpeduncular, suprasellar and sylvian cisterns. Optochiasmatic arachnoiditis can paradoxically develop, while anti-tuberculosis drugs are being administered. Neuroimaging demonstrates multiple enhancing lesions in basal cisterns, particularly in middle cranial fossa, along with intense basal meningeal enhancement. Tuberculous optochiasmatic arachnoiditis is usually with corticosteroids. Thalidomide, methylprednisolone and hyaluronidase have also been tried with variable success[32] (Box 8.2).

BOX 8.2   OPTOCHIASMATIC ARACHNOIDITIS IN TUBERCULOUS MENINGITIS

A young male presented with fever and headache for 2 months, and decreased visual acuity since last 15 days. On examination, meningeal signs were present. Vision was impaired in both the eyes, visual acuity was just perception of light in both eyes, and bilateral pupils were dilated and sluggishly reacting. Fundus examination was suggestive of bilateral optic atrophy. Examination of the cerebrospinal fluid revealed elevated protein, low sugar and lymphocytic pleocystosis. The cerebrospinal fluid was also subjected to GeneXpert MTB/RIF which was positive for mycobacterium tuberculosis. A contrast-enhanced MRI of the brain showed thick exudates and tuberculomas in the optochiasmatic areas (Figure 8.3). This is a typical case of tuberculous optochiasmatic arachnoiditis.

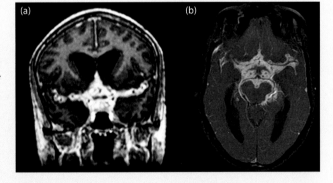

FIGURE 8.3   Contrast-enhanced magnetic resonance imaging of the brain shows thick basal exudates and tuberculomas in the optochiasmatic areas (a and b).

Syphilis

Ophthalmological manifestations are common in syphilis. Common eye complications are scleritis, panuveitis, dacryoadenitis, chorioretinitis, vitritis, keratitis, oculomotor palsies and optic neuropathy.[33] Ocular involvement is generally part of central nervous system involvement. The optic nerve in syphilis is involved in secondary or tertiary stages.[2] The syphilitic optic neuropathy can be unilateral or bilateral, often without involvement of the anterior segment.[2] Syphilitic optic neuropathy presents either as papillitis, chiasmal syndrome, neuroretinitis, optic nerve gumma or optic nerve perineuritis.[34–36] There can also be cortical vision loss. Appropriate tests for the diagnosis of ocular syphilis are fluorescent treponemal antibody absorption assay or the *Treponema pallidum* particle agglutination assay. The non-treponemal tests, like venereal disease research laboratory (VDRL), fail to diagnose late stages of syphilis.[37] Intravenous penicillin G is the drug of choice for all forms of syphilis. Intramuscular benzathine penicillin along with oral probenecid is another option. Newer treatment options include drugs with good cerebrospinal fluid penetration, like ceftriaxone and azithromycin.[38]

Leprosy

Leprosy can have a wide variety of ocular manifestations, like ulcerative keratitis, uveitis, dacryoadenitis, lagophthalmos, cataract and optic nerve damage.[39] The optic nerve damage in leprosy can manifest as papillitis or optic atrophy.[40,41] Treatment of leprosy involves multidrug therapy. Corticosteroids can be used if patient is having optic neuritis.[40]

Bartonellosis (cat-scratch disease)

Bartonella henselae is a gram-negative bacteria, which is known to cause the zoonotic cat-scratch disease.[42] The *Bartonella henselae* organism is transmitted by the infected cats, through bites, licks or abrasions.[42] The cat-scratch disease usually manifests with a flu-like syndrome along with tender lymphadenitis.[43] Ocular involvement is described in 5 to 10% of patients.[44] The ocular involvement in cat-scratch disease is common. There is a gap of about 4 weeks between inoculation and development of ocular complications. Neuroretinitis is the most common and most characteristic ocular complication.[45] Patients can have vision loss, RAPD, color desaturation and visual field abnormalities. The fundus examination shows optic disc edema along with macular star formation. In majority of patients, vision recovers following treatment.[46,47] The indirect fluorescent antibody test, enzyme-linked immunoassay (ELISA), Western blot and polymerase chain reaction (PCR)-based assays are used for the laboratory diagnosis.[42,43] The treatment guidelines are not clear. Usually patients are treated with doxycycline.[48] Alternatively, rifampicin, gentamycin, ciprofloxacin and trimethoprim-sulfamethoxazole have also been used.[49]

Lyme disease

Lyme disease is caused by the spirochete *Borrelia burgdorferi*. The organism spreads by bite of tick ixodes. Three clinical stages of Lyme disease have been described, namely localized, early and late disseminated stages.[50] Optic nerve involvement in Lyme disease usually occurs in early and late disseminated stages. Optic nerve involvement is often bilateral. Optic nerve involvement manifests with papilledema (secondary to meningitis), papillitis, neuroretinitis, optic chiasm involvement and optic atrophy. A two-step approach is required to diagnose Lyme disease. The first step involves the use of ELISA test. If ELISA test is positive, the diagnosis is confirmed by Western blot technique.[50] In patients with neurological involvement, CSF will show pleocytosis and intrathecal antibodies against the organism.[51] Lyme disease with central nervous system involvement is treated with intravenous ceftriaxone.[2]

Brucellosis

Brucellosis is caused by bacteria of *Brucella* species. Human brucellosis is a multisystem disease that can manifest acutely, sub acutely or in chronic course.[52] Ocular involvement is not very common. The ocular manifestations of brucellosis described in the literature are keratitis, uveitis, episcleritis, scleritis, endophthalmitis and optic neuropathy.[53,54] Optic nerve damage, in brucellosis, manifests with optic neuritis or papilledema. Optic nerve involvement is usually part of meningoencephalitis. The diagnosis of brucellosis requires a clinical suspicion along with microbiological confirmation. Brucellosis is treated with doxycycline and rifampicin.[52] The visual prognosis of treated cases is generally good.

Fungal

Cryptococcus

The fungus, *Cryptococcus neoformans*, the causative agent of cryptococcal meningitis, can cause optic neuropathy as well.[2] Cryptococcal meningitis commonly occurs in patients with immunocompromised states. Optic neuropathy may be part of cryptococcal meningitis. The optic neuropathy, in cryptococcal meningitis, results from direct fungal invasion. Other factors responsible for optic nerve damage are raised intracranial pressure and vasculitis of vasa nervorum.[55] A rapid vision loss is mostly attributed to direct infection or inflammation. Slow deterioration of vision is generally attributed to raise intracranial pressure.[56] Diagnosis of cryptococcal meningitis is made if India ink staining, antigen detection using latex agglutination method or culture of cerebrospinal fluid demonstrates the fungus. Treatment requires a combination of amphotericin B and flucytosine/fluconazole. Optic nerve sheath fenestration can be tried in selected patients.

Mucormycosis

Mucormycosis is caused by a group of fungi called mucormycetes. The fungus genera that most frequent affects the human host includes *Mucor, Rhizopus, Absidia* and *Cunninghamella*.[57] This opportunistic fungal infection is mainly seen in uncontrolled diabetic and immunocompromised subjects. Mucormycosis presents as rhino-orbital-cerebral disease. The common clinical features are headache, fever, facial pain and swelling, orbital swelling and proptosis, restricted eye movements and vision loss secondary to optic nerve involvement. Mucormycosis causes infarction or necrosis of the optic nerve.[58,59] Direct invasion of the optic nerve may also occur. Treatment of mucormycosis involves prolonged administration of amphotericin B. Extensive surgical debridement of involved sinuses and orbit are required in many cases[57] (Box 8.3).

BOX 8.3   OPTIC NERVE INVOLVEMENT IN RHINO-ORBITAL MUCORMYCOSIS

A known case of uncontrolled type 2 diabetes mellitus presented with complaints of decreased vision of left eye along with orbital swelling and redness. On examination, vision in left eye was just perception of light, left pupil was dilated and left fundus was hyperaemic. There was also evidence of cranial nerve III, IV, V and VI involvement. The left eye was also swollen and chemosed. Clinically, a diagnosis of left orbital apex syndrome was made.

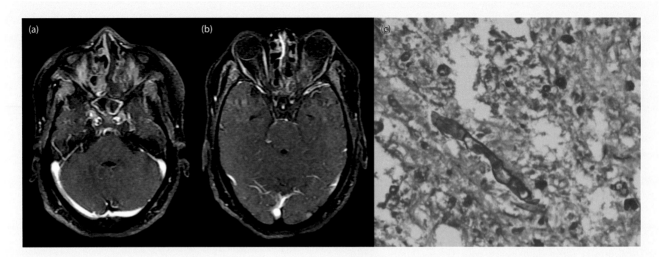

FIGURE 8.4 Contrast-enhanced magnetic resonance imaging shows abnormal contrast enhancement of the paranasal sinuses and left orbital apex (a and b). Hematoxylin and eosin staining show fungal hyphae (c).

MRI of the brain was suggestive of sinusitis and contrast enhancement in left orbital apex and left cavernous sinus. A diagnostic nasal endoscopy was performed; the scraped material was suggestive of fungal hyphae (Figure 8.4).

This classical case suggests that one should think of a fungal etiology whenever dealing with orbital apex/cavernous sinus syndrome in diabetic patient.

Aspergillosis

Aspergillosis is also common in immune compromised state. Aspergillosis varies from noninvasive form to life-threatening invasive form. Optic nerve involvement occurs as a result of extension from aspergillus rhino-sinusitis. Patient presents with facial pain, orbital swelling, rhinorrhea, vision loss and restricted eye movements. Multiple cranial nerves are frequently involved. Aspergillosis can also cause dacryocystitis, periorbital cellulitis, endophthalmitis and vitritis. Definite diagnosis requires biopsy. Microscopic examination shows branching and septate hyphae.[60] Management of invasive rhino orbital aspergillosis requires surgical debridement along with antifungal therapy. Voriconazole is the drug of choice.[60]

Parasitic

Toxoplasmosis

Toxoplasma gondii is an intracellular parasite that affects immunocompromised hosts. Ocular toxoplasmosis typically presents with unifocal retino-choriditis.[2] Other ocular manifestations include multifocal retino-choriditis, scleritis, retinitis and uveitis.[61] Optic nerve involvement manifests with reactive optic disc hyperemia, neuroretinitis, papillitis and isolated anterior optic neuritis.[2,62] Prompt clinical suspicion is needed for an early diagnosis of toxoplasmosis. A positive anti-toxoplasma IgG antibody assay does not confirm the diagnosis; however, a negative serology rules out the possibility of toxoplasmosis. Western blot techniques can be used for antibody detection in aqueous or vitreous humor. A PCR test is used for demonstration of *Toxoplasma* DNA in ocular fluid.[2] A combination of anti-parasitic treatment along with corticosteroids is used for the treatment. The standard anti-parasitic treatment includes pyrimethamine plus sulfadiazine along with folinic acid.[61] Overall visual prognosis, after treatment, is generally good.[62]

Neurocysticercosis

Neurocysticercosis is a common parasitic infection of the brain. In many cases of neurocysticercosis, optic nerve may be involved. Papilledema, chiasmal and retrochiasmal lesions can cause optic nerve damage. Optic nerve may get compressed with enlarging hydrocephalus and raised intracranial pressure.[63] Patients with orbital cysticercosis present with eye pain, proptosis and vision loss. Diagnosis of orbital or ocular cysticercosis is made by orbital sonography. Frequently, orbital neurocysticercosis is part of disseminated neurocysticercosis. Demonstration of scolex within the cysts is pathognomonic of neurocysticercosis. Currently, surgical removal of ocular cysticercosis is the treatment of choice.[64] In some reports, albendazole and corticosteroids were found effective.[65]

Conclusion

A variety of infections, including bacteria, viruses and fungi, can cause optic nerve damage. A direct invasion of the optic nerve by the organism or by the spread of infection from the adjacent structures like meninges, paranasal sinuses and orbits are common pathogenic mechanisms. In setting of recent infection, optic neuropathies can also occur as parainfectious process. Common clinical features are loss of vision, color desaturation, loss of visual field and RAPD. Fever, rash, recent infection, immunocompromised states, uncontrolled diabetes mellitus, simultaneous bilateral involvement, neuroretinitis and presence of a neurological syndrome like multiple cranial nerve palsies are additional features which should lead to a suspicion of infectious optic neuropathy (Table 8.5). A high index of suspicion is needed as timely treatment can lead to the restoration of vision.

TABLE 8.5: Summary of Clinical Features, Diagnosis and Management of Various Infectious Optic Neuropathies

Infectious Agent	Typical Features	History/Examination	Diagnosis	Treatment	Prognosis
Herpes simplex	Optic neuropathy can occur with or without concurrent herpes simplex encephalitis. Optic neuropathy is often associated with acute retinal necrosis syndrome.	Vision loss Floaters Ocular inflammation. Focal areas of retinal necrosis, vitritis and inflammation of anterior chamber. Neuroretinitis Papillitis	Clinical features PCR of vitreous biopsy is confirmatory	Acyclovir 10 mg/kg, three times a day for about 2 weeks. Steroids may be added after 2 days	Prognosis of untreated cases is very poor.
Varicella zoster	Optic neuropathy can occur along with herpes zoster ophthalmicus. It can be associated with involvement of anterior segment, retinitis and vitritis. Acute retinal necrosis syndrome or progressive outer retinal necrosis can occur. Parainfectious optic neuropathy can occur 2 to 6 weeks after chickenpox.	Unilateral or Bilateral vision loss Papillitis Associated vitritis, foci of retinal necrosis	Clinical features suggestive of herpes zoster History of recent chickenpox PCR of CSF, serum and ocular fluid	Retinitis/optic neuritis associated with herpes zoster: Acyclovir 10 mg/kg three times a day for 2 weeks. Parainfectious optic neuropathy: steroids	Prognosis of treated patients is fair. Prognosis of PORN is very poor.
Cytomegalovirus	Associated with HIV/AIDS Typically causes hemorrhagic retinitis Optic neuropathy can occur with or without retinitis	Vision loss Hemorrhagic retinitis Retrobulbar neuritis Optic atrophy	Clinical setting of HIV/AIDS PCR of CSF/serum/ocular fluid	Gancyclovir and foscarnet	Prognosis of untreated cases is poor.
Epstein-Barr virus	Parainfectious optic neuropathy	Vision loss RAPD Papillitis Retrobulbar neuritis Involvement of optic chiasm	Clinical settings EBV serology	Intravenous or oral corticosteroids	Usually good
Measles	Optic neuropathy can occur in the setting of acute measles infection (parainfectious optic neuropathy, can occur along with encephalomyelitis) as well as SSPE.	Vision loss Retrobulbar neuritis If associated with SSPE, cortical vision loss, chorioretinitis, papilledema, papillitis and optic atrophy	Clinical settings CSF anti-measles antibodies	Parainfectious optic neuropathy associated with acute measles can be treated with corticosteroids.	Parainfectious optic neuropathy: good prognosis. Ocular involvement in SSPE: bad prognosis.
HIV	Vision involvement can occur due to direct infection of optic nerve with HIV virus.	Retrobulbar optic neuropathy, papillitis, ischemic optic neuropathy, optic disc pallor	ELISA HIV, other opportunistic infections that can cause vision loss must be ruled out	Anti-retroviral drugs	Guarded
Mycobacterium tuberculosis	Tuberculous optic neuropathy occurs commonly in the setting of tuberculous meningitis. Commonly there is involvement of optic chiasm along with the optic nerve due to inflammation of arachnoid matter; known as optochiasmatic arachnoiditis.	Unilateral or bilateral progressive vision loss Abnormal pupillary reaction. Optic atrophy Signs and symptoms of meningitis	CSF GeneXpert. CSF culture for tuberculosis CSF will show raised protein, low sugar and lymphocytic pleocytosis Evidence of tuberculosis elsewhere Typical neuroimaging abnormalities	Antituberculosis treatment along with corticosteroids	Guarded

(Continued)

TABLE 8.5: Summary of Clinical Features, Diagnosis and Management of Various Infectious Optic Neuropathies *(Continued)*

Infectious Agent	Typical Features	History/Examination	Diagnosis	Treatment	Prognosis
Syphilis	Optic nerve involvement occurs in tertiary or secondary stage. Optic nerve involvement is commonly seen along with central nervous system involvement.	Unilateral or bilateral vision loss. Optic atrophy Neuroretinitis scleritis, panuveitis, dacryoadenitis, chorioretinitis, vitritis, keratitis, oculomotor palsies	Fluorescent treponemal antibody absorption assay or the treponema pallidum particle agglutination assay	Intravenous penicillin G	Timely treatment can improve vision.
Leprosy	Optic nerve involvement in leprosy can be associated with other ocular features like involvement of the cornea, uveitis, dacryoadenitis, lagophthalmos, cataract, involvement of the eyelids.	Vision loss Optic atrophy papillitis	Clinical Skin biopsy Nerve biopsy	Rifampicin Dapsone Clofazimine Corticosteroids	
Bartonella henselae	Neuroretinitis is the most common and most characteristic ocular manifestation of cat scratch disease.	Vision loss Field loss RAPD Optic disc edema along with macular star formation is seen	The indirect fluorescent antibody test, enzyme-linked immunoassay, Western blot, and polymerase chain reaction-based assays	Doxycycline 100 mg twice a day for 4–6 weeks	Good
Lyme disease	Optic nerve involvement occurs in early and late disseminated stages.	Unilateral or bilateral vision loss. Papilledema, papillitis, neuroretinitis, optic atrophy	Serology. ELISA followed by Western blot. CSF: intrathecal antibodies	Ceftriaxone 2 g per day for at least 3 weeks	Good
Brucellosis	Optic neuropathy can occur in the form of optic neuritis or papilledema.	Unilateral or bilateral vision loss History of fever, travel to endemic area, exposure to cattle Associated meningitis	Clinical suspicion, blood culture, serology	Rifampicin plus doxycycline for 6 weeks plus steroids	Good
Cryptococcus neoformans	Optic neuropathy is usually seen in patients suffering from meningitis.	Acute vision loss, or insidious vision loss Papilledema	India ink staining of CSF, antigen detection using a latex agglutination method or culture of CSF	Amphotericin B along with flucytosine/ fluconazole. Optic nerve fenestration	Treated cases can have vision recovery
Mucormycosis	Commonly seen in diabetes and immunocompromised individuals. Optic nerve involvement occurs as a part of rhino-orbital-cerebral disease.	Orbital pain, swelling. Combination of II, III, IV, V and VI cranial nerve palsies	KOH staining and fungal culture of biopsy taken from nasal sinuses	Prolonged course of amphoteric B along with extensive surgical debridement	Poor

Multiple-Choice Questions

1. Which of the following clinical features can suggest a possibility of infectious optic neuropathy?
   a. Presence of neuro-retinitis
   b. Bilateral involvement
   c. Concomitant infection of paranasal sinuses
   d. All of the above

   Answer:
   d. All of the above

2. Which of the following drugs can cause optic neuropathy?
   a. Linezolid
   b. Ethambutol
   c. Quinine
   d. All of the above

   Answer:
   d. All of the above

3. Which of the following viruses is associated with optic neuropathy?
   a. Herpes simplex
   b. CMV
   c. Measles
   d. All of the above

   Answer:

   d. All of the above

4. Which of the following anti-tuberculous drugs can lead to optic neuropathy?
   a. Ethambutol
   b. Streptomycin
   c. Pyrazinamide
   d. Rifampicin

   Answer:

   a. Ethambutol

References

1. Weerasinghe D, Lueck C. Mimics and chameleons of optic neuritis. Pract Neurol. 2016;16(2):96–110.
2. Kahloun R, Abroug N, Ksiaa I, Mahmoud A, Zeghidi H, Zaouali S, Khairallah M. Infectious optic neuropathies: A clinical update. Eye Brain. 2015;7:59.
3. Lau CH, Missotten T, Salzmann J, Lightman SL. Acute retinal necrosis features, management, and outcomes. Ophthalmology. 2007;114(4):756–762.
4. Witmer MT, Pavan PR, Fouraker BD, Levy-Clarke GA. Acute retinal necrosis associated optic neuropathy. Acta Ophthalmol (Copenh). 2011;89(7):599–607.
5. Sergott RC, Belmont JB, Savino PJ, Fischer DH, Bosley TM, Schatz NJ. Optic nerve involvement in the acute retinal necrosis syndrome. Arch Ophthalmol. 1985;103(8):1160–1162.
6. Miller DH, Kay R, Schon F, McDonald WI, Haas LF, Hughes RA. Optic neuritis following chickenpox in adults. J Neurol. 1986;233(3):182–184.
7. Wang AG, Liu JH, Hsu WM, Lee AF, Yen MY. Optic neuritis in herpes zoster ophthalmicus. Jpn J Ophthalmol. 2000;44(5):550–554.
8. Engstrom RE, Holland GN, Margolis TP, Muccioli C, Lindley JI, Belfort R, et al. The progressive outer retinal necrosis syndrome. A variant of necrotizing herpetic retinopathy in patients with AIDS. Ophthalmology. 1994;101(9):1488–1502.
9. Gross JG, Sadun AA, Wiley CA, Freeman WR. Severe visual loss related to isolated peripapillary retinal and optic nerve head cytomegalovirus infection. Am J Ophthalmol. 1989;108(6):691–698.
10. Patel SS, Rutzen AR, Marx JL, Thach AB, Chong LP, Rao NA. Cytomegalovirus papillitis in patients with acquired immune deficiency syndrome. Visual prognosis of patients treated with ganciclovir and/or foscarnet. Ophthalmology. 1996;103(9):1476–1482.
11. Anderson MD, Kennedy CA, Lewis AW, Christensen GR. Retrobulbar neuritis complicating acute Epstein-Barr virus infection. Clin Infect Dis. 1994;18(5):799–801.
12. Frey T. Optic neuritis in children infectious mononucleosis as an etiology. Doc Ophthalmol Adv Ophthalmol. 1973;34(1):183–188.
13. Beiran I, Krasnitz I, Zimhoni-Eibsitz M, Gelfand YA, Miller B. Paediatric chiasmal neuritis—typical of post-Epstein-Barr virus infection? Acta Ophthalmol Scand. 2000;78(2):226–227.
14. Jones J, Gardner W, Newman T. Severe optic neuritis in infectious mononucleosis. Ann Emerg Med. 1988;17(4):361–364.
15. Azuma M, Morimura Y, Kawahara S, Okada AA. Bilateral anterior optic neuritis in adult measles infection without encephalomyelitis. Am J Ophthalmol. 2002;134(5):768–769.
16. Garg RK. Subacute sclerosing panencephalitis. J Neurol. 2008;255(12):1861–1871.
17. Zagami AS, Lethlean AK. Chorioretinitis as a possible very early manifestation of subacute sclerosing panencephalitis. Aust N Z J Med. 1991;21(3):350–352.
18. Serdaroğlu A, Gücüyener K, Dursun I, Aydin K, Okuyaz C, M. Subaşi, M, et al. Macular retinitis as a first sign of subacute sclerosing panencephalitis: the importance of early diagnosis. Ocul Immunol Inflamm. 2005;13(5):405–410.
19. Senbil N, Aydin OF, Orer H, Gürer YKY. Subacute sclerosing panencephalitis: A cause of acute vision loss. Pediatr Neurol. 2004;31(3):214–217.
20. Zako M, Kataoka T, Ohno-Jinno A, Inoue Y, Kon M, Iwaki M. Analysis of progressive ophthalmic lesion in a patient with subacute sclerosing panencephalitis. Eur J Ophthalmol. 2008;18(1):155–158.
21. Berker N, Batman C, Guven A, Ozalp S, Aslan O, Zilelioglu O. Optic atrophy and macular degeneration as initial presentations of subacute sclerosing panencephalitis. Am J Ophthalmol. 2004;138(5):879–881.
22. Colpak AI, Erdener SE, Ozgen B, Anlar B, Kansu T. Neuro-ophthalmology of subacute sclerosing panencephalitis: Two cases and a review of the literature. Curr Opin Ophthalmol. 2012;23:466–471.
23. Larsen M, Toft PB, Bernhard P, Herning M. Bilateral optic neuritis in acute human immunodeficiency virus infection. Acta Ophthalmol Scand. 1998;76(6):737–738.
24. Goldsmith P, Jones RE, Ozuzu GE, Richardson J, Ong EL. Optic neuropathy as the presenting feature of HIV infection: recovery of vision with highly active antiretroviral therapy. Br J Ophthalmol. 2000;84(5):551–553.
25. Sadun AA, Pepose JS, Madigan MC, Laycock KA, Tenhula WN, Freeman WR. AIDS-related optic neuropathy: a histological, virological and ultrastructural study. Graefes Arch Clin Exp Ophthalmol. 1995;233(7):387–398.
26. Beral L, Merle H, David T. Ocular complications of dengue fever. Ophthalmology. 2008;115:1100–1101.
27. Ng AW, Teoh SC. Dengue eye disease. Surv Ophthalmol. 2015;60:106–114.
28. Khairallah M, Kahloun R. Ocular manifestations of emerging infectious diseases. Curr Opin Ophthalmol. 2013;24:574–580.
29. Sinha MK, Garg RK, Anuradha HK, Agarwal A, Singh MK, Verma R, et al. Vision impairment in tuberculous meningitis: Predictors and prognosis. J Neurol Sci. 2010;290(1–2):27–32.
30. Saxena R, Singh D. Tuberculous optic neuropathy. In: Kumar A, Chawla R, and Sharma N, editors. Ocular Tuberculosis [Internet]. Cham: Springer International Publishing; 2017. pp. 95–99.
31. Davis EJ, Rathinam SR, Okada AA, Tow SL, Petrushkin H, Graham EM, et al. Clinical spectrum of tuberculous optic neuropathy. J Ophthalmic Inflamm Infect. 2012;2(4):183–189.
32. Garg RK, Paliwal V, Malhotra HS. Tuberculous optochiasmatic arachnoiditis: A devastating form of tuberculous meningitis. Expert Rev Anti Infect Ther. 2011;9(9):719–729.
33. Peeling RW, Hook EW. The pathogenesis of syphilis: The Great Mimicker, revisited. J Pathol. 2006;208(2):224–232.
34. Smith GT, Goldmeier D, Migdal C. Neurosyphilis with optic neuritis: an update. Postgrad Med J. 2006;82(963):36–39.
35. Parker SE, Pula JH. Neurosyphilis presenting as asymptomatic optic perineuritis. Case Rep Ophthalmol Med. 2012;2012:621872.
36. Smith JL, Byrne SF, Cambron CR. Syphiloma/gumma of the optic nerve and human immunodeficiency virus seropositivity. J Clin Neuroophthalmol. 1990;10(3):175–184.
37. Gaudio PA. Update on ocular syphilis. Curr Opin Ophthalmol. 2006;17(6):562–566.
38. Jay CA. Treatment of neurosyphilis. Curr Treat Options Neurol. 2006;8(3):185–192.
39. Parikh R, Thomas S, Muliyil J, Parikh S, Thomas R. Ocular manifestation in treated multibacillary Hansen's disease. Ophthalmology. 2009;116(11):2051–2057.
40. Lee S-B, Lee E-K, Kim J-Y. Bilateral optic neuritis in leprosy. Can J Ophthalmol. 2009;44(2):219–220.
41. Prabha N, Mahajan VK, Sharma SK, Sharma V, Chauhan PS, Mehta KS, et al. Optic nerve involvement in a borderline lepromatous leprosy patient on multidrug therapy. Lepr Rev. 2013;84(4):316–321.
42. Cunningham ET, Koehler JE. Ocular bartonellosis. Am J Ophthalmol. 2000;130(3):340–349.
43. Biancardi AL, Curi ALL. Cat-scratch disease. Ocul Immunol Inflamm. 2014;22(2):148–154.
44. Carithers HA. Cat-scratch disease. An overview based on a study of 1,200 patients. Am J Dis Child 1960. 1985;139(11):1124–1133.
45. Reed JB, Scales DK, Wong MT, Lattuada CP, Dolan MJ, Schwab IR. Bartonella henselae neuroretinitis in cat scratch disease. Diagnosis, management, and sequelae. Ophthalmology. 1998;105(3):459–466.
46. Chi SL, Stinnett S, Eggenberger E, Foroozan R, Golnik K, Lee MS, et al. Clinical characteristics in 53 patients with cat scratch optic neuropathy. Ophthalmology. 2012;119(1):183–187.
47. Solley WA, Martin DF, Newman NJ, King R, Callanan DG, Zacchei T, et al. Cat scratch disease: Posterior segment manifestations. Ophthalmology. 1999;106(8):1546–1553.
48. Rolain JM, Brouqui P, Koehler JE, Maguina C, Dolan MJ, Raoult D. Recommendations for treatment of human infections caused by Bartonella species. Antimicrob Agents Chemother. 2004;48(6):1921–1933.
49. Margileth AM. Antibiotic therapy for cat-scratch disease: clinical study of therapeutic outcome in 268 patients and a review of the literature. Pediatr Infect Dis J. 1992;11(6):474–478.
50. Hu LT. Lyme disease. Ann Intern Med. 2016;164(9):ITC65–ITC80.
51. Stanek G, Wormser GP, Gray J, Strle F. Lyme borreliosis. Lancet. 2012;379(9814):461–473.
52. Mantur BG, Amarnath SK, Shinde RS. Review of clinical and laboratory features of human brucellosis. Indian J Med Microbiol. 2007;25(3):188–202.
53. Güngür K, Bekir NA, Namiduru M. Ocular complications associated with brucellosis in an endemic area. Eur J Ophthalmol. 2002;12(3):232–237.
54. Abd Elrazak M. Brucella optic neuritis. Arch Intern Med. 1991;151(4):776–778.
55. Cohen DB, Glasgow BJ. Bilateral optic nerve cryptococcosis in sudden blindness in patients with acquired immune deficiency syndrome. Ophthalmology. 1993;100(11):1689–1694.
56. Rex JH, Larsen RA, Dismukes WE, Cloud GA, Bennett JE. Catastrophic visual loss due to cryptococcus neoformans meningitis. Medicine. 1993;72(4):207–224.
57. Nithyanandam S, Jacob MS, Battu RR, Thomas RK, Correa MA, D'Souza O. Rhino-orbito-cerebral mucormycosis. A retrospective analysis of clinical features and treatment outcomes. Indian J Ophthalmol. 2003;51(3):231–236.
58. Mathur S, Karimi A, Mafee MF. Acute optic nerve infarction demonstrated by diffusion-weighted imaging in a case of rhinocerebral mucormycosis. Am J Neuroradiol. 2007;28(3):489–490.
59. Lee BL, Holland GN, Glasgow BJ. Chiasmal infarction and sudden blindness caused by mucormycosis in AIDS and diabetes mellitus. Am J Ophthalmol. 1996;122(6):895–896.
60. Cadena J, Thompson GR, Patterson TF. Invasive aspergillosis: Current strategies for diagnosis and management. Infect Dis Clin North Am. 2016;30(1):125–142.
61. Vasconcelos-Santos DV. Ocular manifestations of systemic disease: Toxoplasmosis. Curr Opin Ophthalmol. 2012;23(6):543–550.
62. Eckert GU, Melamed J, Menegaz B. Optic nerve changes in ocular toxoplasmosis. Eye. 2007;21(6):746–751.
63. Chang GY, Keane JR. Visual loss in cysticercosis: Analysis of 23 patients. Neurology. 2001;57(3):545–548.
64. White AC, Coyle CM, Rajshekhar V, Singh G, Hauser WA, Mohanty A, et al. Diagnosis and treatment of neurocysticercosis: 2017 clinical practice guidelines by the Infectious Diseases Society of America (IDSA) and the American Society of Tropical Medicine and Hygiene (ASTMH). Clin Infect Dis. 2018;66(8):1159–1163.
65. Bajaj MS, Pushker N. Optic nerve cysticercosis. Clin Experiment Ophthalmol. 2002;30(2):140–143.

9

ISCHEMIC OPTIC NEUROPATHIES

Amod Gupta

CASE STUDY

A 50-year-old male, known diabetic and hypertensive, presented with history of visual loss from his right eye upon waking up. The visual loss progressed to 6/24 over a period of 2 days. During these 2 days, the patient appreciated that he was not able to identify objects placed in inferior hemifield of his right eye. The patient denied any pain in eye or head. History of similar episode was present in the left eye 2 years ago. What is the probable diagnosis?

Assessment of a patient presenting with acute vision loss

As discussed in previous chapters, any patient presenting to the ophthalmology emergency or the outpatient service with visual complaints needs to have a quick assessment of the visual loss to draw a differential diagnosis and assess the urgency for intervention to prevent further loss of vision in the ipsilateral eye or the contralateral eye. Similar protocol should be followed in patients with suspected ischemic optic neuropathies (ION). As a quick recap, the history and examination should address the following questions:

1. What is the age/gender of the patient?
2. When did they notice a disturbance in vision? Was it on waking up?
3. Is there any history of myopia or eye surgery?
4. Is the visual loss confined to one eye or both eyes?
5. Is the vision loss painless or painful?
6. Does the eye hurt on moving?
7. What is the severity of visual loss?
8. Was the onset of the symptoms gradual or sudden?
9. What was the course of the vision loss? Was it transient, progressive or remained static since the onset?
10. Was the onset accompanied by headache or pain behind the eyes?
11. What is the medical condition of the patient? Does the patient have any systemic symptoms of fatigue, weight loss and low-grade fever? Is the patient known case of diabetes, hypertension, coronary arterial disease (CAD) or any other systemic disease for which she might be under treatment?
12. Are they a smoker?
13. Do they snore at night?

Let us consider two common case scenarios of acute visual loss presenting to a neuroophthalmologist.

CASE SCENARIO 1

The first clinical scenario is of acute vision loss in male patient above the age of 50 who on waking up in the morning discovers that he has painless progressive blurring of vision or already has a gross loss of vision in one eye. There is no pain on moving the eyes. He is a known diabetic with controlled/uncontrolled hypertension and has smoked in the past. His wife often complains that she is disturbed by his snoring at night. The vision has not recovered since onset.

Quick differential diagnosis in this setting would include a retinal branch or central retinal vein occlusion and ischemic optic neuropathy. Others, less likely though, would include vitreous hemorrhage, a branch or central retinal artery occlusion and retinal detachment.

CASE SCENARIO 2

Another less common case scenario is a woman aged 65 who developed sudden severe loss of vision in one eye accompanied by a severe headache on the ipsilateral side. The patient had been complaining of low-grade fever for several days, not eating well, was easily fatigued and had had difficulty in chewing. She may have had transient obscurations of vision in the past several days.

This patient is most likely to have an ischemic optic neuropathy due to giant cell arteritis that led to an arteritic anterior ischemic optic neuropathy. This is an emergency and no time should be lost as the patient, if left untreated, runs a serious risk of losing vision in the contralateral eye as well.

Common differentials in a patient presenting with acute visual loss are ischemic and inflammatory/demyelinating optic neuropathy (ON). Table 9.1 provides quick clues to the diagnosis of these commonly presenting ON.

Important consideration of the blood supply of the optic nerve head[1]

A brief recap of the blood supply of the optic nerve would help in understanding the ischemic insult to the optic nerve head (Figure 9.1). The anterior-most layer of the optic nerve head, consisting entirely of the retinal nerve fibers as they converge from all over the retina, is supplied by branches from the central retinal artery, the temporal aspect may be supplied by branches of the posterior ciliary artery (PCA) coming from the

DOI: 10.1201/9780429020278-12

TABLE 9.1: Acute Visual Loss due to Optic Neuropathies: Quick Clues to Diagnosis and Treatment

Risk Factor	NA-AION	A-AION	Optic Neuritis
Age	>50 years	>65 years	<50 years
Gender	M > F	F > M	F >> M
Onset	Acute	Acute	Acute
Pain	No	Temporal headache	Retrobulbar pain on moving the eye
Occurrence	10/100,000 population 90% of optic neuropathies	<6% of optic neuropathies	8/100,000 population
Laterality	Unilateral	Unilateral; progress to bilateral 50%	Unilateral, the other eye may get involved
Systemic associations	DM, hypertension, OSA	Giant cell arteritis	Multiple sclerosis
Systemic symptoms	Non-specific	Fatigue, loss of weight, Jaw claudication, temporal headache, temporal tenderness	Ptosis, diplopia, gaze palsy; nystagmus; INO
Visual acuity	6/6 to 6/60	CF-NLP	6/6 to CF
Pupil reactions	RAPD	RAPD	RAPD
Fundus	ODE with hyperemia	Chalky white optic disc	OD may be normal to mild ODE
Visual fields	Inferior nasal/inferior altitudinal defect/central scotomas Respect horizontal meridian	May not be possible Remaining island of vision Altitudinal Respect horizontal meridian	Central/centrocecal scotomas
Imaging study	FFA	FFA	CE MRI
Labs		ESR; C-reactive proteins	AQP4 antibody
Treatment	Corticosteroids +	IV corticosteroids IMT Biologicals	IV corticosteroids

Abbreviations: NA-AION, non-arteritic anterior ischemic optic neuropathy; A-AION, arteritic anterior ischemic optic neuropathy; CF, counting fingers; DM, diabetes mellitus; OSA, obstructive sleep apnea; INO, internuclear ophthalmoplegia; NLP, no light perception; RAPD, relative afferent pupillary defect; ODE, optic disc edema; OD, optic disc; FFA, fundus fluorescein angiography; CE, contrast-enhanced; ESR, erythrocyte sedimentation rate; AQP4 antibody, aquaporin4 antibody; IV, intravenous.

prelaminar region. The prelaminar part is supplied by centripetal branches from the peripapillary choroid, which in turn are drawn mainly from the short PCAs. There is no participation of blood supply from either the choriocapillaris or the central retinal artery in the prelaminar region. The peripapillary choroid that lies between the optic disc margin and the entry site of the short PCAs is a low-pressure system and vulnerable to hemodynamic variations. The laminar part has a rich capillary plexus and gets its blood supply from the centripetal branches from the short PCAs or from the circle of Zinn-Haller whenever present.

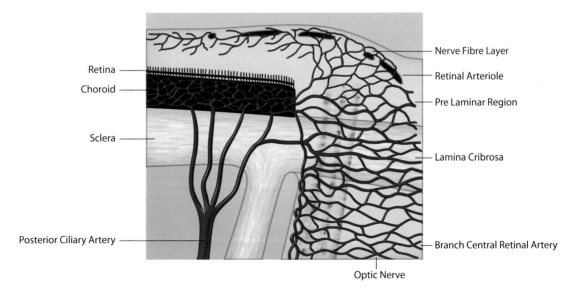

Retina

Choroid

Sclera

Posterior Ciliary Artery

Nerve Fibre Layer

Retinal Arteriole

Pre Laminar Region

Lamina Cribrosa

Branch Central Retinal Artery

Optic Nerve

FIGURE 9.1 Blood supply of the optic nerve head. Schematic representation of blood supply of the optic nerve head. (Reproduced with permission from Hayreh and Publishers. *Glaucoma: Conceptions of a Disease, Pathogenesis, Diagnosis and Therapy.* Eds: Klaus Heilmann and Kenneth T. Richardson. 1978. Georg Thieme Stuttgart.)

Circle of Zinn-Haller is believed to have strict superior and inferior distribution.

The retrolaminar part is supplied by centripetal vessels from the pial plexus formed by recurrent branches from the circle of Zinn-Haller if present or the short PCAs. In addition, pial branches from the central retinal artery also contribute.

Watershed zone
Another aspect of the blood supply is the end-arterial nature of the short post-ciliary arteries right up to the choroidal arterioles. Each PCA supplies a defined sector of the choroid. The area between the two PCAs becomes the watershed zone. An individual has a variable number of the PCAs with a variable site of entry into the choroid. Hence the location of the watershed zone varies. The watershed zone may lie temporal to the peripapillary choroid, nasal to it or the optic disc itself may lie in this zone.

Ischemic optic neuropathies

IONs or stroke of the eye/optic nerve are not infrequent in the ophthalmology clinic presenting with the sudden loss of vision in apparently healthy old individuals. Unlike the inflammatory or demyelinating optic neuropathies that affect the young, the ischemic optic neuropathies occur above the age of 50 years and result from vascular insufficiency. This may be either due to fall in perfusion pressure (non-arteritic anterior ischemic optic neuropathy [NA-AION]) or occlusion of the posterior ciliary arteries (arteritic-anterior ischemic optic neuropathy [A-AION]) that are the main source of blood supply to the optic nerve head. Depending on the anatomical location, vascular insufficiency may result in an anterior ischemic optic neuropathy (AION) or a posterior ischemic optic neuropathy (PION). Table 9.2 gives a broad classification of types of ION.

Clues to diagnose ION
Examination to reach the diagnosis of ION
A brief and quick recap of the correct techniques to record visual acuity, pupil reactions and confrontation visual fields should be done in order since the diagnosis of ischemic optic neuropathies is clinical and can be made correctly only if the following tests are performed in a correct sequence. Once the examining physician has a working differential diagnosis or suspicion of ION in her mind, she should proceed with a systematic ocular examination to reach the clinical diagnosis.

After a quick glance at the face for any gross abnormalities, head posture, gross external eye and adnexal appearance and eye movements, the examiner should proceed to record the visual acuity, pupil reactions and confrontation visual fields in that order (also refer Chapters 1 and 2).

Visual acuity assessment:[2] The commonly available Snellen visual acuity chart is placed at a distance of 6 meters (20 feet).

TABLE 9.2: Classification of ION

a. Anterior ischemic ON
   i. Arteritic AION (A-AION)
   ii. Non-arteritic AION (NA-AION)
b. Posterior ischemic ON
   i. Peri-operative PION
   ii. Arteritic PION
   iii. Non-arteritic PION

Visual acuity (VA) is tested one eye at a time with the other eye occluded. The patient should wear her own glasses if available.

Pupil reactions:[2] Pupil reactions are one of the most critical clinical examinations for patients with optic neuropathies. Pupil reactions are checked in a semi-dark room, patient looking into the distance, a bright pen torch light is shone into the eye from slightly below or temporal away from the visual axis for a duration of 3 seconds and quickly moved to the other eye. The procedure is repeated several times until the examiner is sure of the pupil response. This is known as the swinging flashlight test. Normally as the light is shone into each eye by turn the pupils in both eyes shrink. However, if there is a conduction defect in one of the eyes or there is asymmetric optic nerve involvement, as the light is shone into the abnormal/or more abnormal eye, pupils start dilating in both eyes. The eye is then recorded as having a relative afferent pupillary defect (RAPD).

Confrontation visual field:[2] As a commonly done bedside technique, confrontation test provides a quick clue to the possible site of the pathology in the visual pathways. Sitting at a distance of 1 meter, the examiner compares her own field of vision with that of the patient, asking the patient to count fingers in each of the four quadrants of the visual field.

Neuro-ophthalmological investigations to reach the diagnosis of ION
Perimetry and fundus fluorescein angiography (FFA) can give us a fair idea of the involvement of the abnormalities of blood supply of retina and the anterior part of the optic disc.

Perimetry: Visual field defects are important criteria for the diagnosis of ischemic optic neuropathy. Visual field defects indicate the anatomical site of ischemic or any other pathological insult in the visual pathways from the optic disc to the visual cortex in the occipital lobes. When compared to the standard automated perimetry (SAP) and Goldmann perimetry, a study of confrontation test yielded a sensitivity of nearly 100% for the altitudinal defects and central/centrocecal defects and 76% for the homonymous hemianopia and 50% for the bitemporal field defects thus making confrontation as a quick and highly efficient bedside technique to diagnose ION.[3]

It may not be possible to do a visual field examination in nearly one-fourth of the giant cell arteritis due to poor vision.[4] Moreover, in more than 50% of the eyes with A-AION visual acuity is too poor to perform field testing.[4] Hayreh and Zimmerman, using Goldmann perimeter, found absolute inferior nasal defects (22.4%) much more common than the absolute inferior altitudinal defect (8%) in eyes with NA-AION.[5] In fact, they found an inferior altitudinal defect combined with an absolute inferior nasal defect the most characteristic field defect in NA-AION.[5] The temporal aspect of the optic nerve head falls in the watershed zone of the posterior ciliary circulation making it the most vulnerable area to ischemic insults caused by low perfusion. If the watershed zone falls in the superior temporal part of the optic nerve head, it would produce an inferior nasal defect.[5] Additionally, they found central and centrocecal scotomas in nearly 48.5% of the eyes using an isopter I-2e, 43.8% with I-4e and 29.2% with V-4e.[5] Charting of relative field defects with isopter I-2e that are not seen with I-4e has a functional significance as there is still some visual function present in these areas. Scotomas charted with V-4e are absolute scotomas and in the inferior field pose a challenge in daily activities such as reading, driving or navigation.[5]

It is preferred to use a kinetic perimeter such as Goldmann perimeter for charting the field defects in patients with low vision and in settings wherein the shape of the visual field defect is more informative in localizing the pathology than testing the relative sensitivity of the retina as tested by static perimetry in patients with glaucoma. Depending upon the involvement of the affected PCA/s, the clinical manifestation of GCA may result in anterior or posterior ischemic optic neuropathy, former being the more common manifestation of NA-AION or even the central retinal artery occlusion (CRAO). Visual field defects due to ION respect the horizontal meridian, unlike the chiasmal lesions that respect the vertical meridian. Field defects in arteritic AION include the sector defects, half field defects such as the altitudinal defects inferior being commoner than the superior field or the remaining peripheral island of vision. In a series of 36 patients with giant cell arteritis, most common manifestation was the AION in 20 patients, PION in 10 patients and CRAO in five patients.[4] More than 50% of eyes in this series had visual acuity from counting fingers to no light perception. On the Goldmann perimeter, 11 types of field defects were observed. AION showed either peripheral island, sectoral or altitudinal field defect that almost invariably respected the horizontal meridian except when only an island of vision remained. On the other hand, field testing was possible in all the cases with PION and showed scotomas with or without peripheral defects. Bilaterality was noted in 50% of patients with AION, 31% with PION and 67% with CRAO.

In patients with NA-AION, both central and peripheral visual fields should be obtained at presentation and every 2 weeks thereafter till the optic disc swelling subsides and then monthly till the fields stabilize.[6]

Selecting the perimeter: Goldmann perimeter remained a highly reliable tool to assess the visual field defects especially in patients with poor vision, peripheral visual field defects or gross field defects often encountered in neuro-ophthalmological patients especially those with ION. Principles of kinetic perimetry involve moving a target from a sea of blindness to its first visibility to draw the contour (isopter) of the hill of vision. Kinetic perimetry is a preferred technique in patients with ION as the moving target is easier to see when moved from the blind to the seeing area. Moreover, being a flexible and interactive technique, it is easier on aged patients with ION. The Goldmann perimeter, the manual kinetic perimeter remained the gold standard of kinetic technique in which it was possible to use the variable size of the stimulus and the stimulus intensity on a standard background illumination. Unfortunately, the Goldmann perimeter first introduced in 1946 is no longer manufactured since 2007 and may not be available in more modern neuro-ophthalmological clinics and if available, may be phased out sooner or later. Being an examiner and patients' attention centric technique, the results with this equipment were often not comparable between the clinics and standardization was a challenge. It has been largely supplanted by semi-automatic kinetic Octopus kinetic perimeter first introduced in 1974. A recent study has shown that the Octopus 101 perimeter with the stimulus moving at 5°/second detected all the visual field defects that were detectable with a Goldmann perimeter and nearly 90% of the field defects matched on the two perimeters.[7] A popular perimeter in the ophthalmology clinics is the Humphrey visual field analyzer (HFA) that also sought to replace the Goldmann perimeter and is mostly used for the static perimetry in the central 30°

in patients with glaucoma. This perimeter also offers a kinetic mode. When compared to the Goldmann perimeter, both the HFA3 and the Octopus with the target moving at 5°/second gave similar results but showed larger mean isopter radius compared to the Goldmann perimeter.[8]

FFA: Details are already described in Chapter 3.

Anterior Ischemic Optic Neuropathy

Arteritic-anterior ischemic optic neuropathy (A-AION)
Clinical diagnosis of A-AION
A-AION accounts for less than 10% of patients with ION and is the commonest manifestation of giant cell arteritis, the other less common manifestations being the central retinal artery occlusion and choroidal ischemia.[9,10]

Giant cell arteritis (GCA)

Epidemiology of GCA
GCA is commonly seen in women of northern European descent with wide variations in the incidence in different populations from 0.4/100,000 in people of African descent to 32.8/100,000 in southern Norway.[11] In the past, GCA has been considered uncommon in Indian population. Singh et al. reported a retrospective series of 16 patients with GCA diagnosed in three referral centers in Mumbai (India) over a period of 16 years.[12] Only three of their patients had visual symptoms and none of the patients developed permanent loss of vision.

More recently, Sharma et al.[13] reported on 17 patients seen in a tertiary care institute and reviewed previously reported 55 patients from India and concluded that GCA in Indian population occurs a decade earlier with a male predilection, higher incidence of ophthalmic complications and lower positivity of temporal artery biopsy (TAB).

Clinical features of GCA
Patients above the age of 50 years mostly women present with sudden onset of loss of vision in one eye often accompanied by jaw claudication, temporal headache and scalp tenderness. Visual acuity is usually less than 6/60 in nearly 60% of patients and there may be no perception of light (NLP) in 20%. On examination, there is RAPD and pale to chalky white optic disc edema. If accompanied by a retinal branch, cilioretinal artery or central artery occlusion, there may be pale opacification of the retina. Cherry red spot seen in the fovea in patients with CRAO is absent if there is also an ophthalmic artery occlusion.

Any elderly patient presenting with sudden onset of visual loss must have a high index of suspicion for A-AION. They should have urgent labs that include acute phase reactants such as C-reactive protein, and erythrocyte sedimentation rate (ESR). According to Hayreh et al.,[14] "Clinical criteria, most strongly suggestive of giant cell arteritis include jaw claudication, C-reactive protein above 2.45 mg/dL, neck pain, and an erythrocyte sedimentation rate of 47 mm/hour or more, in that order. C-reactive protein was more sensitive (100%) than erythrocyte sedimentation rate (92%) for detection of giant cell arteritis; erythrocyte sedimentation rate combined with C-reactive protein gave the best specificity (97%)."

An ultrasound (USG) examination of the temporal arteries (TAs) may reveal a characteristic hypoechoic ring, the "halo sign" around the artery lumen, due to inflammation of the vessel wall. With the advances in technology, it is possible to have high-resolution imaging of the entire length of the temporal arteries and TAB may be required if the USG results are inconclusive. It must be kept in mind that the USG signs may be difficult to interpret after 3 days of the start of therapy with corticosteroids.[15]

While systemic symptoms of TA such as scalp tenderness, fatigue and jaw claudication are frequently seen, absence of these symptoms does not rule out TA and is called as "occult temporal arteritis." In a large series, nearly 21.2% of patients with giant cell arteritis and visual loss did not have systemic symptoms.[10]

A delay in investigations may be catastrophic as the other eye gets involved within days to weeks.[16] Mohan et al.[17] reported a case of a 65-year-old man who presented with central retinal artery occlusion in his right eye without any systemic symptoms. ESR was normal. TAs on both sides were palpable, nontender and pulsatile. While the patient was being investigated, 3 days later he reported to the emergency service with left eye central retinal artery occlusion. His visual loss progressed from counting fingers to the light perception within 8 hours. TAB on the left side was found to be consistent with TAs.[17]

While a raised C-reactive protein/ESR is highly sensitive and seen in more than 85% of the patients of TA, yet exceptional cases may occur. This case illustrated that TAB may be indicated even in otherwise asymptomatic elderly patients with CRAO/ION. This patient was seen before the availability of the color Doppler scan. These days USG of TA is a good substitute to provide a quick clue to the possible TA.

A CASE OF A-AION WITH GCA

Dogra et al.[18] reported a 63-year-old man with A-AION in the right eye. The patient had presented with sudden painless loss of vision in the right eye of 2-day duration. He gave history of fever and right-sided temporal scalp tenderness.

There was no perception of light in the affected eye. The right eye pupil reactions revealed an RAPD. Fundus examination showed pale optic disc edema, inferotemporal retinal opacification consistent with a lower temporal branch artery occlusion (Figure 9.2a). On fundus fluorescein angiography, there was hypoperfusion of the optic disc and delayed choroidal perfusion (Figure 9.2b and c). A TAB was done that showed intimal proliferation, a breach in the internal elastic lamina, extravasation of RBCs in the tunica media and mild inflammation consistent with giant cell arteritis (Figure 9.2d). The patient was treated with intravenous pulse steroids and immunosuppressive therapy.

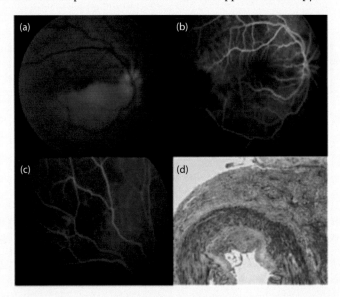

FIGURE 9.2 (a) Optic disc swelling with retinal opacification. On FFA, there is hypoperfusion of the optic disc with delayed choroidal perfusion (b, c). Temporal artery biopsy (d) shows break in the internal elastic lamina, inflammatory cells in the media and intimal thickening. (Reproduced from Dogra et al.[18] No permission required under Creative Commons attribution.)

As discussed above, GCA is one of the commonest causes of A-AION but other vasculitis should also be considered in selected scenarios. The following is a case of A-AION due to ANCA-associated vasculitis (TA).[19]

A 55-year-old woman, presented with sudden-onset bilateral loss of vision for the last 1 week. She had been having fever up to 100°F for the last 6 weeks with a fronto-temporal headache. On examination, she had visual acuity of perception of hand movements (HM+) in the right eye and no light perception in the left eye. There was left eye RAPD. There was no sign of ocular inflammation in either eye. The right eye showed a mild disc swelling with a 1 disc diameter (DD) area of retinal opacification temporal to the optic disc with multifocal gray placoid lesions in the temporal retina and were less than 1 DD in size and located deep to the retinal vessels. The left eye showed pale disc edema with discrete placoid lesions as seen in the right eye (Figure 9.3a and b). On fundus fluorescein angiography (FFA) of the left eye, there was delayed choroidal perfusion and non-perfusion of the optic disc during the dye transit. In the late frames of FFA, the optic disc remained hypofluorescent with some staining of its margins, hyperfluorescence of the placoid lesions and a cattle truck appearance in the major retinal veins (Figure 9.3c and d).

On further questioning, she gave history of jaw claudication for 1 month. There was bilateral scalp tenderness. Doppler USG scanning of the temporal arteries was done, which showed decreased flow in both the temporal arteries. Her hemoglobin was 6.7 g%, ESR was elevated to 70 mm in first hour, platelets were 6,16,000/mm³. Right side TAB was done and she was started on intravenous methylprednisolone (1 g per day for 3 days). The right side TAB showed minimal changes (Figure 9.3g and 9.3h). Since there was a strong suspicion of Temporal arteritis, TAB was repeated on the left side, which showed fibrointimal proliferation, focal break in the internal elastic lamina with minimal inflammation and fibrin in adventitia suggestive of arteritis (Figure 9.3i). During the course of her hospital stay, she developed weakness in bilateral upper and lower limbs over a few days, which was distal more than the proximal and she eventually developed a foot drop. She also had intermittent nasal stuffiness without crust or epistaxis. There was a progressive derangement of renal functions with development of significant proteinuria (24 hours urinary proteins—985 mg) and creatinine increased from normal in the preceding week to 2.67 mg/dL. The kidney was biopsied which was suggestive of pauci-immune focal necrotizing glomerulonephritis with crescents and granulomatous glomerulitis (Figure 9.3k). On pure tone audiometry, she had moderate mixed hearing loss. In view of the rapidly progressive renal failure and mononeuritis multiplex, a possibility of small vessel vasculitis was considered and ANCA(IIF) was done, which was found to be 2+ perinuclear pattern (pANCA 2+) and MPO ELISA was also +ve.

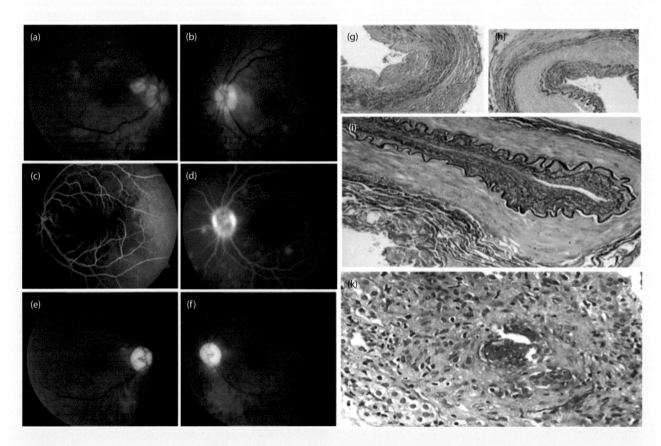

FIGURE 9.3 (a) Mild disc swelling with a 1 DD area of retinal opacification temporal to the optic disc with multifocal gray placoid lesions in the temporal retina of the right eye. The left eye showed similar pale disc edema and discreet placoid lesions (b). On FFA of the left eye, there was delayed choroidal perfusion and non-perfusion of the optic disc during the dye transit. In the late frames of FFA, the optic disc remained hypofluorescent with some staining of its margins, hyperfluorescence of the placoid lesions and a cattle truck appearance in the major retinal veins (c, d). Right-sided temporal artery biopsy (TAB) shows fibrointimal proliferation with intact elastic lamina (g, h). The left TAB shows fibrointimal proliferation left picture (star) and focal break in the internal elastic lamina right picture (arrow) with minimal inflammation and fibrin in the adventitia suggestive of arteritis (i). The renal artery biopsy revealed glomerulonephritis, focal necrotizing (star) with crescents (arrow) and granulomatous glomerulitis (j). After 6 months both discs show pallor (e, f).

Eventually, a final diagnosis of bilateral arteritic-anterior ischemic optic neuropathy (A-AION) due to ANCA-associated vasculitis (AAV) with temporal artery involvement, mononeuritis multiplex and pauci-immune glomerulonephritis was made and she was started on remission induction treatment with intravenous cyclophosphamide pulses according to the European vasculitis study group (EUVAS) regime. She received eight pulses of cyclophosphamide. Azathioprine was used as a remission maintenance agent. Her visual acuity improved to 6/9 in the right eye but remained NLP in the left eye. Her optic disc had turned pale, left more than the right eye (Figure 9.3e and f).

Visual improvement in GCA is very rare. Her systemic symptoms and renal functions improved substantially. There has been no relapse of the systemic disease over 7-year follow-up and she is maintaining her visual acuity in the right eye.

While GCA is a granulomatous inflammation of the large vessels, AAV is a group of necrotizing vasculitis affecting the medium and small vessels.[20] Temporal headache can misleadingly point to a diagnosis of GCA with vastly different outcomes. Pointers toward the AAV with TA involvement in this patient were peripheral neuropathy, otological and kidney involvement. The kidney biopsy findings were consistent with ANCA-associated vasculitis. Histopathological features of the left TAB in our patient cannot help in distinguishing AAV and GCA. There were no giant cells (seen in GCA) noted in the biopsy specimen but there was a break in the internal elastic lamina, which can happen in both the conditions. It is important to differentiate GCA-TA from AAV—TA as the initial choice and duration of immunosuppression is different in both the conditions as has been highlighted in the above case.[12]

Non-arteritic-anterior ischemic optic neuropathy (NA-AION)

The NA-AION is diagnosed by painless loss of vision in an elderly individual with RAPD, optic disc edema and peripheral sectoral hemianopic field defects. A typical patient, usually above the age of 50 years, presents with complaints of sudden-onset, painless loss of vision in one eye. The visual loss is noticed on waking up in the morning and the loss of vision may progress over the hours or even days. The visual acuity in the affected eye may vary from nearly normal to counting fingers. It is highly unusual for a patient with NA-AION to present with NLP. Fundus examination is remarkable for optic disc edema, which may be sectoral. There may be optic disc or peripapillary linear hemorrhages. Other useful clues to reach the diagnosis include the presence of optic disc pallor from a previous episode of the NA-AION in the contralateral eye. While the optic disc cup in the affected eye may appear absent due to disc swelling, an examination of the other eye may show a "disc at risk" characterized by a very small or absent physiological cup.[21]

Presence of a normal cup in the contralateral eye should raise suspicion of an arteritic ION.[22] Optic disc edema may take several weeks for resolution leaving behind a sectoral pallor.[23] On FFA, there is delayed choroidal filling and is seen as the dark watershed zone which may pass through the optic disc (Figure 9.4a and b). Moreover, there is hypoperfusion of the optic nerve head with late staining.

Predisposing factors for NA-AION: The exact pathogenesis of NA-AION is not known, although it is believed that fall in perfusion pressure in small vessels from the PCAs supplying the optic nerve head is responsible. Systemic hypertension in 50% and diabetes in 25% are major risk factors. Dyslipidemia, smoking and coronary artery disease are other common risk factors.[24]

Use of antihypertensive prescription drugs before sleep may trigger NA-AION in predisposed individuals. Nocturnal hypotension by reducing the blood flow to optic nerve head below a critical level especially in those receiving anti-hypertensive drugs may be the final insult in predisposed patients in precipitating NA-AION.[25,26]

The relative risk of obstructive sleep apnea was 4.9 in patients with NA-AION compared with the normal population.[27] More recently, carotid plaque score and intimal-media thickness in hypertensive patients has been found to be a risk for NA-AION. It is likely that similar pathological changes are taking place in arteries supplying the optic nerve that impair the regulation of blood supply to the ONH predisposing the eye to NA-AION.[28]

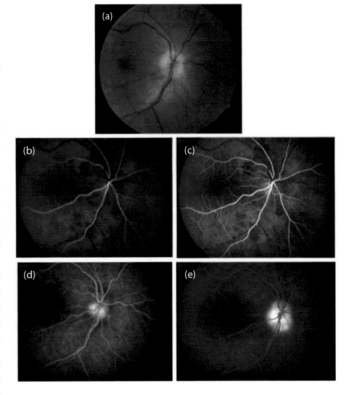

FIGURE 9.4 A 57-year-old man complained of loss of vision in the lower half of his right eye since 10 days. He was a known case of hypertension. Visual acuity was reduced to 6/24 with RAPD. Pale optic disc edema of the optic disc is noted mostly in the upper half (a). FFA study of his right eye shows delayed perfusion of the watershed zone of the choroid which is passing through the optic disc, which is also hypoperfused (upper panel, b–c) and late staining of the optic disc (lower panel, d–e).

Use of drugs like amiodarone, nasal decongestants, tacrolimus or phosphodiesterase-5 inhibitors used for erectile dysfunction may lead to NA-AION.[29–33]

Among the other uncommon reported causes of NA-AION is a case of a young man who stayed for 3 months at an altitude of more than 5400 meters above the sea level.[34]

NA-AION has not been found to increase the risk of stroke in later life.[35]

Recognizing the masquerades: Differential Diagnosis of AION

The most important differential diagnosis of ION is inflammatory ON due to demyelinating disease, a common occurrence in the young, mostly women from 15 to 49 years of age, who typically present with sudden-onset, progressive visual loss in one eye with pain on eye movements. It is critical to differentiate between the NA-AION and ON, as the latter carries a grave prognosis. Commonly, patients of ION are misdiagnosed as ON who live with the fear of developing multiple sclerosis. Patients with ON have significantly reduced vision, defective color vision, RAPD and central/centrocecal visual field defects. The optic disc is normal although some patients may have mild disc edema. It is important to remember that, as they enter the eye, optic nerve fibers lose their myelin sheath the target of the demyelinating inflammation. The inflammation in ON, therefore, is restricted to the retro-ocular segment of the optic nerve while AION mostly affects the optic nerve head. Only less than 10% of ION may have PION. However, atypical cases of ON do occur who do not have pain and have sectoral or altitudinal field defects. In such patients, it may be prudent to do an MRI brain including the optic nerves. Nearly 50% of patients with ON who at presentation show demyelination plaques on MRI develop multiple sclerosis by 5 years of follow-up.[36] Unlike the AION, patients with ON, irrespective of treatment with corticosteroids, start improving visual acuity by 2–3 weeks of the onset and by the end of 1 year 90% have normal vision. In the NA-AION decompression trial, although 43% of eyes recovered ≥3 lines of VA, none recovered normal vision. Likewise, while the pupillary reactions recover in ON in due course, there is no such improvement in the AION.[32]

Other differentials: Other uncommon causes of inflammatory ON that may mimic ION include systemic lupus erythematosus, Sjogren syndrome, Behçet's disease, Lyme disease, Syphilis and Tuberculosis.[36]

Following are cases who presented with acute/hyperacute visual loss brewing a suspicion of ION. However, detailed examination and investigations of these patients revealed a different diagnosis on follow-up.

OCULAR ISCHEMIC SYNDROME

NA-AION PRESENTING WITH RECURRENT EPISODES OF BLURRING OF VISION

A 47-year-old man presented with a 6-month history of episodes of transient loss of vision from the left eye on waking up in the morning. A CT scan and MRI of the brain done elsewhere were normal. Medical history was non-contributory. On examination, he had visual acuity of 6/9 in both eyes with RAPD in the left eye. Fundoscopy of the left eye showed optic disc edema (Figure 9.5a). Diagnosis of Pseudoedema of the optic disc due to buried drusen was ruled out by a normal autofluorescence of the optic disc (Figure 9.5b). Humphrey's VFA (HVF) showed a peripheral lower nasal defect with peripheral low retinal sensitivity in the lower half of the field (Figure 9.5e). Fluorescein angiography showed a patchy delay in the optic disc and choroidal perfusion during dye transit with late fluorescence of the optic disc (Figure 9.5c and d). On Optical coherence topography, the retinal nerve fiber layer (RNFL) analysis showed significant swelling of the superior and temporal peripapillary nerve fibers. The patient was diagnosed as a case of ocular ischemic syndrome. He received oral steroids followed 2 months later by intravitreal injection of dexamethasone implant. Visual fields improved over the next 3 months. Over the next 2 years, the optic disc swelling regressed (Figure 9.5i) and the visual fields improved to near normal with a peripheral lower nasal defect (Figure 9.5f–h).

Transient visual loss may be seen in nearly 15% of patients with the ocular ischemic syndrome (OIS) while 70% of patients with OIS may present with a gradual or sudden loss of vision. OIS results from vascular insufficiency due to atherosclerotic changes in the internal carotid arteries. Optic disc swelling is an uncommon feature of OIS and is characterized by low intraocular pressure, retinal vascular stasis, anterior and posterior segment neovascularization. On FFA, there is marked delay in choroidal filling.[37]

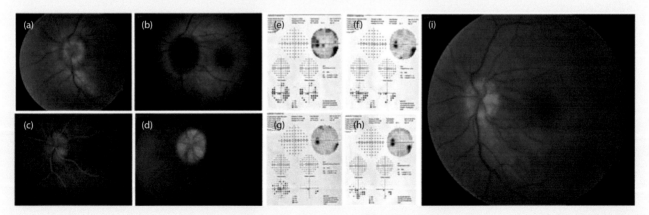

FIGURE 9.5 Fundus photograph of left eye showing optic disc swelling at presentation (a). On fundus autofluorescence, the optic disc was hypofluorescent ruling out buried druse of the optic nerve head (b). The FFA shows very subtle hypoperfusion in superior half (c). Late disc staining (d). HVF showed a peripheral lower nasal defect with peripheral low retinal sensitivity in the lower half of the field (e). Over the next 2 years, the visual fields improved to near normal with a peripheral lower nasal defect (f–h) and the optic disc swelling regressed (i).

CASE OF A-AION MIMICKING MULTIPLE SCLEROSIS

A 47-year-old man presented with a 2-day history of sudden-onset, painless loss of vision in the left eye. His visual acuity was 6/9 in the right eye and hand movements close to face in the left eye. There was left RAPD with optic disc edema (Figure 9.6).

On FFA, there was a significant delay in filling of the peripapillary choroid and complete hypoperfusion of the optic nerve head (Figure 9.6). His blood pressure was recorded 173/105 mm/Hg. His clinical picture was suggestive of A-AION. Review of his past medical records in our institution revealed that he had been diagnosed with multiple sclerosis with left internuclear ophthalmoplegia 17 years ago at the age of 30 years. In this episode, he had shown horizontal nystagmus in left gaze with restriction of the right eye adduction till midline. His MRI brain was reported normal but his brainstem-evoked response audiometry and visual-evoked potential showed an increased conduction defect (right more than left). Rest of the CNS examination and review of systems was normal. He recovered on treatment with intravenous corticosteroids followed by oral steroids. Three years later he became symptomatic again with diplopia and the MRI brain in this episode revealed a hyperintense lesion in the right pons. This episode was also treated with corticosteroids with complete recovery. Four years later he was seen with moderate congestive heart failure (NYHA class III) with pedal edema and was treated with oral diuretics. There is no record of the next 13 years till he was next seen in the current episode with sudden loss of vision in the left eye. There was no clinical evidence of systemic vasculitis in the form of headache, sinusitis, renal, pulmonary, oro-genital ulceration or musculoskeletal and connective tissue involvement. On laboratory investigations his pANCA was positive, ANA-Ab by IFA negative, dsDNA ab were negative, C-reactive protein was 3 mg/L, ESR was 22 mmHg/1st hour; blood urea 46, serum creatinine 0.7, electrolytes and blood counts and hematocrit were normal.

He was diagnosed with A-AION and treated with intravenous/oral corticosteroids without any improvement. At 8 months follow up, his visual acuity was hand movements close to face with RAPD and pale optic disc.

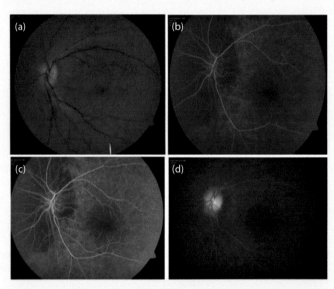

FIGURE 9.6   Fundus examination showing optic disc swelling in the left eye (a). FFA showing a significant delay in filling of the peripapillary choroid and complete hypoperfusion of the optic nerve head and late staining of the disc (b–d).

INTRACRANIAL SPACE-OCCUPYING LESION MASQUERADING AS ISCHEMIC OPTIC NEUROPATHY

A 45-year-old woman presented with sudden-onset progressive loss of vision in the left eye for 6 weeks. She had been having recurrent oral ulcers for the past 18 months. There was a history of holocranial headaches in the past. She was dyslipidemic but her blood sugar levels and blood pressures were normal. Ocular examination showed visual acuity of 6/9 in the right eye and hand motions close to the face in the left eye. The left eye revealed a positive RAPD.

 Fundus examination showed optic disc edema in the right eye and pallor of the left optic disc (Figure 9.7a and b). On FFA of the right eye, there was significant hypoperfusion of the optic disc with staining in the late frames (Figure 9.7c and d). Her confrontation fields were suggestive of inferior altitudinal hemianopia in both eyes. Visual field analysis of the left eye was suggestive of altitudinal hemianopia in the left eye and a residual tunnel field in the right eye. Unusual field defect in the right eye prompted an MRI brain that revealed a cerebellopontine (CP) angle mass lesion suggestive of acoustic schwannoma with the involvement of the midbrain, fourth ventricle and hydrocephalus. She was posted for surgery by the neurosurgeons and was lost to our follow-up. Visual symptoms in CP angle tumors are uncommon who mostly present with hearing loss and tinnitus. Optic disc edema is seen in 8% of cases and is either due to obstructive hydrocephalus or a mass effect from a large tumor. The patient had an unusual presentation of optic atrophy in one eye and optic disc edema in the other eye. Significant hypoperfusion of the optic disc with disc edema, bilateral altitudinal hemianopic field defects on confrontation led to an initial error. We may have been closer to the diagnosis if we had sought a history of deafness/tinnitus.[38]

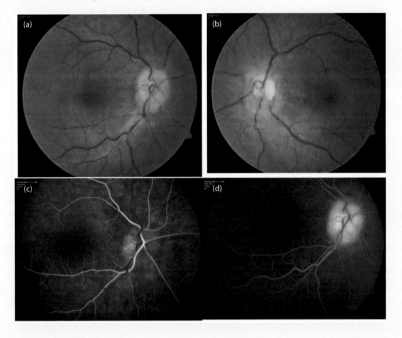

FIGURE 9.7   Fundus examination shows optic disc swelling in the right eye (a), optic atrophy in the left eye (b), hypoperfusion of the right optic disc on FFA (c) and late staining of the right optic disc (d).

Posterior ischemic optic neuropathy

PION is rather an uncommon form of ION compared to NA-AION and the diagnosis is made after all causes of retrobulbar optic neuropathies have been excluded. It may be advisable to ask for a contrast-enhanced MRI to rule out compressive or infiltrative causes of optic neuropathies.[38]

Unlike the NA-AION, there is no edema of the optic disc or splinter hemorrhages in the setting of acute loss of vision, RAPD and the visual field defects. There are mainly three subtypes of PION, namely the perioperative, non-arteritic (NA-PION) and arteritic (A-PION). In a series of 72 patients, perioperative PION was seen in relatively younger patients, was often bilateral and seen frequently after spinal surgery, although it was also seen following a variety of other surgical procedures in relatively older patient who had the usual cardiovascular risk factors.[39] Eyes with PION do not have structural predisposition unlike the NA-AION. Sadda et al. saw small optic discs only in 4% of the eyes in their series.[39] Patients with the NA-PION have otherwise the same risk factors as the NA-AION. Patients with A-PION tend to be older and carry poorer outcome. It is important to rule out GCA in patients older than 50 years. In his series of 43 patients with PION, Hayreh found 12 patients who had A-PION due to GCA.[40] Bilateral PION in a non-surgical setting in the elderly especially those who give a history of headaches should evoke a strong suspicion of GCA. High-dose corticosteroids were not effective in improving the visual outcome in patients with A-PION or the surgical PION.[40]

Perioperative NA-AION

Loss of vision can be a devastating complication of an uneventful non-ocular surgery. The incidence of this complication is quite low after non-cardiac surgery. Among more than 500,000 non-cardiac surgeries conducted at the Mayo clinic, only four patients developed ION.[41] However, from the same hospital the incidence of ION following CABG surgeries was reported as 0.06%.[42] Although the coronary artery bypass grafting (CABG) is performed less frequently now, the incidence of this complication has not changed over the years. Perioperative ION has been estimated as 1.43/10,000 cardiac surgeries/year significantly more than 0.22/10,000 procedures following percutaneous interventions.[43] More than 78% of the perioperative ION were due to isolated CABG.[43] While coronary artery stenosis and stroke are not independent risk factors for ION these were identified as risk factors for perioperative ION.[43] They also identified chronic eye conditions like glaucoma, age-related macular degeneration, hypertensive retinopathy as risk factors for perioperative ION possibly due to dysregulation of blood supply to the optic nerve head in these conditions.[43] Blood loss and low hemoglobin may enhance the risk of ION.[42]

Patients undergoing spinal surgery in prone position under general anesthesia are at a greater risk of developing perioperative PION[44] with the reported incidence of 0.2%.[45]

There is no ophthalmic examination that can predict this complication.[46] Prolonged surgery predisposes the patients to this uncommon complication and the patients may be accordingly advised of this small risk.[46]

A detailed advisory has been issued recently for the attention of the anesthetists to prevent this complication. Patients undergoing spinal surgery should undergo preoperative risk assessment such as anemia, hypertension, diabetes, peripheral vascular disease and tobacco use. The patients should be informed that some of these risk factors if present may increase the risk of perioperative visual loss.[47]

Management of ION

A-AION

A-AION results from granulomatous inflammation of the small arteries supplying the optic nerve head. Any elderly person presenting with the sudden loss of vision accompanied by headache and ION should be suspected to have A-AION and treatment instituted even before the results of labs and TAB become available as the time is of the essence and there is fear of severe visual loss and the other eye involvement.[48,49]

In the presence of visual loss, treatment is initiated with high dose intravenous corticosteroids (methylprednisolone 1–2 g/day) for 2–3 days followed by high dose oral corticosteroids (1–2 mg/kg/day) for the next 4–6 weeks. GCA is highly responsive to corticosteroids with quick relief in the symptoms of headache, jaw claudication and myalgia. Patients require long-term treatment. Recurrence may follow tapering of steroids and should be monitored with periodic ESR and CRP. Hayreh found ESR and CRP as the more sensitive and reliable parameters to follow patients with GCA than the systemic symptoms.[49] They found no set formula to taper or stop the steroids. They could stop steroids only in 7% of their 145 patients with GCA who could maintain their ESR and CRP levels without steroids.[48,50]

For those who lost vision, visual acuity improved in 10% but visual fields recovered only in 4% of patients and continued to worsen in another 4%.[50,51]

Corticosteroid-related adverse reactions may be seen in almost 85% of patients.[51] Methotrexate as a steroid-sparing agent has been used in GCA[48] but it was not found to reduce the cumulative dose of corticosteroids necessary to control GCA.[48,52]

More recently, the role of IL-6 antagonist tocilizumab has been found to be promising.[52]

NA-AION

NA-AION is essentially a clinical diagnosis. There is no evidence that any therapy is effective in improving the outcome. A belief in the early 1990s that NA-AION resulted from compartment syndrome in the optic nerve sheath led to the ischemic optic neuropathy decompression trial, a large prospective interventional trial that studied the effect of optic nerve sheath decompression on the visual outcome in patients with NA-AION. While the decompression of the optic nerve head failed to show any benefit of this intervention, in fact, led to worse visual outcomes, it provided a unique opportunity to study the natural course of NA-AION. In the natural course, nearly 43% of eyes improved visual acuity by three or more lines compared to 33% of the eyes in the intervention group. More importantly, 24% of eyes lost vision in the intervention group compared to 12% in the observation group.[53] Intravitreal injections of corticosteroids, triamcinolone acetonide and anti-VEGF agents have been tried to reduce the optic disc swelling but without any consistent results.[54]

The role of antiplatelet agents, anticoagulants and statins in patients with NA-AION is still controversial. The decision for these agents can be made depending upon the presence of other peripheral signs of thrombosis or atherosclerosis in these patients.

The use of steroids to treat patients with NA-AION remains debatable and there is lack of level I evidence to support its use. In one of the largest series, patients with NA-AION either received oral steroids by choice or declined any intervention. At 6 months from the onset, nearly 70% of eyes with 20/70 or worse VA at presentation who received steroids within 2 weeks of onset had significant improvement of VA versus only 40% of those who did not receive corticosteroids. The visual fields improved by 40% versus 24% at 6 months in the steroid-treated eyes versus not treated eyes.[55] Being a patient choice study, there may have been a potential unrecognized bias in the study.[56] In a recent small, randomized prospective interventional trial from India, there was no difference in the VA at 6 months between the treated and the control group. However, the steroid-treated group did show earlier resolution of the disc and RNFL edema.[56] Apart from being a much smaller study, the current study also excluded patients with diabetes and only two-thirds of their patients had presented within 2 weeks of the onset of symptoms.[56]

To study the practice pattern of treatment offered for NA-AION, it was found that no treatment was offered by neurologists (23%), neuro-ophthalmologists (27%) or the ophthalmologists (33%). Most physicians use aspirin and only 10% use oral steroids.[57]

However, it may be prudent to use steroids in patients with bilateral disease, severe visual loss in the only seeing eye or any suspicion that it may be A-AION.

Conclusion

Ischemic optic neuropathies are an important cause of sudden-onset or acute visual loss. It is important to understand the anatomy of blood supply of the optic nerve to understand the visual field defects. Understanding the temporal profile, clinical features and investigation findings may aid a physician to differentiate ischemic optic neuropathies from inflammatory causes. It is further paramount to recognise arteritic causes of anterior ischemic optic neuropathies which can have fatal consequences if not diagnosed and managed in a timely manner.

Multiple-Choice Questions

1. Which statement regarding the blood supply of the optic nerve is false?
   a. Optic disc head is supplied by posterior ciliary artery.
   b. The peripapillary choroid that lies between the optic disc margin and the entry site of the short PCAs is a low-pressure system and vulnerable to hemodynamic variations.
   c. The laminar part has poor capillary plexus, hence making it vulnerable to ischemic insult.
   d. Circle of Zinn-Haller is believed to have strict superior and inferior distribution.

   Answer:
   c. The laminar part has poor capillary plexus, hence making it vulnerable to ischemic insult.

2. Giant cell arteritis:
   a. Mostly involves men in fourth or fifth decades.
   b. C-reactive protein was around 80% and the erythrocyte sedimentation rate is around 50% sensitive for detection of giant cell arteritis.
   c. An ultrasound examination of the temporal arteries may reveal a characteristic hypoechoic ring.
   d. Visual improvement in GCA is a rule.

   Answer:
   c. An ultrasound examination of the temporal arteries may reveal a characteristic hypoechoic ring.

3. All of the following may masquerade as AION, EXCEPT:
   a. Inflammatory optic neuropathy
   b. Syphilitic optic neuropathy
   c. Behchet's disease
   d. None of the above

   Answer:

   d. None of the above

4. In ocular ischemic syndrome
   a. Transient visual loss may be seen in nearly 95% of patients.
   b. Only 10% of patients with OIS present gradual loss of vision.
   c. Optic disc swelling is an uncommon feature of OIS.
   d. Intraocular pressure is high.

   Answer:

   c. Optic disc swelling is an uncommon feature of OIS.

References

1. Hayreh SS. Ocular vascular occlusive disorders: natural history of visual outcome. Prog Retin Eye Res. 2014;41:1–25.
2. Harper RA. Basic ophthalmology. American Academy of Ophthalmology. 9th ed. 2010; pp. 9–15.
3. Johnson LN, Baloh FG. The accuracy of confrontation visual field test in comparison with automated perimetry. J Natl Med Assoc. 1991;83(10):895–898.
4. Fakin A, Kerin V, Hawlina M. Visual fields in giant cell arteritis (Horton's disease). Translat Neurosci. 2011;2(4):325–330.
5. Hayreh SS, Zimmerman B. Visual field abnormalities in nonarteritic anterior ischemic optic neuropathy: Their pattern and prevalence at initial examination. Arch Ophthalmol. 2005;123(11):1554–1562.
6. Kedar S, Ghate D, Corbett JJ. Visual fields in neuro-ophthalmology. Indian J Ophthalmol. 2011;59(2):103–109.
7. Rowe FJ, Rowlands A. Comparison of diagnostic accuracy between octopus 900 and Goldmann kinetic visual fields. Biomed Res Int. 2014;2014:e214829.
8. Bevers C, Blanckaert G, Keer KV, Fils J-F, Vandewalle E, Stalmans I. Semi-automated kinetic perimetry: Comparison of the Octopus 900 and Humphrey visual field analyzer 3 versus Goldmann perimetry. Acta Ophthalmol. 2019;97(4):e499–e505.
9. Chen JJ, Leavitt JA, Fang C, Crowson CS, Matteson EL, Warrington KJ. Evaluating the incidence of arteritic ischemic optic neuropathy and other causes of vision loss from giant cell arteritis. Ophthalmology. 2016;123(9):1999–2003.
10. Hayreh SS, Podhajsky PA, Zimmerman B. Ocular manifestations of giant cell arteritis. Am J Ophthalmol. 1998; 125(4):509–520.
11. Skanchy DF, Vickers A, Ponce CMP, Lee AG. Ocular manifestations of giant cell arteritis. Expert Review of Ophthalmology. 2019;14(1):23–32.
12. Singh S, Balakrishnan C, Mangat G, Samant R, Bambani M, Kalke S, Joshi VR. Giant cell arteritis in Mumbai. J Assoc Physicians India. 2010;58:372–374.
13. Sharma A, Sagar V, Prakash M, Gupta V, Khaire N, Pinto B, et al. Giant cell arteritis in India: Report from a tertiary care center along with total published experience from India. Neurol India. 2015;63(5):681–686.
14. Hayreh SS, Podhajsky PA, Raman R, Zimmerman B. Giant cell arteritis: Validity and reliability of various diagnostic criteria. Am J Ophthalmol. 1997;123(3):285–296.
15. Schmidt WA. Role of ultrasound in the understanding and management of vasculitis. Ther Adv Musculoskelet Dis. 2014;6(2):39–47.
16. Liu GT, Glaser JS, Schatz NJ, Smith JL. Visual morbidity in giant cell arteritis: Clinical characteristics and prognosis for vision. Ophthalmology. 1994;101(11):1779–1785.
17. Mohan K, Gupta A, Jain IS, Banerjee CK. Bilateral central retinal artery occlusion in occult temporal arteritis. J Clin Neuro-ophthalmol. 1989;9(4):270–272.
18. Dogra M, Singh R, Dogra M. Giant cell arteritis related arteritic anterior ischemic optic neuropathy: Clinico-pathological correlation. Indian J Ophthalmol. 2019;67(1):142.
19. Samanta J, Naidu G, Mittal S, Nada R, Bal A, Singh R, et al. Temporal arteritis revealing antineutrophil cytoplasmic antibody-associated vasculitides: Are the visual outcomes different from giant cell arteritis? Comment on the Article by Delaval et al. Arthritis Rheumatol. 2021 Jul;73(7):1345–1346. doi: 10.1002/art.41698. Epub 2021 Jun 1. PMID: 33605063.
20. Delaval L, Samson M, Schein F, Agard C, Tréfond L, Deroux A, et al. Temporal arteritis revealing antineutrophil cytoplasmic antibody-associated vasculitides: A case-control study. Arthritis Rheumatol. (Malden. Online). 2021;73(2):286–294.
21. Beck RW, Savino PJ, Repka MX, Schatz NJ, Sergott RC. Optic disc structure in anterior ischemic optic neuropathy. Ophthalmology. 1984;91(11):1334–1337.
22. Biousse V, Newman NJ. Ischemic optic neuropathies. N Engl J Med. 2015;372(25):2428–2436.
23. Hayreh SS. Ischemic optic neuropathies—where are we now? Graefes Arch Clin Exp Ophthalmol. 2013;251(8):1873–1884.
24. Hayreh SS. Anterior ischemic optic neuropathy. Clin Neurosci. 1997;4(5):251–263.
25. Hayreh S, Podhajsky P, Zimmerman MB. Role of nocturnal arterial hypotension in optic nerve head ischemic disorders. Ophthalmologica. 1999;213(2):76–96.
26. Hayreh SS, Joos KM, Podhajsky PA, Long CR. Systemic diseases associated with nonarteritic anterior ischemic optic neuropathy. Am J Ophthalmol. 1994;118(6):766–780.
27. Archer Erica L, Pepin S. Obstructive sleep apnea and nonarteritic anterior ischemic optic neuropathy: Evidence for an association. J Clin Sleep Med. 2013;09(06):613–618.
28. Zhu W, Chen T, Jin L, Wang H, Yao F, Wang C, et al. Carotid artery intimal medial thickness and carotid artery plaques in hypertensive patients with non-arteritic anterior ischaemic optic neuropathy. Graefes Arch Clin Exp Ophthalmol. 2017;255(10):2037–2043.
29. Murphy MA, Murphy JF. Amiodarone and optic neuropathy: The heart of the matter. J Neuro-ophthalmol. 2005;25(3):232–236.
30. Fivgas GD, Newman NJ. Anterior ischemic optic neuropathy following the use of a nasal decongestant. Am J Ophthalmol. 1999;127(1):104–106.
31. Gupta M, Bansal R, Beke N, Gupta A. Tacrolimus-induced unilateral ischaemic optic neuropathy in a non-transplant patient. BMJ Case Rep. 2012:bcr2012006718.
32. Campbell UB, Walker AM, Gaffney M, Petronis KR, Creanga D, Quinn S, et al. Acute nonarteritic anterior ischemic optic neuropathy and exposure to phosphodiesterase type 5 inhibitors. J Sex Med. 2015;12(1):139–151.
33. Pomeranz HD. Erectile dysfunction agents and nonarteritic anterior ischemic optic neuropathy. Neurol Clin. 2017;35(1):17–27.
34. Bandyopadhyay S, Singh R, Gupta V, Gupta A. Anterior ischaemic optic neuropathy at high altitude. Indian J Ophthalmol. 2002;50(4):324.
35. Park SJ, Yang HK, Byun SJ, Park KH, Hwang J-M. Risk of stroke after nonarteritic anterior ischemic optic neuropathy. Am J Ophthalmol. 2019;200:123–129.
36. Voss E, Raab P, Trebst C, Stangel M. Clinical approach to optic neuritis: pitfalls, red flags and differential diagnosis. Ther Adv Neurol Disord. 2011;4(2):123–134.
37. Mizener JB, Podhajsky P, Hayreh SS. Ocular ischemic syndrome. Ophthalmology. 1997;104(5):859–864.
38. Grainger J, Dias PS. Case report: Optic disc edema without hydrocephalus in acoustic neuroma. Skull Base. 2005;15(1):83–86.
39. Sadda SR, Nee M, Miller NR, Biousse V, Newman NJ, Kouzis A. Clinical spectrum of posterior ischemic optic neuropathy. Am J Ophthalmol. 2001;132(5):743–750.
40. Hayreh SS. Posterior ischaemic optic neuropathy: Clinical features, pathogenesis, and management. Eye. 2004;18(11):1188–1206.
41. Warner ME, Warner MA, Garrity JA, MacKenzie RA, Warner DO. The frequency of perioperative vision loss. Anesth Analg. 2001;93(6):1417–1421.
42. Nuttall GA, Garrity JA, Dearani JA, Abel MD, Schroeder DR, Mullany CJ. Risk factors for ischemic optic neuropathy after cardiopulmonary bypass: A matched case/control study. Anesth Analg. 2001;93(6):1410–1416.
43. Rubin DS, Matsumoto MM, Moss HE, Joslin CE, Tung A, Roth S. Ischemic optic neuropathy in cardiac surgery: Incidence and risk factors in the United States from the National Inpatient Sample 1998 to 2013. Anesthesiology. 2017;126(5):810–821.
44. Newman NJ. Perioperative visual loss after nonocular surgeries. Am J Ophthalmol. 2008;145(4):604–610.
45. Chang S-H, Miller NR. The incidence of vision loss due to perioperative ischemic optic neuropathy associated with spine surgery: The Johns Hopkins hospital experience. Spine. 2005;30(11):1299–1302.
46. American Society of Anesthesiologists Task Force on Perioperative Visual Loss. Practice advisory for perioperative visual loss associated with spine surgery: An updated report by the American Society of Anesthesiologists Task Force on Perioperative Visual Loss. Anesthesiology. 2012;116(2):274–285.
47. Apfelbaum JL, Roth S, Rubin D, Connis RT, Agarkar M, Arnold PM, et al. Practice advisory for perioperative visual loss associated with spine surgery 2019: An updated report by the American Society of Anesthesiologists Task Force on Perioperative Visual Loss, the North American Neuro-Ophthalmology Society, and the Society for Neuroscience in Anesthesiology and Critical Care. Anesthesiology. 2019; 130(1):13–30.
48. Rucker JC, Biousse V, Newman NJ. Ischemic optic neuropathies. Curr Opin Neurol. 2004;17(1):27–35.
49. Hayreh SS, Zimmerman B, Kardon RH. Visual improvement with corticosteroid therapy in giant cell arteritis. Report of a large study and review of literature. Acta Ophthalmol Scand. 2002;80(4):355–367.
50. Hayreh SS, Zimmerman B. Management of giant cell arteritis. Ophthalmologica. 2003;217(4):239–259.
51. Broder MS, Sarsour K, Chang E, Collinson N, Tuckwell K, Napalkov P, et al. Corticosteroid-related adverse events in patients with giant cell arteritis: A claims-based analysis. Semin Arthritis Rheum. 2016;46(2):246–252.
52. Dejaco C, Brouwer E, Mason JC, Buttgereit F, Matteson EL, Dasgupta B. Giant cell arteritis and polymyalgia rheumatica: Current challenges and opportunities. Nat Rev Rheumatol. 2017;13(10):578–592.
53. Dickersin K, Everett D, Feldon S, Hooper F, Kaufman D, Kelman S, et al. Optic nerve decompression surgery for nonarteritic anterior ischemic optic neuropathy (NAION) is not effective and may be harmful. JAMA. 1995;273(8):625–632.
54. Foroozan R. New treatments for nonarteritic anterior ischemic optic neuropathy. Neurol Clin. 2017;35(1):1–15.
55. Hayreh SS, Zimmerman MB. Non-arteritic anterior ischemic optic neuropathy: role of systemic corticosteroid therapy. Graefes Arch Clin Exp Ophthalmol. 2008;246(7):1029–1046.
56. Saxena R, Singh D, Sharma M, James M, Sharma P, Menon V. Steroids versus no steroids in nonarteritic anterior ischemic optic neuropathy: A randomized controlled trial. Ophthalmology. 2018;125(10):1623–1627.
57. Atkins EJ, Bruce BB, Newman NJ, Biousse V. Translation of clinical studies to clinical practice: Survey on the treatment of nonarteritic anterior ischemic optic neuropathy. Am J Ophthalmol. 2009;148(5):809.

10

INFILTRATIVE OPTIC NEUROPATHIES

Aniruddha Agarwal, Sabia Handa, Vishali Gupta

CASE STUDY

A 68-year-old woman presented with history of decreased vision from left followed by right eye over 15 days duration. Visual acuity was recorded as 6/36 in right eye and the patient could only perceive light from the left eye. Fundus examination revealed presence of optic disc edema with peripapillary hemorrhages and creamy white exudates. Gadolinium-enhanced MRI of the optic nerve and brain showed enlargement and enhancement of bilateral optic nerves and optic chiasma. Multiple T2 hyperintensities with enhancement and restricted diffusion noted at periventricular location. What is the likely diagnosis?

Introduction

Infiltration of the optic nerve is characterized by abnormal yellowish-white mass involving the optic nerve head associated with peripapillary hemorrhages and optic disc edema. Infiltration of the optic nerve head closely mimics other causes of optic disc edema such as raised intracranial tension, ischemic optic neuropathy, toxic and nutritional optic neuropathies.[1,2] However, optic nerve infiltration results in an atypical appearance of the nerve head due to the irregular nodular appearance of the tumor cells. Additional diagnostic tests such as cerebrospinal fluid (CSF) analysis and neuroimaging are relevant in determining the exact cause of the optic nerve abnormality. Features such as retinal vein/artery or combined occlusion, exudates, serous macular detachments and involvement of chiasma, optic tracts and other higher structures strongly favor infiltration of the optic nerve.

A number of primary malignancies such as gliomas can affect the optic nerve. In addition, central nervous system (CNS) lymphoma is also known to infiltrate and involve the optic nerve. Hematological malignancies such as leukemia can also result in involvement of the nervous system and optic nerve. Similarly, inflammatory lesions such as sarcoidosis and tuberculosis (TB) can result in granulomatous infiltration of the optic nerve head and may pose diagnostic challenge in the absence of other associated features.

Infiltrative optic neuropathies are important to identify, as these may be the presenting features of an underlying sinister disease. Various etiologies of this condition are described in the subsequent sections.

Primary tumors of the optic nerve head

Table 10.1 provides differences between classical optic neuritis and infiltrative optic neuropathies.

Optic nerve glioma

Optic nerve gliomas are typically benign indolent tumors, first noted in childhood. These tumors usually represent benign pilocytic astrocytomas (WHO grade I). These tumors are generally sporadic.[3–6] However, a familial preponderance may be noted when associated with neurofibromatosis (NF) type 1.[7–10] In children, gliomas can have an unpredictable clinical course and presenting history.[5,6] In adults, this tumor tends to be highly aggressive and is known as Glioblastoma multiforme (WHO grade IV).[11,12] Histopathologically benign tumors in adults are very rarely reported.

Epidemiology

Optic nerve gliomas comprise 1% of all the intracranial tumors. In children, gliomas represent 2–5% of all brain tumors. Approximately 29% of the optic nerve gliomas are associated with NF1. Among patients with NF1, optic nerve gliomas have been estimated to occur in 14–21% of the cases. Optic nerve glioma usually occurs in the first two decades of life. Females may have a higher preponderance to develop optic nerve gliomas.[3,5,9]

Clinical features

Optic nerve glioma of childhood presents with painless and slowly progressive proptosis associated with vision loss. Most common visual field defect is a central scotoma, but bitemporal field loss may occur if the chiasmal portion of optic nerve gets involved. Optic nerve head may appear edematous, infiltrated with tumor, or it can present in the stage of atrophy. Besides the optic nerve, this tumor can involve the chiasma, hypothalamus and optic tracts.[3,5,11] Patients with NF1 tend to typically have lesser proptosis and visual loss. Bilateral optic nerve gliomas can occur in patients with NF1.[13] Adults with Glioblastoma multiforme typically present with rapidly progressive visual loss, which can be associated with pain.[14]

Radiological features

Magnetic resonance imaging (MRI) of the optic nerve head and brain is the investigation of choice and it shows characteristic fusiform enlargement of the optic nerve. Lesions are usually isointense to hypointense on T1-weighted MRI and hyperintense on T2-weighted MRI. The two characteristic radiologic features seen with optic nerve gliomas are kinking and *double intensity tubular thickening* of the optic nerve. Involvement of the chiasm results in a "dumbbell tumor." This finding is highly characteristic of optic nerve glioma.[15,16] There is increased T2 signal surrounding the nerve due to perineural arachnoid gliomatosis.[17]

Histological and immunohistochemical features

Optic nerve gliomas are low-grade astrocytomas (and not hamartomas as previously thought). Lesions may invade the leptomeninges and result in a desmoplastic reaction consisting of fibroblastic response.[18] These tumors have low cellularity especially away from the main tumor bulk. Lesions with a higher grade on histology show an oligodendroglial response. Histopathological studies performed after tumor excision reveal that in several cases, tumors may remain dormant, fail to recur, or even completely involute despite a positive histological resection margin. This

DOI: 10.1201/9780429020278-13

TABLE 10.1: Differences between Optic Neuritis Related to Demyelinating Diseases and Infiltrative Optic Neuropathy (ON)

	Classical ON (Demyelinating Diseases)	Infiltrative ON
Onset	Acute onset	Acute, subacute onset
Course	Visual recovery starts after 1 month	Progressive visual loss
Pattern of Visual Loss	Central, centrocecal, arcuate	Arcuate, hemianopic
Ophthalmoscopic Findings	75% normal (retrobulbar) Swollen disc in papillitis	Optic disc swollen, elevated
Radiological Findings	Optic nerve enhancement on contrast MRI Findings specific to multiple sclerosis such as T2 hyperintense lesions in periventricular, cortical, juxtacortical space	MRI of the brain and orbit may show meningeal and optic nerve enhancement.
CSF	Elevated protein levels, monoclonal bands	Malignant cells
Additional Findings	Associated neurological signs of brainstem (diplopia, ataxia) and spinal cord involvement (paresthesia, bladder symptoms) may be present	Systemic malignancy in metastatic cases

may be attributed to reactive gliosis. Immunohistochemical studies using cell proliferation markers such as Ki-67 (MIB-1) and p53 may have a prognostic significance, especially in cases where the resection margin is positive. If the resection margin has values of Ki-67 labeling indices similar to the main bulk of the tumor, there may be higher chances of tumor recurrences and growth.[15,19]

Treatment and prognosis
Childhood gliomas are generally benign in their growth pattern. Children with NF1 should be screened for optic pathway gliomas during routine examination from the age of 12 years onward due to their high prevalence in this population.[8–10] Surgical excision should be considered only when there is a cosmetically unacceptable proptosis, progressive deterioration of visual function or radiological proof of tumor extension.[20,21] However, in the presence of chiasmal involvement, surgical intervention cannot be performed. Chiasmal tumors are treated with chemotherapy or radiotherapy.[22] Stereotactic radiotherapy has shown good results in few studies. Glioblastoma multiforme can show rapid spread even after aggressive radiation therapy resulting in high rates of mortality.[23,24]

The prognosis of patients with optic nerve gliomas is probably not much different between those with or without NF1. The mean survival period is reduced when there is involvement of chiasma or hypothalamus, and in patients with Glioblastoma multiforme.

Lymphoma
Lymphoma represents a group of malignant neoplasms of lymphoreticular origin. These tumors are categorized into Hodgkin's and non-Hodgkin's lymphoma. Approximately 10% patients with non-Hodgkin's lymphoma tend to develop CNS involvement, of which 5% develop optic nerve head infiltration.[25,26] Overall, lymphoma is an uncommon cause of optic nerve infiltration, and the clinical presentation and pattern of involvement depends upon the histological sub-type of the disease. In 2015, Kim et al[27] classified the optic nerve infiltration in lymphoma into four categories: (1) primary optic nerve involvement, (2) optic nerve involvement with CNS disease, (3) optic nerve involvement with systemic disease, and (4) optic nerve involvement with primary intraocular lymphoma (PIOL). This classification was developed with an aim to better understand and classify the pathophysiology of the disease and spread of the lesions. These conditions are described in the subsequent sections.

Primary optic nerve involvement
Primary optic nerve involvement with ocular lymphoma without any systemic/CNS lesions are extremely rare. Thus far, only three cases of primary optic nerve involvement in lymphoma have been reported in the literature.[28–30] All the patients were elderly women. Lesions were bilateral in two of these cases. The presenting complaint was decreased visual acuity and visual field loss. CSF analysis was negative for malignant cells in all these cases. The histological diagnosis was B-cell lymphoma in two cases and small cleaved cell lymphoma in one case. It is unknown whether malignant cells in this type of lymphoma arise *de novo* or are actually metastases from a clinically undetected primary tumor. Patients with primary optic nerve lesions are treated with a combination of radiotherapy, corticosteroids and chemotherapy. They can have variable outcomes, ranging from rapid onset of meningeal lymphomatosis leading to death.[27]

Optic nerve involvement with CNS disease
A subset of patients may have concurrent optic nerve and CNS involvement. In a large series of 752 patients from three French hospitals from 1998 to 2014, seven patients were determined to have optic nerve infiltration.[31] These patients present with decreased visual acuity or diplopia with neurological impairment. Optic nerve involvement can occur months to years after CNS disease (even after receiving chemotherapy), or may be the presenting form of the disease.[32–34] While some patients may have a normal fundus on examination, majority have evidence of optic nerve edema. Central retinal arteriolar occlusion as well as concomitant vein occlusion may be present on fundus examination.[35] Bilateral involvement may lead to asymmetric proptosis, especially in T-cell tumors. CSF analysis can show malignant cells in these cases. Neuroimaging shows enhancement of optic nerve, optic chiasma and/or optic tract (Figure 10.1). Rarely, neuroimaging may be completely normal even in the presence of CNS disease. Patients are treated with a combination of intravenous chemotherapy, intrathecal chemotherapy and radiation therapy. The outcomes may range from death within 3 weeks of onset of visual symptoms to several years later.[27]

Optic nerve involvement with systemic disease
A subset of patients with systemic lymphoma may have a positive CSF analysis for malignant cells. However, these patients do not have any evidence of CNS disease (including cranial neuropathies or lesions on neuroimaging). The presenting complaints include decreased visual acuity and field defects. Ocular findings in most of these patients include optic nerve edema with or without peripapillary hemorrhages. There may be conjunctival congestion and lid edema. Proptosis is rarely seen in these cases. Histological diagnosis include Hodgkin's lymphoma, Burkitt's lymphoma, diffuse large B-cell lymphoma and other undifferentiated/mixed lymphocytic/histiocytic tumors.[36–39] Similar to optic nerve lymphomas associated with CNS disease, these may develop

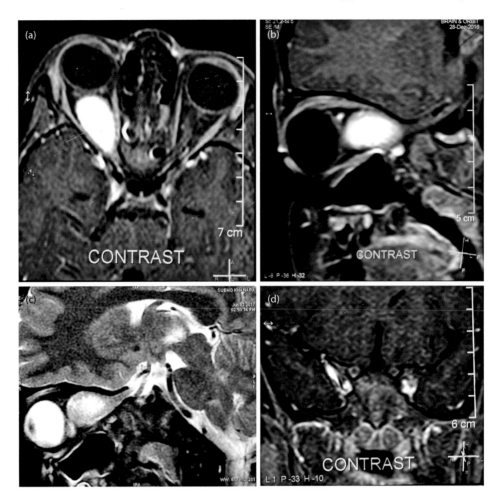

FIGURE 10.1 Gadolinium-enhanced T1-weighted axial (a) and oblique sagittal (b) MR images showing a well-defined homogeneously enhancing orbital intraconal lesion in close proximity with the optic nerve reaching till the orbital apex. Oblique sagittal T2-weighted MR (c) demonstrating its T2 hyperintense nature. Coronal gadolinium-enhanced T1 MR (d) revealing its relationship with the optic nerve. (Figure courtesy: Dr. Santosh G. Honavar, Hyderabad, India.)

while the patient is already on chemotherapy for systemic disease. Therefore, patients with systemic lymphoma who develop decreased visual acuity, and disc edema on fundus examination, must undergo a detailed work-up including CSF analysis and neuroimaging to detect optic nerve head infiltration requiring additional therapy. Treatment for patients in this category includes a combination of radiation, intrathecal chemotherapy and corticosteroids and intravenous chemotherapy.

Optic nerve involvement with primary intraocular lymphoma

PIOL is a malignant involvement of the vitreoretinal tissue and may affect the retina, vitreous or the optic nerve (Figure 10.2). The mechanism of spread of PIOL to the optic nerve is likely by direct extension of the tumor. Clinical examination shows edematous optic disc with exudates, dilated vessels and peripapillary hemorrhages. Treatment for patients in this category includes intravitreal chemotherapy (intravitreal methotrexate/rituximab) and/or systemic chemotherapy.[40,41]

Apart from the above four categories, disc edema in patients with lymphoma could be associated with other conditions such as raised intracranial pressure (ICP), compressive optic neuropathy due to orbital disease, drug-related toxicity (especially vincristine), paraneoplastic disease, infections (such as cryptococcal meningitis/

optic neuritis), or radiation-related. Therefore, a detailed evaluation of these patients is necessary to arrive at the correct diagnosis so that appropriate therapy can be initiated. Often, multiple lumbar punctures and neuroimaging may be necessary. Flow cytometry, polymerase chain reaction (to detect translocations) and interleukin analysis of the CSF may be useful adjunctive diagnostic tools.[27]

Leukemia

Leukemia is a group of hematological malignancies in which the bone marrow is replaced by hematopoietic neoplastic cells. It may involve the optic nerve head by lymphocytic or myelogenous leukemic infiltration as an early or late sequela of CNS leukemia. Optic nerve involvement may be a direct extension of the CNS leukemia, by direct infiltration of the nerve, or can occur passively due to retrolaminar leukemic invasion.[42-46]

Epidemiology

Optic nerve involvement in leukemia signifies presence of CNS leukemia. Optic disc infiltration occurs in about 1.4–9% of patients with acute lymphocytic leukemia (ALL).[46,47] It may occur in chronic lymphocytic leukemia (CLL) as well, typically in association with a hematological relapse.[48-50] In an autopsy series of 384 patients, 18% patients with ALL and 16% with chronic leukemias had optic nerve involvement.[46]

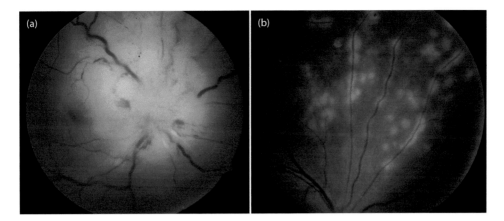

FIGURE 10.2 Optic nerve infiltration in a case of vitreoretinal lymphoma. The optic nerve head appears edematous, elevated and the details of the nerve are totally obscured by the yellowish-white tumor infiltrates. There is significant vascular congestion and venous dilation and tortuosity. There are surrounding flame-shaped as well as blot hemorrhages. In addition, there is diffuse peripapillary whitening of the retina suggestive of retinal ischemia (a). Fundus photograph of the periphery shows subretinal yellow deposits and perivascular infiltrates, characteristic of vitreoretinal lymphoma (b).

Clinical features

The most common manifestation in the leukemic infiltration of optic nerve head is blurring of vision. The loss of vision may be acute, though rarely patients may remain asymptomatic despite optic nerve infiltration.[51] Profound vision loss including no light perception is common. Other symptoms and signs include ocular pain, conjunctival congestion and photophobia. Signs of increased ICP such as sixth cranial nerve palsy may indicate a diffuse meningeal involvement. Ophthalmoscopic examination may reveal optic disc edema with or without hemorrhages. Occasionally, the optic disc may appear normal.[52] Presence of leukemic infiltrates results in the disc to appear creamy white with infiltrates, elevated, with peripapillary dot and blot or flame-shaped hemorrhages, along with serous macular detachment (Figure 10.3). Occlusion of the central retinal artery and vein is common association. Retinal hemorrhages may also be associated with anemia or pancytopenia (Figure 10.4).[52–56]

Optic disc involvement in a patient who has already received chemotherapy heralds a relapse of leukemia. Optic nerves are considered as sanctuaries of leukemic cells and the optic canal may provide a barrier against the penetration of anti-cancer drugs given intrathecally. Therefore, optic disc infiltration is a sinister sign of the disease which needs prompt evaluation and therapy.[49–51,57]

Radiologic features

Neuroimaging including MRI brain is essential to detect various CNS abnormalities related to leukemia such as direct leukemic infiltration, hemorrhages, treatment-related infections, neurotoxicity and secondary malignant tumors. Neuroimaging studies can show either plaque-like deposits or intraparenchymal infiltration of the optic axons or diffuse leptomeningeal-enhancing lesions surrounding the optic nerve. Tubular involvement of the optic nerve can be appreciated on MRI. Extraocular muscles are usually spared.[42,51,57,58]

Treatment and prognosis

In a patient with known disease, prophylactic brain radiation is often administered to prevent a CNS relapse. However, certain areas in the optic nerve may be missed with brain radiation and may harbor leukemic cells that eventually grow resulting in relapse. Although there is no consensus on the management of CNS leukemia, a common approach is to use emergent intrathecal chemotherapy in combination with systemic chemotherapy and external radiation therapy. The visual prognosis for leukemic optic nerve infiltration is generally poor. If the treatment is initiated early, the chances of salvaging vision may be better. Radiation therapy may be particularly helpful in eradicating leukemic cells within the optic canal resulting in better action of the intrathecal chemotherapeutic agents.[43,44,46,47,54,55]

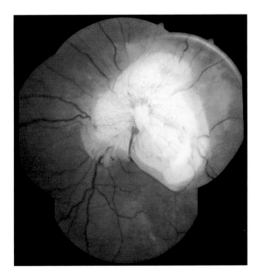

FIGURE 10.3 Optic disc photograph of a young 18-year-old girl diagnosed with acute lymphoblastic leukemia (ALL) and optic nerve infiltration. The optic disc shows raised, voluminous whitish infiltration with fine vessels on the surface and hemorrhages and inferior exudative retinal detachment. The whitish mass is seen extending to the peripapillary area.

Metastasis

Metastasis to the optic disc accounts for 5% of all the intraocular metastasis. Most of the metastatic neoplasms to the optic nerve are carcinomas. Breast and lung are the most common primary

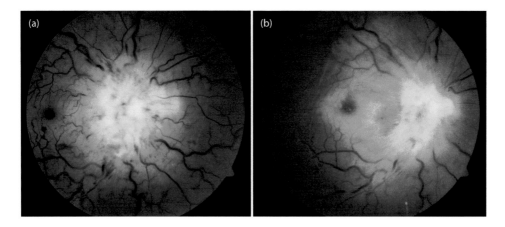

FIGURE 10.4 Optic disc photograph of a 21-year-old male with acute lymphoblastic leukemia (ALL) shows significant optic nerve head edema and elevation, and yellowish-white infiltrates with multiple dot-blot and flame-shaped hemorrhages. There is significant vascular tortuosity and retinal whitening (a). Fundus photograph centered on the macula obtained 3 days later shows perifoveal retinal whitening with a cherry-red spot suggestive of central retinal artery occlusion (b).

neoplasms that account for metastasis to the optic disc.[59,60] Other sites of involvement are the intestines, kidney and prostate.[61–63] However, in 20% patients, the primary site is never determined. Metastatic neoplasm to the optic nerve can occur as a direct hematogenous metastasis to the neural tissue or to the overlying meninges.[64]

Clinical features

Ophthalmoscopic features include optic disc edema that can be seen as diffuse yellowish-white thickening of optic disc with or without flame-shaped hemorrhages. There could be additional features including serous macular detachment, cannon-ball choroidal infiltrates, exophthalmos, retinal hemorrhages, central retinal artery/vein occlusion or rarely a combined artery-vein occlusion.

Radiologic features

Metastatic carcinomas are characteristically isointense or slightly hyperintense on T1-weighted images and hypointense on T2-weighted MRI images. Depending on the primary tumor, the

neuro-radiological features of the metastasis may vary. Additional features on MRI could be hemorrhages, infections and metastatic lesions in the brain.[64]

It is important to differentiate optic disc swelling due to raised ICP from pseudo-papilledema due to metastatic infiltration of optic nerve head. Papilledema is generally bilateral, whereas infiltrative optic neuropathy can be unilateral or bilateral. Fluorescein angiography will show leakage in papilledema, whereas leakage may/may not be present in pseudo-papilledema. In addition, there will be other features of raised ICP like postural headache, sixth nerve paresis and/or focal neurological deficits in papilledema.

Treatment and prognosis

The patient is treated with appropriate chemotherapy for systemic malignancy. External beam radiation is given to the posterior segment of the affected eye. The prognosis of patients with optic disc metastasis is generally poor.

Table 10.2 lists the important differences between various infiltrative optic neuropathies.

TABLE 10.2: Differences between Various Etiologies of Infiltrative Optic Neuropathies

	Optic Nerve Glioma	Lymphoma	Leukemia	Metastasis
Age of presentation	Median age of presentation—6.5 years Glioblastoma multiforme in adults	Fourth to sixth decade	4–5 years (ALL) 65–70 years (CLL)	Fifth to seventh decade
Clinical features	Painless, progressive proptosis and vision loss	Vision loss	Vision loss, ocular pain	Progressive visual loss, features of systemic malignancy
Ophthalmoscopic findings	Optic disc edematous, maybe atrophic in late stages	Optic disc edematous, Vitritis in primary intraocular lymphoma	Creamy white optic disc with infiltrates, elevated with peripapillary hemorrhages	Diffuse yellowish-white thickening of optic disc with or without flame-shaped hemorrhages
Radiological findings	Fusiform enlargement of the optic nerve, kinking and double intensity thickening of optic nerve	Enhancement of optic nerve, optic chiasma and/or optic tract	Plaque-like deposits or intraparenchymal infiltration of the optic axons or diffuse leptomeningeal-enhancing lesions surrounding the optic nerve	Metastatic carcinomas are characteristically isointense or slightly hyperintense on T1-weighted images and hypointense on T2-weighted MRI images

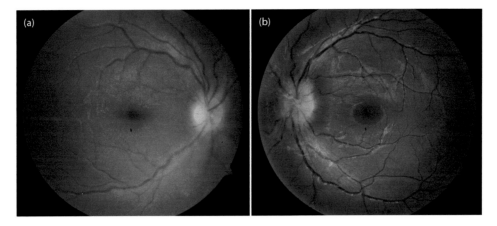

FIGURE 10.5 Fundus photograph of a 30-year-old female with neurosarcoidosis with bilateral decrease in vision (a and b). Fundus photographs reveal bilateral optic disc edema. In addition, there is mild vitritis and focal retinal vasculitis in the right eye (a).

Inflammatory lesions of optic nerve head: Sarcoidosis

Sarcoidosis is an inflammatory multisystem disorder of unknown etiology. Ocular involvement in sarcoidosis is common and can occur at any time during the course of the disease and can even predate the disease. Ocular manifestations vary enormously and include granulomatous or non-granulomatous anterior uveitis, intermediate uveitis, retinal periphlebitis, multifocal choroiditis, papillitis, optic nerve granuloma, lacrimal gland enlargement and, rarely, orbital involvement or scleritis.[65–68]

Optic nerve involvement occurs in 1–5% of the cases and it is the second commonest nerve to be involved after the facial nerve.[69,70] Although optic nerve head involvement is often found in individuals with evidence of systemic sarcoidosis, it can be the initial and even the only sign of this disease. Optic nerve head lesions in sarcoidosis can closely mimic gliomas, especially in children.[71–73] Histologic descriptions have shown infiltration and granuloma formation in the optic nerve head in sarcoidosis. Optic disc edema without granulomatous invasion of the optic nerve head may be seen in patients either with chronic uveitis or with papilledema from CNS sarcoid (Figure 10.5). Occasionally, isolated optic neuropathy (atrophy, optic neuritis, optic disc edema) may occur and may be the first manifestation of neurosarcoidosis.[74]

Treatment of sarcoidosis in general and neurosarcoidosis, in particular, may be extremely difficult. Corticosteroids are the mainstay of therapy; there are no standardized treatment protocols available as yet. Although corticosteroids are very effective in controlling inflammation initially, their long-term use is often associated with significant complications.[70,71] Among patients where chronic steroid usage (≥7.5 mg of prednisone or equivalent daily) is required to control the inflammation, the use of steroid-sparing agents is indicated. Immunosuppressive agents such as hydroxychloroquine, methotrexate, azathioprine, mycophenolate mofetil, or cyclosporine may be useful. Rarely, patients may require biological agents including antagonists of tumor necrosis factor (TNF) such as adalimumab, infliximab or etanercept.[75,76]

Infective lesions of optic nerve head

Tuberculosis
Ocular TB often presents as a diagnostic challenge due to its protean manifestations. Ocular TB can affect various ocular structures resulting in anterior, intermediate, posterior or panuveitis.

Patients with Ocular TB are diagnosed on the basis of positive laboratory evidence of active or latent TB, or radiological evidence of past (or present) active TB in the form of lung parenchymal involvement or presence of lymphadenopathy.[77,78] TB is prevalent in several countries of the world.[79,80] Ocular TB is a predominately a paucibacillary disease that is believed to represent an immune-mediated hypersensitivity reaction to the acid-fast bacilli sequestrated in the ocular tissues, notably the retinal pigment epithelium (RPE).[78,81,82]

Optic nerve involvement is a common complication of ocular TB. It may result from direct mycobacterial infection, by contiguous spread from the choroid or hematogenous dissemination or from a hypersensitivity to the infectious agent. The clinical spectrum of tuberculous optic neuropathy is wide, with papillitis (51.6%), neuroretinitis (14.5%) and optic nerve tubercle (11.3%) being the most common clinical form (Figure 10.6).[83–88] Secondary optic nerve involvement may occur in rare conditions such as pituitary TB.[89]

Optic atrophy in patients on anti-tubercular therapy must be evaluated promptly for ethambutol toxicity.[90] Linezolid is another antimicrobial agent used for the management of TB that can lead to optic atrophy.[91,92]

The management of ocular TB involves the use of anti-tubercular treatment for 9–12 months. The use of adjunctive systemic corticosteroid therapy may help reduce the inflammatory reaction.[79,93,94]

Toxoplasmosis
Ocular toxoplasmosis is one of the most frequent etiologies of infectious posterior uveitis. This condition is caused by the obligate intracellular protozoan parasite *Toxoplasma gondii*. Ocular involvement in toxoplasmosis may result from acquired infection after birth or from the congenital form of the disease. The classical presentation of the disease is a focus of inner retinitis adjacent to an old chorioretinal scar accompanied by dense focal vitritis (*headlight in fog* appearance).[95–97]

Toxoplasma gondii may cause a lesion in the optic disc because of contiguousness or by direct involvement. Optic nerve can become involved even when a retinochoroiditis lesion is located far from the optic nerve. In *toxoplasma papillitis*, the parasite affects the optic disc directly, causing a swollen optic disc with sheathing of the peripapillary veins (Figure 10.7). Diagnosis of ocular toxoplasmosis may be challenging in these cases.[98–100]

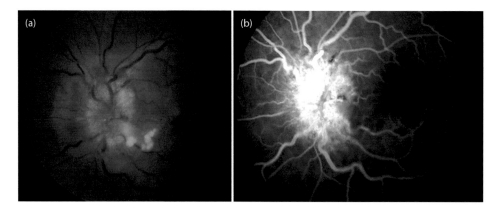

FIGURE 10.6 Optic disc photographs of a 45-year-old female who presented with sudden-onset diminution of vision in the left eye for the past 4 days. Photograph reveals hyperemic disc edema and elevation with surrounding peripapillary fluid and exudation. There is nodular disc elevation suggestive of optic nerve head granuloma (a). Fluorescein angiography (b) shows leakage from the optic nerve head granuloma (b). Her tuberculin skin test was highly positive (30 × 3 mm). There were few paratracheal lymph nodes on contrast-enhanced computerized chest tomography, but no active tubercular lesions. The patient was diagnosed with tubercular optic nerve head granuloma.

The most commonly employed treatment strategy for ocular toxoplasmosis is systemic administration of one or more antibiotics usually given for 4–8 weeks. The patients are treated with a combination of anti-parasitic drugs pyrimethamine (25–50 mg daily orally in one to two doses) and sulfadiazine along with corticosteroids. Trimethoprim-sulfamethoxazole (160–800 mg twice daily orally) is another option that has advantages of low cost, wide availability and tolerability. Clindamycin (300 mg orally four times daily) is often added to triple therapy, which is then referred to as "quadruple therapy."[95,101] The final visual acuity depends basically on the location of the retinal lesion, and not on the involvement of the optic disc.[99,102]

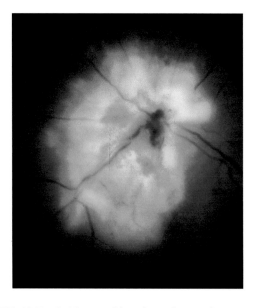

FIGURE 10.7 A 28-year-old male with toxoplasma papillitis and surrounding retinochoroiditis. There is a diffuse optic disc edema and a large whitish area of retinitis with overlying hemorrhages more prominently over the optic disc. There is vascular tortuosity and sheathing suggestive of active inflammation.

Cryptococcosis

Cryptococcus neoformans is the most common cause of fungal optic neuropathy and is related to the HIV-AIDS epidemic.[103] Optic neuritis occurs most commonly with cryptococcal meningitis, and can be unilateral or bilateral. The optic nerve damage may result from direct invasion by the fungus, inflammation, ischemia from vasculitis, increased ICP or a combination of these factors.[103–108]

Cryptococcal infection is characterized by a rapid onset of a few hours to a few days due to rapid and direct invasion of the optic nerve. Commonly, patients are already being treated with amphotericin B and/or fluconazole for cryptococcal meningitis and an increase of the dose can be effective in helping to control the optic nerve involvement. Amphotericin B may be given intravitreally and/or intravenously. This condition carries high systemic and visual morbidity and the prognosis is usually guarded.[107,108]

Conclusion

Various malignancies can lead to infiltration of the optic nerves. Infiltrative optic neuropathies usually cause relentlessly progressive visual symptoms. The classical appearance of an elevated, swollen disc with yellowish/creamy white deposits with or without haemorrhages may not be present in all cases, hence requiring a high index of suspicion in relevant clinical scenarios. Few inflammatory and infectious causes may also cause infiltration of the optic nerve. A systematic clinical approach may help differentiate these causes aiding in early diagnosis and prompt management.

Acknowledgments

The authors have no financial disclosure/proprietary interest. No conflicting relationship exists for any author. The authors report no conflicts of interest. The authors alone are responsible for the content and preparation of this manuscript. We would like to acknowledge efforts of Mr. Arun Kapil, Mr. Sushil Bhatt, and Mr. Nitin Gautam who helped in the acquisition of images for this case.

Multiple-Choice Questions

1. "Dumbbell tumor" refers to one of the following:
   a. Optic nerve meningioma involving the optic nerve head.
   b. Optic nerve glioma involving the optic chiasma.
   c. Optic nerve glioma involving the optic tract.
   d. Optic nerve meningioma involving the optic chiasma.

   Answer:

   b. Optic nerve glioma involving the optic chiasma.

2. The most common tumor metastasizing to optic nerve head in females is:
   a. Adenocarcinoma of kidney
   b. Adenocarcinoma of lung
   c. Adenocarcinoma of ovary
   d. Adenocarcinoma of breast

   Answer:

   d. Adenocarcinoma of breast

3. The most common cranial nerve infiltrated in sarcoidosis is:
   a. Optic nerve
   b. Facial nerve
   c. Trigeminal nerve
   d. None of the above

   Answer:

   b. Facial nerve

4. Leukemic infiltration of the optic nerve is seen most commonly in:
   a. Acute myeloid leukemia (AML)
   b. Acute lymphoblastic leukemia (ALL)
   c. Chronic myelogenous leukemia (CML)
   d. Chronic lymphocytic leukemia (CLL)

   Answer:

   b. Acute lymphoblastic leukemia (ALL)

References

1. Takkar A, Naheed D, Dogra M, et al. Infiltrative optic neuropathies: Opening doors to sinister pathologies. Neuroophthalmology. 2017;41(5):279–283.
2. Birnbaum FA, Meekins LC, Srinivasan A, Murchison AP. A lot of nerve. Surv Ophthalmol. 2020;65(2):272–277.
3. Miller NR. Optic gliomas: Past, present, and future. J Neuroophthalmol. 2016;36(4):460–473.
4. Nair AG, Pathak RS, Iyer VR, Gandhi RA. Optic nerve glioma: An update. Int Ophthalmol. 2014;34(4):999–1005.
5. Rasool N, Odel JG, Kazim M. Optic pathway glioma of childhood. Curr Opin Ophthalmol. 2017;28(3):289–295.
6. Varan A, Batu A, Cila A, et al. Optic glioma in children: A retrospective analysis of 101 cases. Am J Clin Oncol. 2013;36(3):287–292.
7. Eid H, Crevier-Sorbo G, Aldraihem A, Menegotto F, Wilson N. Neurofibromatosis type 1: Description of a novel diagnostic scoring system in pediatric optic nerve glioma. AJR Am J Roentgenol. 2019;212(4):892–898.
8. Peltonen S, Kallionpää RA, Rantanen M, Uusitalo E, Lähteenmäki PM, Pöyhönen M, Pitkäniemi J, Peltonen J. Pediatric malignancies in neurofibromatosis type 1: A population-based cohort study. Int J Cancer. 2019;145(11):2926–2932.
9. Campen CJ, Gutmann DH. Optic pathway gliomas in neurofibromatosis type 1. J Child Neurol. 2018;33(1):73–81.
10. Sylvester CL, Drohan LA, Sergott RC. Optic-nerve gliomas, chiasmal gliomas and neurofibromatosis type 1. Curr Opin Ophthalmol. 2006;17(1):7–11.
11. Bilgin G, Al-Obailan M, Bonelli L, Glasgow BJ, Vinters HV, Arnold AC. Aggressive low-grade optic nerve glioma in adults. Neuroophthalmology. 2014;38(6):297–309.
12. Alvord EC, Lofton S. Gliomas of the optic nerve or chiasm. Outcome by patients' age, tumor site, and treatment. J Neurosurg. 1988;68(1):85–98.
13. Parkhurst E, Abboy S. Optic gliomas in neurofibromatosis type 1. J Pediatr Ophthalmol Strabismus. 2016;53(6):334–338.
14. Nguyen HN, Vo KBH, Howard S, Salamat MS, Rowely H, Robins HI. Vision loss in glioblastoma: Disease mimicking presumed therapeutic toxicity. Neurooncol Pract. 2018;5(4):223–226.
15. Cummings TJ, Provenzale JM, Hunter SB, et al. Gliomas of the optic nerve: Histological, immunohistochemical (MIB-1 and p53), and MRI analysis. Acta Neuropathol. 2000;99(5):563–570.
16. Van Es S, North KN, McHugh K, De Silva M. MRI findings in children with neurofibromatosis type 1: A prospective study. Pediatr Radiol. 1996;26(7):478–487.
17. Seiff SR, Brodsky MC, MacDonald G, Berg BO, Howes EL, Hoyt WF. Orbital optic glioma in neurofibromatosis. Magnetic resonance diagnosis of perineural arachnoidal gliomatosis. Arch Ophthalmol. 1987;105(12):1689–1692.
18. Matsumoto T, Fujii T, Yabe M, Oka K, Hoshi T, Sato K. MIB-1 and p53 immunocytochemistry for differentiating pilocytic astrocytomas and astrocytomas from anaplastic astrocytomas and glioblastomas in children and young adults. Histopathology. 1998;33(5):446–452.
19. Yeung SN, White VA, Nimmo M, Rootman J. Optic nerve gliomas: Role of Ki-67 staining of tumour and margins in predicting long-term outcome. Br J Ophthalmol. 2011;95(8):1077–1081.
20. Spitzer DE, Goodrich JT. Optic gliomas and neurofibromatosis: Neurosurgical management. Neurofibromatosis. 1988;1(4):223–232.
21. El Beltagy MA, Reda M, Enayet A, et al. Treatment and Outcome in 65 Children with Optic Pathway Gliomas. World Neurosurg. 2016;89:525–534.
22. Mohadjer M, Etou A, Milios E, Baden R, Mundinger F. Chiasmatic optic glioma. Neurochirurgia (Stuttg). 1991;34(3):90–93.
23. Uslu N, Karakaya E, Dizman A, Yegen D, Guney Y. Optic nerve glioma treatment with fractionated stereotactic radiotherapy. J Neurosurg Pediatr. 2013;11(5):596–599.
24. El-Shehaby AMN, Reda WA, Abdel Karim KM, Emad Eldin RM, Nabeel AM. Single-session gamma knife radiosurgery for optic pathway/hypothalamic gliomas. J Neurosurg. 2016;125 (1):50–57.
25. Zaman AG, Graham EM, Sanders MD. Anterior visual system involvement in non-Hodgkin's lymphoma. Br J Ophthalmol. 1993;77(3):184–187.
26. MacKintosh FR, Colby TV, Podolsky WJ, et al. Central nervous system involvement in non-Hodgkin's lymphoma: an analysis of 105 cases. Cancer. 1982;49(3):586–595.
27. Kim JL, Mendoza PR, Rashid A, Hayek B, Grossniklaus HE. Optic nerve lymphoma: Report of two cases and review of the literature. Surv Ophthalmol. 2015;60(2):153–165.
28. Strominger MB, Schatz NJ, Glaser JS. Lymphomatous optic neuropathy. Am J Ophthalmol. 1993;116(6):774–776.
29. Behbehani RS, Vacarezza N, Sergott RC, Bilyk JR, Hochberg F, Savino PJ. Isolated optic nerve lymphoma diagnosed by optic nerve biopsy. Am J Ophthalmol. 2005;139(6):1128–1130.
30. Dayan MR, Elston JS, McDonald B. Bilateral lymphomatous optic neuropathy diagnosed on optic nerve biopsy. Arch Ophthalmol. 2000;118(10):1455–1457.
31. Ahle G, Touitou V, Cassoux N, et al. Optic nerve infiltration in primary central nervous system lymphoma. JAMA Neurol. 2017;74(11):1368–1373.
32. Kitzmann AS, Pulido JS, Garrity JA, Witzig TE. Histologic findings in T-cell lymphoma infiltration of the optic nerve. Ophthalmology. 2008;115(5):e1–6.
33. Lee LC, Howes EL, Bhisitkul RB. Systemic non-Hodgkin's lymphoma with optic nerve infiltration in a patient with AIDS. Retina (Philadelphia, Pa). 2002;22(1):75–79.
34. Zelefsky JR, Revercomb CH, Lantos G, Warren FA. Isolated lymphoma of the anterior visual pathway diagnosed by optic nerve biopsy. J Neuroophthalmol. 2008;28(1):36–40.
35. Guyer DR, Green WR, Schachat AP, Bastacky S, Miller NR. Bilateral ischemic optic neuropathy and retinal vascular occlusions associated with lymphoma and sepsis. Clinicopathologic correlation. Ophthalmology. 1990;97(7):882–888.
36. Kim UR, Shah AD, Arora V, Solanki U. Isolated optic nerve infiltration in systemic lymphoma—a case report and review of literature. Ophthalmic Plast Reconstr Surg. 2010;26(4):291–293.
37. Kattah JC, Suski ET, Killen JY, Smith FP, Limaye SR. Optic neuritis and systemic lymphoma. Am J Ophthalmol. 1980;89(3):431–436.
38. Sudhakar P, Rodriguez FR, Trobe JD. MRI restricted diffusion in lymphomatous optic neuropathy. J Neuroophthalmol. 2011;31(4):306–309.
39. Kay MC. Optic neuropathy secondary to lymphoma. J Clin Neuroophthalmol. 1986;6(1):31–34.
40. Akpek EK, Thorne JE, Qazi FA, Do DV, Jabs DA. Evaluation of patients with scleritis for systemic disease. Ophthalmology. 2004;111(3):501–506.
41. Gill MK, Jampol LM. Variations in the presentation of primary intraocular lymphoma: case reports and a review. Surv Ophthalmol. 2001;45(6):463–471.
42. Camera A, Piccirillo G, Cennamo G, et al. Optic nerve involvement in acute lymphoblastic leukemia. Leuk Lymphoma. 1993;11(1–2):153–155.
43. Nikaido H, Mishima H, Ono H, Choshi K, Dohy H. Leukemic involvement of the optic nerve. Am J Ophthalmol. 1988;105(3):294–298.
44. Wallace RT, Shields JA, Shields CL, Ehya H, Ewing M. Leukemic infiltration of the optic nerve. Arch Ophthalmol. 1991;109(7):1027.
45. Rosenthal AR. Ocular manifestations of leukemia. A review. Ophthalmology. 1983;90(8):899–905.
46. Kincaid MC, Green WR. Ocular and orbital involvement in leukemia. Surv Ophthalmol. 1983;27(4):211–232.
47. Ridgway EW, Jaffe N, Walton DS. Leukemic ophthalmopathy in children. Cancer. 1976;38(4):1744–1749.

48. Nagpal BN, Saxena R, Srivastava A, et al. Retrospective study of chikungunya outbreak in urban areas of India. Indian J Med Res. 2012;135:351–358.

49. Salazar Méndez R, Fonollá Gil M. Unilateral optic disk edema with central retinal artery and vein occlusions as the presenting signs of relapse in acute lymphoblastic leukemia. Arch Soc Esp Oftalmol. 2014;89(11):454–458.

50. Ali MJ, Honavar SG. Optic nerve infiltration in relapse of acute lymphoblastic leukemia. Oman J Ophthalmol. 2011;4(3):152.

51. Caty J, Grigorian AP, Grigorian F. Asymptomatic leukemic optic nerve infiltration as presentation of acute lymphoblastic leukemia relapse. J Pediatr Ophthalmol Strabismus. 2017;54:e60–e62.

52. Schocket LS, Massaro-Giordano M, Volpe NJ, Galetta SL. Bilateral optic nerve infiltration in central nervous system leukemia. Am J Ophthalmol. 2003;135(1):94–96.

53. Randhawa S, Ruben J. Leukemic optic nerve infiltration. Ophthalmology. 2017;124(3):277.

54. Shah P, Yohendran J, Lowe D, McCluskey P. Devastating bilateral optic nerve leukaemic infiltration. Clin Experiment Ophthalmol. 2012;40(1):e114–115.

55. Berryman J, Moshiri A, Chang M. Chronic lymphocytic leukaemia presenting as branch retinal artery occlusion and optic disc infiltration. BMJ Case Rep. 2018:bcr 2018227691.

56. Moisseiev E, Ling J, Morse LS. Leukemic optic nerve infiltration complicated by retinal artery and vein occlusions. Retina (Philadelphia, Pa). 2017;37(2):e10.

57. Madani A, Christophe C, Ferster A, Dan B. Peri-optic nerve infiltration during leukaemic relapse: MRI diagnosis. Pediatr Radiol. 2000;30(1):30–32.

58. de Fátima Soares M, Braga FT, da Rocha AJ, Lederman HM. Optic nerve infiltration by acute lymphoblastic leukemia: MRI contribution. Pediatr Radiol. 2005;35(8):799–802.

59. Aghdam KA, Zand A, Sanjari MS. Isolated unilateral infiltrative optic neuropathy in a patient with breast cancer. Turk J Ophthalmol. 2019;49(3):171–174.

60. Hernández Pardines F, Molina Martín JC, Fernández Montalvo L, Juárez Marroquí A. Optic nerve metastasis caused by lung adenocarcinoma. Arch Soc Esp Oftalmol. 2017;92(11):552–554.

61. Yang HS, Jeong HR, Kim CW, Yoon YH, Kim J-G. Histological heterogeneity between primary and metastatic cancer in a pathologic confirmed case of isolated optic disc metastasis of prostate adenocarcinoma. Graefes Arch Clin Exp Ophthalmol. 2013;251(1):375–378.

62. Jamall O, Theodoraki K, Amin S, Verity D, Bates A. Rectal adenocarcinoma: Rare metastasis to the optic nerve. BMJ Case Rep. 2019;12(1):e228090.

63. Lau JJC, Trobe JD, Ruiz RE, et al. Metastatic neuroblastoma presenting with binocular blindness from intracranial compression of the optic nerves. J Neuroophthalmol. 2004;24(2):119–124.

64. Brown GC, Shields JA. Tumors of the optic nerve head. Surv Ophthalmol. 1985;29(4):239–264.

65. Herbort CP, Rao NA, Mochizuki M, members of Scientific Committee of First International Workshop on Ocular Sarcoidosis. International criteria for the diagnosis of ocular sarcoidosis: results of the first International Workshop on Ocular Sarcoidosis (IWOS). Ocul Immunol Inflamm. 2009;17(3):160–169.

66. Acharya NR, Browne EN, Rao N, Mochizuki M, International Ocular Sarcoidosis Working Group. Distinguishing features of ocular sarcoidosis in an International cohort of uveitis patients. Ophthalmology. 2018;125(1):119–126.

67. Kawaguchi T, Hanada A, Horie S, Sugamoto Y, Sugita S, Mochizuki M. Evaluation of characteristic ocular signs and systemic investigations in ocular sarcoidosis patients. Jpn J Ophthalmol. 2007;51(2):121–126.

68. Yang SJ, Salek S, Rosenbaum JT. Ocular sarcoidosis: New diagnostic modalities and treatment. Curr Opin Pulm Med. 2017;23(5):458–467.

69. Mafee MF, Dorodi S, Pai E. Sarcoidosis of the eye, orbit, and central nervous system. Role of MR imaging. Radiol Clin North Am. 1999;37(1):73–87.

70. Graham EM, Ellis CJ, Sanders MD, McDonald WI. Optic neuropathy in sarcoidosis. J Neurol Neurosurg Psychiatry. 1986;49(7):756–763.

71. Elia M, Kombo N, Huang J. Neurosarcoidosis masquerading as a central nervous system tumor. Retin Cases Brief Rep. 2017;11 Suppl 1:S166–S169.

72. Uruha A, Koide R, Taniguchi M. Unusual presentation of sarcoidosis: Solitary intracranial mass lesion mimicking a glioma. J Neuroimaging. 2011;21(2):e180–182.

73. Ng KL, McDermott N, Romanowski CA, Jackson A. Neurosarcoidosis masquerading as glioma of the optic chiasm in a child. Postgrad Med J. 1995;71(835):265–268.

74. Yilmazlar S, Kocaeli H, Korfali E. Primary-isolated optic nerve sarcoidosis. Acta Neurochir (Wien). 2004;146(1):65–67.

75. Fritz D, van de Beek D, Brouwer MC. Clinical features, treatment and outcome in neurosarcoidosis: Systematic review and meta-analysis. BMC Neurol. 2016;16(1):220.

76. Matsou A, Tsaousis KT. Management of chronic ocular sarcoidosis: Challenges and solutions. Clin Ophthalmol. 2018;12:519–532.

77. Gupta V, Shoughy SS, Mahajan S, et al. Clinics of ocular tuberculosis. Ocul Immunol Inflamm. 2015;23(1):14–24.

78. Gupta V, Gupta A, Rao NA. Intraocular tuberculosis—an update. Surv Ophthalmol. 2007;52(6):561–587.

79. Agrawal R, Gunasekeran DV, Grant R, et al. Clinical features and outcomes of patients with tubercular uveitis treated with antitubercular therapy in the collaborative ocular tuberculosis study (COTS)-1. JAMA Ophthalmol. 2017;135(12):1318–1327.

80. Agrawal R, Gunasekeran DV, Raje D, et al. Global variations and challenges with tubercular uveitis in the collaborative ocular tuberculosis study. Invest Ophthalmol Vis Sci. 2018;59(10):4162–4171.

81. Ang M, Vasconcelos-Santos DV, Sharma K, et al. Diagnosis of ocular tuberculosis. Ocul Immunol Inflamm. 2018;26(2):208–216.

82. Nazari Khanamiri H, Rao NA. Serpiginous choroiditis and infectious multifocal serpiginoid choroiditis. Surv Ophthalmol. 2013;58(3):203–232.

83. Davis EJ, Rathinam SR, Okada AA, et al. Clinical spectrum of tuberculous optic neuropathy. J Ophthalmic Inflamm Infect. 2012;2(4):183–189.

84. Invernizzi A, Agarwal A, Di Nicola M, Franzetti F, Staurenghi G, Viola F. Choroidal neovascular membranes secondary to intraocular tuberculosis misdiagnosed as neovascular age-related macular degeneration. Eur J Ophthalmol. 2018;28(2):216–224.

85. Reche-Sainz JA, Gracia García-Miguel MT, Pérez-Jacoiste MA. Papillitis and neuroretinitis of tuberculous etiology. Arch Soc Esp Oftalmol (Engl Ed). 2019;94(7):359–362.

86. Sivakumar P, Vedachalam R, Devy N. Management challenge: Optic disc granuloma in pulmonary tuberculosis. Indian J Ophthalmol. 2018;66(2):301.

87. Majumder AK, Sheth S, Dharani V, Dutta Majumder P. An unusual case of tuberculous optic neuropathy associated with choroiditis. Indian J Ophthalmol. 2019;67(7):1210–1212.

88. Zuhaimy H, Leow SN, Vasudevan SK. Optic disc swelling in a patient with tuberculous meningitis: a diagnostic challenge. BMJ Case Rep. 2017;bcr2017221170.

89. Sohail AH, Bhatti UF, Islam N. Pituitary tuberculoma. J Coll Physicians Surg Pak. 2018;28(6):S97–S98.

90. Jin KW, Lee JY, Rhiu S, Choi DG. Longitudinal evaluation of visual function and structure for detection of subclinical ethambutol-induced optic neuropathy. PLoS ONE. 2019;14(4):e0215297.

91. Han J, Lee K, Rhiu S, Lee JB, Han SH. Linezolid-associated optic neuropathy in a patient with drug-resistant tuberculosis. J Neuroophthalmol. 2013;33(3):316–318.

92. Mehta S, Das M, Laxmeshwar C, Jonckheere S, Thi SS, Isaakidis P. Linezolid-associated optic neuropathy in drug-resistant tuberculosis patients in Mumbai, India. PLoS ONE. 2016;11(9):e0162138.

93. Agrawal R, Gupta B, Gonzalez-Lopez JJ, et al. The role of anti-tubercular therapy in patients with presumed ocular tuberculosis. Ocul Immunol Inflamm. 2015;23(1):40–46.

94. Bansal R, Gupta A, Gupta V, Dogra MR, Bambery P, Arora SK. Role of anti-tubercular therapy in uveitis with latent/manifest tuberculosis. Am J Ophthalmol. 2008;146(5):772–779.

95. Maenz M, Schlüter D, Liesenfeld O, Schares G, Gross U, Pleyer U. Ocular toxoplasmosis past, present and new aspects of an old disease. Prog Retin Eye Res. 2014;39:77–106.

96. Butler NJ, Furtado JM, Winthrop KL, Smith JR. Ocular toxoplasmosis II: Clinical features, pathology and management. Clin Experiment Ophthalmol. 2013;41(1):95–108.

97. Kijlstra A, Petersen E. Epidemiology, pathophysiology, and the future of ocular toxoplasmosis. Ocul Immunol Inflamm. 2014;22(2):138–147.

98. Alipanahi R, Sayyahmelli S. Acute papillitis in young female with toxoplasmosis. Middle East Afr J Ophthalmol. 2011;18(3):249–251.

99. Mikhail MA, Varikkara M. The absence of vitreous inflammation: One more challenge in diagnosing toxoplasma papillitis. BMJ Case Rep. 2013:bcr2013008962.

100. Sandfeld L, Petersen E, Sousa S, Laessoe M, Milea D. Bilateral papillitis in ocular toxoplasmosis. Eye (Lond). 2010;24(1):188–189.

101. Ozgonul C, Besirli CG. Recent developments in the diagnosis and treatment of ocular toxoplasmosis. Ophthalmic Res. 2017;57(1):1–12.

102. Antoniazzi E, Guagliano R, Meroni V, Pezzotta S, Bianchi PE. Ocular impairment of toxoplasmosis. Parassitologia. 2008;50(1–2):35–36.

103. Kresch ZA, Espinosa-Heidmann D, Harper T, Jamie Miller G. Disseminated cryptococcus with ocular cryptococcoma in a human immunodeficiency virus-negative patient. Int Ophthalmol. 2012;32(3):281–284.

104. Cohen DB, Glasgow BJ. Bilateral optic nerve cryptococcosis in sudden blindness in patients with acquired immune deficiency syndrome. Ophthalmology. 1993;100(11):1689–1694.

105. Kestelyn P, Taelman H, Bogaerts J, et al. Ophthalmic manifestations of infections with Cryptococcus neoformans in patients with the acquired immunodeficiency syndrome. Am J Ophthalmol. 1993;116(6):721–727.

106. Portelinha J, Passarinho MP, Almeida AC, Costa JM. Bilateral optic neuropathy associated with cryptococcal meningitis in an immunocompetent patient. BMJ Case Rep. 2014;bcr2013203451.

107. Espino Barros Palau A, Morgan ML, Foroozan R, Lee AG. Neuro-ophthalmic presentations and treatment of cryptococcal meningitis-related increased intracranial pressure. Can J Ophthalmol. 2014;49(5):473–477.

108. Merkler AE, Gaines N, Baradaran H, et al. Direct invasion of the optic nerves, chiasm, and tracts by cryptococcus neoformans in an immunocompetent host. Neurohospitalist. 2015;5(4):217–222.

11

NUTRITIONAL OPTIC NEUROPATHY

**William Sultan, Giulia Amore, Uchenna Francis Nwako,
Stacey Aquino Cohitmingao, Samuel Asanad, Alfredo Sadun**

CASE STUDY

A 40-year-old male, known case of Crohn's disease presented with both eye visual loss, progressive over a period of 4 months. The patient also reported worsening of his gastrointestinal symptoms for past 2 years. The patient was also a known tobacco smoker. Examination revealed visual acuity of 6/36 in right and 6/24 in the left eye. Fundus examination showed optic disc pallor in both eyes. Contrast-enhanced MRI Brain was normal. What is your diagnosis?

Introduction

Nutritional optic neuropathy (NON) is a disorder defined by impairment of the optic nerve caused by deficiency in vital nutrients, vitamins and proteins. Together with toxic and heredo-degenerative metabolic optic neuropathies, they belong to the broader category of metabolic or mitochondrial optic neuropathies (Figure 11.1), sharing mitochondrial dysfunction as the common pathological pathway, which cause loss of selective retinal ganglion cells (RGC) and fibers that constitute the optic nerve. These optic neuropathies are characterized by painless, gradual, progressive, bilateral and symmetrical visual impairment whose defining clinical feature is a central or cecocentral visual field loss. As a consequence, there is also loss of central visual acuity, dyschromatopsia, temporal optic disc atrophy and retinal nerve fiber layer (RNFL) loss, mainly in the papillomacular bundle [1].

Epidemiology

Optic nerve damage, secondary to nutritional deficiencies, is an uncommon cause of optic neuropathy. The incidence is much higher in Africa and South Asia as compared to the other parts of the world.

A variety of micronutrients have been implicated, with the most common being cobalamin (vitamin B12), thiamine (vitamin B1), riboflavin (vitamin B2), pyridoxine (vitamin B6), folic acid (vitamin B9) and copper deficiencies [2]. Additionally, there seem to be several proteins, an insufficient supply of which might also cause RGC and nerve fiber layer loss. These proteins provide sulfur amino acids, in particular, homocysteine and methionine [3].

Many of these associations are still uncertain and mixed deficiencies may coexist in the same patient. In addition to B complex vitamins, an insufficient supply of proteins involved in the metabolism of vitamin B12, like homocysteine and methionine, can lead to a similar nutritional metabolic optic neuropathy, especially in combinations [3].

In developing countries, undernourishment is the most common cause of NON. The prevalence is higher during times of war and famine. Widespread malnutrition can produce the appearance of an epidemic as seen in the case of Cuban epidemic optic neuropathy (CEON). In Cuba, during the early 1990s, more than 50,000 people experienced subacute vision loss and associated peripheral symptoms later in the course of the condition (Figure 11.2a and 11.2b). An international team was invited to help investigate the matter. Several pathogenic hypotheses were put forward, including toxic-nutritional, genetic and infectious causes. In the end, CEON was a combination of NON and exposure to toxins. This was prompted by decreased quantity and quality of food due to the U.S. embargo, in conjunction with toxins, especially methanol in poorly aged rum and tobacco smoke. Vitamin supplementation was subsequently provided to the Cuban population resulting in frank clinical improvement and a dramatic drop in the incidence of NON cases of optic neuropathy [4,5].

Other reports of optic neuropathy outbreaks have been described in a variety of settings: the Tanzania epidemic of 1997 [6] in Jamaica during the early 1900s, in Madrid during the Spanish Civil War and among World War II prisoners [7]. Vitamin deficiencies associated with poor diet have also been reported in Nigeria in conjunction with the chronic ingestion of cassava, which lead to elevated levels of cyanide [2].

In developed countries, prevalence is lower and malnutrition is a rare cause. Nevertheless, some groups of people (the impoverished and alcoholics) are more at risk of developing NON because of poor nutritional intake [8]. The incidence of NON seems to be increasing in the last decades due to vegan diets, anorexia nervosa, gastrointestinal diseases or surgeries, like intestinal resection or gastric bypass, which may result in nutritional malabsorption [9]. No gender, racial or age difference seems to be present in these forms of acquired optic neuropathies [2].

Pathophysiology and risk factors

NON shares a similar clinical presentation with toxic optic neuropathy and hereditary mitochondrial optic neuropathies, which implies that they may share a common pathophysiology. These conditions appear to occur due to defective oxidative phosphorylation, which leads to mitochondrial dysfunction and subsequent loss of optic nerve fibers mainly affecting the papillomacular bundles in the retina. The disparity, however, relates to etiology, the speed of onset and severity of visual impairment [3]. Leber hereditary optic neuropathy (LHON) is likely the most carefully investigated of metabolic optic neuropathies [2] and serves as prototype.

It is interesting to note that all of the vitamins and proteins whose deficiency causes optic damage are crucial for mitochondrial oxidative phosphorylation. The detailed characterization of complex I function affected in cases of LHON/Leigh syndrome mtDNA pathogenic point mutations (11778/ND4, 3460/ND1, 14484/ND6, 14459/ND6) suggests an altered interaction with the

DOI: 10.1201/9780429020278-14

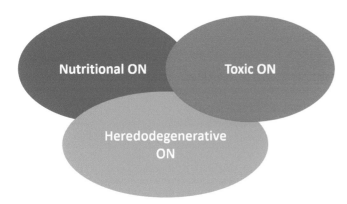

FIGURE 11.1 Categories of metabolic optic neuropathy.

quinone (CoQ) substrate especially in Complex I. This probably induces chronic increase in reactive oxygen species (ROS) and ATP depletion. The subsequent increase in ROS and impairment in ATP production, leads to mitochondrial membrane depolarization and cytochrome C release through the opening of the mitochondrial permeability transition pores (mtPTP). Cytochrome C release activates caspases-9 and 3 in RGC leading to apoptosis (Figures 11.3 and 11.4).

In NON, deficiencies in vitamins B12, B1, B2 and folic acid have most often been implicated [3]. These vitamins act as cofactors to various enzymes in the production of metabolic intermediates—tetrahydrofolate (THF), methionine, homocysteine, cystathionine, cysteine and glutathione. Reduced glutathione is a ROS scavenger which when deficient results in increased accumulation of ROS. Ethanol metabolism can also induce cytochrome p450 (CYP450), mitochondrial uncoupling and subsequent increase in ROS. Other environmental contributors to ROS include smoke, UV exposure, etc.

The question remains as to why these deficiencies target the peripheral nerves and the optic nerve, particularly the papillomacular bundles, leading to symmetrical bilateral central vision loss and peripheral neuropathy.

Two factors play an important role in the energy demands of a given nerve fiber: myelination and caliber.

Small caliber axons and especially long axons, particularly if either unmyelinated (as in the prelaminar retinal nerve fibers) or poorly myelinated (such as C-class long sensory fibers of the peripheral nervous system) are highly susceptible to both energy depletion and ROS accumulation [1].

Furthermore, prelaminar RGC, forming the papillomacular bundle are narrower in caliber and unmyelinated and as such cannot rely on saltatory conduction, thus necessitating higher energy demands, making them particularly susceptible. This causes mitochondria to accumulate in the portion of the optic nerve preceding the lamina cribrosa, while still unmyelinated. The optic nerve head also configures an anatomic "chokepoint," where 1.2 million axons pass through the fixed space of the lamina cribrosa. These anatomo-metabolic peculiarities help to explain why RGC and optic nerve have an increased susceptibility to energy failure and oxidative stress due to both hereditary and acquired mitochondrial dysfunction and why the optic nerve is the "canary in the coal mine" for mitochondrial impairments [11].

The RGC selectivity accounts also for the typical clinical findings of mitochondrial optic neuropathies, consisting of central scotomas and bilateral reduction of central visual acuity, impaired color perception and eventually optic atrophy (OPA).

Risk factors for developing nutritional deficiency optic neuropathy

1. Malnutrition or poor nutrition
2. Strict vegan diet
3. Following bariatric surgery
4. Malabsorption syndromes
5. Inflammatory bowel disease

Clinical features

With some exceptions, nutritional, toxic and hereditary optic neuropathies have very similar clinical presentations as they share a mitochondrial basis of pathophysiology, targeting the papillomacular bundle [2,11]. The main characteristics that

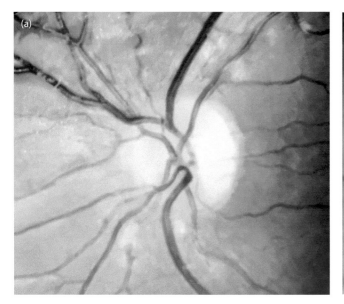

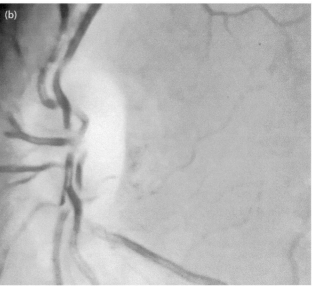

FIGURE 11.2 (a) Thirty-four-year-old Cuban man in CEON epidemic 1993. OS, CF 6' VA OU with central scotomas OU. Photo was taken 15 weeks after vision loss. (b) Thirty-seven-year-old Cuban man in CEON epidemic 1993. OS, 20/400 VA OU with central scotomas OU. Photo was taken 12 weeks after vision loss.

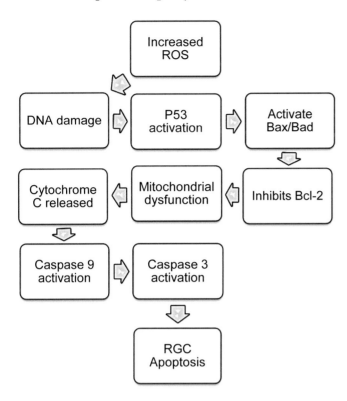

FIGURE 11.3 Outline of RGC apoptotic pathway.

The onset of vision loss is typically painless, bilateral and symmetric. Although it is not rare to observe a mildly asymmetric deficit, especially when the nutritional deficit is recent, the lack of any findings in the other eye would strongly argue against NON.

Progression is usually slow, occurring over several months. It can occur rapidly in rare cases (e.g., thiamine). The extent of visual acuity loss may vary considerably, but visual acuity worse than hand motion is rare. Color perception is severely affected early in the course; as well as contrast sensitivity. Hardy Rand and Rittler (HRR) and Farnsworth D-15 tests are most useful because they identify blue-yellow or red-green deficits, whereas Ishihara assesses red-green defects. The D-15 set is a modification of the Farnsworth-Munsell 100 Hue test. Red cap or color desaturation tests are also symmetrical (Figure 11.5).

Pupillary light reflex is usually maintained or very mildly reduced, but there is usually no relative afferent pupillary defect.

The visual fields are always abnormal, at onset they typically show either a small bilateral central or cecocentral scotoma. Eventually the central scotoma involves the central 5° to 20° surrounding fixation, indicating damage to the macular RGC or to the papillomacular nerve fibers at or within the optic nerve. The cecocentral scotoma extends from the physiological "blind spot" to the point of fixation, typically smaller and dumbbell-shaped. Since the PMB is preferentially affected, a 10-2 visual field provides improved visualization of the visual defect (Figure 11.6).

Rarely, other types of visual field injuries have been reported: paracentral scotomas—involving defects within 20° of the fovea or generalized decreased visual sensitivity.

Ophthalmic fundus findings depend on the duration and extent of the disease. Fundus examination may be completely normal, with the optic disc showing minimal changes such as mild edema or hyperemia. As the disease progresses it typically shows temporal optic disc pallor reflecting papillomacular bundle loss (Figures 11.2a and 11.2b). In longstanding cases, a more generalized OPA may be present.

Optical coherence tomography (OCT) can be a useful tool to assess the degree of RGC damage. It can show variable degrees of RNFL thinning reflecting the OPA, but more specifically, clinicins should look for decreased RGC thickness and volume [12].

should raise suspicion of NON in patients with this presentation after other causes of metabolic optic neuropathies are ruled out include the following:

1. Painless onset of bilateral and symmetric visual loss
2. Slow-progressive course
3. Central or centrocecal bilateral scotoma on visual field testing
4. Decreased RGC thickness observed on optic coherence tomography
5. Decreased color vision

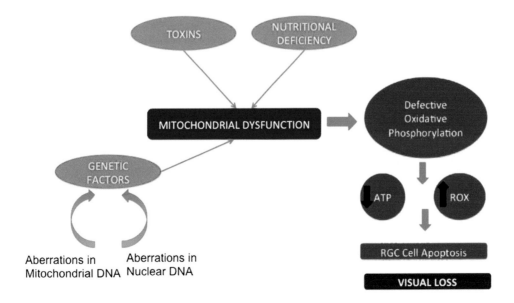

FIGURE 11.4 Schematic representation of visual loss due to mitochondrial dysfunction.

Farnsworth-Munsell 100-Hue Test/2018–12–05

Right eye

Order of color caps entered:

85, 1, 2, 4, 3, 5, 6, 7, 9, 8, 11, 12, 10, 14, 15, 13, 16, 18, 17, 21, 19, 20
22, 23, 24, 29, 25, 27, 28, 26, 30, 32, 31, 34, 35, 33, 36, 37, 38, 40, 39, 42, 41
43, 46, 44, 48, 50, 45, 49, 47, 51, 52, 60, 56, 53, 55, 57, 54, 58, 61, 59, 62, 63
64, 67, 66, 65, 69, 71, 72, 73, 70, 69, 74, 75, 76, 77, 00, 79, 78, 83, 84, 81, 82

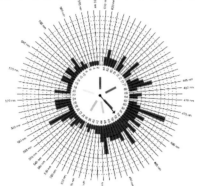

Automatic Evaluation - Classical Method - Individual trays are scored independently
Total error score: 208 - Probably pathologic. Above the 95% confidence level[?] (170 for age 62)
[?]Kinnear PR. Sahraie A. New Farnsworth-Munsell 100 hue test norms of normal observers for
each year of age 5–22 and for decades 30–70. Br J Ophthalmol. 86:1408–1411 (2002)

Automatic Evaluation according Török
Mid-point at cap 53, Bipolarity: 61.18% (0–100%), Selectivity index: 1.33
Color Confusion Index (CCI = $TES_{actual}/TES_{normal}$): 2.22
Pathologic color discrimination, probably diffuse color discrimination error.

Automatic Evaluation - Moment of Inertia Method
Angle: 39.9, Major Radius: 5.7, Minor Radius: 4.8, Total Error Score: 7.4, Selectivity Index:
1.17, Confusion Index: 2.24
Pathologic color discrimination, probably diffuse color discrimination error.
Literature: Vingrys, A.J. and King-Smith, P.E. A quantitative scoring technique for panel tests
of color vision. Investigative Ophthalmology and Visual Science, 1988, 29:50–63.

Farnsworth-Munsell 100-Hue Test/2018–12–05

Left eye

Order of color caps entered:

9, 15, 5, 7, 8, 11, 3, 21, 17, 10, 20, 12, 13, 4, 85, 1, 6, 2, 14, 16, 18, 19
22, 23, 24, 26, 28, 27, 25, 31, 30, 33, 36, 34, 29, 32, 35, 38, 37, 39, 41, 42, 40
47, 46, 44, 43, 49, 45, 56, 53, 51, 50, 48, 52, 60, 55, 63, 61, 57, 54, 58, 62, 59
65, 66, 69, 64, 67, 68, 71, 70, 75, 73, 72, 77, 76, 74, 78, 84, 82, 81, 79, 80, 83

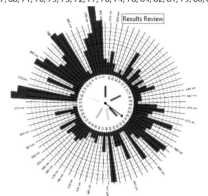

Automatic Evaluation - Classical Method - Individual trays are scored independently
Total error score: 449 - Probably pathologic. Above the 95% confidence level[?] (170 for age 62)
[?]Kinnear PR. Sahraie A. New Farnsworth-Munsell 100 hue test norms of normal observers for
each year of age 5–22 and for decades 30–70. Br J Ophthalmol. 86:1408–1411 (2002)

Automatic Evaluation according Török
Mid-point at cap 9, Bipolarity: 89.41% (0–100%), Selectivity index: 1.89
Color Confusion Index (CCI = $TES_{actual}/TES_{normal}$): 3.64
Pathologic color discrimination, probably deuteranomaly or deuteranopy.

Automatic Evaluation - Moment of Inertia Method
Angle: -55.0, Major Radius: 10.9, Minor Radius: 7.6, Total Error Score: 13.3, Selectivity Index:
1.42, Confusion Index: 4.30
Pathologic color discrimination, probably diffuse color discrimination error.
Literature: Vingrys, A.J. and King-Smith, P.E. A quantitative scoring technique for panel tests
of color vision. Investigative Ophthalmology and Visual Science, 1988, 29:50–63.

FIGURE 11.5 Farnsworth Munsell tests had shown diffuse pathology in color discrimination on OD, and a predominant deuteranomaly on OS in this female NON case.

A ganglion cell complex analysis is useful for identification of decreased RGC thickness in the macula and this may be the earliest indication of disease (Figure 11.7).

Visual-evoked potentials (VEP) may confirm the presence of subclinical abnormalities with reduced P100 amplitude and a normal or near-to-normal latency, although these abnormalities are non-specific [13].

Once suspicion of NON is raised, a detailed history of the types and quantities of food that the patient is consuming is crucial. Evidence of malnutrition (e.g., weight loss, wasting), history of alcoholism or a defined cause for the reduced vitamin level (Crohn's disease, bariatric surgery) should be determined. Other clinical findings may support a diagnosis of nutritional deficiency, including peripheral neuropathy, cutaneous or mucous membrane changes.

It must be emphasized that a complete neurological and medical evaluation is necessary in the presence of systemic manifestations of nutritional deficits.

The diagnosis of NON can be supported by laboratory evidence, including serum vitamin levels and protein concentration when available. Routine laboratory studies such as blood count can help identify specific patterns (e.g., macrocytic anemia with vitamin B12 deficiency).

Nevertheless, it may not be possible to identify a single micronutrient responsible. Multiple deficiencies and other concomitant mechanisms, such as smoke or other toxins, have to be taken into account and detailed carefully, as exemplified by the Cuban epidemic of optic neuropathy [4].

Another controversial entity is the so-called tobacco–alcohol amblyopia [14,15]. This is not common in industrialized countries not withstanding that smoking and alcohol abuse are, pointing out the role of general nutrition. It has been established that cyanide in tobacco can cause toxic effects on the optic nerve. Alcohol on the other hand, appears to produce nutrient malabsorption via gut irritation and liver dysfunction [8]. Chronic alcohol ingestion also induces CYP450 and a subsequent increase in ROS production. Furthermore, many historical cases were in fact Leber's hereditary optic neuropathy precipitated by smoke [16]. Visual symptoms in tobacco–alcohol amblyopia seem to be related to a nutritional deficit or genetic predisposition triggered by smoke and potentially alcohol. The cases related to nutritional deficiency often improve and resolve with adequate nutritional supplementation [17].

Additional investigations

In addition to all the ocular investigations listed above, the following laboratory investigations are recommended:

1. Laboratory tests for serum levels of vitamins B1, B2, B6, B9 and B12.
2. Blood and 24-hour urine heavy metal screening.
3. Genetic testing for heredodegenerative metabolic optic neuropathies (LHON and DOA).
4. Fundus fluorescein angiography showing absence of leakage and inflammation which would help distinguish NON

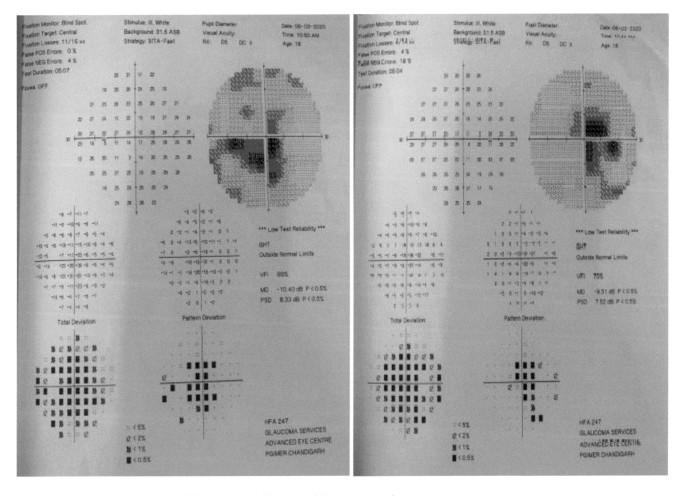

FIGURE 11.6 The 30-2 visual field shows the full extent of the cecocentral scotoma.

from optic neuritis and non-arteritic anterior ischemic optic neuropathy.

5. Dedicated gadolinium-enhanced MRI of the brain and orbit (with fat-suppressed images) to rule out compressive and demyelinating lesions particularly for atypical or asymmetrical presentations. Optic chiasm can be involved in certain mitochondrial disorders.

Differential diagnosis

NON is usually a diagnosis of exclusion, mainly based on history, clinical and paraclinical findings with a high index of suspicion.

Macular disorders may occasionally be mistaken for mitochondrial optic neuropathies since they also cause the loss of central vision. Macular impairments usually are revealed by the presence of metamorphopsia and less severe or absent color vision impairment. Visual fields can show central or paracentral, rather than cecocentral, defects.

Bitemporal scotomas can occasionally mimic the cecocentral scotomas seen in NON although true temporal scotomas, with respect of the vertical meridian, indicate a lesion affecting the optic chiasm in which the macular fibers cross.

Normal tension glaucoma shares similar insidious and bilateral visual acuity loss, although arcuate visual field defects, excavation of the inferior rim and inferior optic nerve thinning may help differentiate it from NON. Multiple studies show an association between OPA1 polymorphisms and normal tension glaucoma.

Other optic neuropathies have to be considered and an MRI of brain and orbits is often essential to exclude compressive and demyelinating lesions.

Optic neuritis may be clinically distinguished from NON as optic neuritis is characterized by pain upon eye movement and visual recovery within weeks, while ischemic optic neuropathy is usually unilateral with edema in the acute stage and diffuse OPA in the chronic stage.

In the few cases of bilateral optic nerve edema, the possibility of increased intracranial pressure (ICP) must be considered. Symptoms of increased ICP may include headache, dizziness, nausea and vomiting.

A careful distinction should be made among the group of mitochondrial optic neuropathies since their presentation is almost identical and the correct identification of the cause of mitochondrial changes management and prognosis.

Beside nutritional, acquired optic neuropathies may be due to toxic exposure. Intoxications may present more acutely with evidences of disc edema and hyperemia at fundus examination. Systemic symptoms may accompany the acute phase, like nausea, abdominal pain and metabolic acidosis after methanol ingestion. The most common toxins are methanol, carbon monoxide, ethylene glycol and nitrosoureas. If heavy metal toxicity is suspected, a 24-hour urine test can be conducted.

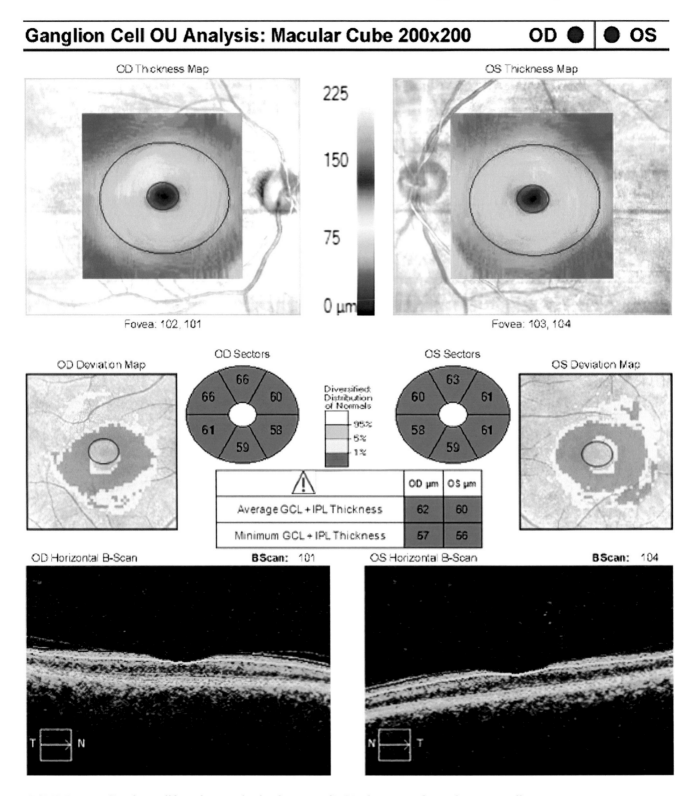

FIGURE 11.7   Ganglion cell layer later in the development of NON shows significant thinning in all regions.

Medication use should be carefully assessed since several antibiotics may cause toxic neuropathy with different mechanisms. The most frequent causes of optic nerve damage are two anti-tuberculosis agents, ethambutol and isoniazid, interfering respectively with mitochondrial oxidative phosphorylation and protein synthesis. Amiodarone toxicity, an antiarrhythmic, is characterized by a prolonged optic disc swelling. Other molecules are the immunosuppressants tacrolimus and cyclosporine.

Since the treatment of toxic neuropathy is discontinuation of the offending agent, a high level of certainty should be established. Accepted criteria that should be present to confirm toxic optic neuropathy are [18]:

1. Symmetric visual loss
2. Scientific plausibility for a causal relationship with the agent
3. Reasonable temporal relationship with clinical dose-response curve
4. Recovery after removal of the offending toxin

A family history of bilateral vision loss may suggest a hereditary optic neuropathy, which should be suspected also in the setting of lack of recovery following appropriate nutritional replacement and toxin elimination. In these cases, it is advisable to exclude the two most common genetic forms of isolated optic neuropathy: Leber's hereditary optic neuropathy (LHON) and dominant optic atrophy (DOA).

LHON is caused by point mutations in the mitochondrial DNA, affecting predominantly young males in their late teens or twenties who experience a sudden onset of severe vision loss. DOA is mainly due to mutations in the nuclear OPA1 gene and affects equally males and females from childhood, with a more indolent course [19,20].

Hereditary optic neuropathies may also be associated with other neurologic and extra-neurological symptoms as part of multisystemic mitochondrial diseases (MELAS, MERRF) or other diseases (Wolfram syndrome, Charcot-Marie-Tooth disease, spinocerebellar ataxias).

Management

The most important measure in approaching NON is the correction of the nutritional deficit and the rebalancing of the patient's nutritional state [21].

A prompt correction with targeted vitamin supplementation is warranted when a specific deficit has been identified. Monitoring of blood levels is useful, when possible, to confirm that values have reached a normal range. Lifelong oral maintenance replacement therapy may be needed in some cases.

In mixed cases, clinicians have to consider the cause of the nutritional deficit, for example, bariatric surgery often causes deficiencies in vitamins B1, B6, B12, folate, vitamin D and several minerals (iron, zinc, magnesium and copper), while people with a vegan diet are more prone to be deficient in B complex vitamins as well as vitamins A, D and E. In these cases, establishing a well-balanced diet plus an oral multi-vitamin supplementation has to be considered.

The cessation of smoking and alcohol use should always be pursued since they can be critical cofactors in worsening visual function or preventing recovery.

Recovery of visual function may take several weeks to months although residual permanent damage to the optic nerve may sometimes persist. Ophthalmologic examinations should be performed to quantify improvement of the visual function every 3–4 weeks and then every 6 months. Visual acuity and color vision should be assessed at each visit and bilateral visual field and OCT examinations should be performed regularly.

Common nutritional deficiencies and related optic neuropathies

Below, we briefly describe the most common nutritional deficiencies.

Vitamin B12

Vitamin B12, together with folic acid, has a critical role in DNA and RNA synthesis. It acts as a cofactor in the regeneration of THF coupled to the conversion of homocysteine to methionine. Vitamin B12 is also important in detoxification of cyanide, generating cyanocobalamin.

Vitamin B12 deficiency is one of the most common nutritional deficits and yet one of the rarest causes of NON with a proven causal relationship. However, a few animal models showed unequivocally demyelination of optic nerve fibers due to toxic levels of cyanide or improper fatty acid synthesis [22].

Vitamin B12 deficiency occurs most frequently in the setting of autoimmune pernicious anemia. Other conditions include damage or surgical resection of the terminal ileum in patients with Crohn's disease, bariatric surgery and a strict uncompensated vegan diet. In addition to optic neuropathy, as described, vitamin B12 deficiency can cause a megaloblastic anemia, glossitis, subacute combined degeneration of the spinal cord and sensory peripheral neuropathy. The optic neuropathy may precede anemia or other neurologic symptoms. An OCT study on 66 children with vitamin B12 deficiency demonstrated that the thickness of the superior RNFL was significantly lower than controls and that average and superior RNFL values were significantly correlated with vitamin B12 levels [23, 24].

Diagnosis relies on vitamin B12 serum levels, which does not always reflect tissue levels. Additional testing for methylmalonic acid (MMA) and homocysteine, intermediates in vitamin B12 and folate metabolism, can be useful in cases with borderline or inconclusive results. Both homocysteine and MMA are usually elevated when vitamin B12 is lacking, while normal MMA and increased homocysteine are consistent with folate deficiency or hereditary homocysteinemia [1].

Prompt recognition and treatment with high-dose oral or intramuscular vitamin B12 or parenteral hydroxycobalamin, converting free cyanide to cyanocobalamin, may reverse existing visual loss as well as prevent further visual deterioration.

Folic acid

Folic acid deficiency is usually due to inadequate dietary intake, malabsorption or in settings of increased requirements, like pregnancy or hemolytic anemia. Folic acid is linked to vitamin B12 metabolism being necessary for the production of THF, which is involved in the detoxification of formate.

The mechanism by which the lack of folic acid leads to optic neuropathy probably relates to mitochondrial dysfunction. Folic acid deficiency may block directly oxidative phosphorylation and also lead to accumulation of formate, which itself blocks electron transport by inhibition of cytochrome oxidase [4,25].

The ophthalmological presentation of optic neuropathy is virtually indistinguishable from vitamin B12 deficiency, except for a more rapid time course. Mouth ulcers are more common than glossitis. Folate levels can be measured in serum and blood examinations may show macrocytic anemia. Oral folate supplementation is recommended.

Vitamin B1

Thiamine is a cofactor for several mitochondrial enzymes and its deficiency results in impaired cellular energy production in animal models [26]. Optic neuropathy in the contest of thiamine deficiency has been reported in association with Wernicke-Korsakoff syndrome, which encompasses two clinical phenotypes. Wernicke encephalopathy is an acute syndrome traditionally occurring in the setting of alcohol abuse and malnutrition or after bariatric surgery; it is characterized by the classic triad of:

1. Encephalopathy
2. Ophthalmoplegia and nystagmus
3. Gait ataxia

Korsakoff syndrome is a chronic dysmnesic condition occurring as a late complication of Wernicke encephalopathy.

The optic neuropathy associated with Wernicke encephalopathy is somehow different from other forms of NON since the visual loss is often acute and disc swelling is a prominent feature in most cases [27]. Other fundus findings are peripapillary telangiectasia and retinal hemorrhages [28]. OCT may show RNFL thickening [29].

Serum and plasma thiamine levels have poor sensitivity and specificity (less than 10% of blood thiamine is contained in plasma) and testing may take several days.

If the suspicion for Wernicke encephalopathy is high, in a context of malnutrition or bariatric surgery, expedited diagnostic testing should be ordered but, since delayed treatment may lead to irreversible neurologic injury, supplementation of thiamine is often given empirically. The recovery of vision is usually complete and dramatic.

Copper

Copper deficiency has recently been associated with optic neuropathy. Pineles and colleagues reported two patients with combined optic neuropathy and myelopathy secondary to copper deficiency [30]. A confounding factor was the concomitant presence of vitamin B12 deficiency, but the authors argue that the visual loss progressed despite correction of vitamin B12 levels and stabilized after copper supplementation. Further evidence is provided by ethambutol optic neuropathy, which occurs in a dose-dependent manner due to the chelation of copper. The mechanism is more complicated but may relate to impaired mitochondrial function secondary to hypocupremia in combination with low levels of zinc and iron [31,32].

Riboflavin, niacin and pyridoxine

Some reports suggest that optic neuropathy may be also associated with deficiencies in riboflavin, niacin and pyridoxine [33], but a causal relationship is uncertain, as these deficiencies are often found in severely malnourished patients, and identification of the specific vitamin deficiency leading to optic neuropathy is difficult.

Conclusion

NONs are rare causes of optic neuropathy characterized by slow progression of bilateral central vision. Clinical history usually contains clues to support the diagnosis of a nutritional deficit and to differentiate it from toxic or hereditary optic neuropathies. A reasonable approach for patients with suspected NON is to exclude alternate etiologies with neuroimaging, obtain vitamin B12 and folate levels and complete blood cell count. If the initial screening is negative and clinical suspicion remains high, it is worthwhile to pursue less common nutritional deficiency optic neuropathies (e.g., thiamine, copper).

Key points

- Nutritional optic neuropathy (NON) and heredodegenerative metabolic optic neuropathies (such as Leber hereditary optic neuropathy [LHON] and dominant optic atrophy

[DOA]) share similar very clinical presentations, which imply that they also share an underlying pathophysiology involving mitochondrial dysfunction with defective oxidative phosphorylation which mainly targets the papillomacular bundles (PMBs) of the optic nerve.
- NON begins as is a diagnosis of exclusion, mainly based on history, clinical and paraclinical findings with a high index of suspicion.
- NON is a rare cause of optic neuropathy characterized by painless, gradual, progressive, bilateral, and symmetrical visual impairment loss with evidence of central or cecocentral scotoma.

Multiple-Choice Questions

1. What type of scotoma occurs in NON?
   a. Ring
   b. Paracentral
   c. Cecocentral
   d. Arcuate

   Answer:

   c. Cecocentral

2. What is the defining clinical symptom of NON?
   a. Painless
   b. Decreased color vision
   c. Symmetric vision loss
   d. All of the above

   Answer:

   d. All of the above

3. Which is a risk factor for NON?
   a. Bariatric surgery
   b. Chronic alcohol use
   c. Inflammatory bowel disease
   d. All of the above

   Answer:

   d. All of the above

4. What is the mechanism of ethambutol optic neuropathy?
   a. Direct cellular toxicity
   b. Copper chelation
   c. Vitamin chelation
   d. ROS production

   Answer:

   b. Copper chelation

References

1. Ianchulev T, Kolin T, Moseley K, Sadun A. Optic nerve atrophy in propionic acidemia. Ophthalmology. 2003;110(9):1850–1854.
2. Pilz YL, Bass SJ, Sherman J. A review of mitochondrial optic neuropathies: From inherited to acquired forms. J Optom. 2017;10(4):205–214.
3. Sadun AA. Metabolic optic neuropathies. In: Seminars in ophthalmology, vol. 17, no. 1. Taylor & Francis; 2002. pp. 29–32.
4. Sadun A. Acquired mitochondrial impairment as a cause of optic nerve disease. Trans Am Ophthalmol Soc. 1998;96:881–923.

5. González-Quevedo A, Santiesteban-Freixas R, Eells JT, Lima L, Sadun AA. Cuban epidemic neuropathy: insights into the toxic–nutritional hypothesis through international collaboration. MEDICC Rev. 2018;20:27–31.

6. Plant GT, Mtanda AT, Arden GB, and Johnson. An epidemic of optic neuropathy in Tanzania: Characterization of visual disorder and associated peripheral neuropathy. J.Neurol.Sci. 1997 145(2):127–140.

7. Hedges III TR, Hirano M, Tucker K, Caballero B. Epidemic optic and peripheral neuropathy in Cuba: A unique geopolitical public health problem. Surv Ophthalmol. 1997;41(4):341–353.

8. Ijaz S, Jackson J, Thorley H, Porter K, Fleming C, Richards A, Bonner A, Savović J. Nutritional deficiencies in homeless persons with problematic drinking: A systematic review. Int J Equity Health. 2017;16(1):71.

9. Moss HE. Bariatric surgery and the neuro-ophthalmologist. J Neuroophthalmology. 2016;36(1):78–84.

10. Sadun AA, La Morgia C, Carelli V. Mitochondrial optic neuropathies: Our travels from bench to bedside and back again. Clin Exp Ophthalmol. 2013;41(7):702–712.

11. Orssaud C, Roche O, Dufier JL. Nutritional optic neuropathies. J Neurol Sci. 2007;262(1–2):158–164.

12. Vieira LMC, Silva NFA, dos Santos AMD, dos Anjos RS, Pinto LAPA, Vicente AR, Borges BICCJ, Ferreira JPT, Amado DM, da Cunha JPPB. Retinal ganglion cell layer analysis by optical coherence tomography in toxic and nutritional optic neuropathy. Neuroophthalmol. 2015;35(3):242–245.

13. Kupersmith MJ, Weiss PA, Carr RE. The visual-evoked potential in tobacco-alcohol and nutritional amblyopia. Am J Ophthalmol. 1983;95(3):307–314.

14. Grzybowski A, Holder GE. Tobacco optic neuropathy (TON)–the historical and present concept of the disease. Acta Ophthalmol. 2011;89(5):495–499.

15. Grzybowski A, Brona P. Nutritional optic neuropathy instead of tobacco–alcohol amblyopia. Canadian J Ophthalmol. 2017;52(5):533.

16. Giordano L, Deceglie S, d'Adamo P, Valentino ML, La Morgia C, Fracasso F, Roberti M, Cappellari M, Petrosillo G, Ciaravolo S, Parente D. Cigarette toxicity triggers Leber's hereditary optic neuropathy by affecting mtDNA copy number, oxidative phosphorylation and ROS detoxification pathways. Cell Death Dis. 2015;6(12):e2021–e2021.

17. Carroll FD. Nutritional amblyopia. Arch Ophthalmol. 1966; 76(3):406–411.

18. Wang MY, Sadun AA. Drug-related mitochondrial optic neuropathies. J Neuroophthalmol. 2013;33(2):172–178.

19. Yu-Wai-Man P, Griffiths PG, Chinnery PF. Mitochondrial optic neuropathies–disease mechanisms and therapeutic strategies. Prog Retin Eye Res. 2011;30(2):81–114.

20. Sadun AA, La Morgia C, Carelli V. Leber's hereditary optic neuropathy. Curr Treat Options Neurol. 2011; 13(1):109–117.

21. Jefferis JM, Hickman SJ. Treatment and outcomes in nutritional optic neuropathy. Curr Treat Options Neurol. 2019;21(1):5.

22. Chester EM, Agamanolis DP, Harris JW, Victor M, Hines JD, Kark JA. Optic atrophy in experimental vitamin B12 deficiency in monkeys. Acta Neurol Scand. 1980;61(1):9–26.

23. Grzybowski A. Problems related to the diagnosis of vitamin B12 deficiency optic neuropathy. Acta Ophthalmol. 2014;92(1):e74–e75.

24. Özkasap S, Türkyilmaz K, Dereci S, Öner V, Calapoğlu T, Cüre MC, Durmuş M. Assessment of peripapillary retinal nerve fiber layer thickness in children with vitamin B 12 deficiency. Childs Nerv Syst. 2013;29(12):2281–2286.

25. Hsu CT, Miller NR, Wray ML. Optic neuropathy from folic acid deficiency without alcohol abuse. Ophthalmologica. 2002;216(1):65–67.

26. Longmuir R, Lee AG, Rouleau J. Visual loss due to Wernicke syndrome following gastric bypass. Semin Ophthalmol. 2007;22(1):13–19.

27. Surges R, Beck S, Niesen WD, Weiller C, Rijntjes M. Sudden bilateral blindness in Wernicke's encephalopathy: Case report and review of the literature. J Neurol Sci. 2007;260(1–2):261–264.

28. Serlin T, Moisseiev E. Fundus findings in Wernicke encephalopathy. Case Rep Ophthalmol. 2017;8(2):406–409.

29. Bohnsack BL, Patel SS. Peripapillary nerve fiber layer thickening, telangiectasia, and retinal hemorrhages in Wernicke encephalopathy. J Neuroophthalmol. 2010;30(1):54–58.

30. Pineles SL, Wilson CA, Balcer LJ, Slater R, Galetta SL. Combined optic neuropathy and myelopathy secondary to copper deficiency. Surv Ophthalmol. 2010;55(4):386–392.

31. Yoon YH, Jung KH, Sadun AA, Shin HC, Koh JY. Ethambutol-induced vacuolar changes and neuronal loss in rat retinal cell culture: Mediation by endogenous zinc. Toxicol Appl Pharmacol. 2000;162(2):107–114.

32. Kozak SF, Inderlied CB, Hsu HY, Heller KB, Sadun AA. The role of copper on ethambutol's antimicrobial action and implications for ethambutol-induced optic neuropathy. Diagn Microbiol Infect Dis. 1998;30(2):83–87.

33. Philipsen WM, Hommes OR. Atrophy of the optic nerve and vitamin B6 deficiency. Ophthalmologica. 1970;160:103–104.

12

INHERITED OPTIC NEUROPATHIES

Hui-Chen Cheng, Jared Ching, An-Guor Wang, Patrick Yu-Wai-Man

CASE STUDY

A 27-year-old male presented with painless progressive loss of vision in the right eye for 6 months duration and left eye for the past 2 years. On ophthalmic examination, the patient was able to count fingers at 6 meters from the right eye and had only perception of light from the left eye. The visual fields were grossly depressed bilaterally. In addition, the patient had bilateral mild sensorineural hearing loss. Gadolinium-enhanced MRI brain and orbits showed bilaterally thinned out optic nerves. What is the probable diagnosis?

Introduction

Inherited optic neuropathies are a genetically heterogenous group of disorders that affect the optic nerve with an estimated prevalence of 1 in 10,000 in the general population (1–4). Although the inheritance pattern may be variable, inherited optic neuropathies share a number of core clinical features including bilateral, symmetrical central visual loss with a central or cecocentral scotoma due to the selective vulnerability of the retinal ganglion cells (RGCs) that constitute the papillomacular bundle (2, 3, 5). Visual failure usually occurs in isolation, but some patients develop more extensive neuromuscular involvement in addition to optic atrophy (OA). The recognition of these syndromic cases requires taking a careful history and examination as this will determine further investigation, including genetic testing. In this chapter, a systemic diagnostic approach for patients with a suspected inherited optic neuropathy is described together with management options.

When to suspect an inherited optic neuropathy

Patients with inherited optic neuropathies tend to present with bilateral, usually symmetrical, visual loss. The onset of visual deterioration can be subacute or insidious and the age of onset varies depending on the underlying cause. In severe and early-onset cases, patients can also develop nystagmus (3). Sequential visual loss is more commonly observed in patients with Leber hereditary optic neuropathy (LHON). In the initial stages of investigation, it is important to exclude other causes of a bilateral simultaneous or sequential optic neuropathy (3). Neuroimaging, for example, may be indicated to exclude compressive, infiltrative or inflammatory pathologies affecting the anterior visual pathway (4). Another important group to consider in the differential diagnosis is a primary retinal dystrophy masquerading as an optic neuropathy since the retinal findings may be subtle with more attention being paid to the coexisting pallor of the optic disc (3). Visual electrodiagnostic

testing can be helpful in these cases to help distinguish retinal dystrophies from optic neuropathies (3, 4).

Classification of inherited optic neuropathies

Having excluded alternative pathologies, inherited optic neuropathies can be divided into three broad categories: (1) isolated OA; (2) syndromic OA with neuromuscular features; and (3) OA as a secondary feature of inherited neurodegenerative diseases (Figure 12.1). In this chapter, we will focus on the three most common inherited optic neuropathies, namely, LHON, autosomal dominant atrophy (DOA) and Wolfram syndrome.

Molecular genetics

Inherited optic neuropathies can be caused by mitochondrial DNA (mtDNA) variants or by variants in nuclear-encoded genes (Tables 12.1 and 12.2) (2, 4). The mitochondrial genome is strictly maternally transmitted whereas nuclear variants can be inherited in a dominant, recessive or X-linked fashion (2, 4). *De novo* mutations in both mitochondrial and nuclear genes have also been reported (4).

The most common inherited optic neuropathy caused by mtDNA mutations is LHON with three primary mutations, m.3460G>A, m.11778G>A and m.14484T>C accounting for ~90% of all cases (4, 5). OA is also a feature seen in other classical mitochondrial phenotypes, such as: (1) the Kearns–Sayre syndrome (KSS) with the development of chronic progressive external ophthalmoplegia (CPEO) and pigmentary retinopathy before the age of 20 years of age; (2) mitochondrial myopathy, encephalopathy, lactic acidosis and stroke-like episodes (MELAS); (3) the syndrome of neuropathy, ataxia and retinitis pigmentosa (NARP); (4) maternally inherited Leigh syndrome (MILS); (5) myoclonic epilepsy associated with ragged-red fibers (MERRF); and (6) mitochondrial neurogastrointestinal encephalopathy (MNGIE) (4–6). The list of nuclear-encoded genes known to cause OA is rapidly growing with *SSBP1* being the latest causative gene reported in the literature (7). OA is the cardinal manifestation as in *OPA1* and *WFS1*, whereas for other causative genes, it is a more variable feature as part of more severe syndromic disease (Table 12.2) (4, 5, 8, 9).

Leber hereditary optic neuropathy (LHON)

The prevalence of LHON has been reported to be between 1 in 31,000 to 1 in 54,000 in Northern Europe and with an estimated incidence of 1 in 1,000,000 in the Japanese population (4, 5, 10, 11). The three most common mtDNA mutations that cause LHON are m.11778G>A in the *MTND4* gene (~60%), m.3460G>A in the *MTND1* gene (~15%) and m.14484T>C in the *MTND6* gene (~15%), with the remainder harboring rarer pathogenic mtDNA mutations (Table 12.1) (5, 10). The three primary mtDNA mutations all affect mitochondrial complex I subunits and they result in disturbed electron flux along the respiratory chain, impairing

DOI: 10.1201/9780429020278-15

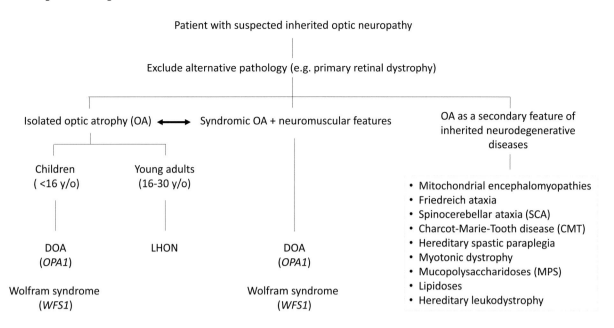

FIGURE 12.1   Diagnostic approach for patients with a suspected inherited optic neuropathy.

oxidative phosphorylation (OXPHOS) and leading to increased levels of reactive oxygen species (ROS) (5, 8). LHON is characterized by incomplete penetrance and a marked predilection for male LHON carriers to lose vision (5, 8). The penetrance varies widely both within and between families. Overall, ~50% of male carriers and ~10% of female carriers will experience visual loss during their lifetime with a peak age of onset in the third decade of life (8, 9).

Typically, disease conversion in LHON is characterized by subacute, painless, central visual loss in one eye, followed by the fellow eye 2–4 months later (5, 9, 10). About 25% of patients may experience bilateral simultaneous optic nerve involvement (9). Visual acuity rapidly deteriorates to 6/60 or worse with significantly impaired color vision and a dense central or cecocentral scotoma on visual field. The optic disc may be hyperemic with peripapillary telangiectasias and vascular tortuosity of the central retinal vessels, but with no leakage on fluorescein angiography (5). Pseudoedema secondary to swelling of the peripapillary retinal nerve fiber layer (RNFL) can be observed both clinically and with optical coherence tomography (OCT) imaging (Figure 12.2) (10). Following this period of swelling, there is thinning of the RNFL layer coincident with RGC loss and the degree of thinning reaches a plateau at 8–10 months after disease conversion (10, 12). From observational studies, disease conversion in LHON may be heralded by swelling of the inferotemporal RNFL, which then spreads to affect other sectors of the optic disc (10, 12–14).

Overall, the visual prognosis in LHON is poor and the majority of patients will become significantly visually impaired (15). The likelihood of spontaneous visual recovery depends on the underlying pathogenic mtDNA mutation, being more likely with the m.14484T>C mutation (37–58%) compared with m.11778G> A mutation (4–25%) (10, 16).

Autosomal dominant optic atrophy (DOA)

DOA is the most common inherited optic neuropathy with an estimated prevalence of 1 in 25,000 in the North of England (17). The majority (50–60%) of patients with DOA harbor mutations in the *OPA1* gene (3q29), which consists of 30 coding exons spreading over

100 kb of genomic DNA (5, 18, 19). *OPA1* mutations cluster in the GTPase domain (exons 8–15) and dynamin central region (exons 16–23), with single base-pair substitutions (69%) representing the most common mutational subtype (5, 20). Most *OPA1* mutations result in premature termination codons and the truncated mRNAs are mostly degraded by protective cellular mechanisms resulting in a reduction in the level of the wild-type protein (5, 20).

OPA1 is highly expressed within the RGC layer and it encodes for a multifunctional transmembrane protein embedded within the mitochondrial inner membrane. *OPA1* regulates OXPHOS by interacting and stabilizing the mitochondrial respiratory chain complexes, thereby facilitating the efficient shuttling of electrons between the complexes (5, 21). *OPA1* also has a role in the regulation of apoptosis and in maintaining the integrity of the mitochondrial genome (5, 22). The pathological hallmarks of *OPA1* mutations are mitochondrial network fragmentation and dysmorphic mitochondria with disorganized cristae and paracrystalline inclusion bodies (5).

Patients with DOA almost invariably present with insidious visual loss in the first two decades of life although there can be pronounced inter- and intra-familial variability in disease severity and progression. The reported visual acuities range from 6/6 to the detection of hand movements. Although the visual prognosis is better compared with LHON, visual acuity does deteriorate with time and the majority of patients will be registered legally blind in later life (5, 23). Most patients have a generalized dyschromatopsia with a central, cecocentral or paracentral scotoma on visual field, consistent with the early involvement of the papillomacular bundle (5, 24). Optic disc pallor is often more marked temporally with more severe thinning of the temporal RNFL in that quadrant (Figure 12.3) (5, 25). Other morphological features that can be observed include saucerization of the neuroretinal rim, peripapillary atrophy and enlarged cup-to-disc ratios greater than 0.5 (24, 26, 27).

Wolfram syndrome

Wolfram syndrome was originally described as an autosomal recessive disorder characterized by diabetes insipidus (DI), diabetes mellitus (DM), OA and deafness (DIDMOAD

TABLE 12.1: Mitochondrial DNA (mtDNA) Variants Identified in Patients with LHON

Disease Name	OMIM# of the Disease	Variant	Associated Gene (OMIM#)
Leber hereditary optic neuropathy (LHON)	535000	*m.11778G>A* *	*MTND4*§ (516003)
		m.11696G>A	
		m.11253T>C	
		m.14484T>C *	*MTND6*§ (516006)
		m.14325T>C	
		m.14568C>T	
		m.14459G>Aᵃ	
		m.14729G>A	
		m.14482C>G/Aᵃ	
		m.14495A>Gᵃ	
		m.14498C>T	
		m.14568C>Tᵇ	
		m.14596A>T	
		m.3460G>A *	*MTND1*§ (516000)
		m.3376G>A	
		m.3635G>Aᵃ	
		m.3697G>A	
		m.3700G>Aᵃ	
		m.3733G>Aᵃ	
		m.4025C>T	
		m.4160T>C	
		m.4171C>Aᵃ	
		m.4640C>A	*MTND2* (516001)
		m.5244G>A	
		m.10237T>C	*MTND3* (516002)
		m.10663T>Cᵃ	*MTND4L* (516004)
		m.12811T>C	*MTND5* (516005)
		m.12848C>T	
		m.13637A>G	
		m.13730G>A	
		m.9101T>C	*MTATP6* (516060)
		m.9804G>A	*MTCO3* (516050)
		m.14831G>A	*MTCYB* (516020)

Source: Reproduced from (4).

* The three most common mtDNA variants that cause LHON have been highlighted in bold.

§ Core genes.

ᵃ These mtDNA variants affecting function. They have been identified in ≥2 independent LHON pedigrees and show segregation with affected disease status. The remaining putative LHON variants have been found in singleton cases or in a single family, and additional evidence is required before pathogenicity can be irrefutably ascribed.

syndrome) in addition to other more variable manifestations, such as renal failure and psychiatric disturbances (28, 29). It is a relatively rare disorder with prevalence figures ranging from 1 in 500,000 to 1 in 770,000 depending on the population studied (30, 31).

The onset of DM is usually in the first decade of life followed by progressive visual loss manifesting in the second decade of life (30). Patients with Wolfram syndrome have a poor visual prognosis and a reduced life expectancy with half of all patients not surviving beyond the third decade of life (28–30, 32). Other reported ocular abnormalities include cataracts, retinal dystrophy, increased optic disc cupping and nystagmus (28, 33). The endocrine defects in Wolfram syndrome arise due to pituitary dysfunction with hypogonadism and DI usually developing in the second decade of life (Figure 12.4) (28). High-frequency sensorineural hearing loss is common (62%) in addition to progressive neurological abnormalities (60%), including cerebellar ataxia, peripheral neuropathy, dementia and psychiatric illness. Urinary tract defects are seen frequently in patients with Wolfram syndrome (60–90%) with ureteric obstruction, atonic bladder, sphincter dyssynergia and incontinence (28, 29). Magnetic resonance imaging (MRI) may demonstrate generalized brain atrophy, particularly in the cerebellum, medulla and pons, absence of signal from the posterior pituitary and thin optic nerves (34).

The majority of patients with Wolfram syndrome harbor recessive mutations in the *WFS1* gene (4p16.1). The latter encodes for a transmembrane endoplasmic reticulum (ER) protein, Wolframin, which plays an important role in regulating ER-mitochondria homeostasis and the flux of calcium between these two organellar components (29). Over 250 pathogenic variants in *WFS1* have been reported, including point mutations, small deletions, insertions and duplications (29, 32). Genetic testing is an important step to confirm the pathogenic mutations and facilitate effective genetic counseling. Multidisciplinary management is particularly important for young children to minimize the complications associated with the multisystemic features of Wolfram syndrome.

Evolving disease classification

Greater access to molecular genetic testing has expanded the phenotypes associated with specific disease-causing genes (i.e., genotypes) (4, 29). It is now apparent that most OA genes can cause both recessive and dominant disease with the features either being limited to OA or with syndromic

TABLE 12.2: Causative Nuclear-Encoded Genes in Patients with Isolated or Syndromic Optic Atrophy

Associated Gene/Locus (OMIM#)	Cytogenetic Location	Inheritance Mode	Isolated Optic Atrophy	Syndromic Optic Atrophy	OMIM# of the Disease
MFN2 (608507)	1p36.22	AD		Optic atrophy + motor and sensory neuropathy (Charcot-Marie-Tooth disease, axonal, type 2A2A; CMT2A2A)	609260
				Optic atrophy + hereditary motor and sensory neuropathy VIA (HMSN6A)	601152
		AR		Optic atrophy + motor and sensory neuropathy (Charcot-Marie-Tooth disease, axonal, type 2A2B; CMT2A2B)	617087
ATAD3A (612316)	1p36.33	AD/AR		Harel-Yoon syndrome: optic atrophy, peripheral neuropathy, delayed psychomotor development, intellectual disability, spastic paraplegia (HAYOS)	617183

(Continued)

TABLE 12.2: Causative Nuclear-Encoded Genes in Patients with Isolated or Syndromic Optic Atrophy *(Continued)*

Associated Gene/ Locus (OMIM#)	Cytogenetic Location	Inheritance Mode	Isolated Optic Atrophy	Syndromic Optic Atrophy	OMIM# of the Disease
				Name of Disease/Associated Phenotype	
NDUFS1 (157655)	2q33.3	AR/XLD		Optic atrophy + multisystem neurological disorder	252010
DNAJC19 (608977)	3q26.33	AR		Optic atrophy + dilated cardiomyopathy with ataxia, type V 3-methylglutaconic aciduria (DCMA syndrome)	610198
OPA1§ (605290)	3q29	AD	+	Optic atrophy + deafness, ophthalmoplegia, myopathy, ataxia, neuropathy (DOA+)	165500/125250
				Optic atrophy + dementia, parkinsonism and chronic progressive ophthalmoplegia (CPEO)	
				Optic atrophy + lethal infantile encephalopathy, hypertrophic cardiomyopathy	
		AR		Behr syndrome: myoclonic epilepsy, progressive spastic paraplegia, dysarthria, extra-pyramidal tract signs, ataxia, urinary incontinence, mental retardation, posterior column sensory loss or muscle contractures (BEHRS)	210000
WFS1§ (606201)	4p16.1	AD	+	Wolfram-like syndrome (WFSL); Wolfram syndrome-like phenotype	614296
		AR	+	Wolfram syndrome 1 (WFS1)	222300
CISD2 (611507)	4q24	AR		Wolfram syndrome 2 (WFS2)	604928
NR2F1 (132890)	5q15	AD		Bosch-Boonstra-Schaaf optic atrophy syndrome	615722
SLC25A46 (610826)	5q22.1	AR		Optic atrophy + motor and sensory neuropathy (Charcot-Marie-Tooth disease, type 6B, HMSN6B, CMT6B)	616505
RTN4IP1 (610502)	6q21	AR	+	Optic atrophy + ataxia, mental retardation, epilepsy (OPA10)	616732
OPA6# (258500)	8q21-q22	AR	+		258500
FXN (606829)	9q21.11	AR		Friedreich ataxia (FRDA)	229300
AUH (600529)	9q22.31	AR		Type I 3-methylglutaconic aciduria, optic atrophy	250950
MTPAP (613669)	10p11.23	AR		Optic atrophy + spastic ataxia (SPAX4)	613672
YME1L1 (607472)	10p12.1	AR		Optic atrophy + sensorineural hearing impairment, ataxia, other CNS symptoms (OPA11)	617302
TMEM126A (612988)	11q14.1	AR	+	Optic atrophy + auditory neuropathy (OPA7)	612989
DNM1L (603850)	12p11.21	AD/AR	+	Optic atrophy + hypoplasia, encephalopathy, myopathy (EMPF1)	614388
TSFM (604723)	12q14.1	AR		Optic atrophy + multisystem neurological disorder	610505
C12orf65 (613541)	12q24.31	AR		Optic atrophy + hereditary spastic paraplegia, peripheral neuropathy (SPG55)	615035
POLG (174763)	15q26.1	AR		Mitochondrial DNA depletion syndrome 4A (Alpers type), optic atrophy	258450
OPA8# (616648)	16q21-q22	AD	+		616648
SPG7 (602783)	16q24.3	AD/AR	+	Optic atrophy + hereditary spastic paraplegia type 7 (SPG7)	607259
ZNHIT3 (604500)	17q12	AR		Progressive encephalopathy with edema, hypsarrhythmia, and optic atrophy (PEHO)	260565
AFG3L2 (104206)	18p11.21	AD	+	Optic atrophy + intellectual disability	
OPA4# (605293)	18q12.2-q12.3		+		605293
C19orf12 (614297)	19q12	AR		Optic atrophy + spastic paraplegia, peripheral neuropathy, cognitive impairment (SPG43)	615043
OPA3 (606580)	19q13.32	AD		Autosomal dominant optic atrophy with early-onset cataract (ADOAC)	165300
		AR		Type III 3-methylglutaconic aciduria (Costeff syndrome)	258501
ACO2 (100850)	22q13.2	AR	+	Optic atrophy + cerebellar degeneration, hypotonia, epilepsy (OPA9)	616289
OPA2# (311050)	Xp11.4-p11.21	XL	+	Optic atrophy + mental retardation, peripheral neuropathy (OPA2)	311050
TIMM8A (300356)	Xq22.1	XLR		Mohr-Tranebjaerg syndrome (MTS)	304700

Source: Reproduced from (*4*).

The causative gene has not yet been identified.

§ Core genes.

Abbreviations: AD, autosomal dominant; AR, autosomal recessive; XL. X-linked; XLR, X-linked recessive; XLD, X-linked dominant.

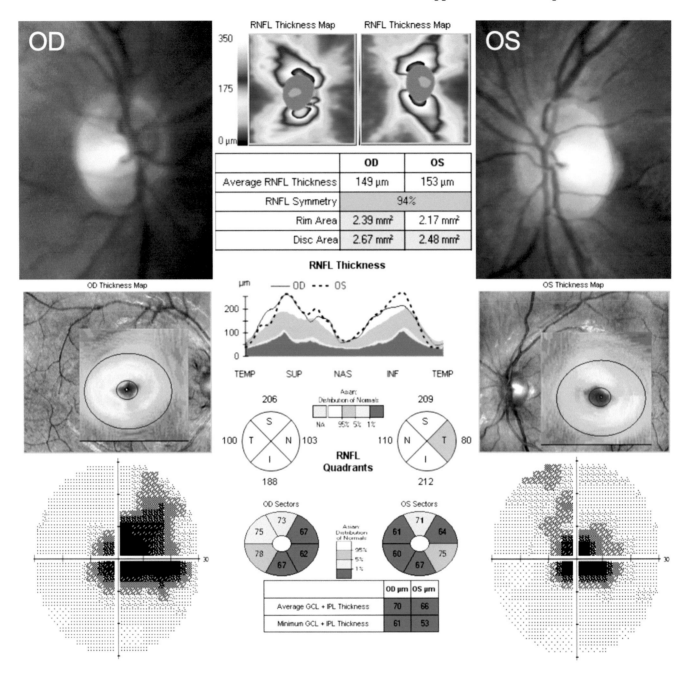

FIGURE 12.2 Ophthalmological features in Leber hereditary optic neuropathy (LHON). A 28-year-old man presented with a 3-week history of sudden-onset blurred vision in both eyes. His visual acuities were 6/60 in his right eye and 4/60 in his left eye. Ishihara color plates were 8/15 and 10/15 plates on the right and left eye, respectively. Visual field testing (Humphrey™ central 30-2) revealed a cecocentral scotoma in the right eye and a central scotoma in the left eye. There was hyperaemia of the right optic disc. OCT showed peripapillary RNFL swelling in the superior and inferior sectors in both eyes. Papillomacular bundle loss was observed on macular ganglion cell layer analysis. Genetic testing confirmed the presence of the pathogenic m.11778G>A mtDNA mutation.

manifestations, in particular involvement of the rest of the central nervous system (4).

LHON-multiple sclerosis (MS) overlap syndrome

Patients with LHON can also develop an MS-like illness (Harding disease) with typical features of demyelination on a brain MRI scan and unmatched oligoclonal bands in their cerebrospinal fluid. However, the pattern of visual loss differs from classical LHON or the typical optic neuritis seen in MS. In LHON-MS, there are recurrent episodes of painless, unilateral visual loss characterized by incomplete visual recovery and progression to registrable blindness in about half of all patients (8, 35, 36). Although a primary mtDNA LHON mutation does not seem to increase the risk of MS, it may modulate the underlying

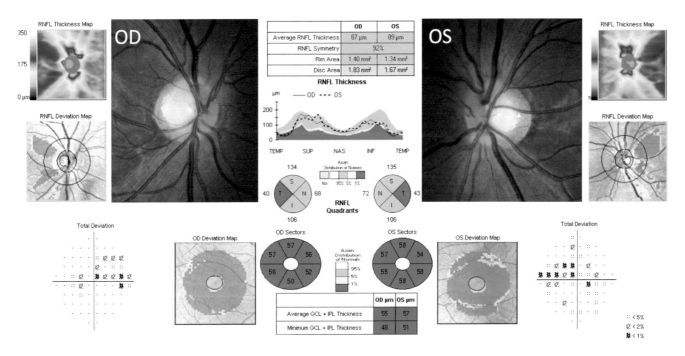

FIGURE 12.3 Ophthalmological features in autosomal dominant optic atrophy (DOA). A 22-year-old man experienced progressive visual loss in both eyes over a period of 1 year. His visual acuities were 6/10 in his right eye and 6/8.6 in his left eye. Ishihara color plates were 11/15 and 9/15 in the right and left eye, respectively. Visual field testing (Humphrey™ central 10-2) showed central scotomas in both eyes. There was temporal optic disc pallor and peripapillary RNFL thinning more prominent in the temporal quadrant. There was marked macular ganglion cell layer thinning in all sectors. Genetic testing identified a pathogenic *OPA1* mutation.

neurodegenerative process in those individuals who are already predisposed to developing MS (8). These observations support the existence of a final common pathway and the importance of mitochondrial dysfunction in the neuronal loss and disease progression seen in demyelinating central nervous system disorders (8).

Childhood LHON

Less than 10% of LHON carriers lose vision before the age of 12 years, but this patient population is clinically relevant as childhood LHON frequently presents atypically and there are often significant diagnostic delays. Children with LHON have been grouped into three subgroups: (1) classical acute (63%); (2) slowly progressive (15%) with visual deterioration over a period exceeding 6 months; and (3) insidious or subclinical (22%) with the child being visually asymptomatic (37). Overall, childhood LHON carries a better visual prognosis with ~40% of patients achieving a final best-corrected visual acuity (BCVA) of 6/12 or better in at least one eye (37). However, given that ~20% of patients only achieved a BCVA of 3/60 in their better seeing eye, parents should be counseled about the poor visual prognosis in LHON and the need for visual rehabilitation (10, 37).

OPA1 spectrum disease

RGCs are particularly sensitive to the deleterious consequences of *OPA1* mutations resulting in optic nerve degeneration and visual loss. In a large multicenter European study, about 20% of *OPA1* carriers developed additional clinical features, including chronic progressive external ophthalmoplegia, sensorineural hearing loss, myopathy, ataxia and peripheral neuropathy (38). As for LHON, DOA can also occur in the context of an MS-like illness (39). These more severe syndromic phenotypes (DOA plus) have been linked with the accumulation of multiple mtDNA deletions, implicating mtDNA instability as a factor contributing to the underlying neurodegeneration (22). Interestingly, there is a higher risk of developing DOA plus with missense mutations involving the catalytic GTPase domain, which points toward a possible dominant-negative effect (22, 38).

WFS1 spectrum disease

Wolfram syndrome was historically defined by the DIDMOAD acronym and it was considered as a recessively inherited disorder. It is now apparent that some *WFS1* mutations are dominant in nature and the phenotype can be milder with patients presenting with isolated OA or OA in combination with sensorineural hearing loss. *WFS1* mutations should therefore be considered in patients with DOA, more so if they are found to be *OPA1*-negative (40, 41).

Optic atrophy in inherited neurodegenerative diseases

OA can also present as a more variable secondary feature of inherited neurodegenerative diseases (Figure 12.1) (5). Friedreich ataxia (FRDA) is the most common form of hereditary ataxia and optic neuropathy, which can be subclinical, is a well-recognized association. FRDA is caused by recessive mutations in the *FXN* gene, which

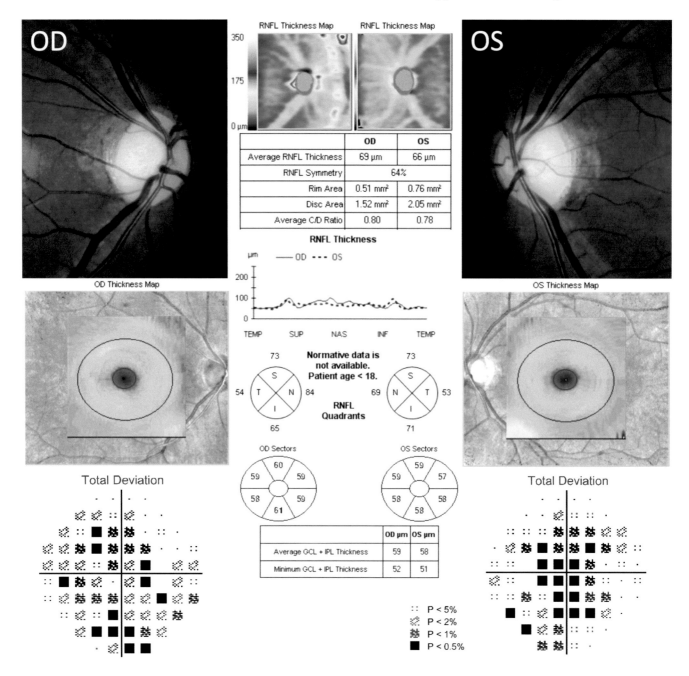

FIGURE 12.4 Ophthalmological features in Wolfram syndrome. A 15-year-old man was diagnosed with Wolfram syndrome at the age of 9 years. His initial presentation was with polydipsia, polyuria and weight loss despite polyphagia. Type 1 diabetes mellitus and optic atrophy developed in the first decade of life. There was no hearing loss and a brain MRI scan was normal. Initially, his best-corrected visual acuities (BCVA) were 6/12 in his right eye and 6/10 in his left eye and Ishihara color testing was 9/15 and 10/15 in the right and left eye, respectively. At the patient's last clinic visit, his BCVA was 6/30 in his right eye and 6/60 in his left eye. Visual field testing (Humphrey™ central 30-2) showed general depression in both eyes. Fundoscopy showed bilateral optic disc cupping with mild temporal pallor of the neuroretinal rim. OCT showed generalized RNFL loss in both the peripapillary and macular regions. Genetic testing identified compound heterozygous *WFS1* mutations.

encodes for a mitochondrial protein involved in the biosynthetic pathways of iron-sulfur clusters. The latter are essential for mitochondrial oxidative phosphorylation being key components of aconitase and the mitochondrial respiratory chain complexes I, II and III (8). Other neurodegenerative diseases that can result in OA are Charcot-Marie-Tooth (CMT) disease and hereditary spastic paraplegia (HSP) caused by *MFN2* and *SPG7* mutations, respectively (8).

Treatment options

The management of patients with inherited optic neuropathies remains largely supportive with visual rehabilitation being essential to maximize the patient's quality of life (42, 43). The neuromuscular deficits in patients with syndromic OA should be managed as part of a multidisciplinary team to prevent these additional comorbidities from worsening the visual impairment (4, 42).

Idebenone is a synthetic, short-chain analogue of ubiquinone, which is responsible for shuttling electrons from complexes I and II directly to complex III (44–46). The current evidence indicates that a subgroup of LHON patients benefits from idebenone and there is a greater likelihood of a positive response when treatment is initiated within the first year of disease onset (44, 47). Idebenone has been approved by the European Medicine Agency (EMA) to treat LHON and the recommended dose is 300 milligrams three times per day (48). Gene therapy based on allotopic expression of wild-type *MTND4* is showing promise for LHON patients carrying the m.11778 G>A mtDNA mutation who are treated within 1 year of disease onset (42, 49, 50). Mitochondrial replacement therapy has been developed to prevent the maternal transmission pathogenic mtDNA mutations, but there are concerns regarding the ethical implications and long-term health implications (42, 51). Treatment strategies for other inherited optic neuropathies besides LHON are still in the preclinical phase of development.

Conclusion

Inherited optic neuropathies are an important cause of blindness in children and young adults. A detailed history and examination are essential to guide the most appropriate investigations when assessing a patient with bilateral OA. It is important to specifically probe for the possibility of other affected family members as this may help point toward a particular mode of inheritance. In addition to OA, some patients can develop more extensive neuromuscular involvement and the relevant medical specialties should be involved when there is a suspicion of extraocular manifestations. Molecular genetic testing is now more widely available and the identification of the underlying genetic defect is a crucial step in providing better counseling to patients and their families. Although, there are limited treatment options for inherited optic neuropathies, several research programs are currently underway worldwide looking at neuroprotective and gene therapy approaches to protect RGCs and improve the visual outcome.

Multiple-Choice Questions

1. Which of the following patients is most likely to have an inherited optic neuropathy?
   a. A 55-year-old man with sudden onset of headaches, vomiting and bitemporal hemianopsia.
   b. A 6-year-old girl with insidious visual loss, bilateral pale optic discs and an electroretinogram showing extinguished cone responses.
   c. A 20-year-old man with rapidly progressive bilateral painless visual loss with dyschromatopsia and dense central scotomas.
   d. A 60-year-old woman with poor diabetic control and hypertension describing sudden-onset unilateral visual loss and an altitudinal visual field defect.

Answer:

c. A 20-year-old man with rapidly progressive bilateral painless visual loss with dyschromatopsia and dense central scotomas.

2. Which of the following descriptions of Leber hereditary optic neuropathy (LHON) is INCORRECT?
   a. LHON is caused by mutations in nuclear-encoded genes.
   b. LHON has a predilection for male carriers to lose vision.
   c. LHON is characterized by subacute, painless, central visual loss and in unilateral cases, the fellow eye becomes involved 2–4 months later.
   d. The optic disc may be hyperemic with peripapillary telangiectasias, but no leakage is seen on fluorescein angiography.

Answer:

a. LHON is caused by mutations in nuclear-encoded genes.

3. Which of the following descriptions of autosomal dominant optic atrophy (DOA) is INCORRECT?
   a. DOA is the most common inherited optic neuropathy in the general population.
   b. The majority of patients with DOA harbor mutations in the *OPA1* gene.
   c. OPA1 is expressed exclusively in the retinal ganglion cell layer.
   d. Patients usually present with insidious visual loss from early childhood.

Answer:

c. OPA1 is expressed exclusively in the retinal ganglion cell layer.

4. Which of the following descriptions of patients with an inherited optic neuropathy is INCORRECT?
   a. The LHON-multiple sclerosis overlap syndrome is characterized by recurrent episodes of visual loss with incomplete visual recovery.
   b. DOA plus is a more severe phenotypic variant of DOA with patients developing additional neuromuscular deficits in addition to optic atrophy.
   c. Friedreich ataxia is the most common form of hereditary ataxia and optic neuropathy is a well-recognized clinical feature in some patients.
   d. Wolfram syndrome is caused by mutations in the *WFS1* gene that encodes for a mitochondrial inner membrane protein.

Answer:

d. Wolfram syndrome is caused by mutations in the WFS1 gene that encodes for a mitochondrial inner membrane protein.

References

1. Yu-Wai-Man P, Griffiths PG, Hudson G, Chinnery PF. Inherited mitochondrial optic neuropathies. J Med Genet. 2009;46(3):145–158.
2. Milea D, Amati-Bonneau P, Reynier P, Bonneau D. Genetically determined optic neuropathies. Curr Opin Neurol. 2010;23(1):24–28.
3. Miller NR, Newman NJ, Biousse V, Kerrison JB. Walsh and Hoyt's clinical neuro-ophthalmology. 6th ed. Philadelphia: Lippincott Williams & Wilkins; 2005.
4. Jurkute N, Majander A, Bowman R, Votruba M, Abbs S, Acheson J, et al. Clinical utility gene card for: inherited optic neuropathies including next-generation sequencing-based approaches. Eur J Hum Genet. 2019;27(3):494–502.
5. Yu-Wai-Man P, Griffiths PG, Chinnery PF. Mitochondrial optic neuropathies—disease mechanisms and therapeutic strategies. Prog Retin Eye Res. 2011;30(2):81–114.

6. Fraser JA, Biousse V, Newman NJ. The neuro-ophthalmology of mitochondrial disease. Surv Ophthalmol. 2010;55(4):299–334.

7. Jurkute N, Leu C, Pogoda HM, Arno G, Robson AG, Nurnberg G, et al. SSBP1 mutations in dominant optic atrophy with variable retinal degeneration. Ann Neurol. 2019;86(3):368–383.

8. Yu-Wai-Man P, Votruba M, Burte F, La Morgia C, Barboni P, Carelli V. A neurodegenerative perspective on mitochondrial optic neuropathies. Acta Neuropathol. 2016;132(6):789–806.

9. Sitarz KS, Chinnery PF, Yu-Wai-Man P. Disorders of the optic nerve in mitochondrial cytopathies: New ideas on pathogenesis and therapeutic targets. Curr Neurol Neurosci Rep. 2012;12(3):308–317.

10. Jurkute N, Yu-Wai-Man P. Leber hereditary optic neuropathy: Bridging the translational gap. Curr Opin Ophthalmol. 2017;28(5):403–409.

11. Ueda K, Morizane Y, Shiraga F, Shikishima K, Ishikawa H, Wakakura M, et al. Nationwide epidemiological survey of Leber hereditary optic neuropathy in Japan. J Epidemiol. 2017;27(9):447–450.

12. Hwang TJ, Karanjia R, Moraes-Filho MN, Gale J, Tran JS, Chu ER, et al. Natural history of conversion of Leber's hereditary optic neuropathy: A prospective case series. Ophthalmology. 2017;124(6):843–850.

13. Barboni P, Savini G, Valentino ML, Montagna P, Cortelli P, De Negri AM, et al. Retinal nerve fiber layer evaluation by optical coherence tomography in Leber's hereditary optic neuropathy. Ophthalmology. 2005;112(1):120–126.

14. Barboni P, Carbonelli M, Savini G, Ramos Cdo V, Carta A, Berezovsky A, et al. Natural history of Leber's hereditary optic neuropathy: Longitudinal analysis of the retinal nerve fiber layer by optical coherence tomography. Ophthalmology. 2010;117(3):623–627.

15. Kirkman MA, Korsten A, Leonhardt M, Dimitriadis K, De Coo IF, Klopstock T, et al. Quality of life in patients with Leber hereditary optic neuropathy. Invest Ophthalmol Vis Sci. 2009;50(7):3112–3115.

16. Lam BL, Feuer WJ, Schiffman JC, Porciatti V, Vandenbroucke R, Rosa PR, et al. Trial end points and natural history in patients with G11778A Leber hereditary optic neuropathy: Preparation for gene therapy clinical trial. JAMA Ophthalmol. 2014;132(4):428–436.

17. Yu-Wai-Man P, Chinnery PF. Dominant optic atrophy: Novel OPA1 mutations and revised prevalence estimates. Ophthalmology. 2013;120(8):1712–1712.e1.

18. Yu-Wai-Man P, Shankar SP, Biousse V, Miller NR, Bean LJ, Coffee B, et al. Genetic screening for OPA1 and OPA3 mutations in patients with suspected inherited optic neuropathies. Ophthalmology. 2011;118(3):558–563.

19. Yen MY, Wang AG, Lin YC, Fann MJ, Hsiao KJ. Novel mutations of the OPA1 gene in Chinese dominant optic atrophy. Ophthalmology. 2010;117(2):392–396.e1.

20. Ferre M, Bonneau D, Milea D, Chevrollier A, Verny C, Dollfus H, et al. Molecular screening of 980 cases of suspected hereditary optic neuropathy with a report on 77 novel OPA1 mutations. Hum Mutat. 2009;30(7):E692–705.

21. Zanna C, Ghelli A, Porcelli AM, Karbowski M, Youle RJ, Schimpf S, et al. OPA1 mutations associated with dominant optic atrophy impair oxidative phosphorylation and mitochondrial fusion. Brain. 2008;131(Pt 2):352–367.

22. Yu-Wai-Man P, Sitarz KS, Samuels DC, Griffiths PG, Reeve AK, Bindoff LA, et al. OPA1 mutations cause cytochrome c oxidase deficiency due to loss of wild-type mtDNA molecules. Hum Mol Genet. 2010;19(15):3043–3052.

23. Cohn AC, Toomes C, Hewitt AW, Kearns LS, Inglehearn CF, Craig JE, et al. The natural history of OPA1-related autosomal dominant optic atrophy. Br J Ophthalmol. 2008;92(10):1333–1336.

24. Yu-Wai-Man P, Griffiths PG, Burke A, Sellar PW, Clarke MP, Gnanaraj L, et al. The prevalence and natural history of dominant optic atrophy due to OPA1 mutations. Ophthalmology. 2010;117(8):1538–1546, 1546.e1.

25. Kim TW, Hwang JM. Stratus OCT in dominant optic atrophy: Features differentiating it from glaucoma. J Glaucoma. 2007;16(8):655–658.

26. Votruba M, Thiselton D, Bhattacharya SS. Optic disc morphology of patients with OPA1 autosomal dominant optic atrophy. Br J Ophthalmol. 2003;87(1):48–53.

27. Fournier AV, Damji KF, Epstein DL, Pollock SC. Disc excavation in dominant optic atrophy: Differentiation from normal tension glaucoma. Ophthalmology. 2001;108(9):1595–1602.

28. Rigoli L, Di Bella C. Wolfram syndrome 1 and Wolfram syndrome 2. Curr Opin Pediatr. 2012;24(5):512–517.

29. Moosajee M, Yu-Wai-Man P, Rouzier C, Bitner-Glindzicz M, Bowman R. Clinical utility gene card for: Wolfram syndrome. Eur J Hum Genet. 2016;24(11).

30. Barrett TG, Bundey SE, Macleod AF. Neurodegeneration and diabetes: UK nationwide study of Wolfram (DIDMOAD) syndrome. Lancet. 1995;346(8988):1458–1463.

31. Kumar S. Wolfram syndrome: Important implications for pediatricians and pediatric endocrinologists. Pediatr Diabetes. 2010;11(1):28–37.

32. de Heredia ML, Cleries R, Nunes V. Genotypic classification of patients with Wolfram syndrome: Insights into the natural history of the disease and correlation with phenotype. Genet Med. 2013;15(7):497–506.

33. Al-Till M, Jarrah NS, Ajlouni KM. Ophthalmologic findings in fifteen patients with Wolfram syndrome. Eur J Ophthalmol. 2002;12(2):84–88.

34. Ito S, Sakakibara R, Hattori T. Wolfram syndrome presenting marked brain MR imaging abnormalities with few neurologic abnormalities. AJNR Am J Neuroradiol. 2007;28(2):305–306.

35. Pfeffer G, Burke A, Yu-Wai-Man P, Compston DA, Chinnery PF. Clinical features of MS associated with Leber hereditary optic neuropathy mtDNA mutations. Neurology. 2013;81(24):2073–2081.

36. Tran M, Bhargava R, MacDonald IM. Leber hereditary optic neuropathy, progressive visual loss, and multiple-sclerosis-like symptoms. Am J Ophthalmol. 2001;132(4):591–593.

37. Majander A, Bowman R, Poulton J, Antcliff RJ, Reddy MA, Michaelides M, et al. Childhood-onset Leber hereditary optic neuropathy. Br J Ophthalmol. 2017;101(11):1505–1509.

38. Yu-Wai-Man P, Griffiths PG, Gorman GS, Lourenco CM, Wright AF, Auer-Grumbach M, et al. Multi-system neurological disease is common in patients with OPA1 mutations. Brain. 2010;133(Pt 3):771–786.

39. Yu-Wai-Man P, Spyropoulos A, Duncan HJ, Guadagno JV, Chinnery PF. A multiple sclerosis-like disorder in patients with OPA1 mutations. Ann Clin Transl Neurol. 2016;3(9):723–729.

40. Majander A, Bitner-Glindzicz M, Chan CM, Duncan HJ, Chinnery PF, Subash M, et al. Lamination of the outer plexiform layer in optic atrophy caused by dominant WFS1 mutations. Ophthalmology. 2016;123(7):1624–1626.

41. Grenier J, Meunier I, Daien V, Baudoin C, Halloy F, Bocquet B, et al. WFS1 in Optic Neuropathies: Mutation findings in nonsyndromic optic atrophy and assessment of clinical severity. Ophthalmology. 2016;123(9):1989–1998.

42. Jurkute N, Harvey J, Yu-Wai-Man P. Treatment strategies for Leber hereditary optic neuropathy. Current opinion in neurology. 2019;32(1):99–104.

43. Yu-Wai-Man P. Therapeutic approaches to inherited optic neuropathies. Sem Neurol. 2015;35(5):578–586.

44. Klopstock T, Yu-Wai-Man P, Dimitriadis K, Rouleau J, Heck S, Bailie M, et al. A randomized placebo-controlled trial of idebenone in Leber's hereditary optic neuropathy. Brain. 2011;134(Pt 9):2677–2686.

45. Klopstock T, Metz G, Yu-Wai-Man P, Buchner B, Gallenmuller C, Bailie M, et al. Persistence of the treatment effect of idebenone in Leber's hereditary optic neuropathy. Brain. 2013;136(Pt 2):e230.

46. Carelli V, La Morgia C, Valentino ML, Rizzo G, Carbonelli M, De Negri AM, et al. Idebenone treatment in Leber's hereditary optic neuropathy. Brain. 2011;134(Pt 9):e188.

47. Barboni P, Valentino ML, La Morgia C, Carbonelli M, Savini G, De Negri A, et al. Idebenone treatment in patients with OPA1-mutant dominant optic atrophy. Brain. 2013;136(Pt 2):e231.

48. Carelli V, Carbonelli M, de Coo IF, Kawasaki A, Klopstock T, Lagreze WA, et al. International consensus statement on the clinical and therapeutic management of Leber hereditary optic neuropathy. J Neuroophthalmol. 2017;37(4):371–381.

49. Yu-Wai-Man P, Newman NJ, Carelli V, Moster ML, Biousse V, Sadun AA, et al. Bilateral visual improvement with unilateral gene therapy injection for Leber hereditary optic neuropathy. Sci Transl Med. 2020;12(573):eaaz7423

50. Newman NJ, Yu-Wai-Man P, Carelli V, Moster ML, Biousse V, Vignal-Clermont C, et al. Efficacy and safety of intravitreal gene therapy for leber hereditary optic neuropathy treated within 6 months of disease onset. Ophthalmology. 2021;128(5):649–660.

51. Newson AJ, Wilkinson S, Wrigley A. Ethical and legal issues in mitochondrial transfer. EMBO Mol Med. 2016;8(6):589–591.

13

NON-ORGANIC VISION LOSS

Ashwini Kini, Mangayarkarasi Thandampallayam Ajjeya, Padmaja Sudhakar

CASE STUDY

An 18-year-old male without any comorbidities presented with sudden-onset visual loss from both eye to no light perception. On examination both pupils were normal in size and were reacting to light. Fundus examination showed normal optic discs in both eyes. When optokinetic drum was rotated in front of patient, optokinetic nystagmus could be elicited. How do you approach patients with like presentation?

Introduction

Non-organic vision loss (NOVL) or functional vision loss (FVL) is abnormal vision or visual fields without an organic pathology. Both terms are used to describe causes of vision loss which is either intentionally feigned or that which occurs under unconscious conditions (i.e., conversion). They may be used as general terms in discussing the diagnosis with the patient without offending or frustrating them. They also serve as an acceptable terminology for documentation in medical records. The diagnosis of NOVL requires the establishment of findings on clinical exam that prove the integrity and functioning of the visual system which is sometimes difficult and time-consuming to establish. NOVL is especially challenging to diagnose when superimposed on organic pathology. But using anatomical rules and basic ophthalmology tools, one can demonstrate integrity of the visual system and confirm the diagnosis of NOVL. It is important to remember that almost anything can present without an organic basis, for example, nystagmus, gaze palsy, ptosis but in this chapter, we will restrict our discussion to cases of visual acuity and visual field loss.

Prevalence of NOVL in a clinic

NOVL patients are often referred to the neuro-ophthalmology clinic after extensive work-up has failed to reveal an underlying cause for poor vision. Overall NOVL has been reported to comprise around 1–5% of the patient population in an ophthalmology clinic (1, 2) and can include both pediatric and adult population. Mean age at presentation is reported around 11–13 years in pediatric group, 40 years in adults with fall in incidence after the sixth decade. There is female predominance in both age groups and around 60–80% cases are bilateral. Visual acuity combined with field loss is found to be the most common presentation in NOVL (3, 4).

Risk factors

A large proportion of these individuals could have underlying stressors, psychiatric disorders, attention deficit hyperactivity disorder (ADHD), somatoform disorders, behavioral/learning disorders or conflicts/disharmony at home. Sexual/physical abuse in children could be risk factor that would need additional attention (4, 5). Likewise, health events (self-limiting illness, operations, injuries) may occur immediately prior to the onset of symptoms. Underlying psychiatric illness is found to be more prevalent in the adult population than the pediatric age group (4). It has also been reported that large proportion of NOVL patients do not have any underlying psychiatric disorder (5–8). According to Newman et al, NOVL is not a diagnosis of exclusion as it is popularly believed but needs examination and tests to determine the same (8, 9). Of note, 15–50% of the patients with NOVL could have underlying visual comorbidities and fall under "non-organic overlay." These cases need to be carefully evaluated and managed in order to not miss a subtle underlying treatable cause (8, 9).

Tests to identify a NOVL in clinic

Initial examination starts even as the patient walks into the clinic. Observing them maneuver around obstacles could give a fair idea on their level of vision. A patient walking into the clinic with sunglasses on is reported as a strong predictor of NOVL provided the patient does not have particular indication for the same like intense photophobia or acute migraine attack (10). Offer a spontaneous handshake either at the beginning of the visit or at the end, intentionally in the blind field (in case of field loss) and observe if patient reaches out without having to turn to look around.

It is important to establish if there is visual acuity loss or visual field loss and also if there is unilateral or bilateral loss. In cases of visual field loss, determine the area of visual field loss, this enables the examiner to tailor the tests necessary for a particular patient. Reduced visual acuity is usually the most common presentation in NOVL. It is always important to rule out organic pathology. Also, binocular visual loss is more difficult to handle and less quantitative maneuvers are available that establish good vision in both eyes (OU).

Tricks on visual acuity tests

The patients referred for NOVL would already have had their vision checked multiple times at other providers and could be frustrated on repeated attempts at the same. Attempts to check or improve the vision while establishing a doctor-patient relationship could be very tricky. This could make patient's lose confidence for the rest of the exam and possibly affect follow-ups in the future. A few ways to do this differently with these group of patients are listed here. Again, these could have variable results and are not foolproof.

Snellen's visual acuity

First step would be to start checking the vision from the smallest letter available on chart, e.g. 20/15 or 6/5 line, keeping affected eye open and good eye closed. Slowly move up the chart. Provide encouragement to the patient for every letter read and for every guess made. This test can be done keeping both eyes open in case of binocular visual loss.

DOI: 10.1201/9780429020278-16

Fogging

Fogging is a test that could be tried in patients with mono-ocular vision loss. This involves gradually fogging the good eye with lenses with an attempt to blur the vision in the good eye and meanwhile asking the patient to read off the vision chart. Hence the patient unknowingly shifts to reading from his "bad eye." At the beginning of the test, the patient is explained that his good eye is being checked to improve vision further and while the test is being performed, holding a light conversation with the patient might distract him from being conscious or aware. Also lenses that when combined are the equivalent of plain glass can be placed over the patient's refraction to suggest that these will magnify the letters on the chart. This might help in those reporting binocular vision losses.

In an ophthalmologist's clinic, the lenses may be used on a phoropter; however, this equipment is unavailable in a neurologist's office and may not always be feasible to do this test. A trial frame with a few loose plus and minus lenses could be kept in the clinic which may be handy in testing in such cases.

Red green glasses

Another trick includes having the patient wear red-green glasses and using red and green letters of gradually increasing size on the Snellen's visual acuity chart. This test is based on the principle that colored lenses allow only similarly colored light to pass through. The eye with the red filter sees only the images that are red and similarly eye with the green filter sees only images that are green. Present this as a color vision test to the patient. Vision in each eye could be checked with reasonable accuracy with this test.

A similar test involves using polarized glasses, with one axis at 90° and the other at 180° in each lens and asking the patient to read a polarized eye chart with some letters perceptible only to one eye or the other.

Stereopsis and visual acuity correlation

Stereopsis tests are based on the principle of binocular fusion and require a particular minimum level of vision to correlate to the degree of stereopsis (Table 13.1) (11). These tests can be administered to the patients without raising suspicion, i.e., Titmus test, Randot test (Stereo Optical Co., Inc., Chicago, IL). These could be used in patients reporting monocular loss and also with binocular loss to some extent (8). Some studies, however, state that commonly used visual acuity estimates based on stereo acuity might overestimate visual acuity (12).

Distance doubling test

Zinkernael reported a close 100% sensitivity and specificity with the distance doubling test which is based on the principle that

TABLE 13.1: Relationship of Stereopsis to Visual Acuity

Stereopsis (arc second)	Visual Acuity	Visual Acuity
40	20/20	6/6
43	20/25	6/7.5
52	20/30	6/9
61	20/40	6/12
78	20/50	6/15
94	20/70	6/24
124	20/100	6/30
160	20/200	20/60

Source: Data modified from Levy NS, Glick EB. Stereoscopic perception and Snellen visual acuity. Am J Ophthalmol. 1974;78(4):722–724.

Note: Table showing relationship of stereopsis to visual acuity in feet and meters.

when vision is checked at a particular distance say around at 20/100 level and then when the distance is reduced to half, by physiology, the patient should be able to read a letter of 20/50 size. Patients with NOVL often will report static, unchanged level of vision despite coming closer to the chart (8, 13).

Using the optokinetic drum (OKN)

The optokinetic drum is a drum with vertical stripes which can be rotated to elicit optokinetic nystagmus in the viewer's eye (pursuit with refixation saccade) (Figure 13.1). In a patient who claims to be unilaterally or bilaterally blind to the extent of no light perception (NLP), light perception (LP) or hand motions, eliciting a nystagmus with OKN drum establishes a vision of at least 20/400. In bilaterally blind, test is conducted with both eyes open and when unilateral, the test is started with both eyes open and the examiner introduces an occluder in front of the good eye during the course of the test to elicit nystagmus in the claimed blind eye (14).

Vertical prism test

This was a novel test first described by Slavin and has proved to be a simple and useful test that can be administered with relative ease in the clinic (15). This involves placing a vertical prism of 4PD base down in front of the good eye. This is useful mostly in patients with mono-ocular vision loss and prior to the test the physician describes to the patient that he will check only his good eye with a prism and he may expect the prism to split the image. The prism placed in front of the "good eye" displaces the image seen with that eye higher up and the original image seen with the "bad eye" lower. This test could be improvised by showing the patient a 20/40 optotype on a Snellen chart at standard distance. If the patient describes seeing two images of similar clarity, the patient has unknowingly

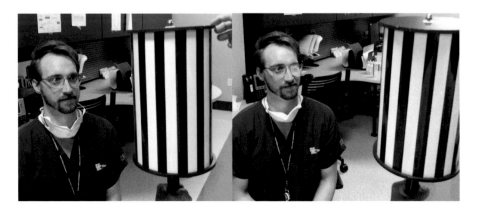

FIGURE 13.1 Eliciting optokinetic nystagmus in binocular and monocular non-organic vision loss.

declared that the vision in his "blind eye" is at least 20/40 or may be even better. Golnik and Lee used this test in three groups of patients, normal, organic and in those referred with "non-organic" vision loss. They conclude that the vertical prism test was fairly accurate and reliable test to identify NOVL and in fact appropriate image response of "one image" was detected in some of their patients referred as NOVL who on further work up were identified with other causes explaining their vision loss (16).

A 4 PD prism may also be placed base out in front of the eye with alleged visual reduction while fixating a 20/40 Snellen letter and diplopia may be elicited to detect NOVL. When the prism is quickly removed if movement of the affected eye is detected by the examiner, an acuity approximately equal to the Snellen letter is likely.

A slight variation of the vertical prism test is done by blocking the affected eye with your finger. Place the vertical prism with its base down splitting the pupil of the good eye. The patient will report seeing two lines of letters with the good eye-monocular diplopia. Ask the patient to read the bottom line (bottom image) and while they do that slide the prism down over the good eye and remove the occlusion from the affected eye. The patient will still report seeing two lines of letters, the bottom line is now seen with the affected eye.

Visual surprise

This is a technique in which a series of Landolt C's are presented to the patient in various orientation, single letter on each time, in total of 32 times. The patient is explained that he has to recognize the pattern or direction of the broken "C" and the time to response is recorded. Following initial presentations of standard "C," an "O" is introduced to the patient and the element of surprise and time to response which should be delayed in a patient with normal vision may help unmask a NOVL. The number of incorrect responses are recorded and the authors report that fewer than three overall correct responses in recognition of pattern suggest NOVL as the probability of getting these right by chance alone (i.e., in a blind person/eyes closed) is <2.5% (17, 18). Practical utility of the test in office setting would be cumbersome and inconclusive.

Using the menace reflex for a response is a test described for detection of NOVL but some practitioners would refrain from using as it would be regarded as an action of threat. Moreover, the perception of motion could be relatively preserved even in cortically blind patients, i.e., Riddoch phenomenon (19), and menace response cannot be used to rule in or rule out NOVL, but in fact some of these patients could have an underlying treatable disorder that could go unchecked (20).

Absence of relative afferent pupillary defect (RAPD)

In a patient reporting poor vision in one eye it would be expected to have a RAPD in that eye if there was an optic neuropathy or a retinal pathology like central retinal artery occlusion.

In a patient displaying unilateral profound vision loss to extent of NLP, an absent RAPD in the presence of normal ophthalmic exam should raise suspicion for NOVL. This would be difficult to assess when the complaint is bilateral or unilateral and with subtle/hemianopic loss. Absence of RAPD may need to be verified using neutral density filters as subtle RAPD can be missed. Absence of RAPD would essentially mean in simple terms either no R, no A, no P or no D. No R means one would not expect to see a RAPD in bilateral and symmetric disease and hence would not be useful in a patient reporting bilateral deficit. No A means the defect is not in the afferent pathway, for example, if the patient complains of diplopia, which is an efferent pathway defect there would not be an RAPD. Similarly no RAPD is seen in cases of media opacities like corneal opacity or cataract. No P, means there is no defect in the pupillary pathway, i.e.,

the issue is either in front of the pupil pathway like refractive error, amblyopia, media opacity or beyond the pupillary pathway, i.e., cortical pathology. Lastly no D, means that no defect detectable either because of anatomic pupillary abnormality or patient is one eyed.

Often it may be difficult to pick up subtle RAPD especially in small, tonic pupils or if there is an anatomic abnormality. Foroozan and Lee mention how an absent RAPD in a structurally normal eye could easily be mislabeled as "faking" in the presence of true underlying cortical visual field deficit that was picked up on formal visual field testing (21). This could be true especially in chiasmal or retrochiasmal lesions which would not have any structural eye abnormality, could have a normal 20/20 vision in both eyes, and not demonstrate RAPD. Also subtle early traumatic lesions could be missed on MRI. Lesions especially of the optic tract are difficult to pick on clinical testing. Sometimes an RAPD and bowtie optic atrophy may be seen on the contralateral side of an optic tract lesion. Optic tract lesions might be difficult to see on MRI and may be picked up on more specific studies either with use of contrast on MRI, PET, SPECT or even with diffusion tensor imaging or tractography (22–25). Clinical presentation and past history could help guide the physician in ordering the right imaging study for the patient.

A useful point to remember is that patients with early LHON may have normal pupil response without RAPD in the background of poor vision and normal eye exam (26). Central scotoma and bilateral involvement are important clues that could prompt genetic testing in these individuals.

Potential acuity meter

The potential acuity meter, or interferometer, can evaluate visual acuity prior to cataract surgery so that patients could be furnished with a realistic visual prognosis pre-operatively. It has a monochromatic light source, which generates interference stripes posterior to the lens, and which are therefore not affected by lenticular opacities. This test can also be used in NOVL (27). The patient is told that the test is designed to circumvent the current eye problem and estimate what the vision would have been like had the illness not occurred. It could measure the visual acuity in monocular or binocular visual complaints.

Mirror test

When distracting the patient by holding a conversation with them, use a mirror that is moved across their field of vision. It is difficult for a patient to resist looking at their own reflection (8).

Visual field: Tunnel vs funnel vision

Visual field abnormalities can be additional evidence of non-organic etiology in some cases. One of the most common visual field deficits encountered in NOVL is a tunnel field, i.e., a constricted visual field restricting usable field to central 5–10 degrees. Normal physiologic visual field is a "funnel" that expands as you move further away from the target. In simple terms, this is the concept by which you could expect to see stars or moon at infinite distances vs seeing a ball at very close range. This concept could be used in patients with unilateral or bilateral constricted fields. Visual field is first checked by confrontation at 1 meter by bringing in your finger from the periphery to the seeing field of the patient in all quadrants to map out the approximate area of visual field. Then move away to around 2 meters or 4 meters (or maximum distance that the examination room allows) and repeat the same. Under normal physiologic fields (and even in patients with constricted fields from an organic cause), the area mapped should expand out, i.e., patient should be able to detect your finger to further periphery as compared to 1 meter (2, 8). A field that fails to expand is suggestive of NOVL.

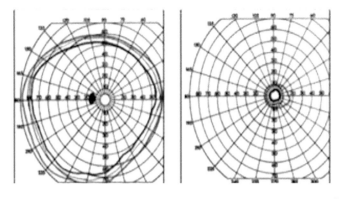

FIGURE 13.2 Goldman kinetic perimetry demonstrating normal visual field and constricted visual fields in NOVL.

Goldman kinetic visual fields administered by a well-trained administrator may be a more reliable technique for assessment. NOVL patients may show a constriction with non-physiologic overlap of isopters. They may claim to see the smaller, less bright object at same place as the larger, brighter test object. A continuous spiral or a jagged inconsistent star pattern may be produced (8) (Figure 13.2).

If there is the privilege of using the automated perimeter, the fields can be checked initially with a smaller target and then repeated with a larger target. However, automated perimetry is generally not helpful in the assessment of NOVL. Poor testing parameters, inconsistent responses and variable testing patterns do not differentiate NOVL from the organic etiology. A "clover leaf" or rarely a square-like pattern mapped out on automated perimetric testing is suggestive but not diagnostic of NOVL (Figure 13.3) (14). In contrast, a central scotoma on

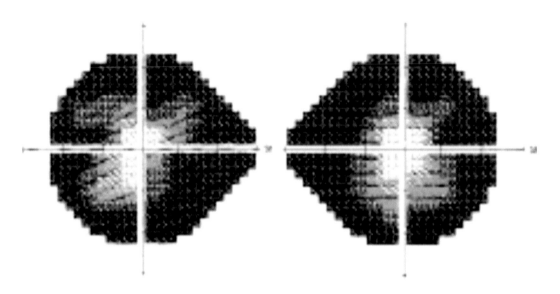

```
CENTRAL 24-2 THRESHOLD TEST

FIXATION MONITOR: GAZE/BLINDSPOT          STIMULUS: III. WHITE
FIXATION TARGET: CENTRAL                  BACKGROUND: 31.5 ASB
FIXATION LOSSES: 0/17                     STRATEGY: SITA-STANDARD
FALSE POS ERRORS:   0 %
FALSE NEG ERRORS:  33 %
TEST DURATION: 07:33

FOVEA: 33 DB
```

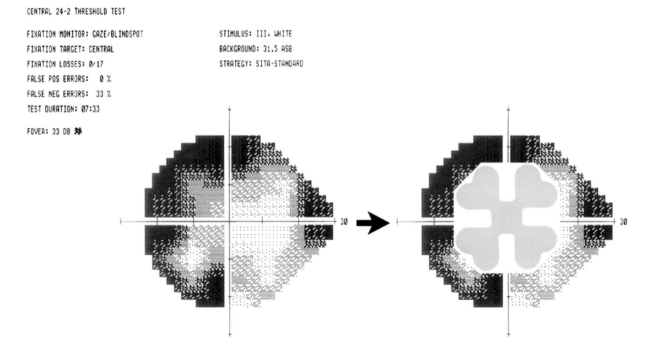

FIGURE 13.3 Automated perimetry demonstrating a square and clover leaf pattern in non-organic vision loss.

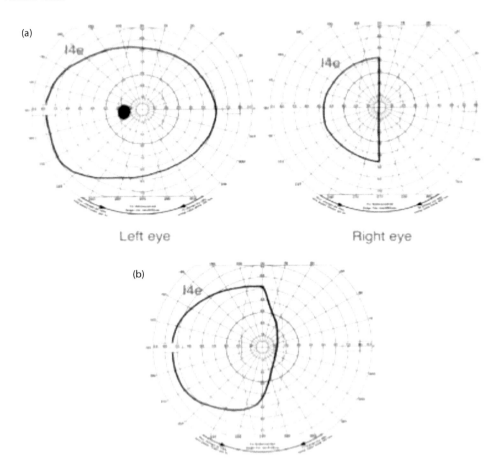

FIGURE 13.4 Monocular visual field testing with Goldman perimetry shows right temporal hemianopia that persists on binocular testing suggesting non-organic visual loss.

field testing is least likely to be from a NOVL (28) and should prompt the clinician to look further for underlying optic nerve or retinal pathology.

Binocular visual field testing

Consider that one eye is truly non-seeing, when a visual field is checked with both eyes open, the good eye will compensate for the missing field of the bad eye. In a patient with NOVL, on binocular field testing the monocular field loss will persist on binocular testing (Figure 13.4). This test could be used even in patient reporting constricted visual field/hemianopic field defect in one eye. On binocular field testing, if the reported defect, i.e., constricted field/hemianopic defect continues to persist, it suggests NOVL as the visual field with the seeing eye alone should practically produce a normal visual field under binocular conditions. The functional status of the good eye could be initially established with a monocular field of that eye prior to binocular testing. Similarly, in the patient with professed severe monocular visual loss, a binocular visual field (with both eyes open) may reveal a non-physiologic constriction or absence of the visual field on the side of the monocular loss, a region clearly seen on prior testing of the good eye alone (Figure 13.5).

The monocular and binocular testing may be done both with confrontation field testing, Goldman kinetic perimetry or automated perimetry.

Test of proprioception

A patient with bilateral NOVL may be asked to touch the tips of both his fingers keeping his eyes open or with one eye (good eye) patched and may be seen to fail this attempt. A bilaterally blind person due to organic causes should be able to do this simple test by principle of proprioception that would be intact (Figure 13.6). Applying the same concept the patient may be told to use their own arm to point in a particular direction and asking them to point with the other arm as to where the first arm is pointing or hold up their own fingers and ask them how many fingers are being held up.

Ancillary testing

VEP and electroretinograms (ERG)

Somers et al. report that pattern visual-evoked potential (pVEP) could detect NOVL in children and help differentiate from organic visual loss (OVL). Visual-evoked potentials of normal and symmetric amplitude and latency in profound monocular visual loss help in diagnosing NOVL. This test could also be useful in a larger group of patients who have non-organic overlay over underlying established vision loss who may exaggerate the extent of vision loss for the purpose of compensation, seeking attention or seeking sympathy (29). VEP could give a gross correlation of the visual status. A VEP of <5.77 uv is closely consistent with legal blindness, i.e.,

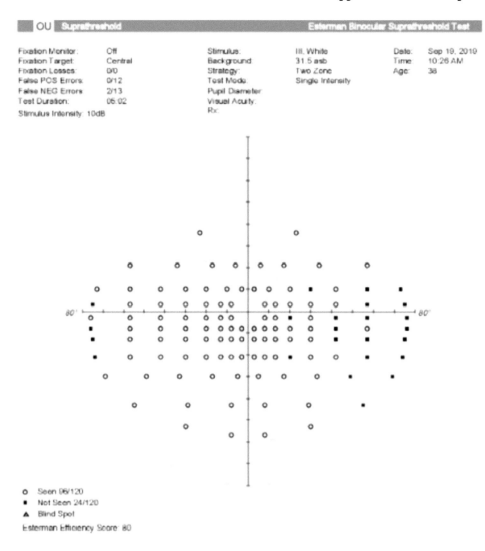

FIGURE 13.5   Esterman's binocular automated perimetry demonstrating right temporal defect in a subject claiming monocular right temporal field loss.

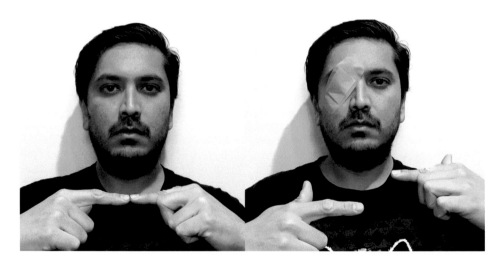

FIGURE 13.6   Demonstrating how to test touching of finger tips of both index fingers in patient reporting binocular and monocular vision loss.

<20/200 acuity and could fairly help reduce suspicion for NOVL (30). Multifocal VEPs may demonstrate normal electrophysiological responses in the region of purported visual loss.

However, an abnormal VEP is less helpful. It is important to note that VEP responses could be volitionally altered by the patient's defocusing. This may be inapparent even to a trained observer. On the other hand, normal VEP responses could be obtained in cortically blind patients (31, 32).

Pattern and multifocal ERG that produce a normal and symmetric response argue against severe organic disease, but an abnormal test is inconclusive. The flash ERG measures the function of predominantly the outer retinal layers. It should be abnormal in a patient with diffuse retinal dysfunction but will be normal in a patient with more distal organic disease such as optic neuropathy, chiasmal neuropathy or retro chiasmal visual dysfunction.

Neuroimaging
Neuroimaging such as CT/MRI head and orbit and vascular imaging such as CTA/MRA head and neck may help rule out compressive or vascular lesions, but negative studies do not establish the diagnosis as functional.

Optical coherence tomography
Optical coherence tomography (OCT) of the optic nerve and retina can identify anatomical pathology involving optic nerve and retina; however, a normal OCT cannot rule out organic causes of vision loss.

How to deal with a NOVL loss in the clinic

It is potentially easy to label a patient with NOVL and this can lead to devastating consequences if the patient actually has an organic underlying cause that was missed. Some of the intracranial mass lesions involving the pituitary or frontal lobe could have a normal structural exam and go undetected on CT scan and non-contrast MRI. A finger confrontation test could have a sensitivity as low as 20% in cases of bitemporal hemianopia and hence an inability to detect a field defect cannot be used to rule out an organic cause. Homonymous hemianopia could be missed in up to around 30% of the patients. Some of the patients with pituitary or frontal lesions could have accompanying psychiatric changes that could also add to the error in judgment.

Kerr et al compared seven different methods of doing a confrontation in the clinic setting including using kinetic and static wiggling finger, use of red target both static and kinetic and concluded that 5 mm kinetic red target moved from peripheral non-seeing field across the field to cross the midline and asking the patient's ability to see and interpret a change in color/hue of the red target had the best sensitivity to pick up a visual field loss from neurologic causes (33, 34).

Scott and Egan in their paper report a patient with persistent poor bilateral acuity but had normal visual field, color vision, contrast sensitivity, stereopsis and structurally normal eye but diagnosed with cone dystrophy after multifocal ERG (34).

Evaluation of NOVL is time-consuming, tedious and potentially frustrating process.

Such patients may need psychiatric evaluation, psychotherapy and management. However, NOVL patients may not have as high an incidence of true psychiatric disease as previously assumed (8).

Jing Ming et al mention that being open to the patient and their family, involving them in the care of the patient and discussing positive tests like a positive response on the OKN drum

help encourage or motivate the patient and the family. An OKN stimulus can be obtained from YouTube and the family can be encouraged to use it at home regularly and acknowledge a daily improvement in the patient's visual status (35). Regular follow-up appointments may work as therapeutic sessions in which the patient's progress can be encouraged and also helps build confidence in the patient rather than just labeling them as functional. Refusing or denying to do any further tests or follow ups and telling the patient "there is nothing else I can do for you as there is nothing wrong" can only frustrate them further. This may make them go to a new physician for a repeat cycle of battery of tests.

Stone mentions in his article that some strategies in approaching a diagnosis of functional deficit could be applied to NOVL also. When the diagnosis is made, explain it to the patient with a name. "Non-organic" is an acceptable term that could be used and tell them it is not unusual or abnormal. Explain it as a processing/wiring/transmission error in the brain and not a structural damage; that their eyes see but is unable to transmit the information to the brain. Thus, use this basis to build confidence in them that their problem is potentially reversible, and they need to re-establish the transmission error (36, 37). Jing Ming et al describe use of transcranial magnetic stimulation and hypnotherapy to essentially increase awareness in the patient about visual perception (35). Stone reports about successful use of propofol for a brief period of sedation, mainly with non-organic motor deficits. He argues that even the brief treatment session builds a sense of confidence in the patient that he is being treated for a "disease," and leads to disinhibition and relaxation (36, 37). However, there is insufficient evidence at this time about the utility, benefits and safety about these procedures and a vast majority could improve on mere suggestion, motivation and encouragement, some of them requiring repeated and frequent appointments in order to build faith (5). This also reduces chances of "doctor shopping" and multiple unnecessary repeated testing. If the patient is a child, first step would be to inform the parents of your findings. In older children, diagnosis could also be discussed with them. Prognosis is good in the pediatric population and in patients with faith in possible chances of reversibility. Somers et al report that though there could be resolution of the visual symptoms, underlying psychiatric issues and psychosocial problems could emerge that could need gentle management. Identification of underlying stressors in children could help with recovery and could be approached and discussed gently during the clinic visits either by individualized interviews with patient and family or from questionnaires that could be filled out without the need for referral to psychiatry (5).

Prognosis

Though the prognosis is good with possible recovery in 80–90%, there is an almost 10–15% chance of recurrence. There is limited literature on the recovery of vision loss and results are variable. Kathol et al in a cohort study of 42 people with functional visual loss (mean age 32 years) found that 45% regained normal visual function while 55% had persistent visual dysfunction at a mean follow-up of 53 months (6, 7). Barris et al. found that 78% of the 45 people in his cohort (mean age 25.9 years) showed improvement or normalization of vision during a mean follow-up of 114 days with the use of a timetable for recovery comprising reassurance and visual exercises (38). Sletteberg et al found that 51% of the 41 people in his group reported good visual function as opposed to 49% reporting poor visual function at a mean follow-up of 2 years (39). The latter two studies also found that those aged under 16 years were more likely to recover normal visual function compared with older people. Somers et al report that though there could be resolution of the visual symptoms, underlying psychiatric issues and psychosocial problems could emerge that could need gentle management (33).

Conclusion

Thus, the role of the ophthalmologist and neuro-ophthalmologist is to establish NOVL and attempt to prove normal visual function. However, this can be difficult and challenging to establish. One should always attempt to understand the potential etiologies or underlying motivation and should never confront the patient. Politely say "I cannot find an explanation" and suggest the possibility of "stress." Once diagnosed, avoid obtaining unnecessary tests or procedures. Overall, records should indicate that there is no organic explanation for the patient's symptoms.

Pitfalls: When OVL can be misdiagnosed as NOVL

1. *Amblyopia*: Amblyopia is the most common cause of monocular blindness. It is unusual for RAPD to be present in unilateral amblyopia, and its presence should prompt to look for alternate etiology.
2. *Retrobulbar optic neuritis*: In the majority of cases, the fundus appears normal. Careful eye exam looking for RAPD will help in the diagnosis, but subtle RAPD might be missed in some cases. Visual field examination will show central scotoma in early cases, but if the disease has progressed there might be only a small island of preserved vision. Imaging with MRI orbit with and without contrast can usually show an enhancing optic nerve on T1 post contrast. Further testing with OCT to demonstrate the progression of loss of nerve fiber layer thickness over time may be used as a marker of loss of function of optic nerve.
3. *Optic nerve glioma*: Gradual, painless, unilateral loss of vision associated with an afferent pupillary defect is a common presentation. Proptosis may or may not be present. The optic nerve head is initially swollen and subsequently becomes atrophic. Imaging with CT and MRI orbits and brain will help in the diagnosis.
4. *Stargardt disease*: It is the single most common inherited single gene retinal disease. It is characterized by macular degeneration that begins in childhood, adolescence or adulthood, resulting in progressive loss of vision that is uncorrectable with glasses. They may also have impaired color vision, delayed dark adaptation, loss of depth perception and peripheral vision that is less affected than central vision. Ophthalmology evaluation will show yellow flecks of lipofuscin deposits in the macula that could be missed on examination.
5. *Autosomal dominant optic atrophy (DOA)*: It is the most common hereditary optic neuropathy. It presents as bilateral slowly progressive loss of vision. Both DOA and a sequel of optic neuritis could show a pale optic nerve. However, a history of presentation and progression could help distinguish between the two. Genetic testing could be pursued for confirmation.
6. *Leber's hereditary optic neuropathy (LHON)*: It is a mitochondrial inherited degeneration of retinal ganglion cells and their axons that predominantly affects young adult males. It can present with acute or subacute loss of central vision mimicking optic neuritis. It typically evolves to very severe optic atrophy. Both eyes may be affected simultaneously or sequentially. In acute stages, fundus examination may show edematous appearance of the optic disc with telangiectatic and tortuous peripapillary vessels. The main features are seen on fundus examination just before or subsequent to the vision loss. Other findings include decreased visual acuity, loss of color vision and cecocentral scotoma on visual field examination. Genetic testing is confirmatory.
7. *Cone dystrophy*: Patients with cone dystrophy present with vision loss, sensitivity to bright lights and poor color vision. It can occur in late teens to the sixties. The fundus exam may be normal in early stages and definitive changes usually occur well after visual loss. Fundus fluorescein angiography, ERG and color vision tests are important tools in the diagnosis of cone dystrophy.
8. *Paraneoplastic syndromes*: Paraneoplastic syndromes include patients with cancer-associated retinopathy (CAR), melanoma-associated retinopathy (MAR) or paraneoplastic optic neuropathy (PON). They often present as bilateral progressive painless vision loss, decreased nighttime vision, worsening color vision, positive visual phenomena and visual field loss. Patients have a normal fundus exam and have normal CT/MRI head. In clinically suspected cases, one should promptly further evaluate by obtaining retinal and optic nerve autoantibodies and ERG.
9. *Visual variant of Alzheimer's*: Posterior cortical atrophy (PCA) is a neurodegenerative syndrome characterized by striking progressive visual impairment and a pattern of atrophy mainly involving posterior cortices. PCA is the most frequent atypical presentation of Alzheimer's disease.
10. *Posterior hemisphere strokes/alexia without agraphia*: Alexia without agraphia is a relatively uncommon condition, which should always be thought in a patient presenting with difficulty in reading with normal visual acuity and normal writing. This is caused by a left occipital lobe lesion with ipsilateral coinvolvement of the splenium of the corpus callosum or adjacent periventricular white matter leading to a disconnection syndrome. Features include right homonymous hemianopia with sparing of key language areas but an inability to access lexical visual information processed in the intact right occipital lobe.
11. *Optic tract lesions*: Lesions especially of the optic tract are difficult to pick on clinical testing or even imaging. Sometimes a RAPD and bowtie optic atrophy may be seen on the contralateral side of an optic tract lesion.
12. *Traumatic optic neuropathy (TON)*: It is a serious vision threatening condition that can be caused by ocular or head trauma. It is caused by either direct penetrating injury to the optic nerve or via indirectly transmitted forces to the nerve from a blunt eye trauma. The vision loss may vary from mild to total blindness. Diagnosis is based on a good clinical history of trauma, direct corelation of vision loss post trauma, a fundus exam (which could be normal), presence of RAPD, imaging which in acute stage could show disruption of the optic canal or compression from edema or hemorrhage.

Multiple-Choice Questions

1. In the distance doubling test, when the vision is checked at a particular distance say at 20/100 level, and then when the distance is reduced to half, the patient should be able to read:
   a. 20/200
   b. 20/50
   c. 20/100
   d. 20/20

   Answer:

   b. 20/50

2. Fogging is a test that may be useful in:
   a. Binocular vision loss
   b. Monocular vision loss
   c. None of the above
   d. Both a and b

   Answer:

   b. Monocular vision loss

3. In a patient who claims to be unilaterally or bilaterally blind to the extent of no light perception (NLP), light perception (LP) or hand motions, eliciting a nystagmus with OKN drum establishes a vision of at least:
   a. 20/400
   b. 20/100
   c. 20/200
   d. 20/20

   Answer:

   a. 20/400

4. A patient with bilateral vision loss may be asked to touch the tips of both his index fingers keeping his eyes closed.
   a. He should be able to do this by principle of proprioception.
   b. He should be able to do this only when he keeps his eyes open.
   c. He will not be able to do this due to bilateral vision loss.
   d. This is possible only in unilateral vision loss and not in bilateral.

   Answer:

   a. He should be able to do this by principle of proprioception.

5. A 60-year-old patient presents with complaints of vision loss in the right eye since last 1 hour. Visual acuity shows 20/20 in each eye, has no RAPD on exam, anterior segment exam and fundus exam are all normal in the clinic. What would you do next?

   a. Diagnose NOVL and plan for follow-up in 6 months
   b. Refer to neuro-ophthalmology for an evaluation of NOVL
   c. Send to ER for stroke evaluation
   d. Refer for an ERG and VEP

   Answer:

   c. Send to ER for stroke evaluation

References

1. Bose S, Kupersmith MJ. Neuro-ophthalmologic presentations of functional visual disorders. Neurol Clin. 1995;13(2):321–339.
2. Schlaegel TF, Quilala FV. Hysterical amblyopia: Statistical analysis of forty-two cases found in a survey of eight hundred unselected eye patients at a state medical center. AMA Arch Ophthalmol. 1955;54(6):875–884.
3. Somers A, Casteels K, Van Roie E, Spileers W, Casteels I. Non-organic visual loss in children: Prospective and retrospective analysis of associated psychosocial problems and stress factors. Acta Ophthalmol. 2016;94:e312–e316.
4. Lim SA, Siatkowski RM, Farris BK. Functional visual loss in adults and children: Patient characteristics, management, and outcomes. Ophthalmology. 2005;112(10):1821–1828.
5. Catalano RA, Simon JW, Krohel GB, Rosenberg PN. Functional visual loss in children. Ophthalmology. 1986;93(3):385–390.
6. Kathol RG, Cox TA, Corbett JJ, Thompson HS, Clancy J. Functional visual loss: II. Psychiatric aspects in 42 patients followed for 4 years. Psychol Med. 1983;13(2):315–324.
7. Kathol RG, Cox TA, Corbett JJ, Thompson HS. Functional visual loss. Follow-up of 42 cases. Arch Ophthalmol. 1983;101(5):729–735.
8. Bruce BB, Newman NJ. Functional visual loss. Neurol Clin. 2010;28(3):789–802.
9. Kathol RG, Cox TA, Corbett JJ, Thompson HS, Clancy J. Functional visual loss: I. A true psychiatric disorder? Psychol Med. 1983;13(2):307–314.
10. Bengtzen R, Woodward M, Lynn MJ, et al. The "sunglasses sign" predicts nonorganic visual loss in neuro-ophthalmologic practice. Neurology. 2008;70(3):218–221.
11. Levy NS, Glick EB. Stereoscopic perception and Snellen visual acuity. Am J Ophthalmol. 1974;78(4):722–724.
12. Sitko KR, Peragallo JH, Bidot S, Biousse V, Newman NJ, Bruce BB. Pitfalls in the use of stereoacuity in the diagnosis of nonorganic visual loss. Ophthalmology. 2016;123(1):198–202.
13. Zinkernagel SM, Mojon DS. Distance doubling visual acuity test: A reliable test for nonorganic visual loss. Graefe's archive for clinical and experimental ophthalmology. 2009;247(6):855–858.
14. Miller NR. Neuro-ophthalmologic manifestations of psychogenic disease. Sem Neurol. 2006;26(3):310–320.
15. Slavin ML. The prism dissociation test in detecting unilateral functional visual loss. J Clin Neuroophthalmol. 1990;10:127–130.
16. Golnik KC, Lee AG, Eggenberger ER. The monocular vertical prism dissociation test. American journal of ophthalmology. 2004;137(1):135–137.
17. Graf MH, Roesen J. Ocular malingering: A surprising visual acuity test. Arch Ophthalmol. 2002;120(6):756–760.
18. Kröger N, Jürgens C, Kohlmann T, Tost F. Evaluation of a visual acuity test using closed Landolt-Cs to determine malingering. Graefes Arch Clin Exp Ophthalmol. 2017;255(12):2459–2465.
19. Finkelstein JI, Johnson LN. Relative scotoma and statokinetic dissociation (Riddoch's phenomenon) from occipital lobe dysfunction. Trans Pa Acad Ophthalmol Otolaryngol. 1989;41:789–792.
20. Vidal Y, Hoffmann M. Improvement of Astatikopsia (Riddoch's phenomenon) after correction of vertebral stenoses with angioplasty. Neurol Int. 2012;4(1):e1.
21. Rod Foroozan MD, Andrew G, Lee MD. Don't get off the track. Surv Ophthalmol. 2018;63 (3):437–444.
22. Al-Zubidi N, Ansari W, Fung SH, Lee AG. Diffusion tensor imaging in traumatic optic tract syndrome. J Neuroophthalmol 2014;34:95–98.
23. Kowal KM, Rivas Rodriguez FF, Srinivasan A, Trobe JD. Spectrum of magnetic resonance imaging features in unilateral optic tract dysfunction. J Neuroophthalmol 2017;37:17–23.
24. Moster ML, Galetta SL, Schatz NJ. Physiologic functional imaging in "functional" visual loss. Surv Ophthalmol. 1996;40(5):395–399.
25. Silverman IE, Galetta SL, Gray LG. SPECT in patients with cortical visual loss. J Nucl Med. 1993;34(9):1447–1451.
26. Wakakura M, Yokoe J. Evidence for preserved direct pupillary light response in Leber's hereditary optic neuropathy. Br J Ophthalmol. 1995;79:442–446.
27. Levi L, Feldman RM. Use of the potential acuity meter in suspected functional visual loss. Am J Ophthalmol. 1992;114(4):502–503.
28. Thompson JC, Kosmorsky GS, Ellis BD. Field of dreamers and dreamed-up fields. Functional and fake perimetry. Ophthalmology. 1996;103:117–125.
29. Jeon J, Oh S, Kyung S. Assessment of visual disability using visual evoked potentials. BMC Ophthalmol. 2012;12:36.
30. Howard JE, Dorfman LJ. Evoked potentials in hysteria and malingering. J Clin Neurophysiol. 1986; 3(1):39–49.
31. Spehlmann R, Gross RA, Ho SU, Leestma JE, Norcross KA. Visual evoked potentials and postmortem findings in a case of cortical blindness. Ann Neurol. 1977;2:531–534.
32. Johnson LN, Baloh FG. The accuracy of confrontation visual field test in comparison with automated perimetry. J Natl Med Assoc. 1991;83(10):895–898.
33. Kerr NM, Chew SSL, Eady EK, Gamble GD, Danesh-Meyer HV. Diagnostic accuracy of confrontation visual field tests. Neurology. 2010;74(15):1184–1190.
34. Scott JA, Egan RA. Prevalence of organic neuro-ophthalmologic disease in patients with functional visual loss. Am J Ophthalmol. 2003;135:670–675.
35. Yeo JM, Carson A, Stone J. Seeing again: Treatment of functional visual loss. Pract Neurol. 2019;19:168–172.
36. Stone J, Edwards M. Trick or treat?: Showing patients with functional (psychogenic) motor symptoms their physical signs. Neurology. 2012;79(3):282–284.
37. Stone J, Hoeritzauer I, Brown K, Carson A. Therapeutic sedation for functional (psychogenic) neurological symptoms. J Psychosom Res. 76(2):165–168.
38. Barris MC, Kaufman DI, Barberio D. Visual impairment in hysteria. Doc Ophthalmol. 1992;82:369–382.
39. Sletteberg O, Bertelsen T, Høvding G. The prognosis of patients with hysterical visual impairment. Acta Ophthalmol 1989; 67:159–163.

Part III

Neuro-Ophthalmology
The Efferent Pathway

14

AN APPROACH TO PUPILLARY DISORDERS
Physiology and Pathology

Sarosh M. Katrak, Azad M. Irani

CASE STUDY

A 24-year-old male presented to the emergency department when he noted that his right pupil was larger in size as compared to the left one. He had history of low-grade fever with myalgia around 10 days back which was managed by local physician as viral fever. On examination, patient had normal visual acuity. His right pupil was dilated and was not responsive to direct and indirect light reflexes. At near vision, however, miosis was noted in both eyes. Fundus showed normal optic disc examination. Rest of the neurological examination was normal. What should be the approach of management in this patient?

The normal pupil

One of the most important parts of the eye isn't a structure at all – it's an open space – the pupil. It is the counterpart of the aperture stop in a camera. It regulates the amount of light falling on the retina and also affects the depth of field. The pupil has two main functions: contraction and dilatation; hence, the size of the pupil is determined by the tone in two opposing muscles. The pupillary constriction is done by circular fibers close to the pupillary margin and dilatation by radially orientated fibers. Based on the amount of ambient light, the size of the pupil is automatically adjusted – the sympathetic system producing dilatation and the parasympathetic producing constriction.

Sympathetic pathways

The first-order neurons of the sympathetic pathways originate in the hypothalamus and descend in the brainstem and spinal cord up to the cervical 8 and thoracic 1 level. The second-order neurons emerge through the ventral roots and join the cervical sympathetic chain, passing through the first thoracic (stellate) ganglion at the apex of the lung. They then ascend uninterrupted before terminating in the superior cervical ganglion. The postganglionic fibers emerge from the superior cervical ganglion and form a plexus in the adventitia of the internal carotid artery (ICA). They ascend with the ICA into the middle cranial fossa where they lie in close relationship to the trigeminal ganglion. They course forward through the cavernous sinus and enter the orbit through the superior orbital fissure in the nasociliary branch of the ophthalmic division of the trigeminal nerve. The pupillary dilator fibers enter the eye with the long ciliary nerves and innervate the radially orientated pupillary dilator fibers (Figure 14.1). Activation of the noradrenergic (mainly alpha-1) adrenoreceptors causes dilatation or mydriasis of the pupil. The sympathetic pathways also contain vasomotor and sudomotor (sweating) fibers which course along the internal and external carotid arteries [1].

Parasympathetic pathways

The pupillary constrictor muscle is innervated by the parasympathetic neurons. The preganglionic fibers originate in the ipsilateral Edinger-Westphal nucleus in the tectum of the midbrain. The fibers course ventrally through the midbrain to emerge in the interpeduncular fossa along with other fibers of the oculomotor nerve. These parasympathetic fibers remain dorsal and superficial throughout the course of the third cranial nerve in the subarachnoid space. Hence, these fibers are more susceptible to extrinsic compression (e.g., posterior communicating artery aneurysm) and relatively protected from ischemic insults as the vasa nervorum lies deep within the substance of the oculomotor nerve. These preganglionic parasympathetic fibers terminate in the ciliary ganglion within the orbit. Postganglionic parasympathetic fibers pass through the sclera as the short ciliary nerves and innervate the pupillary constrictor fibers (Figure 14.2). Activation of its muscarinic (M3) cholinergic receptors produces constriction or miosis of the pupil. An interesting anatomical fact is that only 3–5% of these fibers terminate in the iris sphincter muscle. The remainder terminate in the ciliary muscles

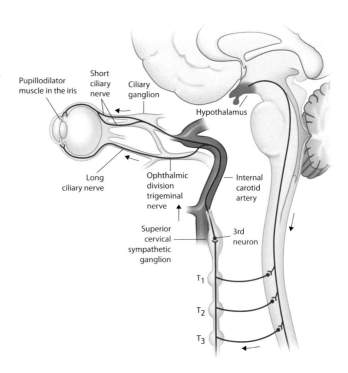

FIGURE 14.1 The sympathetic pathway for pupillary dilatation. (Diagram taken from *Principles of Neural Science*, 4th Edition. Editors, Eric R Kendel, James H Schwartz, Thomas M Jessell, Fig. 45-14, page 905. The McGraw-Hill Companies, Health Profession Divn. Copyright 2000.)

DOI: 10.1201/9780429020278-18

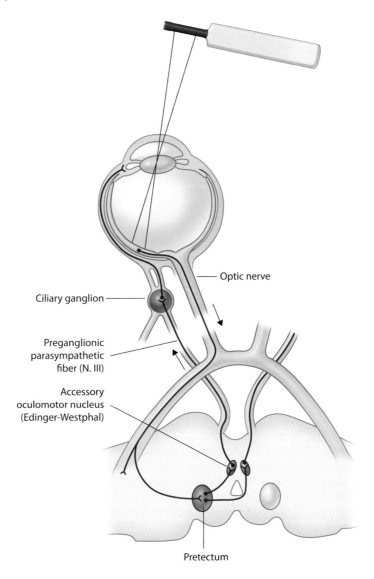

Optic nerve

Ciliary ganglion

Preganglionic
parasympathetic
fiber (N. III)

Accessory
oculomotor nucleus
(Edinger-Westphal)

Pretectum

FIGURE 14.2 The parasympathetic pathway for pupillary constriction. (Diagram taken from *Principles of Neural Science*, 4th Edition. Editors, Eric R Kendel, James H Schwartz, Thomas M Jessell, Fig. 27–5, page 528. McGraw-Hill Companies, Health Profession Divn. Copyright 2000.)

that control accommodation [2]. The importance of this will be discussed later.

When light falls on the retina, it stimulates the retinal ganglion cells, which have a slightly greater density in and around the macula. The axons from this area pass along the optic nerve, traverse the optic chiasma, with decussation of the nasal fibers and then continue along the optic tracts, leaving just before the lateral geniculate body, to terminate on the ipsilateral as well as contralateral pretectal nuclei. Neurons from the pretectal nuclei then project to the ipsilateral, and through a decussation in the posterior commissure, the contralateral Edinger-Westphal nucleus resulting in bilateral pupillary innervation. Thus, a bright light shone in one eye produces a direct (ipsilateral) as well as a consensual (contralateral) pupillary constriction. The response latency between the direct and the consensual pupillary response is in the range of 200–500 ms [3]. This latency has to be kept in mind when performing the "swinging torch light test". When there is an involvement of one optic nerve (e.g., optic neuritis) light shone in the normal eye will produce ipsilateral as well as contralateral pupillary constriction. However, when the torch light is swung to the affected eye, the constricted pupil dilates as the direct light reflex is impaired. This is the basis of detecting a relative afferent pupillary defect (RAPD). This is a very cost-effective method of detecting optic neuritis in the Indian population who have dark irises and detecting a consensual light reflex through the conventional methods is cumbersome and difficult.

The accommodation reflex is the only physiological reflex which produces dysconjugate eye movements. It consists of a triad of miosis, convergence of the eyes and greater convexity of the lens. Without this reflex, one would not be able to read this paragraph clearly. It is elicited by asking the patient to relax and look at a distant object; the patient is then asked to look at the examiner's finger which is kept in the midline 12 inches away.

The abnormal pupil

In clinical practice, abnormalities of interest are anisocoria, abnormal response to light, a tonic accommodative response and abnormal pharmacological responses.

Pupillary abnormalities occur mainly at four anatomical sites. Lesions involve the pupillary constrictor and dilator muscles, the sympathetic and parasympathetic pathways, the afferent visual pathways and the oculomotor nucleus in the midbrain.

Lesions involving pupillary constrictor/dilator muscles

Lesions of the pupillary constrictor/dilator muscles essentially occur within the eye ball. These abnormalities lie in the ophthalmologist's turf. The etiologies are trauma, inflammation, ischemia of the iris, diabetes mellitus, acute glaucoma, cyst or tumors within the eye and rare congenital anomalies. These topics are beyond the scope of this chapter. However, in clinical practice, any pupillary abnormality in isolation warrants an ophthalmologist's opinion.

Lesions involving sympathetic pathways

The sympathetic nerve supply to the eye contains pupillary dilator fibers as well as vasomotor, sudomotor and vasodilator fibers to the face. Hence, in Horner syndrome (HS) there are pupillary as well as non-pupillary signs. The pupillary signs are anisocoria and ipsilateral miosis. Normally during deep sleep, there is miosis and when the subject is suddenly woken up – startle response – there is a reflex dilatation of the pupil in the first 5 seconds because of a sudden increase in sympathetic tone [4]. In HS, this startle response is also lost or there is delayed dilatation beyond 5 seconds (dilatation lag). The non-pupillary signs are ipsilateral subtle ptosis, due to weakness of the Muller's muscle, conjunctival congestion due to paresis of the vasomotor and anhidrosis through involvement of the sudomotor fibers. The latter will involve the full face in a preganglionic lesion. As the postganglionic sympathetic fibers "piggyback" with the nasociliary branch of the ophthalmic division of the trigeminal nerve within the orbit, a postganglionic lesion will produce anhidrosis only in the supraorbital area [1, 5]. Thus anhidrosis of only the supraorbital area of the face is an important pointer to a postganglionic lesion and is commonly associated with ICA dissection.

The causes of HS are many, reflecting the long course of the sympathetic pathway from the hypothalamus to the eye. They are divided into: (1) the central (first-order) lesions from the hypothalamus to the exit of the sympathetic pathways at C8-T1 level of the spinal cord; (2) the preganglionic sympathetic plexus exiting with the C8-T1 ventral roots in the base of the neck up to superior cervical ganglion and (3) the postganglionic sympathetic plexus emerging from the superior cervical ganglion, ascending up the neck with the ICA and ending in the orbit.

The frequency of occurrence is practically equal for lesions of the second- and third-order neurons, each constituting over 40% of cases. Lesions affecting the central neurons are infrequent [6].

Central pathway lesions

The most common etiology of a first-order lesion is the Wallenberg's lateral medullary syndrome [7], an infarct in the posterior inferior cerebellar artery territory. Associated findings are dysphagia (ipsilateral palatal palsy) ipsilateral facial analgesia (involvement of the ipsilateral trigeminal tract) and contralateral analgesia of the trunk and extremities (involvement of the spinothalamic tract), cerebellar ataxia and rotatory nystagmus (involvement of the inferior cerebellar peduncle). As many as 75% of patients with Wallenberg's syndrome demonstrate ipsilateral sympathetic paresis [7, 8]. As the first-order neurons course through the cervical spinal cord, HS may be present in syringomyelia, trauma [5, 9], infectious inflammatory myelitis, vascular malformations, neoplasms and rarely infarction of the spinal cord [10].

The **preganglionic second-order neurons** lie at the base of the neck and ascends up to the superior cervical ganglia located

at the level of bifurcation of the common carotid artery and the angle of the jaw. In a large series of HS, an etiological diagnosis was made in 44% of patients with a preganglionic lesion [6]. The most common etiology was malignant tumors of the apex of the lungs (Pancoast tumor) or metastasis from breast cancer. The Pancoast tumor may also involve the brachial plexus with pain in the shoulder and arm. *Therefore, this tumor should be considered in any patient with a non-traumatic, new-onset HS and shoulder or arm pain, particularly in elderly males who are smokers.* Direct trauma to the spinal cord during forceps delivery may produce a HS together with upper arm palsy (Klumpke palsy) [11].

HS from **postganglionic lesions** can result from a variety of causes. They may occur at the level of the superior cervical ganglion, ICA, cavernous sinus and superior orbital fissure. Of clinical relevance is spontaneous or traumatic ICA dissection. This condition presents with unilateral head and/or neck pain, focal cerebral ischemic symptoms and a HS. Here, anhidrosis is restricted to the distribution of the first division of the trigeminal nerve as mentioned earlier. The rest of the face is spared because the sudomotor fibers travel along the external carotid artery which is not involved in the dissection. *Thus, ICA dissection should be considered in any case with an acute-onset HS with pain in the neck and anhidrosis localized to the supraorbital area.* HS, secondary to lesions of the superior cervical ganglion, are usually seen in trauma. Rarely HS may accompany oculomotor, first division of the trigeminal or abducens nerve palsy in cavernous sinus thrombosis or inflammation of the superior orbital fissure. Approximately two-thirds of cluster headaches may have postganglionic HS [12]. Raeder paratrigeminal neuralgia – a combination of unilateral headache, supraorbital pain and ipsilateral postganglionic HS – is a rare entity and is believed to be a variant of cluster headache [13].

As the pupil contains adrenergic as well as cholinergic receptors, it responds symmetrically to topically applied receptor agonist. Phenylephrine produces 2.5–10% mydriasis, and Pilocarpine produces 1–4% miosis. Failure to respond to normal concentrations of a receptor agonist indicates a receptor blockade. On the other hand, when there is denervation there is a response to minute concentrations of receptor agonists – denervation hypersensitivity. It is important to understand the response of a normal and a denervated pupil to receptor agonists, as this helps to augment the clinical localization in HS. Cocaine blocks 4–10% active reuptake of noradrenaline. Hence, a normal pupil will dilate. In HS, with oculosympathetic palsy, there is no release of noradrenaline from the presynaptic nerve endings. Hence, there is no noradrenaline for reuptake. Therefore, the HS pupil will not dilate. Hence, cocaine confirms the diagnosis of HS but has no localizing value, i.e., whether the lesion involves the central, the preganglionic or the postganglionic neurons [14].

Hydroxyamphetamine displaces 1% noradrenaline at intact sympathetic nerve endings. Therefore, topical application of this agonist produces dilatation of a normal pupil. With central (first-order) and preganglionic (second-order) lesions this agonist releases normally stored noradrenaline from the synaptic vesicles as the nerve terminals are intact. Hence, the pupil dilates. A lesion of the postganglionic (third-order) nerve terminals results in a loss of noradrenaline stores. Thus there is no noradrenaline to be displaced or released and hence no pupillary dilatation. Thus, denervation hypersensitivity has great localizing value in HS and helps to differentiate between central, preganglionic or postganglionic lesions, thereby augmenting the clinical localization [15]. The sensitivity is always better in unilateral lesions. However, the test may be false positive, if the subject "squeezes out" the drops because of a highly sensitive corneal reflex.

Bilateral HS is a rare entity and difficult to prove. There is no anisocoria and the absence of a "control" eye makes pharmacology testing insensitive. Redilatation lag using pupillographic technique or diagnostic imaging systems are the only reliable tests to establish this entity [16, 17]. Diabetes mellitus is one of the commonest causes of bilateral HS. Other rare causes may be amyloidosis, dysautonomia and hereditary sensory autonomic neuropathy [18].

Lesions involving parasympathetic pathways

Damage to the parasympathetic pathways, in contrast to sympathetic lesion, produces a dilated pupil – mydriasis, irrespective of the fact whether the lesion is pre- or postganglionic. Hence, clinical examination suffices, and there is no need for pharmacological testing. The abnormal pupil is dilated and round and shows a poor or absent response to light, both direct and consensual. Besides this, there is no miosis on accommodation. Most of the lesions are preganglionic and occur in the context of oculomotor nerve palsies. In the clinical context, a lot of stress has been put on oculomotor nerve involvement with or without pupillary involvement. In general, the rule is that if the oculomotor nerve palsy is incomplete, then pupillary involvement implies an extrinsic compressive lesion most likely aneurysms of the posterior communicating artery [19]. Anatomical studies [20] help to explain this clinical finding. The pupiloconstrictor fibers lie dorsally and superficially in the oculomotor nerve and are, therefore, prone to compression (Figure 14.3). On the other hand, these fibers are spared in occlusion of the vasa nervorum which lies deep within the oculomotor nerve. Thus in diabetic oculomotor palsy the pupil is spared in 50% of the cases [21]. The pupil may also be spared in the early part of a compressive pathology. Hence, pupils sparing incomplete third nerve palsy needs close monitoring for pupillary involvement. Lastly, any patient with a progressive external ophthalmoplegia with or without pupillary involvement requires neuroimaging to rule out a surgical cause. Oculomotor nerve palsy together with the first division of the trigeminal nerve and abducens nerve indicates involvement at the level of the lateral wall of the cavernous sinus or the superior orbital fissure which is just anterior to it.

Postganglionic lesions occur with involvement of the ciliary ganglion or the short ciliary nerves, usually within the orbit or the eye itself. The clinical features are initially of a large and round pupil which is non-reactive to direct as well as consensual light reflex. Later, the abnormal pupil constricts and acquires an irregular shape. The light reflex is slow, attenuated or even absent. In contrast, the pupil shows an exaggerated miosis during accommodative efforts, i.e., there is a light – near dissociation.

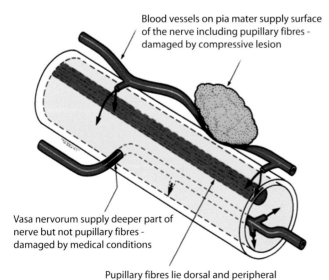

Blood vessels on pia mater supply surface of the nerve including pupillary fibres - damaged by compressive lesion

Vasa nervorum supply deeper part of nerve but not pupillary fibres - damaged by medical conditions

Pupillary fibres lie dorsal and peripheral

FIGURE 14.3 Applied anatomy of the oculomotor nerve.

This exaggerated miosis of the pupil is based on anatomical facts. Only 3–5% of the postganglionic fibers from the ciliary ganglion innervate the circular muscles for pupillary constriction, whereas 95% terminate in the ciliary muscles [2]. After injury to the pupiloconstrictor fibers, these "accommodation" fibers reinnervate the pupillary sphincter muscles. This gives rise to an exaggerated miosis during accommodation, but an impaired/absent pupillary light response [22]. *Thus a "tonic" pupil with a slow, attenuated or even absent light reflex is pathognomonic of damage to the postganglionic parasympathetic fibers.* The etiologies are varied. A unilateral abnormal response usually occurs with a unilateral lesion – trauma, neoplastic, inflammatory and panretinal photo coagulation. Bilateral lesions usually occur with pure autonomic failure associated with amyloidosis, Sjogren's and paraneoplastic syndromes [19]. In many patients, no cause can be found. In such cases, bilateral "tonic" pupils are associated with absence of the deep tendon reflexes and occur in otherwise healthy young adults, commonly females. This – the Holmes-Adie syndrome — is unilateral in approximately 80–90% of cases. It can be progressive, and approximately 10% may become bilateral over each subsequent decade. Such patients may also show subclinical abnormalities of both the sympathetic and the parasympathetic pathways of the autonomic nervous system [23, 24].

Lesions involving visual pathways

Lesions of the visual pathway which produce a pupillary defect are essentially related to the afferent arc of the pupillary light reflex, i.e., the optic nerves. This defect is evident essentially as an RAPD and is detected by the "swinging torch light" test.

There is no pupillary defect in the retrochiasmal visual pathways. The defects are usually superior/inferior quadrantic/hemianopic defects at the chiasmal level and various grades of homonymous hemianopia with involvement of the optic tracts, radiation and occipital visual cortex.

Lesions involving oculomotor nucleus

Lesions involving the oculomotor nucleus are commonly extrinsic compression of the pretectal area of the midbrain, due to pineal tumors or hydrocephalus. Compression of the pretectal nuclei interrupts the pathway for the light reflex without affecting the ventrally placed one for accommodation. This results in the absence of a pupillary light reflex but preserves miosis on accommodation – "light-near" dissociation. The classical Parinaud's syndrome consists of light-near dissociation with normal vision. The other associated signs may be vertical gaze palsy, conversion retraction nystagmus and lid retraction on attempted up-gaze (Collier's sign) [25].

Argyll Robertson pupils

A practically non-existent abnormality nowadays is the Argyll Robertson (AR) pupils, mostly described in tertiary syphilis. AR pupils are usually small and irregular. Again, there is "light-near" dissociation, despite the small size of the resting pupil. The exact site of lesion is not known, but it is assumed to be ventral to the aqueduct in the upper midbrain. Other conditions which may simulate AR pupils include diabetes mellitus, neurosarcoidosis and myotonic dystrophy. "Light-near" dissociation warrants neuroimaging, in spite of the fact that in the majority of cases it may be normal.

In summary, a systemic examination of the pupils will detect the site of abnormality of the pupillary pathways. At times, applied anatomy gives a precise location of the lesion. In view of the multiple etiological factors affecting the pupil, blood studies and neuroimaging may be essential, based on the four main anatomical sites of involvement.

Conclusion

Ophthalmic examination cannot be completed without a detailed pupillary examination. It is paramount to know applied anatomy of the sympathetic and parasympathetic pathways and their impact on the pupillary reflexes in order to understand various pupillary abnormalities. Many etiologioes like trauma, infection, inflammation, ischemia and compression can cause anisocoria. A step-wise approach is required to anatomically localize and characterize the lesion.

Multiple-Choice Questions

1. Pupillary dilator muscles:
   a. Are parasympathetically innervated fibers.
   b. Are radially oriented muscle fibers.
   c. Are located circumferentially around the pupil margin.
   d. The first-order cell bodies originate in Edinger Westphal nuclei.

   Answer:

   b. Are radially oriented muscle fibers.

2. In patients with light near dissociation
   a. Light reflex is preserved.
   b. Near reflex is preserved.
   c. Syphilis is the only cause.
   d. Abnormal pupil is large.

   Answer:

   b. Near reflex is preserved.

3. Which of the following statements is true about a tonic pupil?
   a. It is caused by sympathetic pathway damage.
   b. It is caused by parasympathetic pathway damage.
   c. It is mostly bilateral.
   d. Patients are always asymptomatic.

   Answer:

   b. It is caused by parasympathetic pathway damage.

4. Which of the following statements is true for ansiocoria?
   a. Physiological anisocoria usually does not exceed 2 mm.
   b. Big pupil is abnormal when anisocoria is more in dark.
   c. Small pupil is abnormal when anisocoria is more in dark.
   d. Parasympathetic pathway causes mydriasis by activating the dilator muscles.

   Answer:

   c. Small pupil is abnormal when anisocoria is more in dark.

5. Horner's syndrome
   a. Involves the abnormally large pupil more in dark.
   b. Always associated with ptosis and anhidrosis.
   c. Abnormality of pupillary reaction to light and near occurs.

   d. Alpha 2 adrenergic agonists are one of the pharmacological agents being used to detect Horner's syndrome.

   Answer:

   d. Alpha 2 adrenergic agonists are one of the pharmacological agents being used to detect Horner's syndrome.

6. Pediatric Horner's syndrome:
   a. Additional tests are required to look for abnormalities in in abdomen, chest, neck and brain.
   b. Iris in the affected side appears darker than the uninvolved side – heterochromia.
   c. Klumpke's palsy can be associated with contralateral Horner's syndrome in children.
   d. Wilms tumor is one of the common associations of Horner's syndrome in children.

   Answer:

   a. Additional tests are required to look for abnormalities in in abdomen, chest, neck and brain.

References

1. Bremner FD. Pupillary disorders. In: Kidd DP, Newman NJ and Biousse V, editors. Neuro-ophthalmology. New Delhi: Elsevier, a Division of Reed Elsevier India Pvt. Ltd; 2010;32:264–279.
2. Warwick R. The ocular parasympathetic nerve supply and its mesencephalic sources. J Anat. 1954;88:71–93.
3. Smith SA, Ellis CJ, Smith SE. Inequality of the direct and consensual light reflexes in normal subjects. Br. J Ophthalmol. 1979;63:523–527.
4. Pilley SF, Thompson HS. Pupillary "dilation lag" in Horner's syndrome. Br J Ophthalmol. 1975;59:731–735.
5. Walton KA, Buono LM. Horner syndrome. Curr. Opin Opthalmol. 2003;14:357–363.
6. Maloney WF, Younge BR, Moyer NJ. Evaluation of the causes and accuracy of pharmacologic localization in Horner's syndrome. Am J Ophthalmol. 1980;90:394.
7. Sacco RL, Freddo L, Bello JA, et al: Wallenberg's lateral medullary syndrome. Clinical-magnetic resonance imaging correlations. Arch Neurol. 1993;50:609–614.
8. Kim JS, Lee JH, Suh DC, et al. Spectrum of lateral medullary syndrome. Correlation between clinical findings and magnetic resonance imaging in 33 subjects. Stroke. 1994;25:1405–1410.
9. Kerrison JB, Biousse V, Newman NJ. Isolated Horner's syndrome and syringomyelia. J Neurol Neurosurg Psychiatry. 2000;69:131–132.
10. Kanagalingam S, Miller NR. Horner syndrome: Clinical perspectives. Eye Brain. 2015;7:35–46.
11. Nixon M, Trail I. Management of shoulder problems following obstetric brachial plexus injury. Shoulder Elbow. 2014;6(1):12–17.
12. Dodick DW, Saper J. Cluster and chronic daily headache. Neurology. 2003;60(7):S31–S37.
13. Grimson BS, Thompson HS. Raeder's syndrome. A clinical review. Surv Ophthalmol. 1980;24:199–210.
14. Kardon RH, Denison CE, Brown CK, Thompson HS. Critical evaluation of the cocaine test in the diagnosis of Horner's syndrome. Arch Ophthalmol. 1990;108:384.
15. Thompson HS, Mensher JH. Adrenergic mydriasis in Horner's syndrome: Hydroxyamphetamine test for diagnosis of postganglionic defects. Am J Ophthalmol. 1971;72:472–480.
16. Smith SA, Smith SE. Bilateral Horner's syndrome: Detection and occurrence. J Neurol Neurosurg Psychiatry. 1999;66:48–51.
17. Pellegrini F, Capello G, Napoleone R. Dilation lag in Horner syndrome can be measured with a diagnostic imaging system. Neurology. 2018;90:618.
18. Bremner FD, Smith SE. Pupil findings in a consecutive series of 150 patients with generalised autonomic neuropathy. J Neurol Neurosurg Psychiatry. 2006;77:1163–1168.
19. Rucker CW. The causes of paralysis of third, fourth and sixth cranial nerves. Am J Ophthalmol 1966;61:1293–1298.
20. Kerr FWL, Hollowell OW. Location of pupillomotor and accommodation fibres in the oculomotor nerve: Experimental observations on paralytic mydriasis. J Neurol Neurosurg Psychiatry. 1964;27:473–481.
21. Keane JR. Third nerve palsy: Analysis of 1400 personally examined inpatients. Can J Neurol Sci. 2010;37:662–670.
22. Lowenfeld IE, Thompson HS. The tonic pupil: A re-evaluation. Am J Ophthalmol. 1967;63:46–87.
23. Bacon PJ, Smith SE. Cardiovascular and sweating dysfunction in patients with Holmes-Adie syndrome. J Neurol Neurosurg Psychiatry. 1993;56:1096–1102.
24. Jacobson DM, Hiner BC. Asymptomatic autonomic and sweat dysfunction in patients with Adie's syndrome. J Neuro-Ophthalmol. 1998;18:143–147.
25. Shields M, Sinkar S, Chan W, Crompton J. Parinaud syndrome: A 25-year (1991–2016) review of 40 consecutive adult cases. Acta Ophthalmologica. 2017;95:792–793.

15A

OCULAR MOTOR CRANIAL NEUROPATHIES

Zane Foster, Ashwini Kini, Bayan Al-Othman, Andrew G. Lee

CASE STUDY

A 67-year-old male patient with a medical history notable for coronary artery disease and poorly controlled type 2 diabetes presents to your clinic complaining of acute-onset, painless double vision that began this morning upon awakening. When he later looked in the mirror, he noticed that his eyes were misaligned, which prompted him to consult his physician. On review of symptoms, he reports that he's been having bilateral headaches and feeling a little feverish, on and off for about a week. On examination, the patient's pupils were asymmetric, with the left pupil larger than the right. On motility, the left eye exhibited abduction and elevation deficits. Laboratory workup revealed significantly elevated erythrocyte sedimentation and c-reactive protein. Given that concern was high for giant cell arteritis, the patient was started on high-dose intravenous empiric steroids. Temporal artery biopsy confirmed the diagnosis, and the patient was started on a closely monitored steroid treatment. Within 3 weeks, all of his symptoms resolved.

Introduction

There are two main concerns when evaluating a presumed ocular motor cranial nerve palsy: (1) the topographical localization and (2) the underlying etiology. A clinician should be suspicious of an ocular motor cranial nerve lesion whenever patients complain of binocular diplopia, be it sudden onset or more gradual. Patients with third nerve palsy may also have ptosis or pupil involvement. This chapter describes the history, clinical examination, and evaluation needed to make the diagnosis for ocular motor cranial neuropathies (OMCN).

Initial considerations: History and clinical examination

History

A careful and thorough history should be obtained on all patients with diplopia to establish the onset (e.g., acute, subacute, chronic), associated findings (e.g., pain, numbness, other neurologic deficit), and course (e.g., progressive, resolving, relapsing, static) of the complaint. OMCN produce binocular diplopia. The best way to determine this in the history is to ask the patient if the double vision goes away on closing *either* eye. If the diplopia resolves when closing *either* eye, then it is caused by misalignment of the eyes (binocular). If the diplopia does not resolve on closing either eye, then the lesion can be localized to unilateral monocular or bilateral monocular causes.

Age is one of the most powerful factors that determines prevalence of a disease, and hence in an elderly individual, ischemic

etiologies for OMCN predominate in the acute setting, neoplastic/vascular in subacute and degenerative or benign neoplastic in a chronic setting. In a child, congenital etiologies predominate. In a young individual, we would consider demyelinating or traumatic in acute, infectious, or inflammatory in a more subacute onset. Patients should be questioned regarding trauma, ischemic risk factors (e.g., hypertension, diabetes, hypercholesterolemia), or recent illnesses and infections. A gradual or progressive course points toward etiologies such as history of neoplasm, degenerative, or autoimmune conditions.

Past medical history in older adults should focus on vasculopathic risk factors, previous history of malignancy (including stage and grade), and surgical procedures. Alcohol and smoking history as well as family history may also be important.

Physical examination

External eye examination should include checking for local eye signs (conjunctival congestion, tearing, discoloration, etc.), concomitant proptosis with motor neuropathy (this would localize the lesion to orbit/orbital apex or cavernous sinus), and ptosis (third nerve palsy).

Though OMCN is an efferent pathway deficit, every eye examination begins with checking the afferent pathway and includes visual acuity, color vision, confrontation visual field testing, and pupils. This is because if the patient presents with both an afferent (sensory) deficit and an efferent (motor) deficit, the lesion localizes to the orbit, where both pathways lie together.

Pupillary examination includes examining the afferent pathway (relative afferent pupil defect) as well the efferent pathway (anisocoria). Pupil size and reaction to light should be measured, and the two pupils should be compared. After assessing pupil size, the physician should look for a relative afferent pupillary defect (RAPD) with a swinging flashlight test. In the setting of a fixed, dilated pupil, reverse RAPD can be used to assess the afferent pathways, as the contralateral, nondilated pupil will still constrict when the light is shone into the dilated eye. This could be relevant in a pupil involving third nerve palsy that raises concern for a posterior communicating artery aneurysm (PCom), but a concomitant RAPD (by direct or reverse testing) reduces the chances of a PCom aneurysm and puts the topographical localization of the lesion in the orbit.

The Hirschberg test can be easily performed to estimate ocular deviation. Normally, when a light is shone into the eye, the light reflex appears almost in the center of the pupil of both eyes. If it is off to the side, and if it is asymmetrical, then this indicates ocular deviation. The amount of deviation from the pupillary axis can be used to estimate the ocular deviation in estimated prism diopters.

Next, extraocular motility should be examined with ductions and versions and measurements made in the cardinal positions of gaze as shown to determine if the deviation is worsened when only certain muscles are active (i.e., in one particular gaze) (Figure 15A.1).

DOI: 10.1201/9780429020278-19

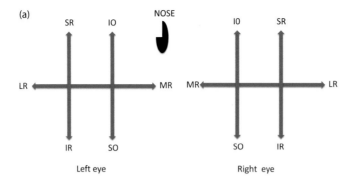

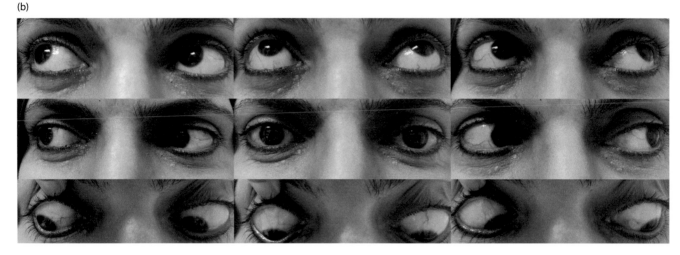

FIGURE 15A.1   Arrow diagram of the cardinal positions of gaze (a) and the cardinal gazes from a healthy individual (b).

Primary and secondary deviations

Primary deviation is the deviation measured with the paretic eye fixating, and secondary deviation is the deviation when the nonparetic eye is fixating. When an ocular misalignment is due to a paresis, the secondary deviation will be greater the primary deviation. This is due to Hering's law of equal innervation: in an attempt to fire the paretic muscle, the brain sends a stronger signal, which carries over to the contralateral, yoked eye, resulting in increased deviation. If the cause is nuclear or infranuclear paresis (more on this later), the deviation will worsen in the direction of action of the paretic muscle. However, in a restrictive pathology, such as thyroid eye disease, the opposite occurs, and the pathologic muscle restricts eye movement, and the deviation worsens in the direction opposite of the affected muscle.

Sometimes patients may have both a fourth and a third nerve palsy at the same time. To test for this, the patient is asked to look down and toward their nose, and the physician should look for a cyclotorting movement of the limbal blood vessels. A normal eye movement is shown in Figure 15A.2. Patients with abnormal torsion movement may show movement of the horizontally oriented blood vessel (arrow) in the roll plane (intorsion or extorsion).

On fundus examination, papilledema should be assessed – a sign that could indicate a raised intracranial pressure, a possible link to a nonlocalizing sixth nerve palsy.

A complete evaluation of all other cranial nerves and a neurologic examination would be necessary to look for signs of conditions that could mimic an OMN (e.g., thyroid eye disease, myasthenia gravis).

Control of oculomotor system

There are three clinically relevant locations of ocular motor control: supranuclear, nuclear, and infranuclear. Lesions can occur in any of these locations, and the differences in presentation allow for clinical localization.

Supranuclear control refers to the higher-order control of the brainstem nuclei, located in the cerebrum (frontal lobe [saccade],

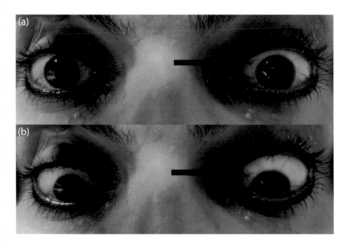

FIGURE 15A.2   Examination of a patient with fourth nerve palsy with or without a concomitant third nerve palsy (a). Look for torsional movement of a limbal blood vessel when you ask the patient to look toward their nose (b).

parieto-occipital-temporal regions [pursuit]). One common supra-nuclear ocular motility disorder is progressive supranuclear palsy (PSP). In the context of ophthalmology, PSP most frequently causes bilateral, conjugate vertical gaze palsy, either upgaze or downgaze, as well as abnormal pursuits and hypometric saccades.[1]

The doll's head maneuver is used to distinguish supranuclear palsy from other infranuclear etiologies. As a supranuclear lesion is in the cerebrum, patients with such a disorder will have an intact vestibulo-ocular reflex (VOR). Another important clue is that diplopia is usually not a complaint in patients with supranuclear gaze disorders despite ocular motility restriction. The palsy is usually conjugate without misalignments.[2] Meanwhile, a nuclear or infranuclear cause of these symptoms would result in an interrupted doll's head reflex.

A nuclear lesion refers to a disruption of the activity of a specific motor nucleus. An infranuclear lesion refers to any structure distal to the nucleus: the nerve fascicle, subarachnoid course of the nerve through the skull and cavernous sinus and then into the orbit, neuromuscular junction, and lastly muscle itself (Table 15A.1).

TABLE 15A.1: Clinical Examination Findings to Help with Localization of the Pathology and Some Named Clinical Pathologies with the Constellation of Findings and the Localization

Signs	Localization
Cranial monitor neuropathy (CMN) with proptosis	Orbit
CMN(efferent) with afferent visual pathway defect-vision/field/relative afferent pupil defect	Orbit/orbital apex
CMN with ocular findings of dilated episcleral vessels, pulsatile proptosis, elevated intraocular pressure	Cavernous sinus/or orbit/think of carotid cavernous fistula
CMN – Sixth with Horner's syndrome	Cavernous sinus
CMN, isolated or combination with V1/V2 involvement	Cavernous sinus
Sixth with concomitant seventh/eighth	Cerebellopontine angle
Bilateral fourth nerve-bilateral hypertropia, worse on gaze to either direction and tilt to either direction	Dorsal midbrain at root exit posteriorly where nerve cross to opposite side. Trauma is a likely cause
Saccades, pursuit, and vergence may be affected but with preserved dolls head maneuver testing	Supranuclear
Weakness of contralateral superior rectus with ipsilateral third nerve palsy	Nucleus of third nerve
Bilateral ptosis or no ptosis (with involvement or sparing of central caudate subnucleus of oculomotor nucleus) in third nerve palsy	Dorsal midbrain at level of superior colliculus, ventral to cerebral aqueduct
Claude syndrome – Complete ipsilateral third nerve palsy with contralateral ataxia and tremor	Fascicular third nerve (concomitant damage to surrounding mesencephalic structures causes specific localization syndromes) with Red nucleus and dentate-rubral fibers
Benedikt syndrome – Complete ipsilateral third nerve palsy with choreiform movements and contralateral hemiparesis	Fascicular third nerve (larger rostral lesions that involve subthalamic nuclei)
Nothnagel syndrome – Complete ipsilateral third nerve palsy with ipsilateral cerebellar ataxia	Fascicular third nerve (larger caudal lesions that involve input to cerebellum)
Weber syndrome – Complete ipsilateral third nerve palsy with contralateral hemiparesis	Fascicular third nerve with anterior cerebral peduncle involved (ventromedial midbrain)
Contralateral superior oblique palsy (fourth nerve is crossed)	Nucleus of fourth nerve, dorsal midbrain, level of inferior colliculus
Ipsilateral horizontal gaze palsy	Nucleus of sixth nerve–pons
Raymond syndrome – Ipsilateral abduction deficit with contralateral hemiparesis. Could have concomitant Internuclear ophthalmoplegia	Fascicular sixth nerve (with involvement of pyramids) localizes to ventral medial pons
Millard Gubler syndrome – Ipsilateral abduction deficit with facial palsy and contralateral hemiparesis	Fascicular sixth with seventh nerve palsy with pyramidal involvement localizes to ventral pons
Foville syndrome – Ipsilateral abduction deficit, facial palsy with hypoesthesia, deafness with gaze palsy and Horner syndrome and contralateral hemiparesis. Can have concomitant internuclear ophthalmoplegia (INO-see below)	Fascicular sixth nerve involvement with concomitant involvement of other cranial nerves including the fifth, seventh, and eighth nerve with pyramidal involvement – localizing to caudal, medial pontine tegmentum
Ipsilateral adduction deficit/lag and contralateral gaze, horizontal dissociated abducting nystagmus producing an internuclear ophthalmoplegia (INO)	Medial longitudinal fasciculus (MLF)
Vertical gaze palsy (conjugate upgaze or down gaze palsy or both)	Vertical Gaze center – Rostral interstitial MLF and Interstitial nucleus of Cajal-tegmentum of midbrain
Parinaud dorsal midbrain syndrome – Limitation of upgaze with convergence retraction nystagmus and lid retraction (Collier sign). Associated light near dissociation	Dorsal midbrain at level of superior colliculus. Upgaze more likely affected as the upgaze centers communicate via posterior commissure VS downgaze – which has bilateral input, hence a larger lesion could theoretically affect downgaze also.
[a]Combination deficits may also occur (e.g., "a one and a half syndrome" (horizontal gaze palsy and INO) or "wall-eyed bilateral INO (WEBINO) or paralytic pontine exotropia"	Various combinations of deficits of pontine structures (e.g., parapontine reticular formation [PPRF], sixth nerve nucleus, MLF) with or without other brainstem signs (e.g., seventh nerve palsy)

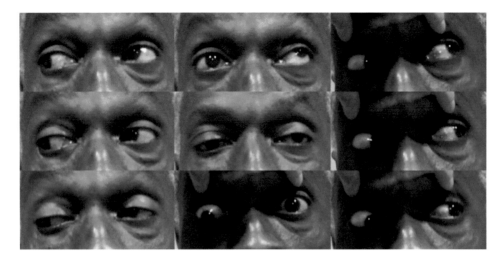

FIGURE 15A.3 This patient demonstrates an isolated, pure nuclear lesion of the left third nerve. On motility examination, he displays bilateral ptosis, ipsilateral exotropia, and hypertropia, with contralateral hypotropia.

The oculomotor nerve[3–6]

The third cranial nerve arises from two nuclei: the somatic oculomotor nucleus and the parasympathetic Edinger-Westphal nucleus. These nuclei control all of the orbital muscles except for the lateral rectus and superior oblique.

The third nerve is rather unique in its pattern of innervation. The Edinger-Westphal nuclei provide parasympathetic innervation to the pupillary sphincters, causing constriction. Both oculomotor nuclei join together inferiorly to form the shared "caudate nucleus," which innervates *both* levator palpebrae. Thus, destruction of the caudate portion will cause bilateral ptosis. The superior rectus is innervated *contralaterally*, meaning destruction of the nucleus itself will cause a *contralateral* elevation deficit (hypotropia). The rest of nuclei have ipsilateral supply to the muscles. Thus an isolated, unilateral, pure nuclear lesion will have a rather unusual presentation of bilateral ptosis, unilateral adduction deficit and hypertropia, and contralateral hypotropia (Figure 15A.3).

Fibers from the oculomotor nuclei and Edinger-Westphal nuclei join together to form the two oculomotor nerves. The somatic fibers travel along the inner portion of the nerve, whereas the parasympathetic fibers travel on the outer surface of the nerve. The third cranial nerve travels through the superior portion of the cavernous sinus before entering the orbit and splitting into a superior and inferior branch. The superior branch innervates the superior rectus and levator palpebrae superioris, whereas the inferior branch innervates the medial and inferior recti, and the inferior oblique. Thus, a distal lesion of the nerve can affect these muscle groups and cause either ptosis with an elevation deficit in the case of the superior branch *or* abduction and elevation of the eye in the case of the inferior branch. Proximal lesions will affect both branches. Because of unopposed action of the lateral rectus and superior oblique, the eye will display the classic "down and out" appearance. However, it also important to know if the patient is fixating with the paretic or normal eye. This could make a difference if the patient has preexisting poor vision in the non-paretic eye, he could attempt to fix with the paretic eye. This can give a false appearance of a deviation in the non-paretic eye rather than the paretic eye and could be misleading.

A loss of parasympathetic fibers traveling on the third nerve will result in mydriasis. As previously noted, the somatic fibers travel along the core of the nerve, whereas parasympathetic fibers travel along the surface of the nerve. This is an important distinction because, depending upon the etiologic cause of the lesion, the patient may lose somatic innervation, parasympathetic innervation, or both. The classic example of an isolated loss of somatic innervation is ischemic, particularly due to diabetes. This will cause damage to the innermost portion of the nerve first, causing a "down and out" eye, but usually without affecting pupillary constriction. Conversely, impingement syndromes such as tumors or aneurysms will affect the outermost, i.e., parasympathetic, fibers first. Thus, it will produce a dilated pupil.

These are not completely specific findings, however, and if the pupil is spared in a third nerve palsy, this does not rule out a compressive etiology.[7] It has been reported that around 15–20% of posterior communicating artery aneurysms present with a pupil-spared nerve palsy.[8] Conversely, an ischemic nerve palsy occasionally involves the pupil. Other studies report that up to 38% of ischemic nerve palsies do, in fact, involve the pupil.[9,10]

The need for neuroimaging in third nerve palsies is determined by the likelihood the patient is suffering a microvascular, ischemic neuropathy. Put simply, Gadolinium-enhanced magnetic resonance imaging (MRI) of the brain and cavernous sinuses and/or MR angiography (MRA) of the intracranial vessels is recommended in all patients with isolated third nerve palsies *except* when the etiology is highly likely to be ischemic (pupils spared, complete, third nerve palsy) due to diabetes or other vasculopathic risk factor (and is improving). Some authors and textbooks therefore recommend that in an elderly patient presenting with atherosclerotic risk factors and a pupil-spared, isolated, complete third nerve palsy can be followed as a presumed ischemic etiology. Neuroimaging according to these authors can be followed clinically for improvement but imaged if atypical course, new symptoms, or lack of improvement occurs.[11,12] Thus, if this type of patient does not improve in 6–8 weeks, or pupil later becomes involved, or if the patient manifests additional symptoms, MRI brain/MRA imaging should be performed at that time. In all other patients: children, young adults, those without atherosclerotic risk factors, those with partial nerve lesions, those with additional nerve lesions, and those with pupillary involvement, neuroimaging with MRI should be routinely performed.[12]

The diagnostic sequence should start with an MRI brain and an MRA with and without contrast. In the acute setting, non-contrast computed tomography (CT) of the head is recommended to exclude subarachnoid hemorrhage followed by a contrast CT angiography (CTA). In a patient with strong suspicion for aneurysm and a negative initial imaging (MRI/MRA and CT/CTA), a catheter angiogram may be performed for confirmation. This recommendation is controversial, however, since MRA detects aneurysms as small as 4 mm, and the risk of rupture of an aneurysm this small is below 2.5%.[13] Forget et al.,[14] however, mention in their paper that over 80% of PCom aneurysms were <10 mm in size, and 40% of these were <5 mm. Thus CTA or MRA could be used as an initial screening test in cases with moderate or low clinical suspicion of aneurysm, however, if the non-catheter angiogram results are negative or equivocal or in cases with higher clinical suspicion, it is recommended to consider a catheter angiogram.

The trochlear nerve[5,15]

The fourth cranial nerve arises from the trochlear nucleus in the midbrain. The trochlear nerve is unique in that not only does it exit dorsally from the brainstem but also it decussates and innervates the contralateral side. However, because it is a purely motor nerve and innervates only one muscle, it is impossible to localize a fourth nerve palsy to the nucleus or fascicle in the absence of any other brainstem signs without imaging studies. Despite this, neuroimaging generally has little clinical value in isolated cases. Many authors and textbooks recommended that clinically isolated fourth nerve palsy can be observed with imaging performed only in patients who do not improve after 3 months of evaluation, or in younger patients who have either a history of cancer or multiple neurological complaints.[12] Neuroimaging in this setting, however, is a practice option.

As the fourth cranial nerve only innervates the superior oblique muscle, damage will result in excyclotorsion and hypertropia of the affected eye. Patients with lesions of this nerve will complain of vertically separated, and often tilted, images. A double Maddox rod test can quantify the degree of tilt (torsion).

The best test to diagnose a fourth neve palsy is the three-step method (Figure 15A.4). First, the hypertropic or hypotropic eye in primary gaze is identified, and its deviation should be measured. Since hypertropia of one eye is equivalent to a contralateral hypotropia, at this stage, deficiency of four muscles could be the cause: the elevators of one eye (inferior oblique and superior rectus) or the contralateral depressors (superior oblique and inferior rectus). Next, deviation is measured in both horizontal gazes. This isolates the elevator muscles from each other – in medial gaze, only the obliques are active; in lateral gaze, only the rectus muscles are active. Finally, the head is tilted to either side, and the deviation is again measured. This isolates the muscles based on cyclotorsion.

The abducens nerve[5,16]

The abducens nucleus is a part of the horizontal gaze center (discussed in detail below), when involved causes a gaze palsy as opposed to a unilateral motility deficit and allows for clinical

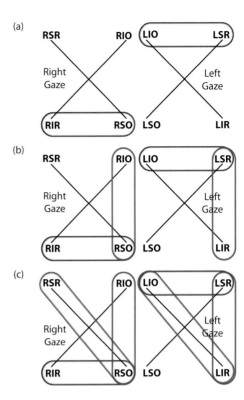

FIGURE 15A.4 A graphical representation of the three-step test. (a) The patient is evaluated in primary gaze. In this example, the left eye is hypotropic, meaning that the right eye is hypertropic. This can result from a deficiency in any of the above muscles circled in black. (b) The patient is asked to look in both directions, which in this case produces an increase in misalignment on left gaze. This isolates the muscles circled in blue, indicating the lesion must lie in those muscles. (c) The patient then tilts his or her head in both directions, which in this case produces an increase in misalignment on right head tilt. This indicates a lesion in the muscles circled in red. Only the right superior oblique (RSO) can produce all of these signs, so the deficiency must be in that muscle.

localization distinct between the sixth nerve and its nucleus. When patients present with a conjugate lateral gaze palsy, this localizes it to the horizontal gaze center, indicating a nuclear lesion.[17] However, if the patient simply has a unilateral abduction deficit in one eye, it is more likely an infranuclear lesion.

The sixth cranial nerve arises from the pons anteriorly at the junction of pons and medulla from the medial aspect and travels through the subarachnoid space, climbs superiorly over the clivus in the Dorellos canal and makes a sharp bend over the petrous temporal bone to pierce the dura. The sharp angled turn by the nerve and its relatively tethered position within the canal makes the sixth nerve susceptible to compression in either elevated intracranial pressure as well as very low intracranial pressures giving rise to a "nonlocalizing sign of sixth nerve palsy." It then enters the cavernous sinus, where it joins with sympathetic fibers. Then it courses through the superior orbital fissure and innervates the ipsilateral lateral rectus muscle. The sixth cranial nerve only innervates the lateral rectus, so damage to this nerve will result in an abduction deficit and/or esotropia of the affected eye.

There are several additional anatomical considerations to consider with the sixth cranial nerve. First, the seventh cranial nerve wraps around the abducens nucleus, so lesions of the abducens nucleus often have seventh nerve involvement. Second, it has the longest course of the three ocular nerves, traveling vertically along the clivus, then turning a full 90 degrees to exit through Dorello's canal. This leaves it very susceptible to stretch and impingement against the rim of the clivus. Any lesion that causes downward displacement of the brainstem, or a change in intracranial pressure, either increase or decrease, can thus result in a sixth nerve palsy. For this reason, a sixth nerve palsy is typically described as "nonlocalizing."[18] In fact, upward of 30% of patients with pseudotumor cerebri may present with a sixth nerve lesion as the only feature of their condition.[19]

Within the cavernous sinus, the sixth nerve lies in close proximity to the internal carotid artery and can be affected early in an arterial pathology (e.g., fistula or aneurysm). Because it also carries sympathetic fibers, lesions at this location often cause a sixth nerve palsy with a concomitant ipsilateral Horner's syndrome. When together, this is called the Parkinson sign and localizes to the cavernous sinus. An exception to this is when sixth nerve palsy and Horner could co-exist, but this time with a pontine lesion, again another region where the sixth nerve lies in close proximity to the descending sympathetic pathway. However in a pontine lesion, in addition to sixth nerve palsy and Horner, we would look additional brainstem symptoms or signs.

Tips on localization

Determining the etiology

When it comes to determining the etiology of the deficit, there are several questions that help to narrow the differential.

1. In an elderly patient, always consider the symptoms of giant cell arteritis (GCA). These include headache (unilateral or bilateral), jaw claudication, polymyalgia rheumatica symptoms, fatigue, night sweats, weight loss, and fever.[20,21] Many patients may have these symptoms but still present to the clinic complaining of diplopia as their primary problem.[5] GCA should be considered in any elderly patient as it is a life and sight-threatening disease that must be treated quickly. A sedimentation rate and C-reactive protein should be ordered to evaluate, whenever GCA is suspected.
2. Is the onset acute or is it more indolent? Acute etiologies include such things as trauma, ischemia, or hemorrhage. In contrast, conditions such as benign neoplastic, thyroid eye disease could be slow progressive and could be associated usually without pain. More aggressive neoplasm could show a more acute progression of symptoms. Aneurysmal compression of nerve could be associated with pain and may be gradually progressive. Guillain-Barre syndrome could present acutely again with single or multiple cranial nerve involvement, unilateral or bilateral. Chronic demyelinating polyneuropathies could occasionally present with motor cranial neuropathy.[22]

3. Are there any other symptoms? Other neurologic symptoms point toward nucleus and brain etiologies, implicating stroke, mass effect, or central nervous system (CNS) demyelinating diseases. Systemic symptoms such as fever and night sweats point toward etiologies such as lymphoma, GCA, or infection. Isolated nerve lesions may be caused by trauma.
4. How old is the patient? If the patient is older, then etiologies such as stroke are far more likely if acute and neoplastic if it runs a more chronic course. If the patient is younger, demyelinating disease, trauma, or hemorrhage is more likely.
5. Is it constant or does it change? The symptoms of myasthenia gravis will worsen throughout the day. Additionally, myasthenia gravis is characterized by *variability and fatigue*, in presentation, with some days worse than others. By contrast, thyroid eye disease will typically be worse upon waking and typically improves as the day progresses.

Lastly, it is important to remember the causes of acute-onset ophthalmoplegia which include myasthenia gravis, Miller Fisher variant of Guillain-Barre syndrome, botulism, brainstem encephalitis, Wernicke encephalopathy, carcinomatous meningitis, or leptomeningeal disease when the ophthalmoplegia is acute, bilateral, or appears to involve multiple cranial nerves.

Conclusion

Despite every advancement in imaging and laboratory studies, the history and physical examination remains the most essential component to properly diagnose every ocular motor cranial neuropathy. Patients will often complain of a singular problem: "I started seeing double," and it is very commonly up to the clinician to elicit additional symptoms and signs such as fever and weight loss in the case of GCA, pupillary findings in ischemic diabetic neuropathy, or the variability and fatigue in myasthenia gravis. Clinicians should have a low index of suspicion for the life-threatening etiologies such as giant cell arteritis or acute stroke and follow-up with confirmation via biopsy or MRI imaging, when appropriate. Physicians should labor to master the associated symptoms and examination techniques, as, depending upon the cause, making a speedy and accurate diagnosis is potentially sight- and lifesaving.

Multiple-Choice Questions

1. A 23-year-old male patient presents with acute double vision and right eye pain. His symptoms began last night after he fell down while riding his bicycle home. He states that his right eye is painful, and it is mildly hyperemic and very teary. When he occludes his right eye, the double vision resolves. Which of the following is the next step in making the diagnosis of binocular versus monocular diplopia?
   a. Slit lamp examination
   b. Fundus examination
   c. Test symptoms with occlusion of either eye
   d. Brain MRI

Answer:

    c.   In order to localize the double vision from the history as monocular or binocular, the symptoms and ocular alignment should be tested with occlusion of *either* eye.

2. A 22-year-old woman has acute, binocular oblique diplopia. Examination reveals a right hypertropia. Which of the following is the next most appropriate step in making the diagnosis of a fourth nerve palsy?

    a. MRI of the head and orbits with contrast

    b. Test pupil

    c. Examine eyelids for ptosis

    d. Measure deviation in right and left gaze and head tilt

Answer:

    d. The three steps of the three-step test are (1) measure the hypertropia in primary gaze; (2) measure the ocular deviation in right and left gaze; and (3) measure the deviation in right and left head tilt. A right hypertropia worse in left gaze and right head tilt suggests a right fourth nerve palsy.

3. A 47-year-old man has hypertension, diabetes, and previous coronary artery bypass graft. He complains of acute painful, drooping of his right eyelid and binocular double vision with a right exotropia and hypotropia. The remainder of the eye and neurologic examination are normal. The pupil is fixed and dilated on the right. A CT of the head was normal. Which of the following is the next most appropriate step?

    a. Outpatient MRI

    b. CT scan of the orbits

    c. Follow-up in clinic in 2 weeks as ischemic palsy

    d. CTA head

Answer:

    d. CTA to look for posterior communicating artery aneurysm. If high clinical suspicion or non-diagnostic CTA then proceed to catheter angiography.

References

1. Friedman DI, Jankovic J, McCrary JA. Neuro-ophthalmic findings in progressive supranuclear palsy. J Clin Neuro Ophthalmol. 1992;12(2):104–9.

2. Danchaivijitr C. Diplopia and eye movement disorders. J Neurol Neurosurg Psychiatry. 2004;75:24–31.

3. Cranial nerves and associated pathways. In: Waxman SG. editor. Clinical neuroanatomy, 29th ed. New York: McGraw Hill; 2020

4. Park HK, Rha HK, Lee KJ, Chough CK, Joo W. Microsurgical anatomy of the oculomotor nerve: Microsurgical anatomy of the oculomotor nerve. Clin Anat. 2017;30(1):21–31.

5. Cornblath WT. Diplopia due to ocular motor cranial neuropathies. Continuum: Lifelong Learning in Neurology. 2014;20:966–80.

6. Remington LA. Cranial nerve innervation of ocular structures. In: Clinical Anatomy and Physiology of the Visual System. Elsevier; 2012. pp. 218–32.

7. Motoyama Y, Nonaka J, Hironaka Y, Park Y-S, Nakase H. Pupil-sparing oculomotor nerve palsy caused by upward compression of a large posterior communicating artery aneurysm. Case report. Neurol Med Chir (Tokyo). 2012;52(4):202–5.

8. Kissel JT, Burde RM, Klingele TG, Zeiger HE. Pupil-sparing oculomotor palsies with internal carotid-posterior communicating artery aneurysms. Ann Neurol. 1983;13(2):149–54.

9. Jacobson DM. Pupil involvement in patients with diabetes-associated oculomotor nerve palsy. Arch Ophthalmol. 1998;116(6):723.

10. Dhume K, Paul K. Incidence of pupillary involvement, course of anisocoria and ophthalmoplegia in diabetic oculomotor nerve palsy. Indian J Ophthalmol. 2013;61(1):13.

11. Lee S-H, Lee S-S, Park K-Y, Han S-H. Isolated oculomotor nerve palsy: Diagnostic approach using the degree of external and internal dysfunction. Clin Neurol Neurosurg. 2002;104(2):136–41.

12. Khaku A, Patel V, Zacharia T, Goldenberg D, McGinn J. Guidelines for radiographic imaging of cranial neuropathies. Ear Nose Throat J. 2017;96(10–11):E23–39.

13. Kupersmith MJ, Heller G, Cox TA. Magnetic resonance angiography and clinical evaluation of third nerve palsies and posterior communicating artery aneurysms. J Neurosurg. 2006;105(2):228–34.

14. Forget TR, Benitez R, Veznedaroglu E, Sharan A, Mitchell W, Silva M, et al. A review of size and location of ruptured intracranial aneurysms. Neurosurgery. 2001;49(6):1322–5.

15. Joo W, Rhoton AL. Microsurgical anatomy of the trochlear nerve: Microsurgical anatomy of the trochlear nerve. Clin Anat. 2015;28(7):857–64.

16. Joo W, Yoshioka F, Funaki T, Rhoton AL. Microsurgical anatomy of the abducens nerve. Clin Anat. 2012;25(8):1030–42.

17. Pierrot-Deseilligny C. Nuclear, internuclear, and supranuclear ocular motor disorders. Handb Clin Neurol. 2011;102:319–31. doi: 10.1016/B978-0-444-52903-9.00018-2. PMID: 21601072.

18. Azarmina M, Azarmina H. The six syndromes of the sixth cranial nerve. J Ophthalmic Vis Res. 2013;8(2):160–71.

19. Krishna R, Kosmorsky GS, Wright KW. Pseudotumor cerebri sine papilledema with unilateral sixth nerve palsy. J Neuroophthalmol. 1998;18(1):53–5.

20. Thurtell MJ, Longmuir RA. Third nerve palsy as the initial manifestation of giant cell arteritis. J Neuroophthalmol. 2014;34(3):243–5.

21. Fytili C, Bournia VK, Korkou C, Pentazos G, Kokkinos A. Multiple cranial nerve palsies in giant cell arteritis and response to cyclophosphamide: A case report and review of the literature. Rheumatol Int. 2015;35(4):773–6.

22. Waddy HM, Misra VP, King RH, Thomas PK, Middleton L, Ormerod IE. Focal cranial nerve involvement in chronic inflammatory demyelinating polyneuropathy: Clinical and MRI evidence of peripheral and central lesions. J Neurol. 1989;236(7):400–405.

15B

NEUROMUSCULAR JUNCTION SYNDROMES AND OCULAR MYOPATHIES

Dan Milea

CASE STUDY

A 48-year-old male presented with history of ptosis of left eye with intermittent double vision for 2-month duration. He noted that his symptoms are worse at the evening time. Bilateral asymmetric ptosis with normal extraocular movements was noted on examination. What is the probable diagnosis?

Background

Neuromuscular junction (NMJ) disorders present with unique symptoms of fluctuating weakness and fatiguability. Depending upon the site of involvement, patients have presynaptic or postsynaptic neuromuscular blockade. Figure 15B.1 highlights the sites of involvement of various NMJ syndromes. While myasthenia gravis (MG) is a classic example of postsynaptic neuromuscular blockade, Lambert Eaton myasthenic syndrome represents a typical presynaptic neuromuscular disorder. Diseases such as botulism and ophthalmoplegia due to snake bite need to be differentiated from these conditions, given the therapeutic implications they have. Chronic progressive external ophthalmoplegia (CPEO) leads on to bilaterally symmetric ptosis and ophthalmoparesis, and oculopharyngeal myopathy involves non-ocular, bulbar or proximal limb musculature in addition.

This chapter gives the insight into NMJ syndromes causing ocular involvement and ocular myopathies.

Ocular myasthenia gravis

Introduction

Myasthenia gravis (MG) is an autoimmune condition in which muscular weakness results from impaired neuromuscular transmission. Most patients with MG will display ocular signs at some point during the evolution of their disease, often at presentation. The muscular signs in MG are typically variable over time, being exacerbated by repetitive contraction and improving on resting. In patients with MG, the acquired acetylcholine receptor antibodies (AChR Abs) block nicotinic AChRs located at the postsynaptic junction, impairing muscular activity. Despite an archetypical clinical presentation in most of cases, MG may at times be difficult to diagnose and, in general, is probably an underdiagnosed condition.[1]

MG shows no geographical or racial predilection, occurring in both sexes, at all ages, although a bimodal distribution of the condition has been described, with a late-life peak between 70 and 75 years.[2] Women seem to be more commonly affected in the group of early-onset cases (before age 40), whereas men predominate in later-onset cases. Childhood MG is rare, although probably more common in Asia.[3]

Depending on the distribution of the motor weakness, MG can affect only the ocular area (causing ptosis and/or diplopia), or can be generalized, becoming a life-threatening condition.[4] It is estimated that a majority (50–85%) of MG patients present initially with isolated ocular symptoms; conversely, most of the patients with generalized disease will present ocular symptoms at some time during the course of the disease.[5] In ocular myasthenia gravis (OMG), weakness is limited to extraocular muscles, levator palpebrae muscles and/or orbicularis oculi muscles, causing diplopia and/or ptosis, without apparent dysfunction of other muscles. Prognosis of OMG is variable; while some studies report low generalization rates (15%),[6] most reports suggest that the majority (50–80%) of patients with initial ocular symptoms will subsequently convert to a generalized form of the disease, mainly within the first 2 years after the initial symptoms.[4,6] MG has been associated with numerous medications,[7] which have been suspected to cause, unmask or worsen the disease (statins, beta-blockers, antibiotics, penicillamine); a formal causal relationship is however questionable in most of the cases.

Ocular myasthenia gravis: Clinical features

OMG can cause any type of ocular motor deficit sparing the pupils. The clinical hallmark of the disease consists of variable symptoms over time; a history of variable weakness or fatigability involving the extraocular muscles and/or the eyelids should raise the suspicion of the disease.

Ptosis, which is the most common ocular sign in OMG, is due to involvement of the levator palpebrae superioris complex; it may be unilateral (Figure 15B.2) or bilateral, occurring more often in association with diplopia, than isolated.[8] Ptosis is typically worse in the evening, or after an effort (e.g., after sustained upgaze). There are several maneuvers aiming to show fatigability and variability of ptosis; the Cogan lid twitch sign is very suggestive, though not pathognomonic of OMG. It is visualized by asking the patient to look down for a few seconds and then to perform a saccade in primary position. The ptotic eyelid in myasthenia overshoots in the latter position and progressively returns to its initial, lower, position. Such an "overactivity" of the levator palpebri muscle may seem surprising in OMG; it has been however suggested that the sign is the result of rapid muscle recovery, after its rest in downgaze position, followed by contraction-related relapse, in primary position. Any form of ptosis can become more severe with fatigue, and therefore, this feature is not characteristic of OMG. However, as a general rule, a history of alternating or recurrent ptosis is strongly suggestive of the condition. The combination of ptosis with orbicularis weakness is virtually diagnostic of MG.

Ophthalmoparesis is the second most common manifestation of OMG[9] but occurs quite rarely as an isolated feature (Figure 15B.3), being often associated with ptosis. The ocular

DOI: 10.1201/9780429020278-20

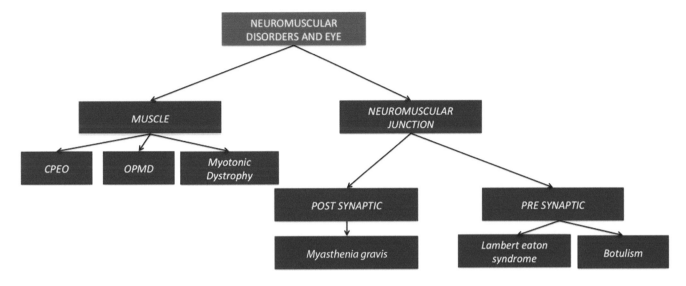

FIGURE 15B.1   Representation of sites of involvement in neuromuscular junction disorders.

motor dysfunction, which can affect any muscle or combination of extraocular muscles, is not specific and can present as any type of ophthalmoplegia, including neurogenic, i.e., resembling a sixth or a fourth nerve palsy. OMG can mimic in reality any ocular motor palsy pattern, including more complex features, such as internuclear ophthalmoplegia,[10] nuclear gaze palsy, one-and-a-half syndrome,[11] complete ophthalmoplegia, etc. Demonstration of fatigability (throughout the same examination or at two successive examinations), especially if associated with unilateral or bilateral ptosis, prompts suspicion of OMG. Fatigability can be demonstrated acutely, by asking the patient to sustain prolonged upward gaze, without blinking, which

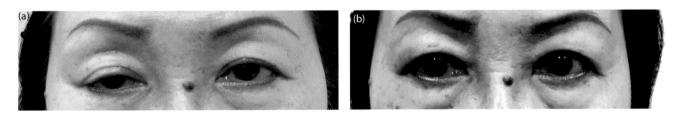

FIGURE 15B.2   Positive ice-test in a patient with confirmed ocular myasthenia gravis. (a) Right ptosis, (b) improving after application of an ice-pack, during 2 minutes, over the eyelid.

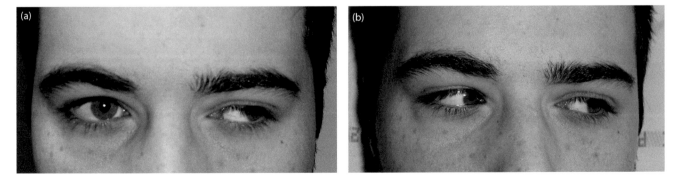

FIGURE 15B.3   Isolated adduction deficit in the right eye in a patient of OMG (a) and recovering completely after injection of edrophonium (b).

may worsen the ocular misalignment and/or ptosis. An appropriate history may reveal symptoms worsening as the day progresses and/or with fatigue and improving after physical rest. Spontaneous remission of the ocular signs, during months or years, is not uncommon. A few following associated signs are not consistent with OMG: pain, anisocoria, abnormal pupillary reactions to light, sensory or visual symptoms.

Orbicularis muscle weakness, associated with ptosis and ophthalmoplegia, is strongly suggestive of OMG. At more advanced stages, orbicularis muscle weakness can cause ectropion, which can be variable over time.[12] Pupils are typically spared in OMG; some pupillometric studies have reported a decrease of various pupillometric parameters (e.g., constriction amplitude, velocity and acceleration),[13] but the clinical assessment of the pupils is always normal.

Diagnosis

Diagnosis of OMG is primarily clinical, supported by serological and electrophysiology data. Clinical examination aims to demonstrate variability or fatigability of the signs, as well as to rule out other differential diagnosis, which may mimic OMG. Last but not least, examination of a patient presenting with OMG needs to evaluate the presence of systemic involvement (weakness of the extensors of the neck, dysphagia, dyspnea, dysarthria, global weakness), which may prompt acute supportive treatment.

Various eye signs have been described in OMG and can aid diagnosis at bed side (Table 15B.1). Enhancement of ptosis can be obtained by lifting one ptotic eyelid, observing the contralateral eyelid for increased ptosis (Figure 15B.4). Lifting or closing one ptotic eyelid reduces the previously increased nervous influx to *both* eyelids (Hering's law) and may result in unmasking infra clinical weakness in the contralateral eyelid. This phenomenon of "enhanced ptosis" is suggestive but not characteristic of OMG. Similarly, prolonged fixation in upgaze (usually during 1–2 min) causes worsening of ptosis. These simple, non-invasive tests are of first choice in the clinic, aiming to reduce the need for intravenous edrophonium (Tensilon) testing. Other tests aim to reverse the clinical signs (most commonly the ptosis), including the ice test and the sleep/rest test. The ice pack test (Figure 15B.2) is a quick, affordable, effective and sensitive clinical method to test variability of ptosis, especially the latter is incomplete. An ice pack is applied on the patient's most ptotic eyelid during 2 minutes, after measuring the palpebral aperture (by blocking the frontalis muscle). Measurements are then repeated, within 10 seconds after removal of the ice pack: improvement of 2mm or more of the ptosis signifies a positive

TABLE 15B.1: Important Eye Signs to Be Examined in a Patient with Myasthenia Gravis

Important Clinical Eye Signs in Myasthenia Gravis	Comments
Enhanced ptosis	Enhancement of ptosis can be obtained by lifting one ptotic eyelid, observing the contralateral eyelid for increased ptosis
Edrophonium/Tensilon Test	Resolution of ptosis on administration of edrophonium
Ice pack test	An ice pack is applied on the patient's most ptotic eyelid during 2 minutes, after measuring the palpebral aperture. Increased opening of the aperture is noted in patients with OMG.
Sleep test	Resolution of ptosis or ophthalmoparesis after sleep or rest with patient's eye closed for a period of about 30 min.
Cogan's lid twitch sign	The patient is told to look straight in primary gaze after looking down for 15 seconds. Rapid overshooting upward movement followed by a down-drift of the upper lid is noted
Peek sign	The eyelids tend to drift apart (with underlying sclera being visible) when the patient is asked to forcefully close his eyelids.

test and strongly suggest MG (Figure 15B.2). The beneficial effect of the cooling is reduced in case of *complete* ptosis. The specificity of this test has been reported as high as 100%, with a sensitivity of 80%.[14] The ice pack test is less effective to evaluate fatigability of an ocular motor abnormality in OMG, compared to evaluation of fatigable ptosis.[15]

Pharmacological, laboratory, electrophysiology and imaging testing

In MG, infusion of intravenous edrophonium chloride (commonly known as the Tensilon test[16]) inhibits activity of the acetylcholinesterase, resulting in an increase in acetylcholine concentration at the synaptic cleft and improvement of the previously deficient muscular function. If the motor deficit is unequivocally reversed after edrophonium infusion, the test is considered as "positive," indicating a high likelihood of OMG. False-positive results have been described in botulism, Guillain-Barre syndrome as well as in other conditions. The sensitivity of the test is considered

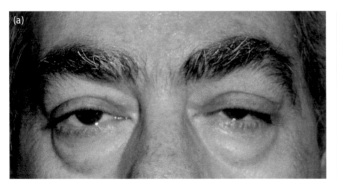 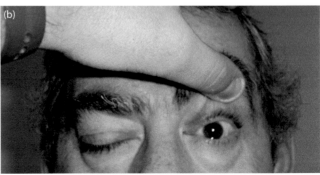

FIGURE 15B.4 Bilateral ptosis in ocular myasthenia gravis (a) and enhanced ptosis in the right eye, after lifting the left eyelid (b).

as high as 90% for MG, when considering ptosis reversal. This test requires an objective evaluation of the improvement, and therefore, the amount of ptosis/ocular misalignment should be documented photographically "before" and "after" the injection. Edrophonium has a quick, short-acting effect: its action begins within the first minute after injection, lasting 5–10 minutes.

Edrophonium can cause multiple side effects related to the increased muscarinic activity, including abdominal cramping, lacrimation, salivation, sweating. Continuous cardiovascular monitoring during its performance is necessary, in order to avoid more serious side effects, such as bradycardia, hypotension, and syncope, sometimes requiring the use of atropine. The Neostigmine test can be used as a safer and easier alternative to edrophonium testing: it is a longer acting drug (30 minutes), allowing a more detailed post-treatment evaluation which is valuable for measuring diplopia, for instance.

Detection of circulating AChR Abs is diagnostic for the disease. Detection of binding AChR Abs is a more sensitive test than the detection of blocking or modulating antibodies. AChR Abs are present only in 50% of OMG (vs 90% in GMG cases) and their levels most often do not correlate with the clinical presentation. Thus, failure to find AChR Abs does not rule out OMG (seronegative MG). However, the presence of AChR Abs has a high value in ruling out a congenital myasthenic syndrome, which is not an autoimmune disease. The presence of binding AChR Abs may be indicative of a higher risk of generalization, but their absence has no prognostic value. In patients without AChR antibodies, other serological tests may be performed. In seronegative patients, muscle-specific kinase (MuSK) antibodies can be detected, especially in patients with GMG; they are very rarely detected in patients with pure OMG.[17] Other antibodies can be detected, such as low-density lipoprotein (LDL)-related receptor-related protein 4 (LRP4), but their clinical value is not yet firmly established. It is considered that in 10% of MG cases, all the above mentioned antibodies are negative (so-called triple negative antibodies). In summary, absence of AChR, which are routinely explored in clinical settings does not rule out OMG, prompting additional investigations for diagnosis.

Electromyography (EMG) and nerve conduction testing may be useful in diagnosing OMG, especially in seronegative cases. In order to increase their diagnostic yield, it is important to discontinue acetylcholinesterase treatments at least 12 hours prior to the examination. Repetitive nerve stimulation studies aim to disclose a decremental response, more easily found in GMG cases (75%) than in OMG cases (less than 50%). Single fiber electromyography (SFEMG) is a very sensitive method (80–90%), exploring the neuromuscular transmission[18] (the presence of abnormal jitter indicating MG); it has the disadvantage of not being easily available.

MG and OMG can be associated with thymoma in 10–30% of cases,[19] its presence having both prognostic and therapeutic implications. Malignant thymomas and other thymic tumors are more rarely associated with OMG. Appropriate imaging (e.g., chest CT) is mandatory in all newly diagnosed cases of OMG and MG since delayed diagnosis of thymoma could lead to a poorer systemic outcome.[20] Conversely, among patients with confirmed thymoma, almost half have an associated autoimmune condition, possibly of paraneoplastic origin. It is assumed that 40% of these patients may have an associated MG. Thymoma-associated MG tends to have a more difficult course and a poorer prognosis.[21]

Differential diagnosis

OMG may mimic any ocular motility dysfunction sparing the pupils, including peripheral cranial nerve palsies (Figure 15B.5),

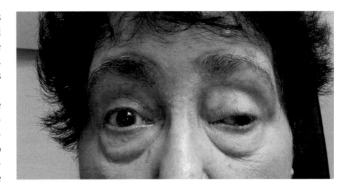

FIGURE 15B.5 Patient with ocular myasthenia, mimicking a left third cranial nerve palsy. The pupils were intact on both sides.

central or internuclear palsies or other conditions affecting the ocular muscles themselves. Conversely, other neurogenic, NMJ or muscular disorders may mimic OMG, such as CPEO, oculopharyngeal dystrophy, botulism, Lambert-Eaton syndrome. OMG can also coexist, based on a common autoimmune pathophysiology, with other conditions affecting the ocular muscles in the orbit, such as thyroid eye disease (TED).

TED can mimic or be associated with OMG. Concomitant presence of thyroid dysfunction is found in up to 13% of patients with MG.[22] As a practical rule, ptosis in a patient with TED suggests the coexistence of MG, prompting further evaluation. Similarly, exotropia in a patient with known TED prompts further evaluation for coexisting OMG (since the most common ocular motor pattern in TED is esotropia, due to the preferential involvement of the medial recti muscles). The symptoms are however different in the conditions: diplopia due to OMG is typically worse in the afternoon, whereas diplopia due to TED is worse in the morning, upon waking. Bilateral eyelid retraction is a common sign in TED; *unilateral* eyelid retraction can be due to TED or can also represent a physiological, compensatory reaction to contralateral ptosis. The latter situation can be revealed by lifting the ptotic eyelid, which will revert the contralateral eyelid retraction (Figure 15B.6). MG can be associated with other immune-mediated conditions, such as rheumatoid arthritis, systemic lupus erythematosus and multiple sclerosis.[9]

Therapeutic management

The goal of OMG therapy is to reduce symptoms of diplopia and ptosis and to prevent progression and generalization. The medical and surgical means to achieve this are nevertheless controversial.[23] Because of the high risk of generalization after OMG, it is usually recommended to manage the treatment in cooperation with a neurologist, especially during the first 2 years of ocular signs, when generalization most often occurs. A symptomatic, non-pharmacological approach can be sometimes very helpful: patching of one eye, use of prisms and/or of ptosis crutches may be temporary solutions. It is mandatory at the initial stage to manage intercurrent infections, which may worsen, temporarily, OMG signs. The patient is also advised to avoid medications (statins, quinolones, aminoglycosides, anesthetics, curariform agents, botulinum toxin) which may interfere with the neuro-muscular junction.

Oral acetylcholinesterase inhibitors may provide temporary symptomatic treatment of ptosis, although their long-term efficacy, dosage and side effects are not completely known. Acetylcholinesterase inhibitors (neostigmine or pyridostigmine) are typically more efficient on ptosis than on ophthalmoparesis, while not improving the risk of subsequent generalization. Pyridostigmine bromide can be

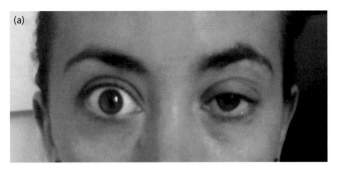
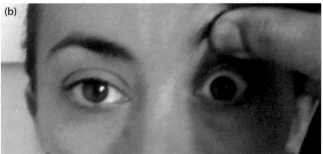

FIGURE 15B.6 Ptosis and contralateral compensatory eyelid retraction in a patient with myasthenia. There is a left ptosis and a right eyelid retraction (a). The right eyelid retraction is compensatory, which can be reversed by suppressing the left ptosis (b).

prescribed at increasing doses up to 90–180 mg/day, if well tolerated. Muscarinic side effects occur very often, such as nausea, abdominal cramps, diarrhea, which can be partly alleviated by the use of oral agents with anticholinergic effect.

Oral steroids are usually the first-line treatment for diplopia, at various regimens (usually 0.5–1 mg/kg/day). Initiation of steroid treatments can sometimes be associated with a temporary worsening of the symptoms, during the first 2 weeks. Similarly, rapid reduction of steroids can exacerbate OMG signs, including generalization. Steroids are usually effective on the OMG signs, but complete, permanent remission without treatment is only rarely obtained. It has been suggested that early initiation of steroids may prevent further generalization of OMG. Unfortunately, no evidence-based medicine recommendations can be made for this purpose, until the release of the results of an undergoing prospective, randomized, controlled study evaluating steroids in newly diagnosed OMG (EPITOME).[24] In the meanwhile, it is accepted that low-dose oral prednisone for OMG has an acceptable side-effect profile, causing only few serious complications (2-year risk, approximately 1%).[25] Thus, corticosteroids are effective[26] possibly reducing generalization.[27] However, formal predictive factors for MG generalization are lacking, including the use of early steroid therapy.[28]

Refractory or generalized MG may be treated, in addition to steroids, with other immunosuppressive agents, either for short-term (intravenous immunoglobulins, plasmapheresis) or long term (azathioprine, methotrexate, cyclosporine, tacrolimus, etanercept, mycophenolate mofetil, rituximab), despite their known systemic potential side-effects.[23]

Recent data suggest that patients with seropositive GMG may benefit from thymectomy, even in the absence of radiologically detectable thymoma. The role of thymectomy in OMG patients is not well defined, even when thymoma is present.[29] Strabismus or eyelids surgery can be indicated in selected cases, displaying long-standing, stable ocular deviations or ptosis.

Lambert-Eaton myasthenic syndrome (LEMS)

LEMS is a very rare presynaptic autoimmune disorder, characterized by the clinical triad associating muscle weakness (commonly fluctuating, mostly affecting proximal muscles), autonomic dysfunction and depressed tendon reflexes. LEMS is usually a paraneoplastic condition associated with small-cell lung cancer, often preceding its diagnosis, but can also occur in isolation. A majority of patients have pathogenic circulating antibodies against the presynaptic P/Q-type voltage-gate calcium channel,

allowing the diagnosis. Although differential diagnosis with MG can be very difficult, the ocular involvement in LEMS is extremely rare. Paradoxically, bilateral ptosis in LEMS has been reported to improve transiently after sustained upgaze.[30] Management of LEMS aims to detect and treat a lung tumor. Its treatment often improves the LEMS symptoms, which can be also treated symptomatically using 3, 4-diaminopyridine phosphate, and sometimes also with pyridostigmine. Immunosuppression, plasmapheresis and high-dose administration of intravenous immunoglobulins may sometimes be required for a better control of the symptoms.

Botulism

Botulism is a very rare, severe, neurological, potentially lethal condition, characterized by flaccid paralysis. It is caused by a neurotoxin released from *Clostridium botulinum* (serotypes A-E), which is an anaerobic, spore-forming, Gram-positive bacillus with a worldwide distribution. Food borne botulism (most commonly type B) is the most frequent form of the disease in the western world. Typically, the first clinical signs are present within 12–36 hours after ingestion of contaminated food. Nausea, vomiting, abdominal pain, diarrhea or constipation are rapidly followed by dysarthria, dysphagia and other oculobulbar signs with a pattern of descending paralysis. Neuro-ophthalmic signs are common, although rarely isolated, including bilaterally dilated pupils, accommodation palsy, ptosis and external ophthalmoplegia. Bilateral involvement of various cranial nerves (commonly the sixth nerve) may occur.[31] If untreated, the condition spreads rapidly, involving respiratory muscles and requiring respiratory assistance. Clustering and the clinical presentation are suggestive of the diagnosis, which requires bacteriological confirmation. The mainstays of therapy include rapid and meticulous intensive care and timely treatment with antitoxin. Survivors usually recover from their neuro-ophthalmic dysfunction, including cranial nerve palsies.

Snake bite

Snake bite is another important cause of myasthenic pattern of weakness involving extraocular muscles specially in tropical and subtropical countries. Snake envenomation may have varied manifestations depending upon the type of toxins. Vasculotoxic snakes initiate consumption coagulopathy and may lead on to spontaneous hemorrhage. Cardiotoxic snakes may cause myocardial damage and arrhythmias. Neurotoxic manifestations include motor weakness and myasthenia like syndrome.

The hallmark of neurotoxic snake bite is a defective neuromuscular transmission. Neurotoxins bind to AChR binding sites producing weakness similar to MG. Traditionally snakes may cause presynaptic or postsynaptic neuromuscular blockade. Cobras are associated with production of post-synaptic neurotoxins and common krait and Russel's viper produce presynaptic toxins.[32]

Usually, the initial manifestation is bilateral ptosis associated with ophthalmoplegia. Further in course palatal, laryngeal and neck muscles may be involved sequentially. This may be also be followed by facial and limb muscle weakness. Proximal muscle weakness occurs in more than half of the neurotoxic snake bites. Pupillary responses are preserved till late. Diaphragmatic weakness and respiratory involvement denote a pre-terminal event. The neuromuscular weakness arising due to snake bite may not respond to edrophonium and has been considered as myasthenic syndrome with atypical findings by some researchers.[33]

Due to variation in site of action, repetitive nerve stimulation test also gives varied results. While decremental response at low frequency stimulation is suggestive of a postsynaptic neuromuscular blockade, low amplitude action potentials, decremental response on high frequency stimulation is representative of presynaptic neuromuscular blockade. Fibrillations may also be seen on electromyography.

Anti-myasthenic agents like neostigmine may transiently improve ptosis. Definitive management involves use of anti-snake venom (ASV).

Sudden-onset ptosis with ophthalmoplegia during monsoon season with progressive neck, facial, limb and diaphragmatic weakness noted on awakening should alert a physician for possibility of snake bite (Case 1).

CASE 1

A 42-year-old male woke up from sleep at midnight with complaints of severe abdomen pain and vomiting. On awakening, he was noted to have bilateral drooping of eyelids associated with inability to hold head. The patient was a mason and had slept on the ground near the construction site on the night of the ictus. General physical examination did not reveal any abnormality. No fang marks over body could be appreciated. Neurological examination suggested ptosis weak neck muscles (both flexors and extensors) and mild proximal muscle weakness (MRC 4/5) (Figure 15B.7a). Sensory examination was normal. Edrophonium test was negative. Possibility of a neuroparalytic snake bite was considered. ASV was administered (200 mL bolus followed by 100 mL every 6 hours). The patient had complete recovery 48 hours following the administration of ASV (Figure 15B.7b).

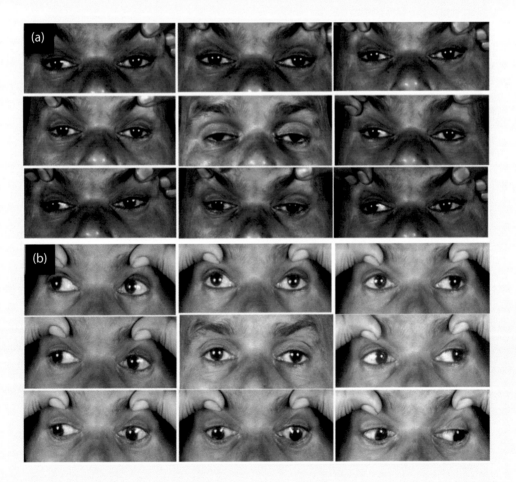

FIGURE 15B.7 Complete ophthalmoparesis with ptosis in a patient with neuroparalytic snake bite (a) Complete recovery of ophthalmoparesis after receiving anti-snake venom (b).

Chronic progressive external ophthalmoplegia

CPEO, caused by mitochondrial DNA mutations, presents typically as progressive (over many years), bilaterally symmetric ptosis and ophthalmoparesis (Figure 15B.8). CPEO is in reality a clinical description, rather than an established diagnosis; it can occur in isolation (affecting only the periocular muscles) or in association with other systemic signs of mitochondrial dysfunction ("CPEO plus"). The association with pigmentary retinopathy, cardiac, and auditory signs is known as the Kearns–Sayre syndrome (KSS), which occurs typically before the age of 20. KSS, which has a poorer outcome, can be associated with elevated cerebrospinal fluid protein, elevated blood lactate/pyruvate and brain abnormalities on MRI. Other CPEOs can present at any age, including in the elderly. Rarely, CPEO can have atypical presentations (such as unilateral or very asymmetric initial presentations) which may raise the suspicion of MG. Ptosis associated with CPEO is almost always inaugural and is very rarely absent during the late, full-blown form of the disease. Typically, the levator palpebri function is reduced in CPEO, as in most ocular myopathies. Ophthalmoparesis associated with CPEO is in most cases bilateral and symmetrical, but it is typically unnoticed by the patients until late stages of the disease, due to the symmetrical involvement, causing little, if any diplopia. Systemic involvement can occur, associating neurological signs [bulbar signs, ataxia, deafness, vestibular signs, encephalopathy and optic atrophy] or endocrinological, cardiac, skeletal involvement).

CPEO diagnosis can be confirmed on muscle biopsy, by showing presence of ragged-red fibers and/or Cox-negative fibers. Their presence is however not always diagnostic since they may exist, at a lower extent, in normally aging patients or in other myopathies. For these reasons, muscle biopsy may at times be equivocal, prompting further mitochondrial DNA analysis or additional testing of the respiratory complexes I-V. CPEO is characterized by a very large heterogeneity, being sporadic in more than 50% of cases. In these sporadic cases, polymerase chain reaction (PCR) can identify *de novo* mitochondrial DNA deletions, which are very rarely transmitted to the offspring. Inherited ocular myopathies are not common; they can be transmitted as autosomal dominant, autosomal recessive or maternally inherited diseases. The most common nuclear DNA mutations in CPEO involve the POLG1 gene, others being less frequent (OPA1, POLG2, twinkle, etc.). They have a common consequence, altering mitochondrial DNA function and structure, the latter being detected by PCR.

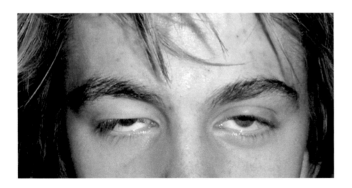

FIGURE 15B.8 Chronic progressive ophthalmoplegia associating long standing, slowly progressive ptosis and ophthalmoparesis.

Other mitochondrial diseases can be associated with ophthalmoplegia, such as MELAS (mitochondrial encephalopathy, lactic acidosis, stroke), MNGIE (mitochondrial neurogastrointestinal encephalomyopathy) and Leigh syndrome (subacute necrotizing encephalomyelopathy).

Oculopharyngeal muscular dystrophy and Steinert's disease

Oculopharyngeal muscular dystrophy (OPMD) differs from CPEO, having an autosomal dominant transmission. Typically, ptosis is an early presenting sign, followed usually years later by ocular motor dysfunction, and/or involvement of non-ocular, bulbar or proximal limb musculature. The hallmark of the disease is the association of ptosis, progressive ophthalmoplegia and dysphagia. Unlike in CPEO, diagnosis does not require a muscle biopsy, but a blood genetic testing, searching for a trinucleotide repeat on chromosome 14.

Myotonic dystrophy type 1 (DM1), also known as "Steinert's disease," is the most common form of adult of adult-onset muscular dystrophy, which affects the eyes. In addition to the classic posterior subcapsular cataract, the eyelids can be affected (ptosis) and more rarely the extraocular eye muscles. As for the other inherited ocular myopathies, the neuro-ophthalmic treatment is most often symptomatic, correcting the ptosis and sometimes performing strabismus surgery to improve the ocular alignment.

Conclusion

NMJ disorders involving the ocular apparatus can be recognized as disorders causing fluctuating, fatigable ptosis and diplopia. In acute settings, botulism and snake bite should be considered as important differentials. In long-standing ophthalmoplegia without diplopia, CPEO should be considered and ocular myopathies present with ophthalmoparesis, and involvement of non-ocular muscles.

Multiple-Choice Questions

1. Which of the following statements is NOT true for myasthenia gravis?
   a. Women are more commonly affected.
   b. In 20–25% initial symptoms are ocular.
   c. Beta-blockers can cause exacerbations of myasthenic symptoms.
   d. Ocular myasthenia gravis can mimic internuclear ophthalmoplegia.

   Answer:

   b. In 20–25% initial symptoms are ocular.

2. All of the following are clinical signs for bed side diagnosis of myasthenia gravis, EXCEPT:
   a. Enhanced ptosis
   b. Peek sign
   c. Sleep test
   d. Impaired ptosis

   Answer:

   d. Impaired ptosis

3. Kearns Sayre syndrome
   a. Is a common cause of ophthalmoplegia in middle-aged females.
   b. Is associated with good outcome in younger children.
   c. Is associated with increased CSF proteins.
   d. Is associated with trinucleotide repeats.

   Answer:

   c. Is associated with increased CSF proteins.

4. Botulism
   a. Is caused by neurotoxins released by *Clostridium difficile* bacteria.
   b. Clinical signs present with first 6 hours after ingestion of contaminated food.
   c. Involvement of bilateral seventh nerves is common.
   d. Accommodation palsy may occur.

   Answer:

   d. Accommodation palsy may occur.

References

1. Vincent A, Clover L, Buckley C, et al. Evidence of underdiagnosis of myasthenia gravis in older people. J Neurol Neurosurg Psychiatry. 2003;74(8):1105–8.
2. Ariatti A, Stefani M, Miceli P, et al. Prognostic factors and health-related quality of life in ocular myasthenia gravis (OMG). Int J Neurosci. 2014;124(6):427–5.
3. Yu YL, Hawkins BR, Ip MS, et al. Myasthenia gravis in Hong Kong Chinese. 1. Epidemiology and adult disease. Acta Neurol Scand. 1992;86(2):113–9.
4. Kupersmith MJ. Ocular myasthenia gravis: Treatment successes and failures in patients with long-term follow-up. J Neurol. 2009;256(8):1314–20.
5. Grob D, Brunner N, Namba T, Pagala M. Lifetime course of myasthenia gravis. Muscle Nerve. 2008;37(2):141–9.
6. Bever CT, Jr., Aquino AV, Penn AS, et al. Prognosis of ocular myasthenia. Ann Neurol. 1983;14(5):516–9.
7. Purvin V, Kawasaki A, Smith KH, Kesler A. Statin-associated myasthenia gravis: Report of 4 cases and review of the literature. Medicine (Baltimore). 2006;85(2):82–5.
8. Colavito J, Cooper J, Ciuffreda KJ. Non-ptotic ocular myasthenia gravis: A common presentation of an uncommon disease. Optometry 2005;76(7):363–75.
9. Kusner LL, Puwanant A, Kaminski HJ. Ocular myasthenia: diagnosis, treatment, and pathogenesis. Neurologist. 2006;12(5):231–9.
10. Jay WM, Nazarian SM, Underwood DW. Pseudo-internuclear ophthalmoplegia with downshoot in myasthenia gravis. J Clin Neuroophthalmol. 1987;7(2):74–6.
11. Davis TL, Lavin PJ. Pseudo one-and-a-half syndrome with ocular myasthenia. Neurology. 1989;39(11):1553.
12. Chang GY, Sole G, Ferrer X. Teaching neuroimages: Reversible ectropion in myasthenia gravis. Neurology. 2010;74(15):1239; author reply.
13. Tsiptsios D, Fotiou DF, Haidich AB, et al. Evaluation of pupil mobility in patients with myasthenia gravis. Electromyogr Clin Neurophysiol. 2008;48(5):209–18.
14. Golnik KC, Pena R, Lee AG, Eggenberger ER. An ice test for the diagnosis of myasthenia gravis. Ophthalmology. 1999;106(7):1282–6.
15. Chatzistefanou KI, Kouris T, Iliakis E, et al. The ice pack test in the differential diagnosis of myasthenic diplopia. Ophthalmology. 2009;116(11):2236–43.
16. Daroff RB. The office Tensilon test for ocular myasthenia gravis. Arch Neurol 1986;43(8):843–4.
17. Bennett DL, Mills KR, Riordan-Eva P, et al. Anti-MuSK antibodies in a case of ocular myasthenia gravis. J Neurol Neurosurg Psychiatry. 2006;77(4):564–5.
18. Cui LY, Guan YZ, Wang H, Tang XF. Single fiber electromyography in the diagnosis of ocular myasthenia gravis: report of 90 cases. Chin Med J (Engl). 2004;117(6):848–51.
19. Mao ZF, Mo XA, Qin C, et al. Incidence of thymoma in myasthenia gravis: a systematic review. J Clin Neurol. 2012;8(3):161–9.
20. Tung CI, Chao D, Al-Zubidi N, et al. Invasive thymoma in ocular myasthenia gravis: Diagnostic and prognostic implications. J Neuroophthalmol. 2013;33(3):307–8.
21. Beydoun SR, Gong H, Ashikian N, Rison RA. Myasthenia gravis associated with invasive malignant thymoma: Two case reports and a review of the literature. J Med Case Rep. 2014;8:340.
22. Osserman KE, Tsairis P, Weiner LB. Myasthenia gravis and thyroid disease: Clinical and immunologic correlation. J Mt Sinai Hosp N Y. 1967;34(5):469–83.
23. Benatar M, Kaminski H. Medical and surgical treatment for ocular myasthenia. Cochrane Database Syst Rev. 2012;12:CD005081.
24. Benatar M, Sanders DB, Wolfe GI, et al. Design of the efficacy of prednisone in the treatment of ocular myasthenia (EPITOME) trial. Ann N Y Acad Sci. 2012;1275:17–22.
25. Bruce BB, Kupersmith MJ. Safety of prednisone for ocular myasthenia gravis. J Neuroophthalmol. 2012;32(3):212–5.
26. Kupersmith MJ, Moster M, Bhuiyan S, et al. Beneficial effects of corticosteroids on ocular myasthenia gravis. Arch Neurol. 1996;53(8):802–4.
27. Kupersmith MJ. Does early immunotherapy reduce the conversion of ocular myasthenia gravis to generalized myasthenia gravis? J Neuroophthalmol. 2003;23(4):249–50.
28. Wong SH, Huda S, Vincent A, Plant GT. Ocular myasthenia gravis: Controversies and updates. Curr Neurol Neurosci Rep. 2014;14(1):421.
29. Mineo TC, Ambrogi V. Outcomes after thymectomy in class I myasthenia gravis. J Thorac Cardiovasc Surg. 2013;145(5):1319–24.
30. Brazis PW. Enhanced ptosis in Lambert-Eaton myasthenic syndrome. J Neuroophthalmol. 1997;17(3):202–3.
31. Simcock PR, Kelleher S, Dunne JA. Neuro-ophthalmic findings in botulism type B. Eye (Lond). 1994;8(Pt 6):646–8.
32. Lewis RL, Gutmann L. Snake venoms and the neuromuscular junction. Semin Neurol. 2004 Jun;24(2):175–9. doi: 10.1055/s-2004-830904. PMID: 15257514.
33. Sanmuganathan PS. Myasthenic syndrome of snake envenomation: a clinical and neurophysiological study. Postgrad Med J. 1998 Oct;74(876):596–9. doi: 10.1136/pgmj.74.876.596. PMID: 10211352; PMCID: PMC2361006.

15C

ORBITAL INFLAMMATORY SYNDROMES

Jaspreet Sukhija, Savleen Kaur

Orbital apex syndromes

CASE STUDY

A 22-year-old woman presented with diminution of vision and inward deviation of the right eye. On examination, right eye pupil was dilated. Visual acuity in right eye was 6/36 and fundus examination revealed disc edema. Right eye proptosis, ptosis with limitation of adduction, and elevation were noted while examining extraocular movements. Examination of the left eye was normal. Contrast-enhanced MRI brain and orbits showed thickening of right optic nerve with T2 hyperintense signal at right orbital apex and anterior cavernous region. How do you approach a patient with such presentation?

Introduction

Orbital inflammation may be either idiopathic or due to a specific inflammatory disease. It may involve different orbital structures, responsible for the different clinical presentations. Recognizing the inflammatory etiology, identifying which structures are involved, and determining the underlying disease are mandatory to establish an adequate treatment.

The term orbital inflammatory syndrome (OIS) classically refers to a benign inflammatory process of the orbit characterized by a polymorphous lymphoid infiltrate along with varying degrees of fibrosis. While OIS classically refers to the inflammation localized to orbital structures, the pathology affecting the orbits may occasionally spread beyond orbits. Depending upon the site of spread, these syndromes are recognized by various nosologies.

Orbital apex disorders

These include three groups of disorders: orbital apex syndrome, superior orbital fissure syndrome (SOFS), and cavernous sinus syndrome (CSS).

Orbital apex syndrome, also known as Jacod syndrome, is an uncommon disorder related to various etiologies involving the orbital apex, including trauma, neoplastic, developmental, infectious, inflammatory as well as vascular causes. It is characterized by ophthalmoplegia; proptosis; ptosis from palsy of cranial nerves (CN) III, IV, and VI; hypoesthesia of the ipsilateral forehead, upper eyelid, and cornea by involvement of ophthalmic (V1) division of the trigeminal nerve; and eventual visual deficit from optic neuropathy. SOFS, also known as Rochon–Duvigneaud syndrome, occurs from a lesion immediately anterior to the apex. It presents similarly to orbital apex syndrome but without the accompanying optic nerve impairment. The term CSS is used when the cavernous sinuses are involved. The clinical symptoms

include hypoesthesia of the cheek and lower eyelid in addition to the signs seen in orbital apex syndrome due to involvement of maxillary (V2) division of the trigeminal nerve. Additionally, CSS may present with oculosympathetic paresis (Horner's syndrome) due to involvement of the sympathetic chain adjacent to the cavernous segment of the internal carotid artery.

Systemic associations of OIS

Differential diagnosis of OIS ranges from idiopathic inflammatory disease to systemic or local inflammatory conditions to other associated conditions such as neoplasm, infection, congenital malformation, or trauma (Table 15C.1).

TABLE 15C.1: Differential Diagonsis of OIS

Systemic associations of OIS

1. Autoimmune thyroid disease
2. Sarcoidosis
3. Wegener's granulomatosis
4. Crohn's disease
5. Systemic lupus erythematosus and other connective tissue diseases
6. Churg–Strauss syndrome, Erdheim–Chester, histiocytosis X
7. Giant cell arteritis

Neoplasm

1. Lymphoma
2. Lymphoproliferative disorders
3. Rhabdomyosarcoma
4. Metastatic disease

Infections

Trauma

History and examination

There are numerous systemic diseases that can be associated with orbital inflammation. Therefore, a proper history and examination should be carried out.

The following points should be kept in mind while taking history of these patients:

1. *Age of patient*
   Children are more susceptible to suffer from an infection, whereas the elderly are more likely to develop neoplasia.
2. *Duration*
   A relatively short duration of hours to days favors infection. An insidious presentation of days to weeks is more characteristic of diseases like thyroid or neoplasia.
3. *History of pain*
   Painful diplopia is seen in myositis.
4. *Associated disease*
   Any features suggestive of history of rheumatologic disease such as systemic lupus erythematosus (SLE) or polyarteritis

DOI: 10.1201/9780429020278-21

nodosa should be asked. History of trauma or insect bites and compromised immune status, for example, due to diabetes, may further point toward infection. Mucor mycosis constitutes a life-threatening emergency and should be suspected in immune-suppressed patients, particularly in those with poorly controlled diabetes.

Some clinical features might point toward a specific etiology. Physical examination of the orbit includes inspection, measurement of exophthalmos, palpation, determination of motility, and auscultation. Changes in the lesion during voluntary valsalva may suggest vascular malformations.

1. Eyelid examination: Position of the eyelid is an important clue in diseases like thyroid which may cause lid retraction.
2. Orbital palpation may reveal orbital mass lesions or define areas of point tenderness. Nontender swelling and mild discomfort are more concerning for neoplasm or specific inflammatory syndromes such as Wegener granulomatosis, whereas severe pain is more suggestive of myositis or orbital cellulitis.
3. Examination of the pupils for relative afferent pupillary defect may point toward optic nerve involvement. Pupillary testing is also performed to evaluate sympathetic and oculomotor innervation.
4. Corneal sensation should be tested to detect involvement of the trigeminal nerve.
5. Ocular motility to be examined next in all directions of gaze.

Investigations and workup

Initial laboratory evaluation may include a complete blood count, electrolytes, thyroid function studies, erythrocyte sedimentation rate, antinuclear antibodies, and antineutrophil cytoplasmic antibodies (ANCA), although ANCA testing may be negative in cases of granulomatosis limited to the orbit. Serum angiotensin-converting enzyme (ACE) and rheumatoid factor assessment should be done. Chest radiographs or computed tomography (CT) should be performed in patients with suspected sarcoidosis. A biopsy is generally not performed as part of the initial evaluation but may be appropriate for atypical cases or those refractory to initial management. When a biopsy is obtained, a variety of histological findings may be present in OIS, including granulomatous inflammation, diffuse infiltrate, tissue eosinophilia, and sclerosis.

Imaging modalities in OIS

CT is the investigation of choice for most orbital surgeons. Magnetic resonance imaging (MRI) can be used where greater soft tissue detail is required. The choice of MRI or CT is determined both by the clinical features of disease and suspected tissue involvement. In evaluations of the optic nerve and nerve sheath, identification of extraorbital extension, or if there is concern about radiation dose, MRI is superior to CT. Contrast agents should typically be used to diminish the fat signal in order to maximize the view of orbital anatomy. Patients in whom a detailed analysis of orbital bone and adjacent sinuses is desired, CT is the imaging modality of choice. Characteristic imaging findings may help differentiate idiopathic inflammatory, thyroid, infectious, and oncologic causes. Imaging findings in OIS will be dependent on the structures involved. Lacrimal gland involvement is often observed as enlargement with ill-defined borders and may occur in isolation or in combination with changes in other orbital structures.[1] Orbital fat, when involved, exhibits diffuse or ill-defined infiltration. Extraocular muscle (EOM) involvement in idiopathic OIS is thickening of the entire muscle from origin to insertion, whereas thyroid eye disease classically spares the tendons. Orbital cellulitis on the other hand is accompanied by evidence of underlying sinus infection on imaging in 75% of cases. Rhabdomyosarcoma is typically accompanied by bony changes that are not present in OIS. Table 15C.2 details the various differentials of orbital inflammation along with key clinical features.

TABLE 15C.2: Important Differentials of Orbital Inflammation

Differential	Pain	Onset	Laterality	Ocular Signs and Symptoms	Imaging Finding
Thyroid-associated orbitopathy	Initial disease pain is rare	Variable	Bilateral may be asymmetric	Lid retraction, lid lag, and muscle involvement most commonly affect the inferior and medial rectus	Tendon sparing multiple enlarged muscles with increased orbital fat
Sarcoidosis	Present	Acute or subacute	May be unilateral or bilateral	Any rectus muscle may be involved; potential involvement of the optic nerve	Hilar lymphadenopathy; diffuse soft tissue mass
Wegener's granulomatosis	Present	Acute	May be unilateral or bilateral	Any rectus muscle may be involved without any specific pattern of involvement	Bone erosion; extraocular muscle involved
Tolosa–Hunt syndrome	Present	Acute	Unilateral	No proptosis Cranial nerve palsies	
Lymphoproliferative orbital disease	Variable	Variable	Unilateral	Mass, swelling, and ptosis	No bony erosion with any extraocular muscle involvement
Metastatic orbital disease	Variable	Variable	Unilateral	Mass, swelling, and ptosis	Bony metastasis, infiltrative process, and obscured landmarks
Orbital cellulitis	Present	Acute	Unilateral	Erythema, chemosis, ptosis, and ocular motility restriction	Decreased orbital fat signals, bony erosions, and sinusitis
IgG4-related orbital disease	Absent, mild to moderate	Chronic	Majority are Bilateral	Chronic noninflammatory lid swelling and proptosis	Isointensity on T1-weighted lesions, hypointensity on T2-weighted lesions, and homogenous gadolinium enhancing lesions

Note: Specific examination points and imaging findings can differentiate separate entities.

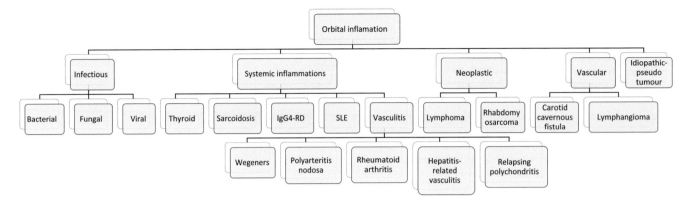

FIGURE 15C.1 Differential diagnosis of orbital inflammation.

Subtypes of OIS

Orbital inflammation can be due to a myriad of etiologies and hence classified accordingly (Figure 15C.1).

Idiopathic orbital inflammation

When the cause of an inflamed orbit cannot be determined, the term idiopathic OIS is applied. The term is used synonymously with nonspecific orbital inflammation (NSOI), also known as orbital inflammatory pseudotumor and idiopathic orbital inflammation.[2] This inflammation can be localized or diffuse. Idiopathic OIS is the third most common orbital disease after thyroid eye disease and orbital lymphoma.[3] It is the most common cause of painful orbital mass in adults.

When localized, inflammation can affect the EOMs (orbital myositis), lacrimal gland (dacryoadenitis), sclera (scleritis), uvea (uveitis), and the superior orbital fissure and cavernous sinus (Tolosa–Hunt syndrome). Optic peri neuritis refers to inflammation around the optic nerve sheath (as opposed to optic neuritis, which is inflammation of the nerve itself). It often involves more than one structure.

Due to a lack of defining criteria, the true incidence of the disorder is difficult to evaluate. Nonspecific inflammation has been shown to account for up to 6.3% of orbital disorders. It represents approximately 5–8% of all orbital masses.[4]

Pathogenesis

The orbital and periorbital tissues are quiet susceptible to inflammation from many conditions. The most commonly studied mechanism is immune-related idiopathic orbital inflammations. Co-occurrence of certain rheumatological disorders such as Wegener's granulomatosis, sarcoidosis, giant cell arteritis, SLE, dermatomyositis, and rheumatoid arthritis further indicate that it is an autoimmune disease. Specific circulating antibodies have not been yet found associated with the condition. Inflammatory cytokines such as interleukin-1 are known to be increased. Immunohistochemical staining of tissue samples demonstrates the presence of toll-like receptors suggesting an abnormal innate immune response may be responsible.

Biopsy is usually reserved for refractory or atypical cases. Histopathology typically shows a mixture of small lymphocytes, plasma cells, and histiocytes and fibrosis.

Histologically there are some subtypes of pseudotumor namely classical orbital pseudotumor, sclerosing orbital pseudotumor, granulomatous orbital pseudotumor, vasculitis orbital pseudotumor, and eosinophilic orbital pseudotumor.[5]

Signs and symptoms

The clinical course may be acute, subacute, or chronic. The lesion is most commonly restricted to the orbit; however, extension into adjacent retro-orbital structures can also be seen.

Clinical features are orbital pain and signs of eyelid swelling, proptosis, ophthalmoplegia, and varying degrees of vision loss. Symptoms of orbital inflammation also depend on involved structures, which can include the lacrimal gland, EOMs, sclera, fat, and optic nerve (Figure 15C.2). Pain is the most common symptom in adult and occurs 58–69% of the time followed by diplopia (31–38%). Periorbital edema/swelling is the most common sign and occurs 75–79.2% of the time followed by proptosis (32–62.5%), EOM restriction (54.2%), red eye (48%), chemosis (29%), decreased vision (20.8%), and ptosis (16.7%). Therefore, physical examination of suspected patients should include lid assessment (retraction/lid lag/lagophthalmos), orbital assessment (proptosis), EOMs (restriction), globe (injection/chemosis), and optic nerve function (visual acuity/color plates/relative afferent pupillary defect). In children, proptosis is typically mild or moderate, visual acuity loss is common, and periorbital swelling tends to be worse in the morning and improve throughout the day. Bilateral involvement is present in approximately 25% of adult patients but in 45% of children.[6-8] Most children also report systemic symptoms, including headache, vomiting, sore throat, or fever. Patients commonly report preceding upper respiratory symptoms or flu-like illness. Pediatric cases show higher rates of uveitis, disc edema, and eosinophilia than adults in conjunction with their orbital inflammation although the overall prevalence of disease is less common in these patients. Presentation may be similar to orbital cellulitis, including acute onset of symptoms over hours to days. Ptosis, chemosis, conjunctival injection, and bilateral presentation point toward a diagnosis of pseudotumor rather than an infection. Overall uveitis maybe underreported in these patients, hence a slit lamp examination is essential in all such cases. The uncommon presentations may include exudative detachment and scleritis.

The disease is also associated with lower socioeconomic status, high body mass index, and use of oral bisphosphonate, lithium, and chemotherapies.[9]

Workup

Laboratory workup is needed to rule out other morbidities. Complete blood count, electrolytes, thyroid function tests, sedimentation rate, antinuclear antibodies, ANCAs, ACE level, rapid plasma regain test, and rheumatoid factor should be done.

CT scan is the preferred method because of its good inherent contrast of orbital fat, muscle, bony structures, and air in the

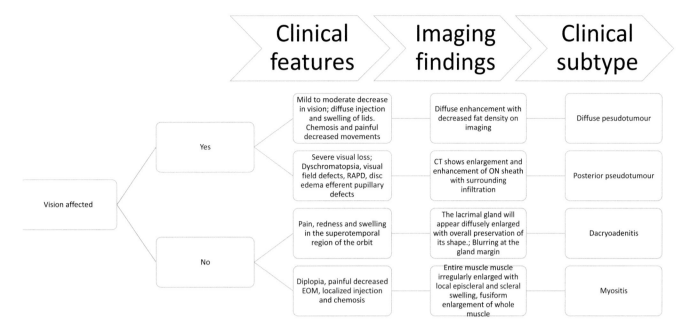

FIGURE 15C.2 The anatomical subtypes of idiopathic orbital inflammation and their clinical presentations, with radiological features.

adjacent paranasal sinuses. MRI is preferred in demonstrating soft tissue changes in the region of the cavernous sinus/superior orbital fissure due to beam hardening and bone streak artifacts seen in CT.[10] Diffusion-weighted images may differentiate inflammation from orbital cellulitis and lymphoid tissue.

Different imaging findings may be observed depending on the clinical subtype involved (Figure 15C.2). In case of myositis, enlargement of the single or multiple EOMs will be seen. Unilateral single muscle inflammation with tendon involvement is the most common. The most frequently involved muscle is the medial rectus followed by the superior rectus, lateral rectus, and inferior rectus. There may be infiltrates throughout the orbital fat bordering the muscle, blurring the margin of the muscle. Inflammatory tissues surrounding an unenhanced optic nerve may demonstrate the classical, "tramline" sign in cases of perineuritis. The cavernous sinus and middle cranial fossa are the two most common locations for intracranial extension. Intracranial involvement can feature abnormal soft tissue in the superior orbital fissure, expansion of the ipsilateral cavernous sinus, and thickening of the meninges contiguous with the orbital inflammation.

Management
Treatment is largely with steroids, which is the first-line treatment for these patients. Eighty percent of patients respond well to prolonged high-dose oral corticosteroid therapy with a long and slow taper. Oral doses are started at 1–1.5 mg/kg daily with a slow taper over 4–8 weeks. Response is typically rapid, with dramatic symptom improvement within 24–48 hours. A small number of cases will spontaneously resolve. Nonsteroidal anti-inflammatory medication may be used in conjunction with steroid therapy or as monotherapy in mild cases. Recurrence is more likely with bilateral disease. Pediatric patients also respond well to steroid treatment, and biopsy is typically undertaken only in cases where the patient has a poor response to an initial trial of steroids. Steroid-sparing agents may be considered earlier in patients with OIS that are found to have uveitis. Refractory

patients may receive radiation therapy as well as steroid-sparing agents.[11,12,13] A wide range of interventions in adults not responding to steroids have been reported, including cyclophosphamide, methotrexate, intravenous immunoglobulin, cyclosporine, biologic agents including rituximab and infliximab, radiation, and surgical debulking.[14]

Course and outcome
A single unilateral episode generally recovers fully without any long-term sequelae. Uveitis is associated with recurrent disease and residual impairment. Severe disease, bilateral involvement, or recurrent disease may also lead to permanent loss of visual acuity along with residual proptosis or strabismus in some patients. Severe acute complications such as orbital compartment syndrome may compromise blood flow to the optic nerve. Forty percent of biopsy-proven cases can relapse. Figure 15C.3 outlines the steps in workup and management of a case of pseudotumor.

Orbital inflammation related to thyroid eye disease
Thyroid eye disease is the most common cause of orbital inflammation in adults and has been found to account for nearly 60% of cases of orbital inflammation in the 21- to 60-year-old age-group.[15] The active inflammatory phase of thyroid eye disease is characterized by orbital discomfort, periocular and conjunctival edema and redness, and progression in proptosis, strabismus, or optic neuropathy. Clinically, it can be identified by clinical features of lid retraction. In contrast to myositis, EOM enlargement in thyroid is characterized by sparing of the tendon, which may be a useful sign on CT and MRI. Involvement of the insertions and irregular borders of the EOMs is usually a sign of myositis.

Orbital inflammation related to sarcoidosis
Sarcoidosis is a multisystem granulomatous inflammatory disease that affects the respiratory tract, skin, and eyes. Ocular involvement is reported in up to 50% of affected patients and is characterized by noncaseating granulomas of the conjunctiva, uveitis, optic neuropathy, or orbital involvement of the lacrimal

Adequate history- Similar episodes in the past/chronicity and duration of disease. Trauma, infection, systemic disorders (including cancer and immunological compromise)

Baseline work up-CBC and cultures, Radiologic evaluation of orbit and sinus (CT) Rule out- Thyroid orbitopathy, (Thyroid function test), Sarcoidosis: (ACE, lysozyme and chest radiograph); Wegener's granulomatosis; (ANCA studies, Pulmonary and renal function evaluation.)

For presumed idiopathic orbital inflammatory syndrome initial treatment. Systemic prednisone 1.0-1.5 mg/kg per day for 1-2 weeks with taper over 5-8 weeks

Recurrence or no response; consider biopsy for definitive diagnosis (+steroid sparing agents)

If biopsy findings are consistent-restart systemic steroid with slower taper

If steroid intolerant, non-responsive or dependent consider radiation therapy lowdose external beam irradiation, typically 1500-2000 cGy fractionated over 10 days

Surgical debulking if the lesion is easily accessible or if there is a severely progressive and disabling clinical course

FIGURE 15C.3 Outline for workup of a patient with pseudotumor.

gland, EOM, or fat. The lacrimal gland is the most common site of involvement, in 42–63% of patients, followed by orbit, eyelid, and lacrimal sac. Relatively nontender inflammation of the lacrimal glands points toward a sarcoidosis. Diagnosis can be made by conjunctival and/or lacrimal gland biopsy. Serum ACE, if elevated, may be helpful in diagnosing sarcoidosis. Treatment involves steroids and sometimes methotrexate or other immunosuppressive medications.[16–18]

Orbital inflammation related to systemic granulomatous disorders

Wegener's granulomatosis is a systemic vasculitis of small vessels that typically affects the renal and respiratory systems. Ocular involvement is demonstrated in up to 50% of involved patients, and Wegener's granulomatosis is the diagnosis in 15% of scleritis patients. Orbital involvement includes mass lesions, pain, epiphora, and diplopia. Treatment requires both systemic corticosteroids and other systemic medication such as cyclophosphamide.

Erdheim–Chester is a systemic non-Langerhans histiocytic xanthogranulomatous inflammatory disease with variable orbital involvement ranging from mild impairment of function to devastating loss of visual acuity secondary to mass effect.

The Tolosa–Hunt syndrome is a painful ophthalmoplegia with variable CN involvement including motor, sensory, and oculosympathetic pathways localizing to the region of the cavernous sinus or superior orbital fissure.

Localized OIS may occur in the lacrimal gland, EOMs, or optic nerve sheath. The typical acute presentation of dacryoadenitis includes pain, enlargement of the lacrimal gland, an S-shaped ptosis of the upper eyelid, and tenderness to palpation. Inflammatory disease of the lacrimal gland may also present in a subacute or chronic form in which a painless mass appears in the region of the lacrimal fossa.

IgG4-related orbital disease

IgG4-related disease (IgG4-RD) is a lymphoproliferative disease which affects different organs. The largest series of patients come from Japan, where the disease was first described. Average patients are middle aged, and orbital disease affects men and women equally. Orbital involvement presents with a variety of clinical features namely sclerosing dacryoadenitis, myositis with nerve enlargement, eosinophilia, pachymeningitis, systemic involvement, and sclerosing orbital inflammation. Those patients thought to have IgG4-related ocular disease have more frequent systemic symptoms, less conjunctival involvement, and more commonly develop sclerosis than other patients with OIS. Involvement of EOMs or orbital soft tissue is also associated with proptosis. EOM involvement may cause pain, diplopia, restrictive strabismus (less common than in Graves' orbitopathy), and enlargement of the infraorbital canal/bone. The inferior rectus muscle is the most commonly affected EOM, followed by the superior rectus–levator complex, lateral rectus, medial rectus, inferior oblique, and superior oblique muscles.

Diagnostic criteria include a dense lymphoplasmacytic infiltrate with elevated IgG41/IgG1 plasma cell ratio, storiform fibrosis, and obliterative phlebitis. Serum IgG4 may or may not be elevated. Pediatric cases have also been reported. They are less likely to respond adequately to steroid therapy alone and may require other agents such as methotrexate or rituximab.[19–21]

Orbital inflammation related to herpes zoster

Herpes zoster ophthalmicus can be triggered by reactivation of varicella zoster virus that is dormant in the trigeminal nerve ganglia. Reactivation of varicella zoster virus can be triggered by aging, an immunocompromised host, trauma, surgery, iatrogenic immunosuppression, tuberculosis, syphilis, and radiation therapy. Majority of patients with herpes zoster ophthalmicus have ocular complications, including blepharitis, keratoconjunctivitis, iritis, scleritis, and acute retinal necrosis. Ophthalmoplegia was found in 3.5–10.1% of two large herpes zoster ophthalmicus series. Among the cases with extraocular nerve palsies, oculomotor nerve palsy is the most frequent and abducens nerve palsy is the second most frequent.[22,23]

Orbital involvement in ophthalmic zoster is extremely rare but reported. It can occur due to extensive vasculitis, hemorrhage, perineuritis, and inflammatory cell infiltrate affecting all orbital contents

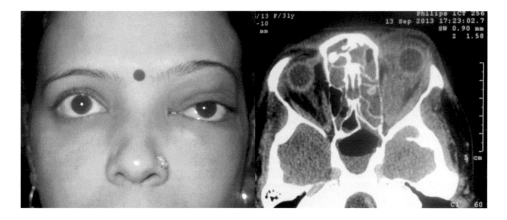

FIGURE 15C.4   A 31-year-old female diagnosed as orbital cellulitis. She presented with left eye painful proptosis and lid erythema. Imaging revealed diffuse inflammation with fat stranding in preseptal, intraconal, and superomedial extraconal region, as well as the ethmoid sinuses. (Image courtesy: Dr Usha Singh, Professor, Oculoplasty services, Advanced Eye Centre, PGIMER, India.)

including the EOMs and the optic nerve.[23] Histopathological studies have demonstrated significant perivascular and perineural inflammation of the ocular tissues, including the optic nerve, cavernous sinus, superior orbital fissure, and retina.

Orbital inflammatory signs in these patients include acute orbital myositis, perioptic neuritis, or dacryoadenitis, without zoster rash.[24] A number of cases presenting as orbital apex syndrome have been reported. Herpes zoster ophthalmicus preceded the ophthalmoplegia as orbital apex syndrome by a mean interval of 9.5 days in one such series. Sixty-five percent of these cases recovered completely or partially after antiviral and steroid therapy, although anisocoria remained in most cases.[25] Authors suggest combined antiviral and steroid therapy should be effective in cases of orbital apex syndrome if the steroid therapy is used for at least 4 months.[26] Ophthalmoplegia and optic neuritis are rare but are responsive to antiviral or steroid treatment. Suspicion of orbital invasion should be kept within 14 days after onset of herpes zoster ophthalmicus.

Orbital inflammation related to sino-orbital infections

Orbital cellulitis is a potentially life-threatening disease often associated with antecedent sinus disease, dental procedures, or trauma and is typically accompanied by fever and leukocytosis. These patients need hospitalization for intensive, broad-spectrum intravenous antimicrobial therapy pending identification of the inciting organism.

Due to close proximity of the paranasal sinuses to the orbit, contiguous spread of infection might occur, especially in immunocompromised hosts. Most common of these infection are fungal. It is potentially fatal due to spread to middle cranial fossa via superior orbital fissure and optic canal; with mortality of up to 80%.[27] The most common presenting features include pain, proptosis, and extraocular movement restriction (Figure 15C.4).

Imaging features of sino-orbital diseases are nonspecific and may be confused with varied orbital pathologies, most commonly idiopathic orbital inflammatory disease. CT scan usually reveals a heterogeneous, enhancing mass with density similar to EOMs. Concomitant sinus disease has been reported in 60–90% of patients by various authors.[28] MRI provides better details of the posterior orbit, optic canal, and cavernous sinus. Subtle signs of sinus involvement, such as enhancement of the sinus lining and focal hypointense areas within it, may be picked up on MRI.

Vigorous antifungal therapy is needed in such cases. Exenteration has been recommended by some authors in all patients with retrobulbar and apical involvement.[29]

Conclusion

Orbital inflammation may be caused by a myriad of causes like infections and various systemic diseases. While the term OIS specifically refers to a benign inflammatory cause of inflammation of the orbit, the pathology may often spread to structures beyond the orbit like cavernous sinus and superior orbital fissure affecting other cranial nerves as well. Recognising systemic associations may aid in the holistic management of a patient with OIS.

Multiple-Choice Questions

Orbital inflammation

1. Which of the following clinical features differentiate pediatric pseudotumor from adults?
   a. More frequent involvement of the lacrimal gland in children.
   b. More frequent constitutional symptoms such as headache, fever, vomiting, and peripheral eosinophilia in children.
   c. Greater resistance to steroid therapy in adults.
   d. More pain in children.

   Answer:
   b. More frequent constitutional symptoms such as headache, fever, vomiting, and peripheral eosinophilia in children.

2. The most frequently involved extraocular muscle in Graves' ophthalmopathy is the:
   a. Inferior rectus
   b. Lateral rectus
   c. Superior rectus
   d. Medial rectus

   Answer:
   a. Inferior rectus

3. A 7-year-old boy presents with a 3-day history of progressive proptosis, injection, and pain of the left eye. He is systemically well with normal temperature. White blood cell count is normal, and emergent orbital computed tomography (CT) scanning reveals superonasal orbital infiltration with bony erosion. The diagnosis that must be excluded at this point is:
   a. Bacterial orbital cellulitis
   b. Optic nerve glioma
   c. Frontal sinus mucocele
   d. Rhabdomyosarcoma

Answer:

   d. Rhabdomyosarcoma

4. Computed tomography (CT) scan findings that differentiate orbital pseudotumor from Graves' ophthalmopathy include:
   a. Enlargement of multiple extraocular muscles
   b. Enlargement of EOM tendons
   c. Unilateral involvement
   d. Pain

Answer:

   b. Enlargement of EOM tendons

5. All of the following disorders may be associated with a clinical presentation indistinguishable from typical inflammatory orbital pseudotumor, EXCEPT:
   a. Systemic lupus erythematosus (SLE)
   b. Polyarteritis nodosa
   c. Wegener's granulomatosis
   d. Sarcoidosis

Answer:

   d. Sarcoidosis

References

1. Gordon LK. Orbital inflammatory disease: A diagnostic and therapeutic challenge. Eye (Lond). 2006;20(10):1196–1206.
2. Weber AL, Romo LV, Sabates NR. Pseudotumor of the orbit: Clinical, pathologic, and radiologic evaluation. Radiol Clin North Am. 1999;37:151–168.
3. Yuen SJ, Rubin P. Idiopathic orbital inflammation: Ocular mechanisms and clinicopathology. Ophthalmol Clin N Am. 2002;15:121–126.
4. Li Y, Lip G, Chong V, Yuan J, Ding Z. Idiopathic orbital inflammation syndrome with retro-orbital involvement: A retrospective study of eight patients. PLoS One. 2013;8:e57126.
5. Fujii H, Fujisada H, Kondo T, Takahashi T, Okada S. Orbital pseudotumor: Histopathological classification and treatment. Ophthalmologica. 1985;190(4):230–242.
6. Yuen SJ, Rubin PA. Idiopathic orbital inflammation: Distribution, clinical features, and treatment outcome. Arch Ophthalmol. 2003;121(4):491–499.
7. Schmidt J, Pulido J, Matteson E. Ocular manifestations of systemic disease: Antineutrophil cytoplasmic antibody-associated vasculitis. Curr Opin Ophthalmol. 2011;22(6):489–495.
8. Mottow LS, Jakobiec FA. Idiopathic inflammatory orbital pseudotumor in childhood. Clinical characteristics. Arch Ophthalmol. 1978;96:1410–1417.
9. Jacob MK. Idiopathic orbital inflammatory disease. Oman J Ophthalmol. 2012;5:124–125.
10. Kline LB, Hoyt WF. The Tolosa-Hunt syndrome. J Neurol Neurosurg Psychiatry. 2001;71:577–582.
11. Espinoza GM. Orbital inflammatory pseudotumors: Etiology, differential diagnosis, and management. Curr Rheumatol Rep. 2010;12:443–447.
12. Mendenhall WM, Lessner AM. Orbital pseudotumor. Am J Clin Oncol. 2010; 33:304–306.
13. Jacobs D, Galetta S. Diagnosis and management of orbital pseudotumor. Curr Opin Ophthalmol. 2002;13:347–351.
14. Rubin PA, Foster S. Etiology and management of idiopathic orbital inflammation. Am J Ophthalmol. 2004;138(6):1041–1043.
15. Dutton JJ. Orbit and lacrimal gland. In: Yanoff M, Duker JS, editors. Ophthalmology. St. Louis: Mosby, Inc.; 2004. pp.729–743.
16. Liu D, Birnbaum AD. Update on sarcoidosis. Curr Opin Ophthalmol. 2015;26(6):512–516.
17. Demirci H, Christianson MD. Orbital and adnexal involvement in sarcoidosis: Analysis of clinical features and systemic disease in 30 cases. Am J Ophthalmol. 2011;151(6):1074–1080.e1.
18. Prabhakaran VC, Saeed P, Esmaeli B, et al. Orbital and adnexal sarcoidosis. Arch Ophthalmol. 2007;125(12):1657–1662.
19. Stone JH, Zen Y, Deshpande V. IgG4-related disease. N Engl J Med. 2012;366(6):539–551.
20. Wallace ZS, Khosroshahi A, Jakobiec FA, et al. IgG4-related systemic disease as a cause of "idiopathic" orbital inflammation, including orbital myositis, and trigeminal nerve involvement. Surv Ophthalmol. 2012;57(1):26–33.
21. Wu A, Andrew NH, McNab AA, et al. IgG4-related ophthalmic disease: Pooling of published cases and literature review. Curr Allergy Asthma Rep. 2015;15(6):27.
22. Womack LW, Liesegang TJ. Complications of herpes zoster ophthalmicus. Arch Ophthalmol. 1983;101(1):42–45.
23. Marsh RJ, Cooper M. Ophthalmic herpes zoster. Eye (Lond). 1993;7(Pt 3):350–370.
24. Bak E, Kim N, Khwarg SI, Choung HK. Case series: Herpes zoster ophthalmicus with acute orbital inflammation. Optom Vis Sci. 2018;95(4):405–410.
25. Sanjay S, Chan EW, Gopal L, et al. Complete unilateral ophthalmoplegia in herpes zoster ophthalmicus. J Neuroophthalmol. 2009;29(4):325–337.
26. Kurimoto T, Tonari M, Ishizaki N, et al. Orbital apex syndrome associated with herpes zoster ophthalmicus. Clin Ophthalmol. 2011;5:1603–1608.
27. Shamim MS, Siddiqui AA, Enam SA, Shah AA, Jooma R, Anwar S. Craniocerebral aspergillosis in immunocompetent hosts: Surgical perspective. Neurol India. 2007;55:274–281.
28. Adulkar NG, Radhakrishnan S, Vidhya N, Kim U. Invasive sino-orbital fungal infections in immunocompetent patients: A clinico-pathological study. Eye. 2019;33(6):988–994.
29. Mauriello JA Jr, Yepez N, Mostafavi R, Barofsky J, Kapila R, Baredes S, et al. Invasive rhinosino-orbital aspergillosis with precipitous visual loss. Can J Ophthalmol. 1995;30:124–130.

15D

CONGENITAL CRANIAL DYSINNERVATION DISORDER

Ramesh Kekunnaya, Mayank Jain

CASE STUDY

A 12-year-old girl presented with bilateral congenital, non-progressive external ophthalmoplegia with bilateral ptosis. The patient had a compulsory chin-up position and face turn. Extraocular movement examination revealed restricted extraocular movements with marked limitation to elevate the eye above the midline. How do you approach patient with such symptom complex?

Introduction

The term congenital cranial dysinnervation disorder (CCDD) was coined to encompass congenital, sporadic, non-progressive, or familial abnormalities of cranial musculature that results from developmental abnormalities of one or more cranial nerves with primary (absence of normal innervation) or secondary (aberrant innervation by other nerves) muscle dysinnervation (1). CCDD can be broadly categorized into three groups; those affecting vertical motility, disorders affecting horizontal motility, and those affecting predominantly facial weakness (Table 15D.1). Conditions included under the umbrella term of CCDD are namely congenital fibrosis of extraocular muscle (CFEOM), congenital ptosis, Duane retraction syndrome (DRS), Duane radial ray syndrome (DRRS), Brown syndrome, horizontal gaze palsy with progressive scoliosis (HGPPS), hereditary congenital facial palsy (HCFP), and Möbius syndrome (2).

Etiological factors

Previously, it was believed that these disorders were primarily due to myopathy of extraocular muscles (3). However, recent studies have shown that the above-mentioned disorders are largely

TABLE 15D.2: Various Mutations in CCDD Targeting Different Neuronal Functions

Gene Transcription	Microtubule Function	Receptor Signaling
• SALL4	• KIF21A	• CHN1
• PHOX2A	• TUBB3	• ROBO3
• HOXA1		
• HOXB1		

neuropathies rather than myopathy (4, 5). After birth, the axons of three cranial nerves destined to innervate the six extraocular muscles of each eye migrate along a pre-determined path. However, the factors guiding the ocular motor axons to their exact muscle targets are still poorly understood. Pathology arising due to the axonal misguidance leads to aberrant innervation of these muscles, resulting in various phenotypes (6, 7). Genes responsible for transcription, microtubule function, and receptor signaling (Table 15D.2) have been identified, and their mutation is responsible for various dysinnervation syndromes (2, 8). A summary of inheritance patterns and causative genes identified in different CCDD phenotypes are enlisted in Table 15D.3.

Congenital fibrosis of extraocular muscle

Clinical features

CFEOM is identified by the presence of bilateral congenital, non-progressive external ophthalmoplegia which may be complete or incomplete associated with severe bilateral ptosis. Initially thought to be a primary myopathy involving fibrosis of muscles around the eye, recent studies enumerate this entity as myopathy secondary to aberrant innervation of extraocular muscles (5, 9). Eyes are infraducted below the midline due to marked limitation of elevation and poor *Bell's* phenomenon. This is usually associated with limitation of depression, adduction, and variable

TABLE 15D.1: Classification of Various Congenital Cranial Dysinnervation Disorders

Congenital Cranial Dysinnervation Disorder (CCDD)		
Predominantly Vertical Disorder of Ocular Motility	**Predominantly Horizontal Disorder of Ocular Motility**	**Disorder of Facial Weakness**
• Congenital fibrosis of the extraocular muscles	• Duane retraction syndrome	• Congenital facial palsy
• Brown syndrome	• Duane radial ray syndrome	• Möbius syndrome (with abduction deficit)
• Congenital ptosis	• Horizontal gaze palsy with progressive scoliosis	

TABLE 15D.3: Inheritance Pattern and Associated Genes Identified in Various Disorders

Disorder	Genes Associated	Inheritance
CFEOM Type 1	*KIF21A*	Autosomal dominant
CFEOM Type 2	*ARIX* (previously called *PHOX2A*)	Autosomal recessive
CFEOM Type 3	*TUBB3*	Autosomal dominant
	KIF21A	
DRS	*CHN1*	Autosomal dominant
	SALL4	Autosomal dominant
	HOXA1	Autosomal recessive
DRRS	*SALL4*	Autosomal dominant
HGPPS	*ROBO3*	Autosomal recessive

DOI: 10.1201/9780429020278-22

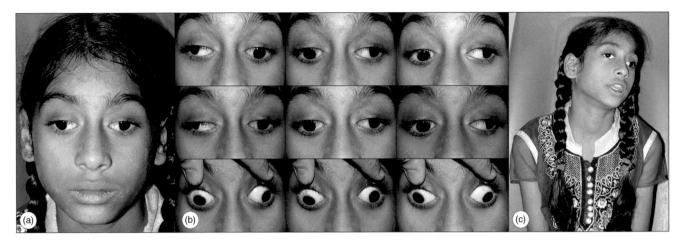

FIGURE 15D.1 (a) CFEOM Type 1 with bilateral ptosis and exotropia. (b) Nine-gaze collage showing limited extraocular movements with marked limitation to elevate the eye above the midline. (c) An anomalous head posture is adopted by the child with chin elevation and face turn for reading distant optotypes.

limitation of abduction. The patient has a compulsory chin-up position and face turn as shown in Figure 15D.1. Children may show *digitilo-palpebral* sign, in which the child uses finger, palm, or dorsum of the hand to elevate the ptotic eye. In these cases, the contralateral eye is usually amblyopic. Force duction test (FDT) is usually positive for restriction for all extraocular muscles.

Etiological classification and genetics
CFEOM Type 1
Also known as "Classical CFEOM," it presents with chin up position; orthotropic, esotropic, or exotropic eyes and inability to elevate the eyes above the midline. Convergence is seen on attempted elevation, simultaneous abduction on attempted horizontal gaze, and *Marcus Gunn jaw-winking* phenomenon are few of the synkinetic movements due to aberrant axonal routing as oculomotor nerve may be absent or hypoplastic. Due to high astigmatism seen in these patients, amblyopia is usually present. Patients show normal intelligence, but neurological abnormality can be associated infrequently. Inheritance is autosomal dominant with complete penetrance. Missense mutations in *KIF21A* gene, encoding a kinesin microtubule-associated motor protein, mapped to chromosome 12cen is largely responsible (10).

CFEOM Type 2
Clinical features are usually similar to the classical CFEOM, but the eyes are usually in exotropic position. High-resolution magnetic resonance imaging (MRI) has shown absent cranial nerve III and IV in CFEOM 2 patients. In some patients, the muscles supplied by oculomotor nerve viz. superior rectus, levator palpebrae superioris, inferior rectus, and medial rectus, and that supplied by trochlear nerve viz. superior oblique were found to be small, fibrotic, and thin strand-like (11). Autosomal recessive inheritance with complete penetrance is observed, frequently associated with history of parental consanguinity. The *ARIX* gene (previously called *PHOX2A*) encodes a transcription factor that is specifically involved in the determination of the noradrenergic neuronal phenotype. In an animal model, loss of function mutations has resulted in the loss of III and IV cranial nerves (12).

CFEOM Type 3
Patients in this subtype do not present with all the classical features of CFEOM and variable phenotypes such as bilateral or unilateral involvement, variable motility defects ranging from complete ophthalmoplegia (eyes fixed in hypo- and exotropic position) to less disabling and asymptomatic presentations with the ability to elevate eye above midline in some family members. Autosomal dominant inheritance with incomplete penetrance and variable expressivity is seen. The responsible gene has been mapped to chromosome 16 (13). *TUBB3* gene mutations are the most commonly found mutations in CFEOM3 (14). Mutations in the *KIF21A* gene are also responsible for a few cases (8).

Differential diagnosis
Major differential diagnoses are chronic progressive external ophthalmoplegia (CPEO) and ocular myasthenia. Table 15D.4 enlists the important differentiating features.

TABLE 15D.4: Differentiating Features between CPEO, Ocular Myasthenia and CFEOM

	Chronic Progressive External Ophthalmoplegia	Ocular Myasthenia	Congenital Fibrosis of Extraocular Muscle
Nature of disease	Progressive	Variable progression	Non-progressive
Diurnal variation	Absent	Present	Absent
MRI orbit – Extraocular muscle	Bright internal signal on T1	No bright internal signal on T1	Small EOM +/−Bright internal signal on T1
Others	• Mitochondrial cytopathy • Onset in second decade • Ragged red fibers on muscle biopsy	• Variable onset • Fatigability present • Positive ice pack test	• Aberrant innervation of muscles • Autosomal dominant and autosomal recessive inheritance

Treatment

Non-surgical management

Correction of refractive errors and appropriate management of amblyopia are important. Crutch glasses can be used to relieve the ptosis and prevention of ametropic amblyopia; however, this is only a temporary measure. At times, this should be the only treatment if surgery is contraindicated. Topical lubricants are prescribed in patients with poor *Bell's* phenomenon to prevent the cornea from exposure keratopathy.

Surgical management

Strabismus surgery is always done first, and the ptosis correction is planned later. This is because it is important to improve *Bell's* phenomenon prior to ptosis correction surgery, and secondly, the lid position may change after surgery on extraocular muscles. Recession of fibrosed horizontal rectus muscles is done to align the eye in the primary position. Larger than usual doses are kept while recessing the muscles as small recessions do not generally help. Bilateral inferior rectus recession can alleviate the chin-up position. Anterior segment ischemia can occur post-operatively, as more than two rectus muscle surgery in an eye is a known risk factor (15). Lid surgery for correction of ptosis may be contraindicated due to increased risk of corneal exposure in cases of poor *Bell's* phenomenon.

Duane retraction syndrome

Clinical features

DRS is characterized by a combination of variable restrictions in ductions, globe retraction, palpebral fissure height changes, overshoots, and variable letter patterns (V/Y/X/A). Type 1 DRS classically show limitation of abduction, narrowing of palpebral fissure on adduction, retraction of the globe on adduction associated with either upshoot or downshoot of the adducted eye (Figure 15D.2). The child may have an anomalous head posture. Other ocular findings may include nystagmus, ptosis, and epibulbar dermoid.

Classification

DRS is clinically characterized by dysinnervation of the lateral rectus. Huber classified DRS based on electromyography study. Type 1 with limitation of abduction, Type 2 with limitation of adduction (Figure 15D.3), and Type 3 with limitation of both abduction and adduction (16). Clinically, Type 1 is the most commonly encountered retraction syndrome, with a female preponderance of around 57%. It is important to understand that esotropia, exotropia, and orthotropia can be found in any of the subtypes of DRS. Up to 15% of the cases presents with bilateral involvement (17, 18).

Etiology

Apart from the dysinnervation of the lateral rectus muscle, different other causes such as abducens nucleus hypoplasia, absence of abducens nucleus, or absence of abducens nerve have been identified.

Genetics

CHN1 gene is responsible for encoding signaling molecule α2-chimaerin and its mutation, or overexpression of wild-type α2-chimaerin results in stalling of axons of third cranial nerve with aberrant branching. Mutation of *CHN1* gene can result in familial or isolated DRS. *SALL4* is another identified gene in Duane's phenotype. *HOXA1* genes are responsible for transcription encoding which is critical for hindbrain development and its mutation results in bilateral DRS, deafness, and autism (8, 19, 20).

Differential diagnosis

1. *Sixth nerve palsy* – see Table 15D.5.
2. *Infantile esotropia* – Presence of large angle esotropia with an absence of abduction limitation on *Doll's* eye maneuver. Patching of either eye in a small child is usually helpful to observe full motility of horizontal extraocular muscles.
3. *Möbius syndrome* – Retraction syndrome associated with facial nerve palsy characterized by mask-like facies.

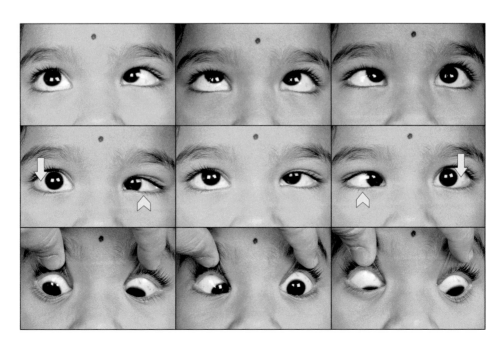

FIGURE 15D.2 Bilateral Duane restriction syndrome showing bilateral limitation of abduction (arrow) and retraction of the globe with the eye in adduction, characterized by narrowing of the palpebral fissure (arrowhead).

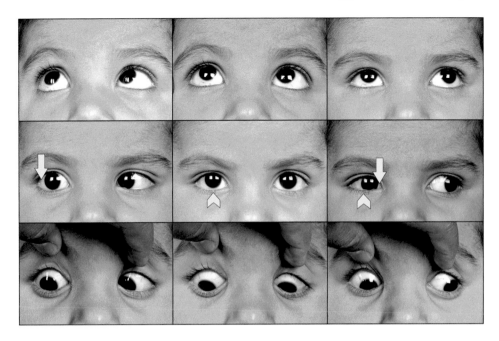

FIGURE 15D.3 Nine-gaze collage of a child with Type 3 DRS showing limitation of abduction and adduction of the right eye (arrow). Note the narrowing of right palpebral fissure in primary position (arrowhead), which narrows further with the eye in adducted position and widens with the eye in the abduction.

4. *Congenital oculomotor apraxia* – Impaired horizontal gaze in which a child is unable to generate horizontal saccades, subsequently resulting in head thrusting past the fixation target.

Treatment

Correction of refractive error is an essential component of nonsurgical management of DRS, and treatment of amblyopia should be initiated where possible. To decide for surgical correction, the following points should be assessed prior:

1. Deviation in primary position
2. Quantification of limitation of abduction
3. The severity of globe retraction
4. Overshoots present in adduction

It is crucial to note that the patients with orthotropia in the primary position and good binocular function need not undergo any

TABLE 15D.5: Differentiating Features of Duane Retraction Syndrome and Sixth Nerve Palsy

Features	Duane Retraction Syndrome	Sixth Nerve Palsy
1. Type of strabismus	Restrictive	Paralytic
2. Saccades	Restrictive type	Floating saccades
3. Primary position deviation	Disproportionately smaller deviation to the abduction limitation	Much larger and proportional to abduction limitation
4. Binocularity	Difficult, with poor convergence ability	Possible, with good convergence ability
5. Globe retraction	Present	Absent
6. Vertical deviations	Present as upshoot or downshoot	Absent

surgery (Figure 15D.4). Horizontal deviations can be managed by unilateral or bilateral medial rectus recession. Lateral rectus recession can be performed in cases of exo-DRS.

Resection of horizontal muscles is rarely performed and should be religiously avoided as it increases the retraction of the globe and causes significant narrowing of the palpebral fissure.

Upshoot or downshoot in adduction can be corrected by lateral rectus Y-split combined with the recession of horizontal rectus muscles. Globe retractions can be tackled with the differential recession of medial and lateral rectus of the affected eye. Abduction limitation can be improved slightly with superior rectus muscle transposition alone to lateral rectus.

Duane radial ray syndrome

DRRS (Okihiro syndrome) comprises unilateral or bilateral Duane syndrome (Type 1 or 3) with unilateral or bilateral radial dysplasia. The most common defect seen is hypoplasia of thumb which can range from hypoplasia of the thenar eminence to a phocomelic limb as seen in cases of thalidomide ingestion during pregnancy (1). The associated features include pigmentary disturbance, anal stenosis, atrial septal defect, hearing impairment, renal anomalies, external ear malformations, and facial asymmetry (21). Autosomal dominant inheritance with *SALL4* gene mutation is responsible for DRRS phenotype.

Congenital Brown syndrome

Clinical features

It is clinically identified by an inability to elevate the affected eye in adduction along with the widening of the palpebral fissure in adducted position (Figure 15D.5). Hypotropia may be present in the ipsilateral eye with increasing severity of this disease.

Etiology

It is also known as "Superior oblique sheath syndrome" and initially thought to be due to short anterior tendon sheath of

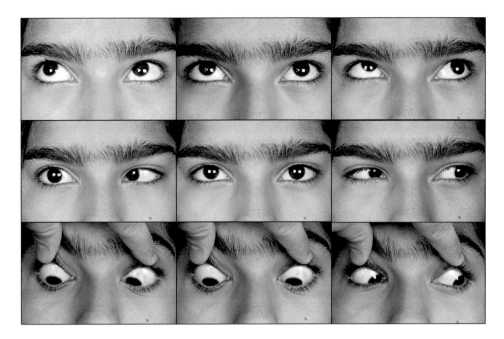

FIGURE 15D.4 Right eye DRS Type 1 with orthotropia in primary position. Note that there is a minimal retraction and no overshoot of left eye in the adducted position. This patient was advised against any surgical correction to improve right eye abduction.

superior oblique as described by Brown (22). However, subsequent studies disproved this fact. Congenital Brown syndrome can result from tendon-trochlear abnormality due to persistent embryonic trabeculae between superior oblique and trochlea. Absence of trochlear nerve or nucleus can result in abnormal development of axons of the fourth nerve (23). This will cause a lack of innervation or paradoxical innervation of superior oblique from the fibers of the oculomotor nerve. This abnormal innervation causes hypoplastic superior oblique with taut and immobile tendon through the trochlea (24, 25). Co-contraction of both inferior and superior oblique results in widening of palpebral fissure in adduction, as the functional origin of both the muscles is anterior to the equator (26). Acquired Brown syndrome can be due to a structural abnormality in the trochlea or tendon sheath, which does not form a part of CCDD.

Genetics
Congenital Brown syndrome often occurs sporadically but several familial cases have been reported in the literature including identical twins (27, 28). Brown syndrome is mostly unilateral with around 10% of the cases being bilateral and no sexual preference is usually seen (29).

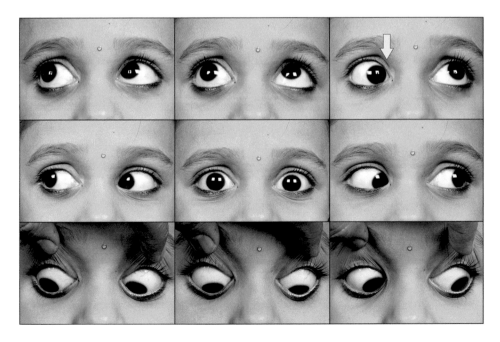

FIGURE 15D.5 Brown syndrome in a child showing limitation of elevation of the right eye, characteristically seen more in adduction (arrow).

Differential diagnosis

1. *Inferior oblique paresis*: Presence of superior oblique overaction with inferior oblique paresis pattern on Parks three-step test. Compensatory head tilt, A-pattern, and absence of restriction on FDT differentiate it from the Brown syndrome.
2. *Mono-elevation deficit*: Restriction in elevation in both adduction and abduction along with component of ptosis or pseudoptosis.
3. *Blowout fracture*: History of trauma with complaints of paresthesia and signs of enophthalmos is present. Restriction in elevation is more marked in abduction than in adduction.
4. *Thyroid eye disease*: Restriction in elevation is more marked in abduction than in adduction along with other signs such as lid lag, lid retraction, and lateral flaring of the upper lid.
5. *Fat adherence syndrome*: History of extraocular muscle surgery, especially inferior oblique. Also, restriction in elevation is more marked in abduction than in adduction.

Treatment

Orthotropia or small deviation in primary position, presence of binocular fusion, and absence of anomalous head posture warrants no surgical intervention. Observation plays a vital role in such cases as spontaneous resolution has been reported (30). If no intervention is planned, it is important to monitor any threat to binocularity and acuity caused by decompensation. Surgery is indicated in the following circumstances; hypotropia in primary position, anomalous head posture, diplopia, and downshoot of the eye in adduction. Choice of procedures depends upon the degree of tightness on FDT. Surgery can vary in graded weakening of superior oblique, like posterior tenotomy, posterior tenectomy, Z tenotomy, recession, split-lengthening procedures, and spacer tenotomy (including silicone expander and chicken suture lengthening). These procedures can be combined with ipsilateral inferior oblique recession (to counteract post-operative IO overaction) or contralateral superior rectus recession. Complications largely include superior oblique palsy, persistent vertical deviation in primary position, downshoot in adduction, limitation of downward movement, scarring, and foreign body extrusion (31).

Möbius syndrome

Clinical features

Möbius syndrome is a non-progressive disease characterized by congenital facial and abducens nerve paralysis (Figure 15D.6). Dysphagia, limb malformations, cranial dysmorphism, Poland anomaly (hypoplasia of the pectoralis minor muscle), and mental retardation may be observed (32). Esotropia is commonly seen with variable convergence. *Bell's* phenomenon is usually preserved, but nystagmus and ptosis are not commonly seen (33). Difficulty in feeding and tracheobronchial aspiration are the main issues encountered in infancy. With advancing age, inexpressive face and developing speech disorders lead to difficulty in social adaptation (34).

Etiology

Möbius syndrome has been associated with the use of misoprostol, thalidomide, ergotamine, and cocaine; therefore, a hypoxic or ischemic insult in the first trimester of pregnancy has been a suggested mechanism. Most common etiology is absence or

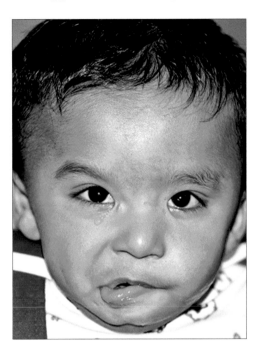

FIGURE 15D.6 Mobius syndrome. Absence of facial features of the left side is seen. Left sixth nerve palsy was also present in this child.

hypoplasia of the central brain nuclei. Other possible reasons are destructive degeneration of the central brain nuclei, peripheral nerve involvement, and myopathy. However, MRI anomalies have not been documented in a few cases with no structural brain or venous anomalies (35). A wide spectrum of clinical features and various cranial nerve involvements directs our understanding that Möbius syndrome is a developmental disorder of the brainstem.

Genetics

Most cases are sporadic, with no family history, but few cases of autosomal dominant, autosomal recessive, and X-linked recessive inheritance have been documented in the literature. Cytogenetic anomalies at loci 1p22 and 13q12.2-13 have been found, but no specific gene has been attributed to the disorder yet.

Differential diagnosis

Congenital sixth nerve palsy, infantile esotropia, and DRS can simulate Möbius syndrome presenting as large angle esotropia with variable lateral rectus limitation, but none of these is associated with facial nerve palsy. Other differentials are HGPPS, oculomotor apraxia, and congenital myotonic dystrophy.

Treatment

Appropriate refractive error correction and amblyopia management is imperative in any strabismus. Aggressive patching can prevent suppression of either eye, and the child may have benefit of basic binocular vision. Prevention of corneal exposure due to poor eye closure is also important. Botulinum toxin injection administered in medial rectus muscle can prevent contracture if given early in life. Bilateral medial rectus recession along with vertical rectus muscles transposition to lateral rectus can provide sufficient abduction force to align eyes in primary gaze. Surgeries are usually performed as a staged procedure because responses to surgical dosage are better calibrated.

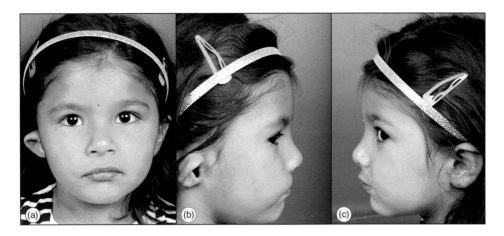

FIGURE 15D.7 (a) Right-sided hereditary congenital facial palsy. (b) Right profile showing the absence of nasolabial fold, hypoplasia of facial bones with right microtia (deformed pinna) compared to the left side (c).

Horizontal gaze palsy with progressive scoliosis (HGPPS)

Congenital HGPPS is an autosomal recessive condition in which individuals are born with a restriction of horizontal gaze, coinherited with progressive scoliosis, which may begin as early as first year of life. The responsible gene for this rare condition has been mapped to chromosome 11q23-q25. *ROBO3* is an important gene for axonal guidance that guides the hindbrain axons in crossing the midline. *ROBO3* mutation results in uncrossed motor and sensory projections in patients with HGPPS culminating in bilateral gaze palsy (19). MRI of affected cases have revealed a normal corpus callosum, cerebrum, and cerebellum; flattening of the pons and medulla, with midline medullary cleft (8). Patients have interneuron medial longitudinal fasciculus dysinnervation, and uncrossed, dorsal column and corticospinal tracts as there is axonal pathway disruption (36).

Hereditary congenital facial palsy (HCFP)

It is characterized by bilateral but an asymmetric isolated facial weakness (Figure 15D.7) that is distinct from Möbius syndrome; as there is no restriction of ocular motility. HCFP is usually autosomal dominant inherited. Studies have shown poorly developed facial nerve roots and reduced number of neurons within the facial nerve nuclei. Two genetic loci, namely HCFP1 and HCFP2 have been identified, but the causative genes are still not defined yet (37).

Hereditary congenital ptosis (HCP)

It is defined as an isolated drooping of the upper eyelid with no other significant ocular features. Bilateral involvement is more common, though asymmetrical. The severity of ptosis in HCP can range from mild to severe. Currently, two loci are mapped by linkage analysis. PTOS1, an autosomal dominant locus on chromosome 1 and PTOS2, is an X-linked locus (38, 39).

Conclusion

CCDD encompasses various congenital and sporadic abnormalities of cranial musculature resulting from developmental anomalies. CFEOM, congenital ptosis, DRS, DRRS, Brown syndrome, HGPPS, HCFP and Mobius syndrome are the conditions included under this umbrella term. Classical clinical features and key neuro-ophthalmic examination findings may help in differentiating these complex syndromes.

Multiple-Choice Questions

1. In congenital fibrosis of extraocular muscle, what is/are the primary pathology?
   a. Fibrosis of extraocular muscle
   b. Congenital agenesis of extraocular muscle
   c. Aberrant innervation of extraocular muscle
   d. Congenital agenesis of cranial nerve/nucleus

   Answer:

   c and d.   Aberrant innervation of extraocular muscle and Congenital agenesis of cranial nerve/nucleus.

2. Reason for retraction of the globe in Duane retraction syndrome is:
   a. Congenital microphthalmia.
   b. Amblyopia leading to deprivation of stimulus for the eye to grow.
   c. Abnormal head of lateral rectus which contracts and retracts the globe.
   d. Co-contraction of horizontal rectus muscles.

   Answer:

   d.   Co-contraction of horizontal rectus muscles.

3. Treatment of Brown syndrome includes:
   a. Superior rectus recession
   b. Inferior rectus resection
   c. Superior oblique weakening
   d. Inferior oblique strengthening

   Answer:

   c.   Superior oblique weakening

4. The Möbius syndrome affects which of the following cranial nerves?
   a. Fifth and sixth nerves
   b. Sixth and seventh nerves

c. Third and fourth nerves
d. Third and sixth nerves

Answer:

b. Sixth and seventh nerves

References

1. Gutowski NJ, Bosley TM, Engle EC. 110th ENMC International Workshop: The congenital cranial dysinnervation disorders (CCDDs): Naarden, The Netherlands, 25–27 October, 2002. Neuromuscular Disorders. 2003;13(7):573–8.
2. Gutowski NJ, Chilton JK. The congenital cranial dysinnervation disorders. Arch Dis Child. 2015;100(7):678–81.
3. Apt L, Axelrod RN. Generalized fibrosis of the extraocular muscles. Am J Ophthalmol. 1978;85(6):822–9.
4. Assaf AA. Bilateral congenital vertical gaze disorders: Congenital muscle fibrosis or congenital central nervous abnormality? Neuro-Ophthalmol. 1997;17(1):23–30.
5. Brodsky MC, Pollock SC, Buckley EG. Neural misdirection in congenital ocular fibrosis syndrome: Implications and pathogenesis. J Pediatr Ophthalmol Strabismus. 1989;26(4):159–61.
6. Matsuo R, Yamagishi M, Wakiya K, Tanaka Y, Ito E. Target innervation is necessary for neuronal polyploidization in the terrestrial slug Limax. Dev Neurobiol. 2013;73(8):609–20.
7. Traboulsi EI. Congenital cranial dysinnervation disorders and more. J AAPOS. 2007;11(3):215–7.
8. Engle EC. The genetic basis of complex strabismus. Pediatr Res. 2006;59(3):343–8.
9. Demer JL, Clark RA, Engle EC. Magnetic resonance imaging evidence for widespread orbital dysinnervation in congenital fibrosis of extraocular muscles due to mutations in KIF21A. Invest Ophthalmol Vis Sci. 2005;46(2):530–9.
10. Heidary G, Engle EC, Hunter DG. Congenital fibrosis of the extraocular muscles. In: Seminars in ophthalmology. Informa Healthcare USA, Inc. vol. 23/1; 2008. pp. 3–8.
11. Bosley TM, Abu-Amero KK, Oystreck DT. Congenital cranial dysinnervation disorders: A concept in evolution. Curr Opin Ophthalmol. 2013;24(5):398–406.
12. Nakano M, Yamada K, Fain J, Sener EC, Selleck CJ, Awad AH, Zwaan J, Mullaney PB, Bosley TM, Engle EC. Homozygous mutations in ARIX (PHOX2A) result in congenital fibrosis of the extraocular muscles type 2. Nat Genet. 2001;29(3):315–20.
13. Doherty EJ, Macy ME, Wang SM, Dykeman CP, Melanson MT, Engle EC. CFEOM3: A new extraocular congenital fibrosis syndrome that maps to 16q24. 2-q24. 3. Invest Ophthalmol Vis Sci. 1999;40(8):1687–94.
14. Tischfield MA, Baris HN, Wu C, Rudolph G, Van Maldergem L, He W, Chan WM, Andrews C, Demer JL, Robertson RL, Mackey DA. Human TUBB3 mutations perturb microtubule dynamics, kinesin interactions, and axon guidance. Cell. 2010;140(1):74–87.
15. Sener EC, Taylan Sekeroglu H, Ural Ö, Öztürk BT, Sanaç AS. Strabismus surgery in congenital fibrosis of the extraocular muscles: A paradigm. Ophthalmic Genet. 2014;35(4):208–25.
16. Huber A. Electrophysiology of the retraction syndromes. Br J Ophthalmol. 1974;58(3):293.
17. Ahluwalia BK, Gupta NC, Goel SR, Khurana AK. Study of Duane's retraction syndrome. Acta Ophthalmol (Copenh). 1988;66(6):728–30.
18. Kekunnaya R, Negalur M. Duane retraction syndrome: Causes, effects and management strategies. Clin Ophthalmol (Auckland, NZ). 2017;11:1917.
19. Chilton JK, Guthrie S. Axons get ahead: Insights into axon guidance and congenital cranial dysinnervation disorders. Dev Neurobiol. 2017;77(7):861–75.
20. Engle EC. Oculomotility disorders arising from disruptions in brainstem motor neuron development. Arch Neurol. 2007;64(5):633–7.
21. Kohlhase J, Heinrich M, Schubert L, Liebers M, Kispert A, Laccone F, Turnpenny P, Winter RM, Reardon W. Okihiro syndrome is caused by SALL4 mutations. Hum Mol Genet. 2002;11(23):2979–87.
22. Brown HW. Congenital structural muscle anomalies. In: Strabismus ophthalmic symposium. CV Mosby. 1950. pp. 205–36.
23. Kaeser PF, Kress B, Rohde S, Kolling G. Absence of the fourth cranial nerve in congenital Brown syndrome. Acta Ophthalmol. 2012;90(4):e310–3.
24. Papst W, Stein HJ. Etiology of the superior oblique tendon sheath syndrome. Klin Monbl Augenheilkd. 1969;154(4):506.
25. Ellis FJ, Jeffery AR, Seidman DJ, Sprague JB, Coussens T, Schuller J. Possible association of congenital Brown syndrome with congenital cranial dysinnervation disorders. J AAPOS. 2012;16(6):558–64.
26. Lorenz B, Brodsky MC, editors. Pediatric ophthalmology, neuro-ophthalmology, genetics: Strabismus-new concepts in pathophysiology, diagnosis, and treatment. Berlin, Heidelberg: Springer Science & Business Media; 2010.
27. Katz NN, Whitmore PV, Beauchamp GR. Brown's syndrome in twins. J Pediatr Ophthalmol Strabismus. 1981;18(1):32–4.
28. Kenawy N, Pilz DT, Watts P. Familial unilateral Brown syndrome. Indian J Ophthalmol. 2008;56(5):430.
29. Kaban TJ, Smith K, Orton RB, Noel LP, Clarke W, Cadera W. Natural history of presumed congenital Brown syndrome. Arch Ophthalmol. 1993;111(7):943–6.
30. Dawson E, Barry J, Lee J. Spontaneous resolution in patients with congenital Brown syndrome. J AAPOS. 2009;13(2):116–8.
31. Velez FG, Velez G, Thacker N. Superior oblique posterior tenectomy in patients with Brown syndrome with small deviations in the primary position. J AAPOS. 2006;10(3):214–9.
32. Verzijl HT, van der Zwaag B, Cruysberg JR, Padberg GW. Möbius syndrome redefined: A syndrome of rhombencephalic maldevelopment. Neurology. 2003;61(3):327–33.
33. Oystreck DT, Engle EC, Bosley TM. Recent progress in understanding congenital cranial dysinnervation disorders. J Neuroophthalmol. 2011;31(1):69.
34. Albayrak HM, Tarakçı N, Altunhan H, Örs R, Çaksen H. A congenital cranial dysinnervation disorder: Möbius' syndrome. Türk Pediatri Arş. 2017;52(3):165.
35. Jacob FD, Kanigan A, Richer L, El Hakim H. Unilateral Möbius syndrome: Two cases and a review of the literature. Int J Pediatr Otorhinolaryngol. 2014;78(8):1228–31.
36. Jen JC, Chan WM, Bosley TM, Wan J, Carr JR, Rüb U, Shattuck D, Salamon G, Kudo LC, Ou J, Lin DD. Mutations in a human ROBO gene disrupt hindbrain axon pathway crossing and morphogenesis. Science. 2004;304(5676):1509–13.
37. Verzijl HT, Van der Zwaag B, Lammens M, Ten Donkelaar HJ, Padberg GW. The neuropathology of hereditary congenital facial palsy vs Möbius syndrome. Neurology. 2005;64(4):649–53.
38. Engle EC, Castro AE, Macy ME, Knoll JH, Beggs AH. A gene for isolated congenital ptosis maps to a 3-cM region within 1p32–p34.1. Am J Hum Genet. 1997;60(5):1150.
39. McMullan TF, Collins AR, Tyers AG, Robinson DO. A novel X-linked dominant condition: X-linked congenital isolated ptosis. Am J Hum Genet. 2000;66(4):1455–60.

16

INFECTION-ASSOCIATED OCULAR CRANIAL NERVE PALSIES

Hardeep Singh Malhotra, Imran Rizvi, Neeraj Kumar, Kiran Preet Malhotra, Gaurav Kumar, Manoj K. Goyal, Manish Modi, Ravindra Kumar Garg, Vivek Lal

CASE STUDY

A 50-year-old male, an uncontrolled diabetic, presented with diplopia and headache for 2 months. Examination revealed left eye mild proptosis, ptosis, and complete ophthalmoplegia. Contrast-enhanced MRI of the brain showed iso- to hypointense mass involving the paranasal sinuses and extending into the left orbit and the adjoining cavernous sinus. What is the next step to manage this patient?

Introduction

Infections can involve both afferent as well as efferent pathways of the visual system. Infections involving the afferent system (viz. infectious optic neuropathies) have already been dealt with; in this chapter, we shall be discussing about infection-associated ocular cranial nerve palsies. Ocular cranial nerves include nerves that innervate the muscles controlling the movements of extraocular muscles of the eye, and these include the third cranial nerve (oculomotor), the fourth cranial nerve (trochlear), and the sixth cranial nerve (abducens). It is important to understand their anatomical localization because of predilection of infectious agents toward specific regions. Ophthalmoplegia can be caused either directly by the infectious agent or indirectly due to its complication/s. Wide spectrum and limited literature restricts the account on prevalence of infectious ophthalmoplegia. In one of the largest personal case series published, Keane JR studied 979 patients of varied etiologies presenting with multiple cranial nerve palsies. Only 10% of all causes were attributed to infectious causes in this series (1).

Important anatomical considerations

Before proceeding further, let's take a look at some important anatomical considerations. Figure 16.1 shows a simplified depiction of the pathway of ocular cranial nerves. Isolated involvement of an individual ocular cranial nerve may occur anywhere along its course starting from the brainstem root exit to innervation-specific extraocular muscles (EOM) in the orbit. It is intuitive that infections involving orbits, retroorbital area, superior orbital fissure, cavernous sinus, subarachnoid space, and nerve root exit zones may cause, in isolation or combination, infranuclear ocular nerve palsies. Similarly, involvement of nuclei in the brainstem may cause nuclear cranial nerve palsies while involvement of higher-order pathways controlling ocular nuclei or the cerebrum may lead to supranuclear palsies.

The close proximity of the ocular cranial nerves at the cavernous sinus and orbital apex, and within the orbits, predisposes them to simultaneous affliction on most occasions. Thus, infections which directly or indirectly involve these anatomical substrates are likely to present with multiple ocular cranial palsies.

Certain infectious etiologies are peculiar to the dangerous area of face, mouth, and teeth. These are more likely to cause orbital infections leading to orbital cellulitis and orbital pericellulitis. The infections of paranasal sinuses often involve the superior orbital fissure, the orbital apex, and the cavernous sinuses because of contiguous spread. As the sinuses are usually affected by fungal or bacterial infections, these are a common cause of cavernous sinus syndrome or orbital apex syndrome. It is important to know that few infectious agents might have predilection towards involvement of specific cranial nerves or their pathways, hence helping in diagnosing them.

Specific anatomical substrates
Orbits
Orbit is a conical structure that contains the globe, EOMs, tendinous and ligamentous attachments, vessels, ocular cranial nerves, lacrimal gland, fat, and connective tissue (2). Periosteum of seven bones surrounds the orbit and an extension of the periosteum, the orbital septum, covers the anterior margin of the orbit, and attaches itself over the tarsal plates (Figure 16.2).

The periosteum and the orbital septum form a barrier restricting the access of any infectious or inflammatory process into the globe. An inflammatory reaction limited to anterior of the septum, i.e., involving skin or the subcutaneous tissue of the eyelid is termed as pre-septal or periorbital, and the one that is posterior to the septum is described as post-septal (Figure 16.3). The most common origin of pre-septal inflammation is spread via facial or dental structures and of post-septal infections is from paranasal sinuses through the lamina papyracea. Further, the extensive valve-less venous supply around the orbits allows the spread of infection from the soft tissues of face, teeth, and paranasal sinuses. The infection can, similarly, spread to the cavernous sinuses or other intracranial structures.

Orbital apex
The posterior most end of the pyramid shaped orbit is called the apex of the orbit. As depicted in Figure 16.2, the four orbital walls converge here at the craniofacial junction leaving two orifices situated in the sphenoid bone (2). The optic nerve and the ophthalmic artery pass through the optic canal and the four recti muscles take their origin from the tendinous annulus of Zinn. Other structures passing through the annulus of Zinn are the superior and the inferior branches of oculomotor nerve, the abducens nerve, and the nasociliary nerve, which pass through the middle portion of the superior orbital fissure (Figure 16.4).

The orbital apex syndromes can be recognized by the involvement of these structures in varied combinations of ophthalmoparesis (due to ocular nerve/s involvement) and visual diminution

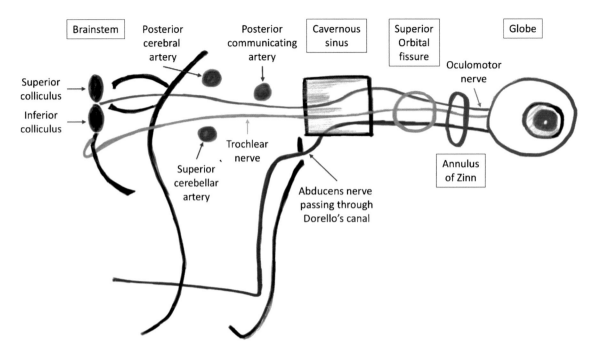

FIGURE 16.1   Simplified depiction of ocular (oculomotor, trochlear, and abducens) cranial nerve pathways.

(due to optic nerve involvement). Other important clinical pointers suggesting involvement are proptosis, ptosis, relative afferent pupillary defect, chemosis, anisocoria, optic disc edema, and absence of corneal sensation.

Cavernous sinus

The cavernous sinus is a dural venous sinus, one on either side, situated on the body of sphenoid bone of the brain extending from the medial end of superior orbital fissure to the petrous portion of the temporal bone (3). It is related to pituitary gland and sphenoid sinus medially and to the temporal bone laterally. Importantly, the ocular motor nerves, trigeminal nerve, and internal carotid

artery pass through the cavernous sinuses. While oculomotor, trochlear, and trigeminal (V1/2) nerves travel through the lateral walls of cavernous sinus, the abducens nerve and the postganglionic sympathetic nerve fibers travel through the core of the cavernous sinus (Figure 16.5).

While it was Jefferson who initially classified it into anterior, middle, and posterior, Ishikawa in 1996 expanded the classification depending upon important anatomical landmarks and structures passing through it. The cavernous sinus is a vulnerable site owing to its connection to orbits anteriorly and sphenoid sinus medially which allows the spread of infection through the paranasal route (4). The presence of loose areolar

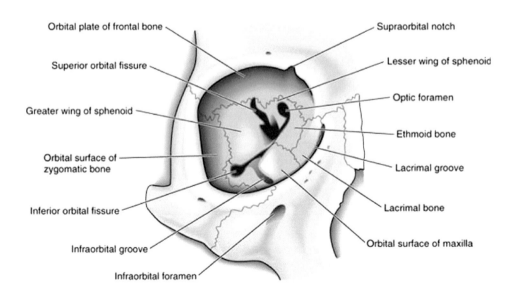

FIGURE 16.2   Anatomy of the orbit.

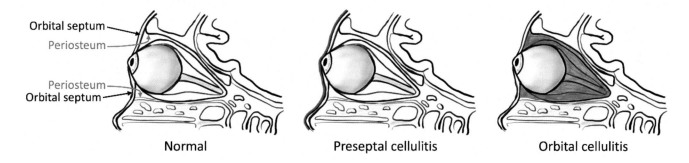

FIGURE 16.3 Depiction of pre-septal (shaded as red) and post-septal inflammation (shaded as red) in context of orbital septum.

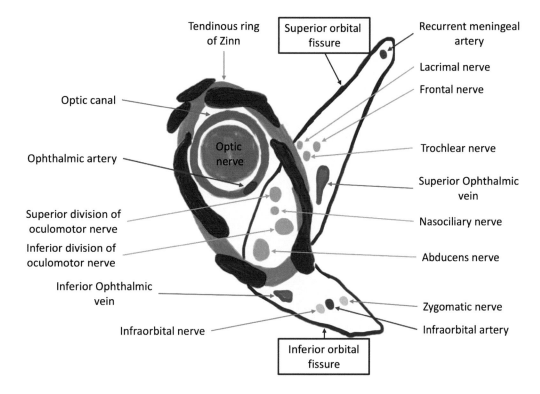

FIGURE 16.4 Depiction of contents, and their relationship, of the superior orbital fissure.

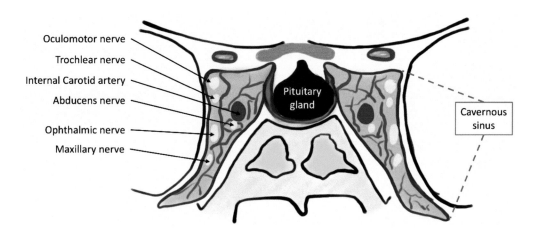

FIGURE 16.5 Structure of the cavernous sinus.

tissue containing emissary veins in the dangerous area of face allows the spread of infection from this area to cavernous sinus. Connection between the two sides allows an easy bilateral involvement leading to involvement of both cavernous sinuses. Involvement of cranial nerves III, IV, V (1), and VI in varied combinations point toward cavernous sinus involvement. Rarely, facial nerve involvement may be seen in cavernous sinus involvement (5).

Approach to a patient with infection-associated ocular cranial nerve palsies

Infection is an important differential in patients presenting with ophthalmoparesis, painful, or otherwise. Frontal headache, peri-orbital, and orbital pain are common and may range from moderate to severe intensity. Diplopia is the most common presenting symptom in patients with ocular cranial neuropathy due to the asymmetrical involvement of ocular cranial nerves. Eyelid swelling, chemosis, conjunctival congestion, induration of skin, proptosis, periorbital, and orbital pain, further suggest an involvement of local orbital structures. Diplopia/ophthalmoparesis associated with oculo-sympathetic paralysis (Horner's syndrome) or involvement of trigeminal nerve suggests an involvement at the level of cavernous sinus. Angio-invasive causes involving the cavernous sinus (e.g., fungal infection) may in addition involve internal carotid artery and cause stroke in the respective territory. Additionally, it is important to ascertain the history of constitutional symptoms like fever, weight loss, etc. Table 16.1 highlights the important historical and clinical components that should be enquired to localize the syndrome anatomically. History of recent infection, diabetes mellitus, immunosuppressive therapy, organ transplant, HIV-infection, tuberculosis, recent dental surgery, facial or head trauma, intracranial surgery, etc. should raise the suspicion of ophthalmoparesis possibly arising as a result of infection.

Table 16.2 summarizes clues that may aid in recognition of involved etiological agent in a given case of painful ophthalmoparesis.

TABLE 16.1: Important Historical Highlights for Anatomical Localization

Important Points in History	Important Considerations Depending upon the Sign/Symptom
Painful Ophthalmoplegia - Diplopia with/without ptosis	Ascertain whether: • Unilateral/bilateral • Asymmetrical/symmetrical
Associated cranial nerve involvement	Establish anatomical location: • Orbits • Orbital apex • Cavernous sinus • Petrous apex • Subarachnoid space
Associated proptosis, eyelid swelling, conjunctival chemosis, suggestion of local involvement	Establish anatomical location: • Orbit/orbital apex/ anterior cavernous sinus Look for source of infection: • Face/dental/nose paranasal sinuses

Investigation protocol should include a complete blood count, erythrocyte sedimentation rate (ESR), C-reactive protein (CRP), renal and hepatic status: all attempts should be made to rule out diabetes mellitus, connective tissue disorders, other granulomatous inflammatory conditions, and malignancy in suitable clinical scenarios. Usually, the initial imaging done is either an ultrasonography (USG) of the orbit or contrast-enhanced computed tomography (CECT) of the orbits. Dedicated fat-suppressed, gadolinium-enhanced magnetic resonance imaging (MRI) of orbits, cavernous sinus, and brain with MR angiography of the intracranial and neck vessels should be sought, depending upon the patient's clinical presentation. Detailed cerebrospinal fluid (CSF) analysis may be required whenever intracranial spread or meningeal involvement is suspected. Vitreous biopsy may be helpful in patients with associated cellular reaction/vitritis. Imaging of thorax/abdomen/pelvis (CT or FDG-PET) may be required in select cases (Table 16.3).

Infectious etiologies causing direct involvement of ocular nerves

The common etiologies of infectious ophthalmoplegia are enumerated in Table 16.4.

Fungal infections

Mucormycosis

Mucormycosis is a relatively rare (usually not more than 10% of Aspergillosis) but fatal fungal infection with high potential of causing mortality and significant morbidity. Four genera of mucorales are associated with human disease (*Rhizopus, Mucor, Absidia,* and *Cunninghamella*). Rhino-orbito-cerebral form is one of the common manifestations of mucormycosis. Other clinical syndromes are pulmonary, gastrointestinal, cutaneous, and disseminated forms. Initial human infection is either secondary to inhalation of sporangiospores or inoculation of wound. Immunocompromised individuals are at highest risk of contracting the infection. Uncontrolled diabetes mellitus, deferoxamine therapy, anti-neoplastic administration, malignancy, burns, and trauma pose a higher risk of developing mucormycosis.

Mucormycosis are angio-invasive and are notorious to invade the vessels due to the presence of an enzyme, elastase. This property, however, either because of difference in the prevalence or due to higher activity of elastase in aspergillus, is comparatively more frequently seen in Aspergillosis. Angio-invasive nature along with ability of bone destruction plays a major role in their virulence. Importantly, extension beyond the sinuses may occur even with intact bony sinus walls. Once the organism becomes tissue invasive, it first invades the internal elastic lamina of the blood vessels, then lymphatics and later veins. Raised intraorbital pressure, in addition, may contribute to obliteration of vascular lumen leading to incomplete or complete blockade. Arterial occlusion leads to tissue necrosis causing ischemic infarction and extensive endothelial venous damage, which may further culminate in hemorrhagic necrosis (6).

An untreated mucormycosis in a susceptible host is almost always fatal. Main clinical features include rapidly declining vision, ophthalmoparesis with ptosis, proptosis, periorbital edema, and facial edema. Pansinusitis is often seen. Orbital apex

TABLE 16.2: Clues to Aid in Etiological Diagnosis

Clues		Suspected Etiology
Immunocompromised state/ post-organ transplantation/ Diabetes mellitus	→	HIV, CMV, VZV, Tuberculosis, Toxoplasmosis, Cryptococcosis, Aspergillosis
Orbital fracture/ infection or procedure involving face, teeth, mouth or nose	→	*Staphylococcus aureus, Streptococcus pneumoniae, Pseudomonas aeruginosa,* Fungi
Infection or procedure involving nose or paranasal sinuses	→	*Mucormycosis, Aspergillosis,* Bacterial infections viz. *Staphylococcus aureus*
Febrile encephalopathy with suggestion of increased intracranial pressure	→	Tuberculosis, Cryptococcosis, *Herpes simplex*
Febrile illness with rash	→	*Varicella zoster,* Herpes zoster ophthalmicus

Abbreviations: HIV: Human Immuno-deficiency Virus; CMV: Cyto Megalo Virus; VZV: Varicella Zoster Virus

syndrome, cavernous sinus syndrome, and intracranial spread, per se, are not uncommon. Involvement of intra-cavernous ICA causing stroke in the involved territory may be seen. Mucormycosis can also cause an invasive orbital cellulitis and is associated with high mortality.

Varied degrees of opacification of paranasal sinuses may be seen on imaging. Fungal (Mucor, Aspergillus) sinus involvement is characterized by nodular mucosal hypertrophy but is not associated with air-fluid level unless secondary bacterial infection is associated. CT may reveal bony erosion, necrosis, palatal erosion, and obliteration of sinuses. Contiguous involvement of orbits, orbital apex, cavernous sinuses, and brain may be

seen. Soft tissue swelling may be seen as a hyperdense lesion. On MRI, the lesions are usually isointense on T1-weighted (T1-W) images and hyperintense on T2-weighted (T2-W) images (T2-W images may show variable signal intensity; in some cases, the lesion may be isointense on T2-W images as well) (Figure 16.6). The lesions show variable enhancement on gadolinium administration. Dural/pachymeningeal enhancement may also be seen. Biopsy of the involved sinus or dura is needed to confirm the diagnosis.

Histopathological examination reveals large non-septate mycelial filaments, which branch at right angle with features of inflammation and angioinvasion (Figure 16.7). Varied degrees of

TABLE 16.3: Battery of Investigations in Painful Ophthalmoplegia

Essential Workup

Complete blood count with ESR
Thyroid, liver, and renal function tests
Blood sugar and glycated Hemoglobin (HbA1c)
CRP
Mantoux/tuberculin skin test
Blood culture: Bacterial, fungal
X-ray: Chest
Serological testing of HIV/syphilis
Serum galactomannan
ANA, ENA
Vasculitis screen
USG orbits
Plain and contrast CT nose, paranasal sinuses, and orbits
Gadolinium-enhanced fat-suppressed MRI of orbits, cavernous sinus, and brain
Examination of cerebrospinal fluid for protein, sugar, total, and differential cell count
Cerebrospinal fluid culture, GeneXpert for tuberculosis, India ink staining, fungal culture

Individualized Workup for Select Patients, as Applicable

Culture: Bacterial and fungal culture from lesions, viral culture from skin lesions
Vitreous biopsy/PCR of aqueous or vitreous
Contrast-enhanced CT thorax, abdomen, pelvis
FDG-PET

TABLE 16.4: Common Causes of Infectious Ocular Nerve Palsies

Fungi

Mucormycosis
Aspergillus
Cryptococcus
Candidiasis

Bacteria

Staphylococcus aureus
Streptococcus
Pseudomonas aeruginosa
Aeromonas hydrophila
Eikenella corrodens
Mycobacterium tuberculosis
Treponema pallidum

Viruses

Herpes simplex virus 1 and 2
Varicella zoster virus
Cytomegalovirus
Human immunodeficiency virus
West Nile virus
Chikungunya
Dengue

Parasites

Cysticercosis
Toxoplasma
Toxocara

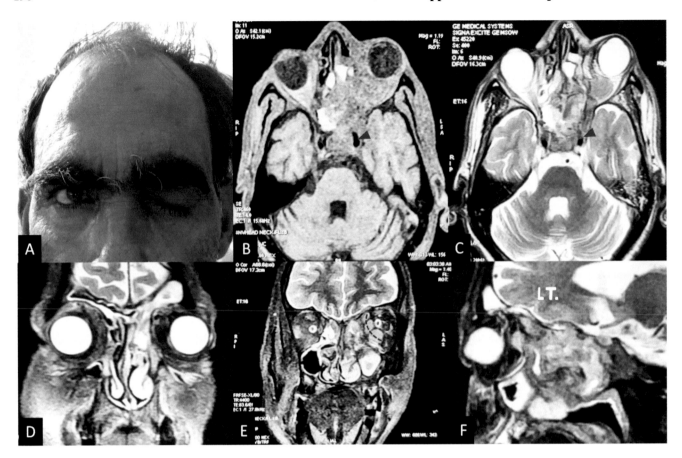

FIGURE 16.6 A 50-year-old male, an uncontrolled-diabetic, presented with left ophthalmoplegia (a) and history of headache for 2 months. Axial sections of MRI of the brain show iso- to hypointense mass involving the paranasal sinuses and extending into the left orbit and the adjoining cavernous sinus, encasing the internal carotid artery (arrowhead), on T1-W (b) and T2-W (c) sequences. The hypertrophic nasal turbinates, pan-sinus involvement (left > right), and the extension into the orbit with swelling of the medially placed extraocular muscles (dashed-curve) with inferolateral displacement of the left globe can be appreciated on T2-W coronal (d, e) and sagittal (f) sequence.

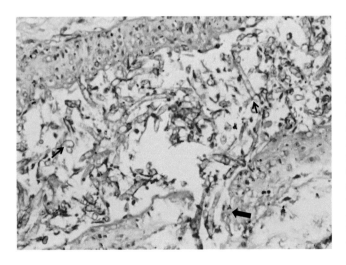

FIGURE 16.7 Photomicrograph depicting a large vessel showing broad fungal hyphae with occasional branching at right angles (arrows) in the lumen. The vessel wall shows rupture with invasion of fungal hyphae (block arrow) (Hematoxylin & Eosin, 200×).

neutrophilic infiltration, necrosis, and hyphae may be seen on histopathological examination. Many a times the hyphae may not be prominent and special stains are needed to demonstrate fungal elements (7).

Combined surgical debridement, diagnostic, or debulking in nature, with antifungal therapy should be considered for treatment. Amphotericin-B (AmB, conventional type) is the only consistently effective agent in mucormycosis (1.5 mg/kg/day). Liposomal and lipid complex preparations are considered superior, less toxic, and allow for a higher dose (up to 10 mg/kg/day). Other drugs which can be used in patients intolerant to AmB are posaconazole, isavuconazole, and echinocandins (salvage therapy). Oral posaconazole is recommended (600 mg on day 1 followed by 300 mg once a day) as a step-down therapy. For better outcomes, early institution of anti-fungal therapy (started within a week) is recommended. A discernable clinical benefit may take several weeks; the duration of therapy, thus, needs to be individualized.

The mortality rate of rhino-orbito-cerebral mucormycosis is approximately 50%, or even higher, depending on the patient's immune status, and the promptness and type of treatment delivered (6).

Aspergillosis

Invasive Aspergillosis is an opportunistic infection of granulocytopenic patients and common predisposing factors include diabetes mellitus, immunosuppressive or steroid therapy, and alcoholism. Singularly, mucormycosis is very selectively associated with diabetes mellitus, while aspergillosis is common in patients with granulocytopenia. Aspergillus fumigatus (followed by Aspergillus flavus) is the usual organism causing invasive fungal infection. Central nervous system (CNS) is one of the most commonly involved sites (ranging from 10% to 40%) and is associated with a high mortality rate. Frequent route of infection is inhalational and spread to CNS is either contiguous from orbits or paranasal sinuses, or hematogenous from a distant primary source like lungs (8).

Aspergillus galactomannan enzyme immunoassay, beta-D-glucan detection, and polymerase chain reaction (PCR) based tests may not be absolute or conclusive. The sensitivity and specificity of galactomannan assay and PCR borders 80%. The utility of beta-D-glucan is best reserved to determine invasiveness of a fungal infection as this is not specific for Aspergillus and shares positivity with other invasive fungal infections. CT of paranasal sinuses and orbits may suggest involvement in the form of hyperdensity and bony erosion. It, however, should be noted that even extensive parenchymal forms of aspergillosis may not accompany obvious bony erosion. Gadolinium-enhanced MRI often reveals a polylobulated abscess (hypointense on T1-W; hyperintense on T2-W images) with significant peripheral enhancement; inflammation of the surrounding soft tissue can be noted, in addition. Involvement of surrounding paranasal sinuses, meninges, and bone is usually seen. Angioinvasion is another important feature of this fungus, somewhat greater than mucormycosis. Interestingly, a few patients may have a T2-W hypointense signal which is postulated to be a result of ferromagnetic fungal deposits (like iron, zinc, manganese, etc.) or due to methemoglobin (in the wall of the capsule or the macrophages). A central intermediate signal may be noted on T2-W images, suggestive of coagulative necrosis (Figure 16.8). Mycotic aneurysms have been noted with aspergillosis as a result of direct spread from paranasal sinuses to proximal part of circle of Willis or through hematogenous spread (9).

Histopathological confirmation should always be attempted by obtaining the relevant specimen, tissue, or fluid. Minimally invasive approaches like FESS are often useful in obtaining sphenoidal biopsy. Acute angles branching fungal hyphae with tissue invasion are seen (Figure 16.9). Fungal culture provides the most certain evidence of aspergillosis, but treatment must not be delayed pending a culture report. The practice guidelines for the diagnosis and management of aspergillosis by Infectious Diseases Society of America (IDSA) do not recommend a routine antifungal susceptibility testing of isolates (10).

Aggressive surgical debridement along with systemic voriconazole or a lipid formulation of AmB is advised for use in invasive Aspergillus fungal sinusitis. While voriconazole is advised for primary therapy in CNS aspergillosis, lipid formulations of AmB are reserved for refractory patients or those intolerant to voriconazole. Monotherapy with echinocandins is not recommended and they should be reserved for salvage therapy alone. A prolonged course of amphotericin B exceeding 2 g is often needed to control the infection. In cases with recurrence or persistent disease, itraconazole 200–400 mg/day may be added; in such patients, therapeutic drug monitoring can help in achieving appropriate levels. It is advisable that all patients be followed up every 3–4 months with nasal endoscopy or CT of nose and paranasal sinuses to look for recurrence (11).

Bacterial infections

Bacterial infections implicated in orbital cellulitis

Across all age groups, *Staphylococcus aureus* and *Streptococci* species are the commonest bacteria causing orbital and cavernous sinus involvement. The most commonly isolated organisms in children are α- or non-hemolytic streptococci, group A β-hemolytic streptococci, *S. aureus*, and *Haemophilus influenzae*. Polymicrobial infections are common. Commonly implicated anaerobic bacteria include Aeromonas hydrophila, *Pseudomonas aeruginosa*, and *Eikenella corrodens* (12,13).

These bacterial infections commonly involve orbits causing pre-septal or post-septal orbital cellulitis. Orbital cellulitis refers to the infectious-inflammatory process involving ocular adnexa within the orbit posterior to the orbital septum (14). Involvement of structures anterior to orbital septum (skin and the soft tissue around the eye) by the infectious process is termed as periorbital cellulitis or pre-septal cellulitis (Figure 16.3).

Extension of infection usually occurs through the paranasal sinuses (approximately 60–70% in adult patients) either though contiguous spread due to the thin lamina papyracea or by causing septic thrombophlebitis of connecting valve-less veins. Hematogenous spread may also be seen. Posterior extension of these infections may cause orbital apex syndrome and cavernous sinus thrombosis. Orbital trauma, nasolacrimal, or dental infections and procedures should always be borne in mind. Fever and leukocytosis are common in the pediatric age group. Clinically, presence of eyelid swelling with or without erythema, conjunctival chemosis, ophthalmoparesis, and proptosis with painful eye movement helps to consider a diagnosis of orbital cellulitis. Involvement and inflammation of optic nerve may cause diminution of visual acuity and optic disc edema. Eye is usually tender to touch, but tenderness and erythema are usually lesser as compared to periorbital cellulitis (Figure 16.10) (15).

Presence of proptosis, ophthalmoparesis, and decreased visual acuity are clinical pointers favoring a diagnosis of orbital cellulitis over periorbital cellulitis. The extent of complications in terms of an increasing risk of vision loss and systemic morbidity, and the level of urgency to intervene can be had by stages as classified by Chandler et al. (16). This classification groups the complications into five stages, namely (1), inflammatory edema (pre-septal cellulitis) (2), orbital cellulitis (3), subperiosteal abscess (4), orbital abscess, and (5) cavernous sinus thrombosis.

Although screening can be done in suspected patients using USG, CECT is often necessary to assess the sinuses, orbits, and intracranial extension. CT is often considered to be the initial investigation of choice due to its ability to decipher the bony orbits, EOMs, optic nerves, intraconal area, and fat. Generally, a localized, homogenous elevation of periorbital tissue with opacified sinuses can be seen along with inflammatory changes in the orbits. Subperiosteal abscess can be made out, if present (Figure 16.11). Gadolinium-enhanced MRI may be necessary to look for intracranial extension in some cases and to delineate the orbital soft tissues and visual pathways in selected cases (13).

Complications occur when the spread of infection occurs to the surrounding anatomical structures. Subperiosteal abscess, orbital abscess, and intracranial extension may occur in untreated cases. Early diagnosis and prompt treatment can help in avoiding the spread of infection; antibiotics remain the

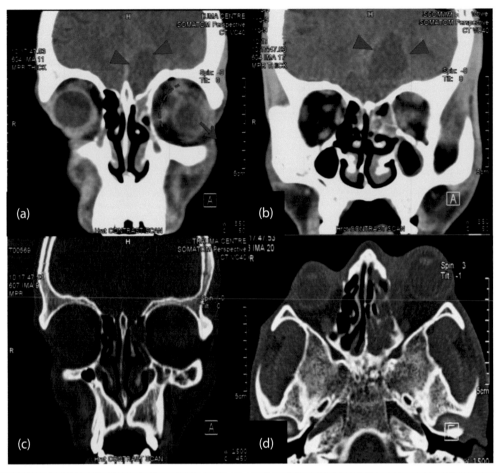

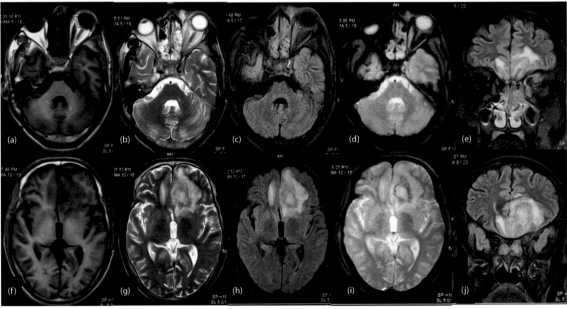

FIGURE 16.8   Set 1: Computed tomography (coronal sections) of the orbits and paranasal sinuses (a, b) show mucosal thickening of the turbinates along with swelling of the medially placed extraocular muscles (dashed-curved) leading to inferolateral displacement of the globe (arrow). Note is made of a hypodense lesion (arrowheads) suggesting an intracranial extension of infection. On bone-window (coronal and axial sections), bony erosion can be appreciated at the level of ethmoid sinus (c) as well as the proptosis of the eye (d). **Set 2:** MRI of the same patient shows involvement of the paranasal sinuses, orbits and brain parenchyma that is hypointense on T1-W (a, f) sequence and hyperintense (with heterogeneity) on T2-W (b, g), FLAIR (c, e, h, j) and GRE (d, i) sequences. Note is made of a hypointense rim especially on GRE sequence (i) suggesting the presence of ferromagnetic substance/s associated with the lesion having extended from the paranasal sinuses.

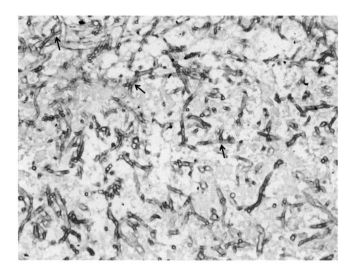

FIGURE 16.9 Photomicrograph of tissue invaded by numerous thin fungal hyphae with dichotomous branching at acute angles (arrows) (Periodic Acid Schiff, 200×).

mainstay of treatment. In resistant cases, debridement and other surgical procedures may be required. Broad spectrum regimens covering organisms like *S. aureus* (including methicillin-resistant *S. aureus*), *Streptococcus pneumoniae*, other *Streptococci*, as well as gram-negative bacilli are usually used along with coverage for anaerobes when an intracranial extension is suspected. Supportive management with analgesics and anti-inflammatory agents should be done.

Mycobacterium tuberculosis (15)

Tuberculosis is a global health problem, specifically so for the developing nations. Mycobacterium tuberculosis bacilli reach CNS primarily through the hematogenous spread. In initial stages of infection, small meningeal, subpial, or subependymal tuberculous lesions are formed which may remain dormant for years together, and later, usually due to immunological alterations, the growth or rupture of lesions produces symptoms of frank CNS tuberculosis.

Intracranial manifestations of tuberculosis are complex. Common clinical syndromes include tuberculous meningitis (TBM), tuberculomas, and abscess formation. Thick gelatinous exudates in the basal cisterns, often encasing brainstem and cerebellum, in TBM are responsible for features of increased intracranial pressure (ICP) and non-communicating hydrocephalous. Border-zone reaction occurs in the parenchymal tissue below the exudates causing parenchymal changes in the underlying brain tissue. Accompanying vasculitis and necrotizing arteritis occurs in the vicinity of circle of Willis.

Around 20–30% patients develop varied cranial nerve palsies. Involvement of cranial nerves occur due to ischemia (secondary to vascular compression/strangulation), nerve entrapment in the basal exudates, or as a false localizing sign due to increased ICP in 17–40% of cases. Cranial nerves commonly involved are the second, third, fourth, sixth, and seventh cranial nerves. Sixth cranial nerve is the most commonly involved cranial nerve, frequently occurring as a result of an increased ICP or brainstem involvement. Bilateral sixth nerve involvement is also common. Third nerve is next commonly involved ocular cranial nerve. Isolated trochlear nerve involvement has

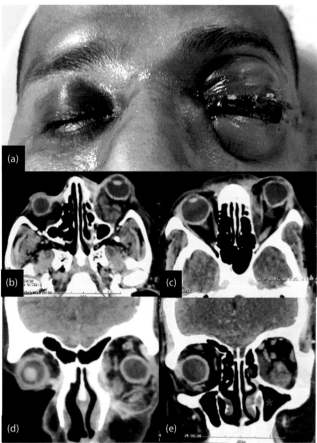

FIGURE 16.10 A 30-year-old gentleman, an undiagnosed diabetic, presented with proptosis, periorbital swelling and ophthalmoplegia of 4-days duration (a). Axial sections of computed tomography (b, c) depict gross proptosis, edematous intraorbital contents, and formation of abscess (arrowhead) with lateral displacement of the muscle cone. The edematous extraocular muscles are better appreciated in the coronal sections (d, e). On the basis of microscopy and culture, this patient was diagnosed as having bacterial cellulitis. Note should be made of clean paranasal sinuses (*) that is not the norm in patients with fungal cellulitis. Pure mucosal hypertrophy, without fluid-air levels, in fungal infections (not complicated by bacterial infection) also serves as a pointer toward fungal involvement vis-à-vis bacterial involvement of sinuses, if any.

also been reported in literature. Encasement secondary to basal arachnoiditis or direct involvement of brainstem due to tuberculomas, infarction, or edema are the commonly implicated hypothesis. Formation of tuberculomas at other strategic sites too might lead to ophthalmoparesis. Kapadia et al. reported tuberculomas in cavernous sinus in a 48-year-old woman presenting with ophthalmoparesis (17). Other ocular signs like internuclear ophthalmoplegia have also been noted in isolated case reports. Tubercular abscess may also cause ophthalmoplegia due to direct compression or increased ICP.

Another important cause of cranial nerve involvement in CNS tuberculosis is believed to be hypertrophic pachymeningitis. Fibrosis and thickening of dura matter due to granulomatous inflammation in tuberculosis may cause entrapment of cranial nerves depending upon the site of involvement (18).

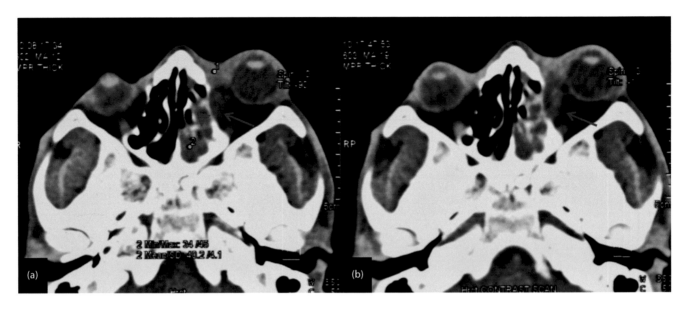

FIGURE 16.11   Computed tomography (a) of the orbit of a patient with Aspergillosis depicts the bony breach at the level of ethmoid sinus (arrowhead) and the resultant subperiosteal abscess (arrows) that shows mild peripheral contrast enhancement (b).

An abnormally thickened dura can be seen in many other infectious, inflammatory, and neoplastic conditions; histopathological confirmation, therefore, is needed to make a definitive diagnosis.

Cranial nerve involvement is associated with poor outcomes in patients with TBM, and it has been noted that age >25 years, history of vomiting, altered sensorium, hemiparesis, diplopia, papilledema, signs of meningeal irritation, severe functional disability, presence of optochiasmatic arachnoiditis, hydrocephalous, CSF protein >2.5 g/L, and CSF cell count >100/mm³ seem to predict cranial nerve involvement (19). Gadolinium-enhanced MRI of the brain is required in most situations. Intense enhancement of meninges, especially in the basal regions, is typical of TBM. It is often associated with ventricular enlargement or hydrocephalous. Infarcts may be seen along with segmental occlusion and beading along the vessels of the circle of Willis.

The appearance of tuberculoma on MRI depends upon whether the lesions are caseating or not (Figure 16.12). The non-caseating granulomas are hypointense on T1-W and hyperintense on T2-W images and shows homogenous enhancement on gadolinium. Caseating tuberculomas are hypo- or isointense on T1-W and T2-W images and may have a solid or a liquified center. Varied amount of perilesional edema may be seen. Liquefaction appears hypointense centrally and hyperintense on T2-W scans with peripheral hypointense rim representing the capsule. Thick ring enhancement is seen on administration of gadolinium.

Tuberculin skin test has a low sensitivity and its performance often depends on patient's age, endemic conditions, vaccination-status, nutritional and immune status, dose, and technique of administration. Definitive diagnosis of TBM is made on detection of tubercle bacilli in CSF. Lymphocytic-predominant pleocytosis, increased proteins, low sugar (<2/3 corresponding blood sugar), and raised adenosine deaminase (ADA) levels are other suggestive signs. Molecular techniques like nucleic acid amplification methods, PCR-based methods, and chemical assays help to increase the diagnostic yield. Treatment with four drugs (Isoniazid, Rifampicin, Pyrazinamide, and Streptomycin

(preferred by World Health Organization [WHO] over ethambutol; prevents visual loss and increases efficacy of the regimen) for 2 months followed by two drugs for 7–10 months is recommended, along with steroids.

Treponema pallidum

Syphilis is a sexually transmitted disease caused by a spirochete bacterium *Treponema pallidum*. Neurosyphilis is a reemerging entity and develops in 5% of the syphilis patients. The CNS may be involved in any stage of syphilis infection from few weeks to several years after the initial infection. Early neurosyphilis is rarely diagnosed but syphilitic meningitis, the earliest manifestation, may occur within 2 years of initial infection. It is during the phase of early symptomatic neurosyphilis that the cranial neuropathies and ocular involvement is commonly seen. The diagnosis of neurosyphilis is most often made in the tertiary stage. With concomitant HIV-infection, neurosyphilis usually presents as a more fulminant disease (20).

Rarely, it can present as single or multiple cranial nerve palsy. Unilateral third nerve involvement has been reported in only a handful of cases. Takakura et al. also reported unilateral complete ophthalmoplegia in a patient of meningovascular syphilis in 2004 (21). Jordan et al. reported a case of bilateral oculomotor palsy due to neurosyphilis (22). Widespread meningeal thickening and strategic granulomatous inflammation, during meningovascular syphilis and acute syphilitic meningitis, may result in compression and ischemia of the cranial nerve rootlets. Small vessel vasculitis may also occur during meningovascular syphilis causing nerve infarction. Gummatous neurosyphilis causing cranial nerve compression may be the cause in the tertiary stage of neurosyphilis (23). Hypertrophic pachymeningitis has also been reported as a cause of cranial nerve involvement (24).

MRI of the brain may show signs of pachymeningitis, sulcal or basal meningitis, cranial nerve enhancement, parenchymal changes, and infarct. Cerebral gummas arising from dura or pia matter in close connection with cranial nerves may be observed. Serological tests are diagnostic. At least one treponemal and

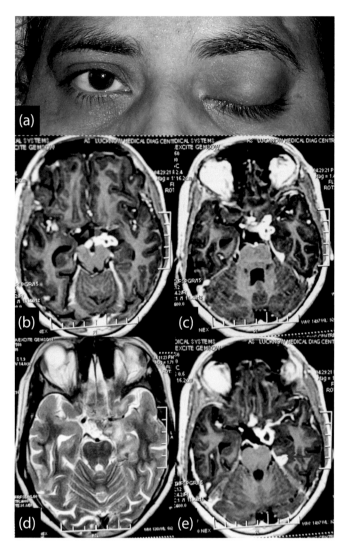

FIGURE 16.12 A 42-year-old woman presented with ophthalmoparesis involving the left eye (a) with history of anti-tuberculosis treatment for 7 weeks. Gad-enhanced axial sections show a conglomerate lesion at the level of left cerebral peduncle (b) and left cavernous sinus (c). T2-W axial section (d) and Gad-gadolinium enhanced sequence (e) at the corresponding level depict basifrontal and medial temporal involvement with meningeal enhancement along with another tuberculous lesion abutting the tentorium cerebelli (arrow).

one non-treponemal test should be sufficient to diagnose syphilis. Non-treponemal tests (semi-quantitative in nature: Venereal Disease Research Laboratory [VDRL] or rapid plasma reagin [RPR]), should be specified quantitatively in titers since the disease activity may correlate with the titers. The specificity of treponemal tests (*Treponema pallidum* hemagglutination test [TPHA], fluorescent treponemal antibody absorption test [FTA-ABS], and *Treponema pallidum* particle agglutination test [TPPA], immunoassays) ranges from 64% to 95%. Positive CSF and blood testing for treponema pallidum particle agglutination and VDRL may suggest the diagnosis of Neurosyphilis. Attempts must always be made to look for concomitant HIV-infection or a concomitant immunocompromised state. Intravenous crystalline penicillin-G 3-4 million units every 4 hours or intramuscular procaine penicillin-G 2.4 million units once a day with probenecid (500 mg orally four times a day) for 10–14 days is the treatment of choice. Other alternatives, especially when penicillin allergy is present, include parenteral ceftriaxone (2 mg/day) for 10–14 days and doxycycline (200 mg orally twice a day) for 3–4 weeks.

Viral infections

Varicella zoster virus (VZV)

Primary infection with VZV leads to viremia and rash commonly known as chicken pox. Along with this, seeding of multiple dorsal root ganglia might occur, reactivation of which causes Herpes Zoster (HZ). Various neurological complications have been reported to be occurring with HZ infection. The most common cranial nerves involved in HZ infection are cranial nerves VII, VIII, IX, and X. Ophthalmic complications may be seen when HZ occurs in the ophthalmic division of trigeminal (V1) nerve (25). Common ocular complications of herpes zoster ophthalmicus (HZO) include keratitis, scleritis, iritis, retinal necrosis, glaucoma, and optic neuritis. Ophthalmoplegia though uncommon, has been reported with HZO (20). While the exact incidence is not clear, it has been contemplated that only 5–31% of all HZ patients go on to develop ophthalmoplegia (26). The encroachment of inflammation from ophthalmic division of trigeminal to ocular cranial nerves, as they pass through cavernous sinus/superior orbital fissure, is thought to be the cause (26).

Edgerton in his extensive review of 2250 patients of HZO noted that ocular motor paralysis is indeed not related to the severity of pain or the degree of affection. Commonly, ophthalmoparesis occurs after skin eruption; this may, however, appear simultaneously in some patients. In Edgerton's series, oculomotor nerve was the most commonly involved nerve, that too in different denominations viz. total/ partial/ pupillary involving/ pupillary sparing, followed by the abducens nerve. Isolated pupillary palsy and paralysis of accommodation was observed by him in a couple of patients. While isolated transitory trochlear nerve palsy is rare in HZO, simultaneous involvement of III, IV, and VI nerve has been noted (27). Haargaard et al. also noted isolated ocular nerve palsies in four of their 110 immunocompetent patients of HZO (28). Bilateral cranial nerve palsies are rare unless cavernous sinus is involved.

Ocular cranial nerve palsies usually follow cutaneous eruptions and rash, and are often, though not always, self-limiting. Though the final word has not been said about the mechanism, a direct cytopathic damage by the virus or a vasculopathy secondary to viral replication has been postulated. While the diagnosis is primarily clinical, PCR positivity in CSF or the presence of specific antibodies in the CSF may be supportive; analysis of the fluid may also be done in patients developing ocular symptoms along with vesicular rash.

Neuroimaging may suggest abnormal enhancement of the recti and oblique muscles or soft tissue swelling in the orbit or orbital apex or cavernous sinus depending upon the cause.

Oral antiviral therapy for 7–10 days should be given to avoid complications in patients with HZO. Choice of antiviral therapy is debatable. Some authors prefer valacyclovir or famciclovir to acyclovir because of ease of dosing and better bioavailability. The route of administration of anti-viral therapy is also debatable; while oral route is usually preferred, some authors have recommended intravenous therapy in order to achieve early virostatic plasma levels. As a rule of thumb, patients where retinal, optic, or parenchymal brain involvement is anticipated, or there are suggestions of the same, intravenous acyclovir and valacyclovir should be used. Concomitant use of antivirals with corticosteroids has been recommended in order to reduce viral load and neuroinflammation. Complete or near-complete resolution is usually seen; it, though, may occur over a wide period ranging from 2 weeks to 1½ years (29,30).

REPRESENTATIVE CASE

A 45-year-old female presented with severe pain in the distribution of ophthalmic division of trigeminal nerve. Her complete examination on the day of presentation was normal. Detailed investigations including non-contrast CT head (Figure 16.13a), contrast-enhanced MRI brain (Figure 16.13b), CT angiography (Figure 16.13c), and CSF analysis were normal. On Day 3 of symptom onset, she developed maculopapular rash in the trigeminal nerve distribution (Figure 16.13d) suggestive of HZO. She was initiated on oral Valacyclovir (in a dose of 1 gm thrice a day). On Day 6, she developed diplopia due to right lateral rectus palsy (Figure 16.13e). She was given a short course of oral steroids; she recovered completely in 3 weeks.

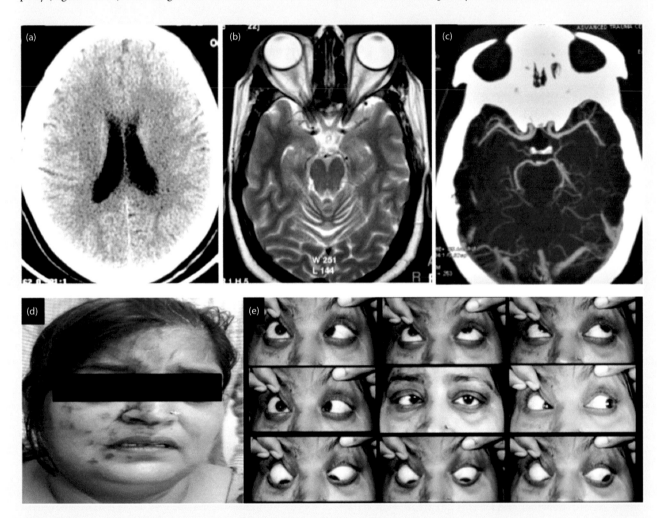

FIGURE 16.13 Normal non-contrast CT head (a), normal contrast-enhanced MRI brain (b), normal CT angiography (c). A maculopapular rash in the distribution of trigeminal nerve (d) can be seen. Right lateral rectus palsy on nine-gaze photography (e).

HIV

HIV-mediated opportunistic infections may cause ocular cranial nerve involvement in many ways. In patients with of AIDS and ocular involvement, neuro-ophthalmic manifestations occur in around 8–15% and only 4% patients have ocular cranial nerve palsies. A small set of patients may have ocular cranial nerve involvement as the earliest presenting symptom. Thus, ocular cranial nerves can be involved either in isolation or in varied combinations. Various opportunistic infections like toxoplasma, cryptococcosis, varicella zoster, cytomegalovirus (CMV), and tuberculosis may cause ocular cranial nerve palsy due to direct infiltration of cranial nerves, meningeal or parenchymal inflammation, or increased ICP. Other associated conditions like progressive multifocal leukoencephalopathy and CNS or orbital lymphoma may also lead to diplopia or ophthalmoparesis because of compression, inflammation or due to increased ICP. Ocular cranial nerves have also been seen to be involved as a part of cavernous sinus syndrome or orbital apex syndrome in patients with strategically placed eosinophilic granulomas (31). Immune-mediated cranial neuropathy has also been reported during the phase of seroconversion in patients with HIV infection.

Patients with HIV infection under long-term highly active anti-retroviral therapy (HAART) may also develop abnormalities in the function of otherwise structurally normal EOMs. Orbital MRIs of these patients may be similar to that of patients with chronic progressive external ophthalmoplegia (CPEO). Pineles et al. described five adult patients with CPEO-like presentation and history of >10 years of HAART. Although, the EOM volume was preserved on orbital MRI, bright signal was observed on T1-W images. The pathophysiology of this condition is debatable. Skeletal myopathy due to HAART therapy or direct muscle infiltration by the virus has been postulated (32). MRI brain and orbits may be suggestive of inflammation, mass lesion related to opportunistic infection or lymphoma. Isolated cranial nerve enhancement has also been seen.

Serological testing for HIV and quantification of CD-4 counts should always be done is suspected patients; besides helping in staging these patients, CD-4 counts also aid in ruling in (or out) the likelihood of opportunistic infections. While HAART is quintessential in all patients affected by HIV, appropriate treatment of the associated opportunistic infection is equally important.

Dengue

Dengue is a mosquito-borne single-stranded RNA virus belonging to the genus *Flavivirus* and endemic in tropical climatic regions. While dengue fever is common, neurological manifestations can be mild to life-threatening. Neurological manifestations can broadly be divided into encephalitis/encephalopathy, neuromuscular, and neuro-ophthalmic complications. Neuro-ophthalmic presentations include dengue maculopathy, optic neuropathy, retinal vasculopathy, and ocular cranial nerve palsies. Oculomotor nerve followed by abducens nerve may be involved. Few reports also describe ophthalmoparesis occurring with dengue-related, immune-mediated Guillain-Barre syndrome (GBS). These complications are generally thought to be due to an immune-mediated phenomenon; however, a few authors believe that direct CNS invasion of the virus may be responsible (33).

Ophthalmoparesis secondary to hemorrhagic complications of dengue has also been reported in the literature. Increased ICP has been noted in various dengue-related neurological complications secondary to strategic intracranial bleeds, pituitary apoplexy, encephalitis, etc. All these conditions may cause diplopia due to involvement of various cranial nerves depending on the site and nature of the lesion.

In early stages, the detection of NS-1 antigen or RNA by reverse transcription (RT)-PCR and viral culture may be appropriate. Serological tests detecting dengue-specific antibodies (IgM) are fruitful during the first 3–10 days of disease onset. Thrombocytopenia may not necessarily be seen in patients with neurological complications. If possible, CSF analysis should be done whenever neurological involvement is suspected, and specific antigens/antibodies should be looked for. Treatment is usually symptomatic and supportive. Maintaining adequate hydration is the key. In patients showing signs of plasma leakage, early fluid resuscitation is warranted. Hemorrhagic complications deserve appropriate management depending on the site

and magnitude of involvement. In cases where immune-mediated process is suspected, immunoglobulins and judicious use of corticosteroids should be considered (33).

Parasitic infections

Cysticercosis

Infestation of the cyst form of *Taenia solium*, and rarely *Taenia saginata*, causes cysticercosis. Subcutaneous tissue, skeletal muscle, brain, and eyes are common sites of infestation. Ocular or adnexal involvement may occur in 13–46% of cases with multiple site involvement, but isolated adnexal cases are uncommon.

With an exception of inferior oblique muscle any EOM may be involved by cysticercosis. While there is no specific predilection of cysticercosis toward any muscle, various series have shown predilection of cysticercosis toward medial rectus, inferior rectus, or superior rectus. Direct muscle infiltration is common, and increased ICP secondary to either large cysts or strategically located cysts may also cause isolated cranial nerve palsies. Few case reports with neurocysticercosis (NCC) mimicking cavernous sinus syndrome have been reported (34). The cysts may further enlarge causing compressive effects or may show an inflammatory reaction. The presentation may, hence, simulate an orbital apex syndrome due to the same (35).

Most common symptoms are diplopia due to restricted ocular mobility, proptosis, or ptosis. Restriction of mobility has been often noted in the direction opposite to the muscle involved, but restriction can also be noted in the direction of the involved muscle (36). Signs of inflammation like pain on eye movements may accompany the presentation especially in those who inadvertently have been given cysticidal medications. Liberation of toxic products occurring as a result of death of larvae is presumed to be the cause of inflammation.

Enzyme-linked immunotransfer blot has been recommended over enzyme-linked immunosorbent assays (using crude antigen) for the diagnosis of patients suspected of NCC (37). Well-defined cystic lesion with a scolex is often visible, pending degeneration, on CT, MRI, or USG. The muscle containing the cyst is enlarged and may show signs of inflammation. MRI of orbits may show diffuse muscle enlargement with signs of soft tissue inflammation (Figure 16.14). MRI of the brain may reveal NCC in various stages of evolution, in addition to ocular lesions. The presence of a cystic lesion differentiates the condition from other differentials like thyroid ophthalmopathy.

Albendazole can be used for EOM cysticercosis provided the following prerequisites are fulfilled. First, an ocular B-scan should be done to rule out the presence of cysticerci in the vitreoretinal space and those closely abutting the optic nerve or optic canal. Prior surgical excision is warranted by a minimum of 6 weeks, if a decision on the use of albendazole has been taken. Second, multiple cysticerci suggest a potential case of dissemination; thus, caution needs to be exercised to prevent a cardiac nodal block or seizures by getting the necessary investigations (ECG, ECHO, MRI of the brain with SPGR-GAD) done (38). More often than not, brain imaging is done as a part of initial evaluation itself, but the cardiac assessment is conveniently missed. Excellent results have been seen due to increased drug bioavailability owing to vascularity of EOM. Because of possibility of inflammatory reaction of the dying larva, steroids should be initiated a few days before and administered simultaneously along with anti-helminthic therapy. Corticosteroids also help by preventing muscle fibrosis.

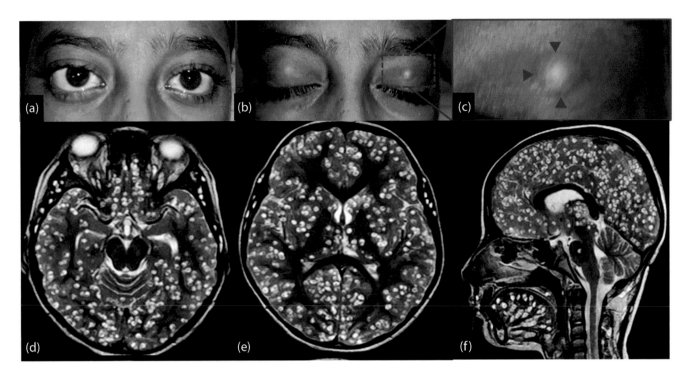

FIGURE 16.14 Clinical images of a 12-year-old boy show proptosis and eyes fixed in convergent gaze (a). Of note is the presence of a small swelling/bleb over the left eyelid (b, c) providing an insight into the possible etiology (cysticercus; proven histologically). T2-W axial (d, e) and sagittal (f) sections show bilateral orbital myocysticercosis along with cysticerci-studded brain parenchyma; involvement of the tongue can also be seen.

While more than half of patients fully respond to medical therapy, surgical removal of intramuscular cysts has been attempted in resistant cases. The procedure is surgically challenging, and inherent dangers include muscle injury and postoperative fibrosis. A bothersome residual restriction of movements with diplopia in extreme position of gaze may require surgical intervention in these few cases.

Toxoplasma gondii

Toxoplasma gondii is an obligate intracellular protozoan parasite that causes both congenital and acquired infections. Cats are definitive hosts; it gets transmitted by ingestion of raw food or undercooked meat, contaminated water, vertical transmission (maternal-fetal), or infected transplants. It is a common opportunistic infection in AIDS and can present with variable manifestations depending on the organs involved. It is considered to be a fatal and severe infection in immunodeficient hosts. Common systemic clinical manifestations are fever, headache, lymphadenopathy, rash (maculo-papular), arthralgias, and myalgias; even immunocompetent hosts may present with these symptoms. Immunodeficient individuals may present with encephalitis, pneumonitis, myocarditis, and other signs of disseminated infection.

CNS infection occurs when the parasite invades a breached blood–brain barrier, or when due to hematogenous spread, tachyzoites present in the blood invade the vascular epithelium to replicate inside the CNS. Toxoplasma has a predilection toward involvement of basal ganglia, corticomedullary junction, cerebral white matter, and the periventricular regions. Isolated ocular cranial nerve involvement or cavernous sinus involvement by toxoplasma has only been demonstrated in small case series or isolated case studies. Mwanza et al. noted ocular motor palsies in

26% of 166 patients with HIV having neurological symptoms (39). Liu et al. described cavernous sinusitis due to toxoplasmosis in a diabetic patient presenting with ocular cranial nerve palsy along with trigeminal and facial nerve palsy (40). Available treatment options include trimethoprim/sulfadiazine, pyrimethamine/sulfamethoxazole, and clindamycin.

Involvement of ocular nerves as a complication of different infections

While direct infiltration by an infectious etiology may lead to ocular cranial nerve palsy, many a times the involvement is indirect due to a complication caused by the infectious agent. Hydrocephalus and increased ICP are caused by many infections like tuberculosis, cryptococcosis, bacterial meningitis, toxoplasmosis, etc. Increased ICP may present with unilateral or bilateral cranial nerve palsy (usually abducens nerve due to its long intracranial course or compression against the petrous ligament). Secondary vasculitis may be caused by some infections like tuberculosis, syphilis, cryptococcosis, etc. which may cause ischemia of brain parenchyma or of cranial nerves causing their affection. Some infections like tuberculosis may lead to the development of hypertrophic pachymeningitis causing entrapment of cranial nerves in various combinations.

Post-infectious involvement of ocular cranial nerves

Cranial nerve involvement has been well described as post-infective syndromes. Some infections may trigger an immune response as a result of antigenic/molecular mimicry leading to inflammation of the cranial nerve. A form of recurrent abducens palsy has been considered to be because of a post-infectious trigger due to various infections like Varicella zoster, Epstein-Barr virus, CMV, or *Coxiella burnetii* (41). Many times, the ocular cranial nerve are involved in post-infective demyelinating syndromes as a variant of GBS. Miller Fischer variant is observed in nearly 5% of GBS patients and presents as a triad of ophthalmoparesis, ataxia, and areflexia. Elevated anti-GQ1b IgG antibody titers are well known in MFS. Carbohydrate structure of various causative organisms (like *Campylobacter jejuni*, *Mycoplasma pneumonia*, *H. influenzae*) may mimic a ganglioside causing molecular mimicry and resultant damage.

Conclusion

Infection-associated cranial nerve palsies can occur either as a direct result of multiple infections ranging from fungal to parasitic or as a complication of different infections. Age at the time of presentation and the presence of comorbidities seem to be the most important determinants in shortlisting or predicting the etiology. An appropriate workup along with prompt institution of treatment, medical *versus* surgical, is the key to prevent a residual impairment or mortality.

Abbreviations

- ADA: Adenosine deaminase
- AIDS: Acquired immunodeficiency syndrome
- ANA: Anti-nuclear antibodies
- CECT: Contrast-enhanced computed tomography
- CMV: Cytomegalovirus
- CNS: Central nervous system
- CRP: C-Reactive protein
- CPEO: Chronic progressive external ophthalmoplegia
- CSF: Cerebrospinal fluid
- EOM: Extraocular muscle
- ESR: Erythrocyte sedimentation rate
- FDG-PET: Fluoro-deoxy-glucose positron emission tomography
- FESS: Functional endoscopic sinus surgery
- FTA-Abs: Fluorescent treponemal antibody absorption test
- GBS: Guillain-Barre syndrome
- HAART: Highly active anti-retroviral therapy
- HZ: Herpes zoster
- HZO: Herpes zoster ophthalmicus
- ICA: Internal carotid artery
- ICP: Intracranial pressure
- IDSA: Infectious Diseases Society of America
- MFS: Miller Fischer syndrome
- MRI: Magnetic resonance imaging
- RNA: Ribonucleic acid
- RPR: Rapid plasma reagin
- T1-W: T1-weighted sequence
- T2-W: T2-weighted sequence
- TBM: Tuberculous meningitis
- TPHA: *Treponema pallidum* Hemagglutination test
- TPPA: *Treponema pallidum* Particle Agglutination test
- USG: Ultrasonography
- VDRL: Venereal Disease Research Laboratory
- VZV: Varicella zoster virus

Multiple-Choice Questions

1. Which of the following statements is true regarding fungal cavernous sinus syndromes?
   a. Mucormycosis is the most common cause in immunocompetent individuals.
   b. Mucormycosis is more angioinvasive than Aspergillosis.
   c. Fungal sinus involvement is commonly associated with air-fluid levels on imaging.
   d. Histopathological examination of mucormycosis reveals large non-septate mycelial filaments, which branch at right angle.

   Answer:
   d. Histopathological examination of mucormycosis reveals large non-septate mycelial filaments, which branch at right angle.

2. Invasive aspergillosis
   a. Is an opportunistic infection of granulocytopenic patients.
   b. Common predisposing factors include alcoholism.
   c. Aspergillus fumigatus (followed by *Aspergillus flavus*) is the usual organism.
   d. All of the above.

   Answer:
   d. All of the above.

3. Which of the following statements is INCORRECT regarding orbital cellulitis?
   a. *Streptococci* species are the commonest bacteria implicated.
   b. *Eikenella corrodens* are commonly implicated anaerobic bacteria.
   c. Refers to involvement of structures anterior to orbital septum.
   d. None of the above.

   Answer:
   c. Refers to involvement of structures anterior to orbital septum.

4. Which of the following are NOT the predictors of cranial nerve involvement in patients with tubercular meningitis?
   a. Hydrocephalous
   b. Age < 10 years
   c. Presence of optochiasmatic arachnoiditis
   d. Cerebrospinal fluid cell count > 100/mm^3

   Answer:
   b. Age < 10 years

References

1. Keane JR. Multiple cranial nerve palsies: Analysis of 979 cases. Arch Neurol. 2005;62(11):1714–7.
2. Turvey TA, Golden BA. Orbital anatomy for the surgeon. Oral Maxillofac Surg Clin N Am. 2012;24(4):525–36.

3. Yoshihara M, Saito N, Kashima Y, Ishikawa H. The Ishikawa classification of cavernous sinus lesions by clinico-anatomical findings. Jpn J Ophthalmol. 2001;45(4):420–4.

4. Bhatkar S, Goyal MK, Takkar A, Mukherjee KK, Singh P, Singh R, et al. Cavernous sinus syndrome: A prospective study of 73 cases at a tertiary care centre in Northern India. Clin Neurol Neurosurg. 2017;155:63–9.

5. Ramanand Y, Sidhu TS, Jaswinder K, Sharma N. An atypical presentation of cavernous sinus thrombosis. Indian J Otolaryngol Head Neck Surg. 2007;59(2):163–5.

6. Riley TT, Muzny CA, Swiatlo E, Legendre DP. Breaking the mold: A review of mucormycosis and current pharmacological treatment options. Ann Pharmacother. 2016;50(9):747–57.

7. Blitzer A, Lawson W, Meyers BR, Biller HF. Patient survival factors in paranasal sinus mucormycosis. Laryngoscope. 1980;90(4):635–48.

8. Fernandes YB, Ramina R, Borges G, Queiroz LS, Maldaun MVC, Maciel Jr JA. Orbital apex syndrome due to aspergillosis: Case report. ArqNeuropsiquiatr. 2001;59(3B):806–8.

9. Marzolf G, Sabou M, Lannes B, Cotton F, Meyronet D, Galanaud D, et al. Magnetic resonance imaging of cerebral aspergillosis: Imaging and pathological correlations. PLoS ONE [Internet]. 2016;11(4): e0152475.

10. Patterson TF, Thompson GR, Denning DW, Fishman JA, Hadley S, Herbrecht R, et al. Executive summary: Practice guidelines for the diagnosis and management of aspergillosis: 2016 Update by the Infectious Diseases Society of America. Clin Infect Dis Off Publ Infect Dis Soc Am. 2016;63(4):433–42.

11. Arora V, Nagarkar NM, Dass A, Malhotra A. Invasive rhino-orbital aspergillosis. Indian J Otolaryngol Head Neck Surg. 2011;63(4):325–9.

12. Chaudhry IA, Shamsi FA, Elzaridi E, Al-Rashed W, Al-Amri A, Al-Anezi F, et al. Outcome of treated orbital cellulitis in a tertiary eye care center in the middle East. Ophthalmology. 2007;114(2):345–54.

13. Chaudhry IA, Al-Rashed W, Arat YO. The hot orbit: orbital cellulitis. Middle East Afr J Ophthalmol. 2012;19(1):34–42.

14. Tsirouki T, Dastiridou AI, Ibánez Flores N, Cerpa JC, Moschos MM, Brazitikos P, et al. Orbital cellulitis. SurvOphthalmol. 2018;63(4):534–53.

15. Baiu I, Melendez E. Periorbital and orbital cellulitis. JAMA. 2020;323(2):196–6.

16. Chandler JR, Langenbrunner DJ, Stevens ER. The pathogenesis of orbital complications in acute sinusitis. Laryngoscope. 1970;80(9):1414–28.

17. Kapadia S, Patrawalla A. Extrapulmonary tuberculosis presenting as a cavernous sinus syndrome: Case report with review of existing literature. IDCases. 2014;1(4):97–100.

18. Shobha N, Mahadevan A, Taly AB, Sinha S, Srikanth SG, Satish S, et al. Hypertrophic cranial pachymeningitis in countries endemic for tuberculosis: Diagnostic and therapeutic dilemmas. J Clin Neurosci. 2008;15(4):418–27.

19. Raut T, Garg RK, Jain A, Verma R, Singh MK, Malhotra HS, Kohli N, Parihar A. Hydrocephalus in tuberculous meningitis: Incidence, its predictive factors and impact on the prognosis. J Infect. 2013;66(4):330–7.

20. Piura Y, Mina Y, Aizenstein O, Gadoth A. Neurosyphilis presenting as cranial nerve palsy, an entity which is easy to miss. BMJ Case Rep. 2019;12(2): e226509.

21. Takakura Y, Yamaguchi Y, Miyoshi T. [Neurosyphilis presenting the left total ophthalmoplegia: A case report]. Rinsho Shinkeigaku. 2004;44(4–5):296–8.

22. Jordan K, Marino J, Damast M. Bilateral oculomotor paralysis due to neurosyphilis. AnnNeurol: Official Journal of the American Neurological Association and the Child Neurology Society. 1978;3(1):90–3.

23. Seeley WW, Venna N. Neurosyphilis presenting with gummatous oculomotor nerve palsy. J NeurolNeurosurg Psychiatry. 2004;75(5):789.

24. Hassin GB, Zeitlin H. Syphilitic cerebral hypertrophic pachymeningitis: Clinicopathologic studies in a case. Arch. Neurol. Psychiatry. 1940;43(2):362–71.

25. Harthan JS, Borgman CJ. Herpes zoster ophthalmicus-induced oculomotor nerve palsy. J Optom. 2013;6(1):60–5.

26. Arda H, Mirza E, Gumus K, Oner A, Karakucuk S, Sırakaya E. Orbital apex syndrome in herpes zoster ophthalmicus. Case Rep Ophthalmol Med. 2012;2012:1–4.

27. Edgerton AE. Herpes zoster ophthalmicus: Report of cases and a review of the literature. Trans Am Ophthalmol Soc. 1942;40:390–439.

28. Haargaard B, Lund-Andersen H, Milea D. Central nervous system involvement after herpes zoster ophthalmicus. Acta Ophthalmol (Copenh). 2008;86(7):806–9.

29. Sanjay S, Chan EW, Gopal L, Hegde SR, Chang BC-M. Complete unilateral ophthalmoplegia in herpes zoster ophthalmicus. J Neuro-Ophthalmol Off J North Am Neuro-Ophthalmol Soc. 2009;29(4):325–37.

30. Jun L, Gupta A, Milea D, Jaufeerally F. More than meets the eye: Varicella zoster virus-related orbital apex syndrome. Indian J Ophthalmol. 2018;66(11):1647.

31. Wells CD, Moodley AA. HIV-associated cavernous sinus disease. South Afr J HIV Med. 2019;20(1):1–7.

32. Pineles SL, Demer JL, Holland GN, Ransome SS, Bonelli L, Velez FG. External ophthalmoplegia in human immunodeficiency virus-infected patients receiving antiretroviral therapy. J AAPOS. 2012;16(6):529–33.

33. Carod-Artal FJ, Wichmann O, Farrar J, Gascón J. Neurological complications of dengue virus infection. Lancet Neurol. 2013;12(9):906–19.

34. Whitefield L, Crowston JG, Davey C. Cavernous sinus syndrome associated with neurocysticercosis. Eye. 1996;10(5):642–3.

35. Sekhar GC, Lemke BN. Orbital cysticercosis. Ophthalmology. 1997;104(10):1599–604.

36. Pandey PK, Chaudhuri Z, Sharma P, Bhomaj S. Extraocular muscle cysticercosis: A clinical masquerade. J Pediatr Ophthalmol Strabismus. 2000;37(5):273–8.

37. White AC, Coyle CM, Rajshekhar V, et al. Diagnosis and treatment of neurocysticercosis: 2017 clinical practice guidelines by the Infectious Diseases Society of America (IDSA) and the American Society of Tropical Medicine and Hygiene (ASTMH). Clin Infect Dis. 2018;66:1159–63.

38. Pandey S, Malhotra HS, Garg RK, Malhotra KP, Kumar N, Rizvi I, Jain A, Kohli N, Verma R, Sharma P, Uniyal R. Quantitative assessment of lesion load and efficacy of 3 cycles of albendazole in disseminated cysticercosis: A prospective evaluation. BMC Infect Dis. 2020;20(1):1–2.

39. Mwanza J-C, Nyamabo LK, Tylleskär T, Plant GT. Neuro-ophthalmological disorders in HIV infected subjects with neurological manifestations. Br J Ophthalmol. 2004;88(11):1455–9.

40. Liu J, Zhang B, Cui L, Zhao T, Sheng Zhang R, Liu H, Du H, Gao J, Fang S. Toxoplasmosis presenting with multiple cranial nerve palsies and cavernous sinusitis: A case report. Neurol Asia. 2019;24(2):171–3.

41. Gonçalves R, Coelho P, Menezes C, Ribeiro I. Benign recurrent sixth nerve palsy in a child. Case Rep Ophthalmol Med. 2017;2017.

Part IV
Higher Visual Pathways

17

AN APPROACH TO A PATIENT WITH GAZE DISORDER

P. Vinny Wilson

CASE STUDY

A 33-year-old woman presented with holo-cranial headache and diplopia of 10 days duration. On examination, best corrected visual acuity was noted to be 6/6 in both eyes. Fundus examination showed normal optic discs bilaterally. Skew deviation with mild vertical misalignment of eyes was noted. Pupillary reflexes were normal and light-near dissociation was noted. Upgaze restriction was present and convergence-retraction nystagmus was observed on an attempted upgaze. Other extraocular movements were normal. What is the clinical syndrome in question?

Introduction

The human eye can resolve only a small area of vision with fine details; the region focused on the fovea. The peripheral retina designed to detect motion cannot resolve with clarity. The eyes have to move constantly to ensure that the point of the interest requiring detailed resolution is always focused on the fovea. Nature has devised a sophisticated mechanism by way of supranuclear gaze control to make this possible.

Mechanisms of gaze

Six systems of supranuclear gaze namely the saccadic system, the smooth pursuit system, the vestibular system, the optokinetic system, the fixation system, and the vergence system ensure that the desired target is always focused on the fovea. These systems of supranuclear gaze may be triggered by the retina (optokinetic and smooth pursuit systems), vestibular apparatus (vestibular system), or may be voluntary (saccadic system). Smooth pursuit and vergence systems are primarily involuntary. Smooth pursuit tracks the moving target in the horizontal or vertical plane, while the vergence system tracks the target in an anteroposterior axis. The optokinetic and vestibular systems keep the target focused on fovea when the head is in motion [1].

Visual fixation is an active process. Active modulation of three types of small eye movements, namely microdrifts, microsaccades and microtremors occurring in horizontal, vertical, and torsional directions are essential for visual fixation. To enable visual fixation, saccades are tonically inhibited by higher cortical centers by activating omnipause cells in the brainstem.

Common final pathway

Various systems of supranuclear control of gaze act through the same set of motor neurons and extraocular muscles. These set of neurons are often referred to as the final common pathway. The

brainstem converts what begins as a retinal visual signal, proprioceptive impulse, volitional, and vestibular information into commands for vertical and horizontal eye movements by coding the information into signals for oculomotor nerves (cranial nerves III, IV and VI). The final destination for the horizontal gaze circuits lies in parapontine reticular formation (PPRF) in the brainstem. PPRF further projects to the abducens nuclear complex comprising the abducens nucleus and interneurons, namely the medial longitudinal fasciculus (MLF). MLF interconnects the ipsilateral abducens nucleus with the contralateral medial rectus nucleus. Similarly, cells in the rostral interstitial MLF (riMLF) in midbrain project to the oculomotor nuclei (obliques, superior and inferior recti) to produce conjugate vertical movements [1, 2] (Table 17.1, Figure 17.1).

Saccades

When a novel object appears in the visual field, our eyes generate a quick movement to bring this novel target on the fovea (saccade). The word saccade comes from the French term "saquer," which refers to flicking the reins of a horse. Saccades are rapid, brief conjugate eye movements that are characterized by their ballistic nature and high velocity (400–800°/s). These redirect our line of gaze, for example, when visually scanning a landscape. Saccades have traditionally been classified based on the behavioral context in which they are generated. Thus, a reflexive saccade is executed when a novel stimulus attracts enough attention for it to be focused on the fovea, like a new patient with hemiballismus entering the consultation room. Voluntary saccades generated by an internal decision are further divided into memory-guided, predictive, endogenous saccades and antisaccades [2, 3].

Several electrophysiological and inactivation studies have shown that interparietal sulcus corresponds to the generation of reflexive saccades, while the frontal eye fields (FEFs) and supplementary eye fields appear to be involved in generating voluntary saccades. Both frontal and parietal areas project to the superior colliculus directly and indirectly via basal ganglia. FEF and superior colliculus in turn project to the contralateral PPRF and riMLF to generate contralateral saccades, while vertical saccades require simultaneous activity in bilateral FEF or superior colliculi [4,5] (Figure 17.2).

Conjugate saccadic movements require that the mechanical resistance of the orbit, which is elastic by nature, be overcome. The brainstem translates multiple cortical inputs into signals for the oculomotor nerves. These input signals are coded for desired velocity and final position. The velocity command is the pulse, while position command is the step. The pulse can also be considered to be the phasic component giving the torque needed to overcome the viscous drag of the orbital tissues, with the step being the tonic component giving the torque required to overcome the elastic recoil forces. The velocity command (*pulse*) is executed by the burst cells (PPRF and riMLF), which is converted into position command (*step*) by mathematical integration of the velocity-coded signal into a position-coded information. The neural integrator(NI) performs this mathematical function that helps in the smooth coordination between the velocity and the position commands [6] (Table 17.1,

DOI: 10.1201/9780429020278-25

TABLE 17.1: Neural Integrators, Omnipause and Burst Neurons

Substrate	Horizontal Saccade	Vertical Saccade	Location
Omnipause neurons	Nucleus raphe interpositus	Nucleus raphe interpositus	Pons
Burst neurons	Parapontine reticular formation(PPRF)	Rostral interstitial medial longitudinal fasciculus (riMLF)	Pons (horizontal saccade) Midbrain (vertical saccade)
Neural integrators	Nucleus propositus hypoglossi Medial vestibular nucleus	Interstitial nucleus of cajal	Medulla/Pons (horizontal saccade) Midbrain (vertical saccade)
Cranial nerves	III and VI	III and IV	Mid brain and pons

Figure 17.3). Neural substrates corresponding to the saccadic gaze deficits they produce are listed in Table 17.2.

The pursuit system

Unlike the saccadic system, the smooth pursuit system tracks a target that is in motion. An apt example would be tracking a bird flying across the sky. The smooth pursuit system cannot follow objects moving faster than 30–40°/s. Objects moving faster than 40°/s elicit saccades.

The smooth pursuit system is driven by the visual motion sensed by the striate cortex. In an animal experiment with monkeys, the perceived motion was first processed in the middle temporal (MT) and medial superior temporal (MST) areas in the superior temporal sulcus. Oculomotor signals from here project to the dorsolateral pontine nuclei in the brainstem from where the fibers decussate to the vestibulocerebellum. Signal then passes to the vestibular nuclei from where the fibers decussate again to reach the final common pathway of the oculomotor nuclei. **The smooth pursuit pathway, therefore, decussates twice generating pursuits to the ipsilateral side of its cortical origin** [7, 8] (Figure 17.4). Vertical pursuits follow a similar pathway until the vestibular nuclei, from where the fibers project to the riMLF [9]. Various lesions in the neuraxis and their corresponding pursuit abnormalities are listed in Table 17.3.

The vestibular, optokinetic and vergence systems

The *vestibular system* is activated to maintain objects of interest on fovea during brief head motions, achieved by compensatory reciprocal eye movements with velocity matching head motion. This eye movement, termed the vestibulo-ocular reflex (VOR), is produced by the labyrinth, vestibular nuclei and flocculonodular lobe of the cerebellum. The *optokinetic nystagmus system (OKN)* takes over from the vestibular system when the head movements are of large amplitude and too rapid. The pathways are similar to that of the smooth pursuit system. The *vergence system* kicks into play during the depth tracking of an object like a cricket batsman watching a delivered ball fast approaching toward him. The vergence system has its origins in the parietal, occipital and frontal regions [7, 10]. OKN abnormalities and their associated disorders are shown in Table 17.4.

Examination in gaze disorder

Testing for saccades

Observe the patient as they fixate their gaze on a stationary object. Show two targets to the patient, one displayed straight ahead and another displayed in the peripheral field. Ask the patient to move their gaze rapidly back and forth between the

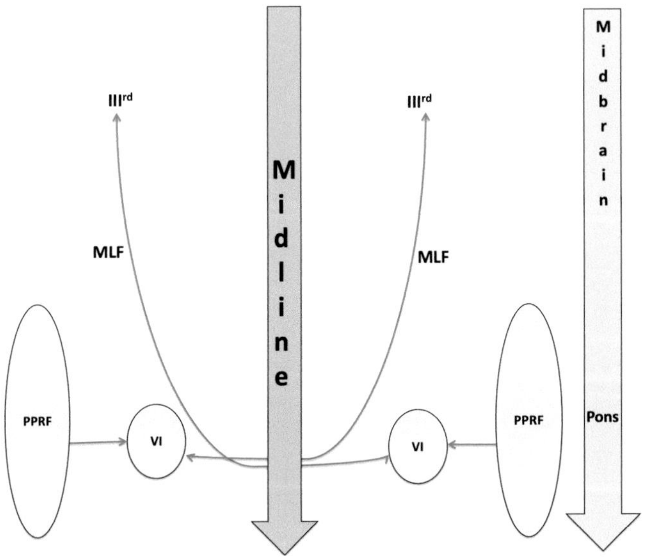

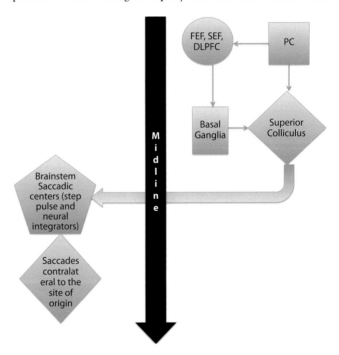

FIGURE 17.1 Schematic diagram depicting internuclear connections between the abducens and third nerve nuclei. *Abbreviations*: PPRF, para pontine reticular formation; VI, abducens nucleus; MLF, medial longitudinal fasciculus; IIIrd, third nerve nucleus.

FIGURE 17.2 Schematic diagram depicting saccadic pathway. *Abbreviations*: PC, parietal cortex; FEF, frontal eye field; DLPFC, dorsolateral prefrontal cortex; SEF, supplementary eye field.

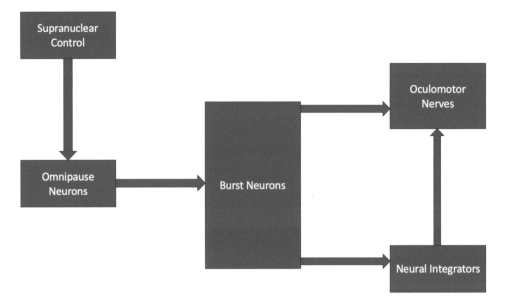

FIGURE 17.3   Schematic diagram depicting pulse, step and neural integrator.

displayed targets. An example of targets would be the examiner's nose and the examiner's finger from an outstretched hand. Alternatively, the quick phases induced by the optokinetic drum or tape also assess the saccadic eye movements. While observing the saccades, the parameters studied are latency (time to onset of saccades), velocity (slow or fast), accuracy (overshoot or undershoot), saccadic intrusions and antisaccades. Typically, saccades should begin within 250 milliseconds. An undershoot of 10% of centrifugal saccade and an overshoot of 10% of the centripetal saccade are normal but should disappear after four or five repetitions [7].

Testing for smooth pursuits

Bedside examination of the smooth pursuit system involves instructing the patient to track a pencil tip held at 1 m distance and moved with a uniform speed (40°/s or slower) while keeping the head stationary. The patient should be able to fixate on the target. Alternatively, movement of optokinetic stripes can be used to assess pursuit represented by the initial phase of the evoked nystagmus. The examiner observes the amplitude, velocity, direction and smoothness of the pursuit movements. Corrective saccades should be sought which may indicate an inappropriate smooth pursuit gain. Smooth pursuit movements that are markedly asymmetric suggest a structural lesion [7].

TABLE 17.2: Gaze Deficits and Localization

Deficit	Localization
Hypermetric saccades	Cerebellum
Isolated horizontal saccadic paresis	Pons (PPRF)
Isolated vertical saccadic paresis	Midbrain (riMLF)
Isolated vertical gaze-evoked nystagmus	Midbrain
Internuclear ophthalmoplegia	Medial longitudinal fasciculus (MLF)
Convergence retraction nystagmus	Midbrain

Testing for vergence

Convergence or depth tracking movements can be tested by comparing ocular alignment in two gaze conditions. Instruct the patient to fixate his vision on a pencil held at 1 m followed by slowly moving the pencil toward the patient's nose. The point of

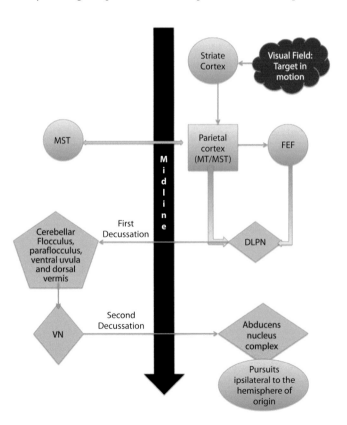

FIGURE 17.4   Schematic diagram depicting the smooth pursuit pathway. *Abbreviations*: MT, middle temporal area; MST, medial superior temporal area; FEF, frontal eye fields; DLPN, dorsolateral pontine nuclei; VN, vestibular nucleus.

TABLE 17.3: Lesions Causing Smooth Pursuit Abnormalities

Lesion	Abnormality
Frontal lobe	Impaired ipsilateral smooth pursuit of targets moving in a predictable fashion
Bilateral occipital lesions	Abolishes smooth pursuit
Parietal lesion	Decreases amplitude and velocity ipsilaterally
Posterior cerebral cortex	Unilateral smooth pursuit deficits for targets moving toward the side of lesion (directional deficit) and bidirectional deficit in estimating the speed of moving target in visual hemifield contralateral to lesion
Thalamic hemorrhage	Ipsilateral smooth pursuit deficits
Unilateral midbrain lesion	Ipsilateral smooth pursuit deficits
MLF lesion	Impaired vertical smooth pursuit
Pontine lesion	Ipsilateral smooth pursuit deficits
Cerebellar flocular or vermal lesions	Impairment of pursuit on the involved side

maximum convergence is where one or both eyes lose fixation and deviate outward. This distance is usually 8–10 cm and usually increases with age [7].

Testing for optokinetic nystagmus (OKN)

OKN is tested clinically by utilizing a drifting visual stimulus across the patient's visual field. At the bedside an optokinetic drum or a tape achieves the necessary stimulus. Alternatively, one may use mobile phone/tablet applications available for this purpose. The optokinetic reflex is composed of two stages. In the first stage, the eye begins to move toward the moving scene rapidly attaining a fast velocity of movement through the smooth pursuit system. The second stage is that of an optokinetic afternystagmus, where the eye jerks back to acquire a new moving target. The examiner should watch for direction and symmetry of the response [7, 10].

Testing for vestibulo-ocular reflex (VOR)

VOR is a type of conjugate eye movement, which moves the eye equal and opposite to the head movement. The VOR is classified into vertical, horizontal and torsional types. Head impulse test is used to test VOR. Examiner holds patient's head between both hands, asks the patient to fixate on a target in front of his eyes, followed by very rapidly turning the patient's head horizontally approximately 20–30°. Rapid reflex conjugate eye movements opposite in direction to the head movements are noticed in healthy subjects. Intact VOR ensures that the eyes maintain their relative position, irrespective of the head movements. VOR thus enables the target to be always centered on the fovea. Video-based head impulse testing allows for more accurate quantification of the VOR deficit. In an unconscious patient, eye movements directed opposite to passive head movements indicate that the VOR pathway from the medulla to pons or midbrain is intact. In

TABLE 17.4: Abnormalities of Optokinetic Nystagmus

Abnormality	Disorder
Symmetrically reduced OKN gain	Progressive supranuclear palsy
Asymmetrical OKN gain	Unilateral vestibular or parieto-occipital lesion
Reversed OKN	Congenital nystagmus

awake patients with limited or absent volitional eye movements, the examiner should observe whether the reflex ocular excursions are greater than the volitional excursions. When the reflex excursions are greater, the lesion causing the gaze disturbance must lie rostral to the brainstem centers mediating the reflex [11].

The head shaking visual acuity test is used to assess the VOR in awake patients who have full-range eye movements. Patients are asked to read aloud the smallest line possible on the Snellen's chart followed by shaking the head quickly (>1 cycle/s). During the shaking maneuver, the patient is asked to read the same line backward. If the visual acuity deteriorates by at least two lines, the VOR is bilaterally deficient. The caloric test uses thermal convection currents to stimulate the semi-circular canals. The patient's neck is flexed at 30°, thereby placing the horizontal canals in the vertical plane. Having ensured that the tympanic membrane is intact, the right external auditory canal is irrigated with 10–50 ml of ice water. A normal response in an awake patient (occurring within minutes) is an ipsilateral slow conjugate deviation, followed by contralateral quick phases resulting in nystagmus. In the comatose patient, the quick phases are absent. Failure of eye deviation suggests disruption of the ipsilateral VOR. After a pause of 5 minutes, the same procedure is repeated on the left side. Ice water is instilled in both ears simultaneously to test the integrity of downgaze. Warm water is instilled in both ears to test upgaze [7, 11].

The cancellation or suppression of VOR is a mechanism by which the VOR is inactivated in response to a situation where the target is moving in the same direction of the head motion. An intact VOR is a prerequisite to test for cancellation of VOR. Cancellation of VOR can be tested by asking the patient sitting on a wheelchair to fixate on the extended thumbs of the patient's outstretched arms with palms together in front of him. As an assistant rotates the wheelchair, the examiner looks for any refixation saccades. Such corrective refixation saccades during this test are indicative of impaired suppression of the VOR. This deficit usually occurs along with the smooth pursuit abnormalities and generally localizes the lesions to the cerebellum or cerebellar pathways. Alcohol, anticonvulsants, and sedatives can also impair suppression of the VOR by their effects on the cerebellum. Testing for VOR suppression is best avoided if VOR itself is not preserved, as it may spuriously appear normal [7, 11].

Testing for fixation

Ask the patient to gaze at a stationary object. In a normal person, the eyes should remain still. Examiner observes for eye movements that take the eyes off the target, for example, a fast jerky eye movement (saccadic intrusions) or slow drifts followed by fast corrective saccades (nystagmus). One may have to observe for at least 10–15 minutes to detect their presence. Minimal amplitude saccadic intrusions, easily missed by the untrained observer, can be picked up by watching the retinal vessels through an ophthalmoscope. In dedicated centers, oculography and video oculography can be used to detect these defects in gaze fixation with higher sensitivity [7].

Approaching gaze disorder

Patients of gaze disorder may present with blurred vision, decreased visual acuity or oscillopsia. Gaze disorders selectively involve some components of gaze (viz. saccades, smooth pursuit, OKN, vergence, VOR) or directions of gaze (horizontal or vertical), while sparing others. Substantial deductions can be made by careful observation of the resulting patterns. As a thumb rule, it

TABLE 17.5: Localization, Clinical Manifestations and Etiologies in Supranuclear Gaze Abnormalities

Deficit	Lesion	Clinical Manifestation	Causes
Horizontal gaze	Fronto-mesencephalic	• Tonic deviation ipsilateral to lesion • Saccadic palsy contralateral to lesion • Doll's eye maneuver and caloric tests intact	Vascular (most common) Neoplasm Demyelinating
	Occipito-mesencephalic	• Pursuit palsy ipsilateral to lesion • Saccadic system intact • Doll's eye maneuver and caloric tests intact	Demyelinating Vascular Neoplasm
	Brainstem at the level of abducens nucleus	• Gaze palsy ipsilateral to lesion • Doll's eye maneuver and caloric tests abnormal	Demyelinating Vascular Neoplasm
Vertical gaze	Dorsal areas of rostral midbrain on both sides	• Tonic upward deviation (oculogyric crisis) • Tonic downward deviation • Paralysis of upgaze	Parkinsonism Phenothiazines Thalamic hemorrhage Metabolic encephalopathy Pineal gland tumors
Internuclear ophthalmoplegia	MLF (INO)	• Impaired adduction ipsilateral to the lesion and nystagmus of the contralateral abducting eye • +/– Skew deviation • Convergence/VOR usually preserved	Multiple sclerosis Vascular Tumor
	MLF + PPRF +/– abducens complex (one-and-half syndrome)	• No horizontal eye movements except abduction (with nystagmus) of the eye contralateral to lesion • VOR affected	
	MLF + PPRF + VII nerve nucleus (eight-and-half syndrome)	• One and half syndrome plus facial palsy	
	MLF + PPRF + bilateral VII nerve nucleus (fifteen-and-half syndrome)	• One-and-half syndrome plus facial diplegia	
	Bilateral MLF (wall-eyed bilateral INO, WEBINO)	• Bilateral features of INO • Exotropia	

helps to remember that via descending modulations from supra-nuclear structures, horizontal eye movements are controlled in the pons. In contrast, vertical and torsional eye movements are controlled in the midbrain [1]. Vergence eye movements mediated by midbrain are involved far less commonly in gaze disorders. When an infra-nuclear pathology (e.g., Myasthenia Gravis) mimics a supranuclear gaze disorder, a preserved VOR and/or vergence movements may be a pointer to the latter. Common lesions causing gaze palsies include cerebral infarcts and hemorrhages, demyelinating lesions, multiple sclerosis, tumors, Wernicke's encephalopathy, metabolic disorders and neurodegenerative disorders such as progressive supranuclear palsy (PSP) [1, 12]. Localization, clinical manifestations and etiologies in supranuclear gaze abnormalities are listed in Table 17.5.

The following questions help in narrowing down the possibilities in a patient with gaze disorder:

a. Is the patient in a coma?
b. Is the eye movement abnormality conjugate?
c. Is it a gaze deviation or gaze deficit?
d. Is the VOR preserved?
e. Is there a fixation defect?
f. Are there associated movement disorders?

Scenario 1

The patient is conscious and presents with conjugate gaze deviations.
The examiner should look for a recognizable pattern.

a. *Horizontal Gaze Deviation*

Horizontal conjugate gaze deviations are most often due to frontal lobe or pontine lesions. VOR should be checked in all patients.

When VOR Is Preserved
A preserved VOR in a patient with horizontal conjugate gaze deviation points to a lesion rostral to the pons. In frontal lobe lesions, the patient looks toward the lesion, away from hemiparesis (Prevost or Vulpian sign) [13, 14]. Strokes, the most common frontal lobe lesions resulting in gaze deviations are often transient. Prolonged gaze deviations suggest pre-existing frontal lobe damage while sustained gaze deviations are often due to large strokes affecting post-Rolandic cortex or subcortical frontoparietal areas [14]. Saccadic and pursuit abnormalities may follow transient gaze deviations. Abnormalities in saccades tend to be contralateral (single decussation of pathways), while pursuit abnormalities are ipsilateral (double decussation of pathways).

In contrast to infarcts, epileptogenic lesions in frontal lobe cause episodic gaze deviations that make eyes look away from the lesion, especially in the first 10 seconds after seizure onset. Gaze deviations due to epileptogenic lesions tend to be transient, lasting for the duration of the focal seizure. Sustained deviation of the gaze toward the side of hemiparesis (wrong way eyes) points to deep hemorrhages, particularly in the medial thalamus [15]. Rarely isolated acute PPRF lesions in pons can cause the eyes to deviate contralaterally with loss of all rapid eye movements (saccades and quick phases of nystagmus) ipsilaterally. The gaze holding ability, smooth pursuit and VOR are preserved in these lesions. This is referred to as *dissociated ipsilateral horizontal conjugate gaze palsy* [7].

When VOR Is Impaired
When VOR is impaired in a patient with conjugate horizontal gaze palsy, the lesion lies within the pons. Gaze deviations from pontine lesions are far less common than those caused by cerebral or thalamic lesions. Most pontine lesions tend to manifest with gaze deficits more than gaze deviations. When pontine lesions cause gaze deviations, the eyes look toward the hemiparetic side [16]. Saccadic, pursuit and optokinetic abnormalities are usually evident toward the side of the lesion. Horizontal gaze-evoked nystagmus may be noted. Vergence movements are usually spared. This constellation, where the majority of the components of gaze are affected, is referred to as *non-dissociated ipsilateral horizontal gaze palsy* [7]. Due to the proximity of facial nerve fibers, an ipsilateral facial palsy often accompanies the abducens nuclear lesion. Pontine hemorrhage, multiple sclerosis or rarely a space-occupying lesion are the usual suspects. Bilateral horizontal gaze palsies may result from bilateral lesions. "16 syndrome" refers to bilateral horizontal gaze palsy and facial diplegia as a result of midline tegmental pontine hemorrhage or multiple sclerosis [7]. When the gaze palsy is asymmetric where the adducting eye is more restricted than the abducting eye, the lesion usually involves MLF on one side and abducens nucleus on the opposite side (*pseudo-horizontal gaze palsy*). *Congenital paralysis of horizontal gaze associated with progressive scoliosis* usually affects all components of gaze (conjugate saccades, pursuit, optokinetic and vestibular eye movements) but relatively spares convergence [17].

b. *Vertical Gaze Deviation*

Acute vertical gaze deviations result from midbrain lesions. VOR is invariably impaired. Sustained downgaze deviation suggests dorsal midbrain damage. A dilated third ventricle from acute hydrocephalus may compress on the dorsal midbrain to cause the *setting sun sign* [18]. If a shunt is in situ, a shunt malfunction should be suspected. The mass effect resulting from a thalamic hemorrhage or infarct may cause a similar sustained downward gaze deviation. Transient upgaze deviation may occur just before fainting or seizures. Episodic upgaze deviations are also seen in oculogyric crisis or may be psychogenic in origin. Sustained upgaze deviations are seen in profound hypoxia or ischemia of pontine tegmentum [19, 20].

Scenario 2

The patient is conscious and presents with conjugate gaze deficits but without gaze deviations.
Unlike readily visible gaze deviations, gaze deficits have to be elicited by the examiner. Gaze deficits may show a directional preponderance (horizontal, vertical) or may selectively involve one component of gaze while sparing the other (saccadic paresis, smooth pursuit paresis, OKN, VOR or vergence). Bilateral lesions and PSP can cause omnidirectional gaze deficits.

a. *Horizontal Conjugate Gaze Deficits*

In all patient of horizontal gaze deficits, the VOR should be tested.

When VOR Is Preserved
All causes of transient gaze deviations may eventually show gaze deficits when gaze deviations disappear. Important causes

include congenital oculomotor apraxia or acute unilateral cerebral lesion, often an infarct or hemorrhage. The patient typically shows deficits in shifting gaze in the direction opposite to the lesion. Pursuits usually recover faster than saccades [21].

When VOR Is Impaired
When VOR is impaired, a pontine lesion should be considered. Convergence mediated by midbrain is usually intact. Medial longitudinal fasciculus is often involved (one-and-half syndrome). Some important causes include Wernicke's encephalopathy, Gaucher's disease, anticonvulsant toxicity and Tay-Sachs disease [22]. Bilateral lesions produce gaze deficits in both directions. Bilateral lesions are often the result of toxic, metabolic and degenerative causes. Infra-nuclear non-CNS causes like Fisher's syndrome, Botulism, Myasthenia gravis may mimic horizontal gaze deficits [23].

b. *Vertical Conjugate Gaze Deficits*

Preferential involvement of vertical gaze points to a lesion in the midbrain or rostral to it. Upward pursuit pathways decussate in the posterior commissure before projecting to the final common pathway. A lesion in the posterior commissure thus causes upward gaze palsy. Fibers for the downward gaze pass ventral to the cerebral aqueduct and are therefore spared in posterior commissural lesions. Testing for VOR further helps to narrow down the localization. Important causes are listed in Table 17.6.

When VOR Is Preserved
When VOR is preserved in vertical gaze deficit, the lesion is usually rostral to the midbrain. The most common cause of acute vertical gaze deficit is a thalamic infarction as a part of basilar artery stroke. Thalamic hemorrhage, encephalitis and hydrocephalus are other important causes of acute vertical gaze deficits. When the vertical gaze deficit is chronic, PSP and Creutzfeldt-Jakob disease are important considerations in older individuals. Wilson's disease, Whipple disease and Niemann-Pick disease type C should be considered in younger patients [22, 24].

When VOR Is Impaired
An intrinsic midbrain lesion or extrinsic compression from large hydrocephalus, thalamic or pineal lesions should be considered. Dorsal midbrain lesions impair upgaze selectively (Parinaud's

TABLE 17.6: Vertical Gaze Deficits

Hydrocephalus
Midbrain infarct/hemorrhage
Thalamic infarct/hemorrhage
Progressive supranuclear palsy
Niemann-Pick disease
Gaucher's disease
Wilson disease
Tay-Sachs
Kernicterus
Maple syrup urine disease
Barbiturates
Carbamazepine
Neuroleptic agents
Multiple sclerosis
Whipple disease
Syphilis

syndrome) while a ventral midbrain lesion restricts downgaze preferentially [25]. Myasthenia gravis and inflammatory extra-ocular myopathy may mimic a supranuclear vertical gaze deficit.

c. *Saccadic Deficits*

Saccadic deficits may manifest as saccadic delay, hypometric saccades, slow saccades or lateropulsion of saccades.

Impaired Initiation of Saccades

Do the eyes promptly generate saccades after commands? A lesion anywhere in the saccadic pathway (Figure 17.2) may result in abnormally increased saccadic latency. Frontal or superior collicular injury delay saccades contralateral to the side of the lesion. Pontine lesions impair saccades to the side of the lesion. In ocular motor apraxia and Huntington disease, ability to generate saccades is strikingly impaired. They have difficulties in making horizontal and vertical saccades to command while reflex saccades (vestibular and OKN) are preserved. Patients often employ head thrusts or eye blinks to generate saccades especially during initial stages of the disease [26].

Hypometric Saccades

Do the eyes move accurately to the new target? Are saccades *hypometric*? Is there correction of the saccade to target, and is this correction accurate? Hypometric saccades fall short of the target and are conclusively abnormal if they occur consistently in one direction. Hypometric saccades are usually contralateral to the cerebral hemispheric lesion and ipsilateral to the cerebellar cortical lesion [26].

Lateropulsion of Saccades

A triad consisting of (i) overshoot of ipsiversive saccades, (ii) undershoot of contraversive saccades and (iii) ipsiversive deviation of vertical saccades along an oblique trajectory may be seen in lateral medullary infarcts [7, 27].

Slow Saccades

Do the eyes move slowly during the trajectory from the initial position to the target position? While testing saccades, one should not be able to follow with one's own eye the full trajectory of a voluntary saccade, due to the very fast speed of normal saccades. It is important to examine vertical and horizontal saccades independently. Slow saccades may result from damage to excitatory burst neurons. Predominant slowing of horizontal saccades is seen in spinocerebellar ataxia 2 (SCA 2). Slow saccades may be present in SCA7, Parkinson disease, Huntington disease, PSP, Alzheimer disease, Whipple disease, Amyotrophic lateral sclerosis, AIDS-associated dementia, Wilson disease, Ataxia telangiectasia and Gaucher disease [28]. The causes of slow saccades are listed in Table 17.7.

d. *Smooth Pursuit Deficits*

Pursuit pathways originating in the cerebral hemispheres undergo double decussation before they reach the final common pathway. The eye movements unable to track the slowly moving target may resort to catch up saccade to compensate for the low velocity. Lesions in parieto-temporal lobe, frontal lobe and cerebellar flocculus produce ipsiversive smooth pursuit deficits. Damage to vestibulocerebellum, rostral pons, unilateral tegmental damage to caudal pons and ventral medulla result in contraversive pursuit deficits (Table 17.3).

TABLE 17.7: Slow Saccades

Huntington disease
Progressive supranuclear palsy (PSP)
Spinocerebellar ataxia
Whipple disease
Niemann-Pick disease
Gaucher's disease
Wilson disease
Creutzfeldt-Jakob disease
Tetanus
Anticonvulsants
Benzodiazepines
AIDS
Alzheimer's disease

Scenario 3

The patient is conscious and presents with gaze fixation abnormalities.

Saccadic intrusions interfere with macular fixation of the object of interest (Table 17.8). It usually represents an omnipause cell dysfunction manifesting in disinhibition of excitatory burst neurons. The examiner should seek answers to the following questions when evaluating saccadic intrusions:

- Is it nystagmus?
- Is it causing symptoms?
- What is the amplitude?
- Is there an inter-saccadic interval?
- What is the axis of intrusion?
- Are eyelids fluttering and eyes converging too?

Saccadic intrusions resulting from disinhibited burst cell firing are always fast. Nystagmus, on the other hand, is characterized by an initial slow or smooth eye movement that may be followed by a fast corrective eye movement [7].

Square wave jerks are small-amplitude intrusions that take the eyes off the target followed by a corrective saccade. An intersaccadic interval is always present. Square wave jerks may normally appear in young individuals and the elderly. When their amplitude is more than 1° to 2°, an underlying pathology is suggested. Square wave jerks seldom produce symptoms [7].

Macro square wave jerks are square wave jerks with larger amplitude (20°–40°). They often result due to dysfunction in the cerebellar outflow. An inter-saccadic interval is always present. Macro square wave jerks tend to be symptomatic. Macro square wave jerks are seen in multiple sclerosis, cerebellar hemorrhage, multiple system atrophy and chiari malformation [7].

TABLE 17.8: Saccadic Intrusions

With inter-saccadic interval

- Square wave jerks (usually asymptomatic)
- Macro square wave jerks

Without inter-saccadic interval

- Ocular flutter
- Opsoclonus

Ocular flutter appears as rapid to-and-fro horizontal saccades that cross the midline. The intersaccadic interval is typically absent. Patients often complain of transient visual disturbances as "jiggling," "wavy" or "shimmering." Post-infectious and para-neoplastic syndromes may present with ocular flutter [7].

Opsoclonus is often referred to as *saccadomania* due to the nature of saccades that show large amplitude bursts in all directions. The intersaccadic interval is absent. They are always symptomatic. Opsoclonus persists during eye closure and sleep. Dysfunctional omnipause neurons leading to disinhibition of burst neurons may explain the underlying pathological mechanism. Opsoclonus, in conjunction with myoclonus, is seen as a paraneoplastic syndrome arising from neuroblastoma in children and tumor (small cell lung carcinoma and breast cancer) in adults [7].

Brief periods of eye movements that resemble ocular flutter but accompanied by convergence and eyelid flutter are likely to be a *voluntary flutter*. Voluntary flutter cannot be sustained for long durations [7].

Scenario 4

Non-conjugate supranuclear deficits in a non-comatose patient.

Unlike conjugate supranuclear deficits, Non-conjugate eye movement disorders manifest commonly with double vision. These include internuclear ophthalmoplegia (*INO*), *Skew deviation, One-and-half syndrome and Dorsal midbrain syndrome*. Non-CNS disorders mimicking supranuclear gaze deficits are an important consideration (Table 17.9).

a. *Horizontal Non-Conjugate Gaze Deficits*

Internuclear Ophthalmoplegia
Lesions in medial longitudinal fasciculus that connects the abducens nucleus on one side and contralateral oculomotor nucleus result in a dysconjugate gaze palsy, where on the side of the MLF lesion, adduction palsy reveals itself. At the same time, the abducting eye shows monocular nystagmus. Nystagmus appears to be an adaptive process that helps the fellow eye overcome the adducting weakness. The adduction weakness becomes evident when the patient is asked to perform large amplitude saccades or during optokinetic testing using a tape or drum. Vertical saccades and convergence are usually preserved in pontine lesions. Bilateral INO is often a consequence of multiple sclerosis or ischemic lesions. Exotropia accompanying bilateral INO where both eyes have deviated laterally is termed as *wall-eyed bilateral INO*

TABLE 17.9: Peripheral Causes Mimicking Supranuclear Gaze Disorder

Acute

- Fisher's syndrome
- Botulism
- Myasthenia gravis

Chronic

- Myasthenia gravis
- Chronic progressive external ophthalmoplegia
- Oculopharyngeal dystrophy
- Myotonic dystrophy
- Graves' disease

(*WEBINO*) [29]. Many non-CNS conditions may mimic INO. These include Guillain-Barre syndrome, thyroid orbitopathy, orbital pseudotumor, Fisher syndrome. Abetalipoproteinemia causes atypical INO, where the adducting eye shows nystagmus.

One-and-Half Syndrome
Conjugate gaze palsy to one side ("one") and impaired adduction on looking to the other side ("and a half") is termed one-and-half syndrome, leaving abduction of one eye as the only possible horizontal movement. The abducting eye shows nystagmus. Convergence and vertical eye movements are usually spared. When facial palsy and ocular bobbing accompany one-and-half-syndrome, it is termed *8 and ½ syndrome*. When facial diplegia occurs with one-and-half-syndrome, it is called *15 and ½ syndrome*. Complete bilateral horizontal gaze palsy with facial diplegia is known as *16 syndrome*. Common causes of the one-and-half syndrome are multiple sclerosis, neuromyelitis optica, strokes, basilar artery aneurysms and AV malformations [30]. Myasthenia gravis and Fisher syndrome may mimic one-and-half syndrome.

b. *Vertical Non-Conjugate Gaze Deficits*

Vertical INO
Vertical upgaze palsy with monocular paresis of downgaze on the side is referred to as a vertical one-and-half syndrome. Another variation is the impairment of all forms of downward rapid eye movements and smooth pursuit movements accompanied by monocular paresis of elevation. Bell phenomenon and all types of horizontal movement are preserved. Meso-diencephalic infarction involving bilateral riMLF is the usual culprit.

Skew Deviation
Vertical malalignment resulting from supranuclear deficits is termed skew deviation. Mechanism underlying skew deviation may be an imbalance of otolith inputs, which ascend via MLF to the oculomotor nuclei. When skew deviation varies in different gaze positions, a medullary lesion is indicated. Peripheral vestibular disease may cause the contralateral eye to be in a higher position. Lateral pontomedullary lesions cause the ipsilateral eye to be lower. An MLF lesion and posterior commissure lesions cause the ipsilateral eye to be higher. Posterior commissure lesion may be accompanied by slowly alternating skew deviation. Transient skew deviations are seen with migraine, vertebrobasilar ischemia, astrocytoma, transient ischemia and epilepsy. When skew deviation presents with head tilt, an alternate cover test should be done. If alternate cover test causes a reversal of the direction of skewed eyes (ocular counter roll), an ocular tilt reaction (head tilt, skew deviation, ocular counter-roll) is confirmed. Ocular tilt reaction suggests a central lesion affecting central utricular pathways. Myasthenia gravis, thyroid ophthalmopathy and superior oblique palsy may cause vertical strabismus mimicking skew deviation. Eyes are usually not rotated in skew deviation, unlike the causes leading to vertical strabismus. Eye rotation is best tested by Maddox rods. Bielschowsky head-tilt test is often negative [7, 31].

Dorsal Midbrain Syndrome
Parinaud syndrome is classically described by the triad of upgaze palsy, convergence retraction nystagmus and pupillary hyporeflexia. Patients may complain of difficulty looking up, blurred near vision, diplopia, oscillopsia and there may be associated neurological symptoms. Vertical diplopia is classically seen and can be very disabling to the patient. The most debilitating symptom is the inability to elevate the eyes, often causing a compensatory

chin-up position. Poor pupillary constriction to light but preserved constriction with convergence indicates compression of fibers mediating light reflex as they pass through the posterior commissure while sparing the fibers for accommodation that traverse more ventrally. Another component of the triad of Parinaud syndrome is convergence–retraction nystagmus which is characterized by an irregular, jerky nystagmus, associated with convergence and retraction of both eyes, especially on attempted upgaze. Convergence retraction nystagmus is a highly localizing sign for dorsal midbrain lesion. Multiple sclerosis, compression by mass in the pineal region, dilatation of the third ventricle, lesions in posterior commissure and midbrain infarction must be considered [25].

Scenario 5

Gaze disorders in a comatose patient.
Voluntary saccades and smooth pursuit movements are absent in comatose patients. Reflex and spontaneous eye movements often help localize the lesion.

a. *Tonic Eye Deviation*

Lesions above and below ocular motor decussation (between midbrain and pons) cause different patterns of gaze deviations. For lesions above the decussation, the eyes deviate toward the lesion (away from hemiparesis). Vestibular stimuli drive the eyes across the midline. For lesions below the decussation, the eyes deviate contralateral to the lesion (toward the hemiparesis). Contralesional eye deviation though typical of pontine lesions may also occur with thalamic lesion and rarely with hemispheric lesions (wrong way eyes). Seizure activity may cause intermittent eye deviation. Initial eye deviation in seizure is contralateral to the lesion. Toward the end of the seizure, the gaze may drift back to the side of the lesion. Thalamic and dorsal midbrain lesions may cause the

TABLE 17.10: Ocular Bobbing and Ocular Dipping

Type	Initial Vertical Movement (Direction/Phase)	Etiology
Typical Ocular bobbing	Down/Fast	Pontine tumor/ hemorrhage/infarct Extra-axial mass Encephalitis
Atypical ocular Bobbing	Down/Fast	Cerebellar hematoma Metabolic encephalopathy
Reverse ocular Bobbing	Up/Fast	Metabolic encephalopathy
Ocular dipping	Down/Slow	Anoxic encephalopathy Post status epilepticus
Reverse ocular dipping	Up/Slow	Metabolic encephalopathy Viral encephalitis

eye to deviate down tonically. Tonic upward deviation of eyes in a comatose patient may be due to hypoxic-ischemic damage [32].

In all cases, reflex eye movements (doll's head maneuver or caloric stimulation) should be tested. Pontine lesions may abolish horizontal reflex eye movements while sparing vertical responses. Selective impairment of vertical reflex eye movements may indicate a lesion in the midbrain or bilateral MLF. In a comatose patient with intact reflex eye movements, the brainstem is likely to be structurally intact.

b. *Spontaneous Eye Movements*

Spontaneous eye movements observed in a comatose patient include *Ocular bobbing, Ocular dipping, Reverse ocular bobbing, Reverse ocular dipping* and *Ping pong gaze* [33]. The typical characteristics are described in Table 17.10. Ping pong gaze or periodic alternating nystagmus (PAG) is a slow and regular conjugate

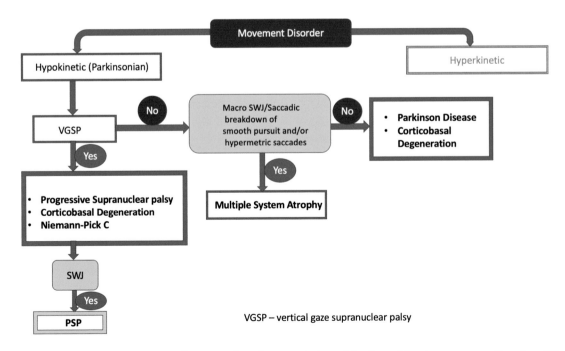

FIGURE 17.5 Flowchart depicting approach to gaze disorders coexisting with a hyperkinetic movement disorder. *Abbreviations*: SCA6, spinocerebellar ataxia 6; AOA, ataxia with oculomotor apraxia; AT, ataxia telangiectasia.

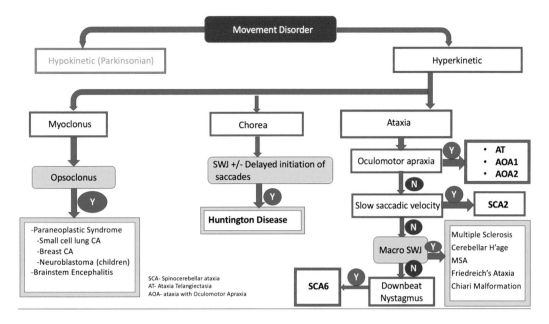

FIGURE 17.6 Flowchart depicting approach to gaze disorders coexisting with a hyperkinetic movement disorder. *Abbreviation*: VGSP, vertical gaze supranuclear palsy.

eye movement that is rigorously horizontal and perfectly pendular. Presence of PAG is a clinical indicator of bilateral cortical damage with preserved brainstem function. The subsequent disappearance of PAG in the same patient indicates that irreversible brainstem damage has already occurred [34].

Scenario 6

Gaze disorder accompanied by a movement disorder.
Various hyperkinetic and hypokinetic movement disorders show supranuclear disorders of gaze [26]. The resulting pattern comprising of the type of movement disorder (chorea, ataxia, dystonia, bradykinesia) and selective gaze abnormality (vertical or horizontal gaze palsy, saccadic, fixation or pursuit abnormalities) can narrow down the differential diagnosis [28]. An algorithm to wade through the complex maze of gaze disorder in the setting of movement disorder is shown in Figures 17.5 and 17.6.

Many treatable diseases manifest with supranuclear gaze disorders (Table 17.11). A systematic approach will ensure that a potentially treatable condition is not missed by the skilled clinician.

TABLE 17.11: Abnormal Eye Movements due to Metabolic Disorders

1. Wernicke's encephalopathy
2. Abetalipoproteinemia
3. Wilson disease
4. Kernicterus
5. Lipid storage diseases
   - Tay-Sachs
   - Adult-onset hexosaminidase A deficiency
   - Niemann-Pick type C
   - Gaucher's disease
6. Aminocidurias
   - Maple syrup urine disease
   - Hyperglycinemia

Conclusion

The main aim of gaze is to keep the object of interest on the fovea in order to have the highest resolution of the image being viewed. The six cardinal systems involved in the supranuclear gaze are the saccadic system, the smooth pursuit system, the vestibular system, the optokinetic system, the fixation system and the vergence system. A thorough knowledge about the final common pathway helps to understand the clinical features caused by various lesions at the key anatomical sites.

Multiple-Choice Questions

1. Gaze fixation is a function of:
   a. Burst cells
   b. Neural integrator
   c. Medial longitudinal fasciculus
   d. Medial lemniscus

   Answer:

   b. Neural integrator

2. Which of the following statements is true about saccades?
   a. Saccades are rapid dysconjugate eye movements.
   b. The velocity command is executed by the neural integrators.
   c. The position command is the pulse, while velocity command is the step.
   d. Supplementary eye fields are involved in generating voluntary saccades.

   Answer:

   d. Supplementary eye fields are involved in generating voluntary saccades.

3. Prevost sign is:
   a. Impaired vestibuloocular reflex in a patient with conjugate horizontal gaze palsy in pontine lesions.
   b. The patient looks toward the lesion, away from hemiparesis in frontal lobe lesions.
   c. Bilateral horizontal gaze palsy and facial diplegia as a result of midline tegmental pontine hemorrhage.
   d. None of the above.

   Answer:
   b. The patient looks toward the lesion, away from hemiparesis in frontal lobe lesions.

4. Which of the following statements is NOT true?
   a. Fibers for the downward gaze pass ventral to the cerebral aqueduct.
   b. Posterior commissural lesions cause downward gaze palsy.
   c. The most common cause of acute vertical gaze deficit is a thalamic infarction.
   d. None of the above.

   Answer:
   b. Posterior commissural lesions cause downward gaze palsy.

5. The difference between square wave jerks (SWJ) and ocular flutter is:
   a. SWJ is due to leaky integrator while ocular flutter is due to burst cell dysfunction.
   b. SWJ is due to burst cell dysfunction while ocular flutter is due to leaky integrator.
   c. SWJ has inter-saccadic interval while ocular flutter doesn't.
   d. SWJ doesn't have inter-saccadic interval while ocular flutter does.

   Answer:
   c. SWJ has inter-saccadic interval while ocular flutter doesn't.

References

1. Vinny PW, Lal V. Gaze disorders: A clinical approach. Neurol India. 2016; 64:121–128.
2. Kennard C. Disorders of higher gaze control. Handb Clin Neurol. 2011;102:379–402.
3. Walker HK, Hall WD, Hurst JW, editors. Clinical methods: The history, physical, and laboratory examinations. Oxford: Butterworth-Heinemann; 1990.
4. Nachev P, Kennard C, Husain M. Functional role of supplementary and pre-supplementary motor areas. Nat Rev Neurosci. 2008;9:856–869.
5. Pierrot-Deseilligny C, Muri RM, Ploner CJ, Gaymard B, Rivaud-Pechoux S. Cortical control of ocular saccades in humans: A model for motricity. Prog. Brain Res. 2003;142:3–17.
6. Sparks DL. The brainstem control of saccadic eye movements. Nat Rev Neurosci. 2003;252–264.
7. Brazis PW, Masdeu JC, Biller J. Localization in clinical neurology. Philadelphia: Wolter Kluwer Health/Lippincott Williams and Wilkins; 2011.
8. Pierrot-Deseilligny C, Gaymard B. Smooth pursuit disorders. Baillieres Clin Neurol. 1992;1:435–454.
9. Petit L, Haxby JV. Functional anatomy of pursuit eye movements in humans as revealed by fMRI. J Neurophysiol. 1999;82:463–471.
10. Papanagnu E, Brodsky MC. Is there a role for optokinetic nystagmus testing in contemporary orthoptic practice? Old tricks and new perspectives. Am Orthopt J. 2014;64:1–10.
11. Perez-Fernandez N, Gallegos-Constantino V, Barona-Lleo L, Manrique-Huarte R. Clinical and video-assisted examination of the vestibulo-ocular reflex: A comparative study. Acta Otorrinolaringol Esp. 2012;63:429–435.
12. Lloyd-Smith Sequeira A, Rizzo JR, Rucker JC. Clinical approach to supranuclear brainstem saccadic gaze palsies. Front Neurol. 2017;8:429.
13. Goodwin JA, Kansu T. Vulpian's sign conjugate eye deviation in acute cerebral hemisphere lesions. Neurology;1986;36(5):711.
14. Fruhmann Berger M, Pross RD, Ilg U, Karnath HO. Deviation of eyes and head in acute cerebral stroke. BMC Neurol. 2006;6:23.
15. Kernan JC, Devinsky O, Luciano DJ, Vazquez B, Perrine K. Lateralizing significance of head and eye deviation in secondary generalized tonic-clonic seizures. Neurology. 1993;43(7):1308–1310.
16. Pedersen RA, Troost BT. Abnormalities of gaze in cerebrovascular disease. Stroke. 1981;12:251–254.
17. Bosley TM, Salih MAM, Jen JC, et al. Neurologic features of horizontal gaze palsy and progressive scoliosis with mutations in *ROBO3*. Neurology. 2005;64(7):1196–1203.
18. Boragina M, Cohen E. An infant with the "setting-sun" eye phenomenon. CMAJ. 2006;175(8):878.
19. Hayman M, Harvey AS, Hopkins IJ, Kornberg AJ, Coleman LT, Shield LK. Paroxysmal tonic upgaze: A reappraisal of outcome. Ann Neurol. 1998;43(4):514–520.
20. Nakada T, Kwee IL, Lee H. Sustained upgaze in coma. J Clin Neuroophthalmol. 1984:35–38.
21. Schweyer K, Busche MA, Hammes J, et al. Pearls & oysters: Ocular motor apraxia as essential differential diagnosis to supranuclear gaze palsy: Eyes up. Neurology. 2018;90(10):482–485.
22. Koens LH, Tijssen MA, Lange F, Wolffenbuttel BH, Rufa A, Zee DS, de Koning TJ. Eye movement disorders and neurological symptoms in late-onset inborn errors of metabolism. Mov Disord. 2018;33:1844–1856.
23. Liu DTL, Li C, Lee VYW. Internuclear ophthalmoplegia. Arch Neurol. 2006;63(4):626.
24. Martin WRW, Hartlein J, Racette BA, Cairns N, Perlmutter JS. Pathologic correlates of supranuclear gaze palsy with parkinsonism. Parkinsonism Relat Disord. 2017;38:68–71.
25. Shields M, Sinkar S, Chan W, Crompton J. Parinaud syndrome: A 25-year (1991–2016) review of 40 consecutive adult cases. Acta Ophthalmol. 2017;95(8):e792–e793.
26. Lal V, Truong D. Eye movement abnormalities in movement disorders. Clin Park Relat Disord. 2019;1:54–63.
27. Kommerell G, Hoyt WF. Lateropulsion of saccadic eye movements: Electrooculographic studies in a patient with Wallenberg's syndrome. Arch Neurol. 1973;28(5):313–318.
28. Termsarasab P, Thammongkolchai T, Rucker JC, et al. The diagnostic value of saccades in movement disorder patients: A practical guide and review. J Clin Mov Disord. 2015;2:14.
29. Virgo JD, Plant GT. Internuclear ophthalmoplegia. Practical Neurology. 2017;17:149–153.
30. Xue F, Zhang L, Zhang L, Ying Z, Sha O, Ding Y. One-and-a-half syndrome with its spectrum disorders. Quant Imaging Med Surg. 2017;7(6):691–697.
31. Tudor KI, Petravić D, Jukić A, Juratovac Z. Skew deviation: Case report and review of the literature. Semin Ophthalmol. 2017;32(6):734–737.
32. Johkura K, Komiyama A, Kuroiwa Y. Vertical conjugate eye deviation in postresuscitation coma. Ann Neurol. 2004;56: 878–881.
33. Mehler MF. The clinical spectrum of ocular bobbing and ocular dipping. J Neurol Neurosurg Psychiatry. 1988;51(5):725–727.
34. Yang SL, Han X, Guo CN, Zhu XY, Dong Q, Wang Y. A closer look at ping-pong gaze: An observational study and literature review. J Neurol. 2018;265(12):2825–2833.

18

A CLINICAL APPROACH TO ABNORMAL EYE MOVEMENTS

M. Madhusudanan

CASE STUDY

A 15-year-old girl presented with intermittent jerky movements of body and frequent dropping of things held in her hands for 1 month. For 15 days prior to presentation the patient was noted to be less coherent, confused and inattentive. Parents also noted presence of involuntary jerky movements of eyes while talking to her for long duration. On examination visual acuity, fundus examination and extraocular movements were normal. Rapid, chaotic, conjugate, jerky multidirectional eye movements were noted. The patient had prominent startle myoclonus. Cerebellar signs were present. What is the anatomical localization of the patient's symptom complex?

Introduction

The function of eye movements is to bring visual stimuli to the fovea and hold them there, during head movements or movement of the stimuli by themselves.

Abnormal eye movements that disrupt steady fixation are of two main types: pathological nystagmus and saccadic intrusions. The key difference between nystagmus and saccadic intrusions lies in the initial eye movement that takes the eye of the visual target. Thus, for nystagmus, the initial movement is a slow drift (or "slow phase") as opposed to an initial inappropriate rapid movement that interrupts the fixation in saccadic intrusions.

There are two types of eye movement systems—a slow eye movement system and a rapid eye movement system.

- The slow eye movement systems include visual fixation, vestibular, optokinetic, smooth pursuit, the neural integrator and vergence systems.
- The saccadic system is the rapid eye movement system. It serves to move the eyes rapidly to bring an image of an object of interest directly onto the fovea.
- Nystagmus is a disorder of the slow eye movement system and always has a slow phase.
- Disorders of rapid eye movement system cause unintended saccades or *saccadic intrusions. They have no slow phase.*

Nystagmus

Nystagmus is defined as a disorder of ocular posture characterized by a rhythmic, repetitive, oscillation of the eyes.

Nystagmus is generally of two types: jerk nystagmus and pendular nystagmus:

- Jerk nystagmus has a slow phase drift followed by a rapid corrective saccade in the opposite direction.
- Pendular nystagmus refers to a sinusoidal oscillation with slow phases in both directions and no corrective saccades.

Examination of nystagmus should include looking for:

- Spontaneous nystagmus
- Nystagmus after avoiding fixation
- Nystagmus after provocative testing: These tests are usually done when the nystagmus is not observed spontaneously.
  - Head-shaking nystagmus
  - Hyperventilation-induced nystagmus
  - Vibration-induced nystagmus
  - Other provocative tests like valsalva maneuver, nystagmus induced by sound (Tullio phenomenon), nystagmus induced by pressure over the tragus (Hennebert's sign, etc.)
- Positional nystagmus

Spontaneous nystagmus

Look for the type of nystagmus, direction of the slow and fast phase, the position of the globe in the orbit where the nystagmus is seen or exaggerated, whether there is a null zone and whether nystagmus is direction changing or not. Looking at the velocity of the slow component gives some clue regarding the localization of the nystagmus (Figure 18.1).

Nystagmus after avoiding fixation

Nystagmus amplitude should be looked for before and after avoiding fixation. The effect of fixation on the nystagmus can be determined at the bedside by observing the change in intensity of the nystagmus when the patient is looking through Frenzel glasses. These glasses consist of +30-diopter binocular lenses that prevent visual fixation. Another easy bedside method is to look for the effect of fixation by viewing the nystagmus with an ophthalmoscope focused on the optic disk or retinal vessels of one eye while the patient covers and uncovers the fixating eye (the direction of the nystagmus is reversed when it is viewed through an ophthalmoscope).[1]

Another bedside method to avoid fixation is a "pen light cover" test; here a bright light from a torch is shown to one eye effectively blocking the fixation of that eye and closing the other eye. Look for the aggravation of the nystagmus.[2]

Nystagmus caused by peripheral disturbances increases when fixation is removed, whereas in central lesions, the nystagmus is not affected by avoiding fixation. If the intensity of the nystagmus and the velocity of its slow phase are increased by covering the fixating eye, it suggests a peripheral vestibular disorder.

Head-shaking nystagmus

Head-shaking nystagmus (HSN) can be assessed using either a passive (by the examiner) or active (by the patient) head-shaking maneuver. The patient's head is pitched forward by approximately 20° to bring the horizontal semicircular canals (HCs) into the plane of stimulation, and then the head is shaken horizontally in a sinusoidal fashion at a rate of about 2–3 Hz with an amplitude of 20° for 15 seconds.[3] HSN is most commonly seen following unilateral peripheral vestibulopathy. In peripheral vestibulopathy, the slow phase is directed to the paretic ear, fast

DOI: 10.1201/9780429020278-26

Types of nystagmus depending on the velocity of slow component

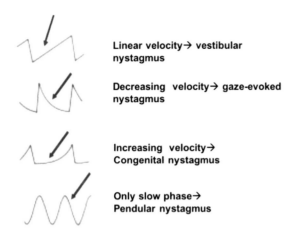

Linear velocity→ vestibular nystagmus

Decreasing velocity→ gaze-evoked nystagmus

Increasing velocity→ Congenital nystagmus

Only slow phase→ Pendular nystagmus

FIGURE 18.1 The velocity of slow phase of the various types of nystagmus.

component to the opposite side. In contrast, patterns of HSN in central vestibular disorders may vary. It may take the form of "perverted nystagmus" (nystagmus occurs in planes other than that being stimulated), disproportionally strong HSN in response to weak head-shaking or strongly biphasic HSN.[4] The central type of HSN suggests lesion in the uvula, nodulus and inferior tonsil.

Hyperventilation-induced nystagmus

To assess hyperventilation-induced nystagmus (HIN), subjects are asked to hyperventilate for about 30 seconds, taking an average of one deep breath per second. HIN can be seen in both central as well as peripheral vestibular disorders. HIN can be elicited in patients with lesions on the vestibular nerve (e.g., an acoustic neuroma or cholesteatoma), neurovascular compression of the VIII nerve, compensated peripheral vestibulopathies, perilymph fistula or in central lesions like multiple sclerosis, cerebellar degeneration and lesions at the craniocervical junction.[5] HIN beating to the side of reduced hearing loss may be a useful sign of cerebellopontine angle (CPA) tumors.[5]

Positional testing

Positional nystagmus refers to the nystagmus that develops in association with changes in the position of the head in relation to gravity. Both peripheral and central vestibular disorders may produce positional nystagmus. The positional nystagmus is mostly paroxysmal in peripheral vestibular disorders, and is almost always observed in benign paroxysmal positional vertigo (BPPV), which is ascribed to otolithic debris that becomes detached from the maculae of the otolithic organs and enters one of the semicircular canals.[6] The patterns of positional nystagmus in BPPV differ according to the canal affected.

Rarely, the positional nystagmus can be seen in central lesions such as tumors near floor of the fourth ventricle and in lesions involving the inferior cerebellar vermis.[7,8] This central positional nystagmus (CPN) may be either paroxysmal or persistent. Prominent positional nystagmus in the absence of vertigo should also make one suspect a central pathology.[9]

Nystagmus in various disease states

Nystagmus in vestibular disorders

Nystagmus can be seen in peripheral as well as central vestibulopathies. Peripheral vestibulopathy suggests a lesion in the labyrinth or vestibular nerve and central vestibulopathy suggests a lesion in the vestibular nuclei or their connections.

Nystagmus due to peripheral vestibular disorder

Peripheral vestibular nystagmus due to a unilateral peripheral lesion consists of either a horizontal-rotary or purely horizontal nystagmus. Nystagmus due to peripheral lesion does not change in direction with gaze to either side, although it increases in amplitude with gaze in the direction of the fast phase and decreases in amplitude with gaze away from the fast phase (Alexander's law) (Video 18.1). In contrast, acute central vestibular disorders, such as infarction or hemorrhage of the brainstem or the cerebellum, cause spontaneous nystagmus that changes its direction with a change in the direction of gaze. However, in some patients with medullary stroke, nystagmus may be present only when the patient is gazing in one direction, thereby appearing similar to a peripheral vestibular nystagmus (pseudovestibular nystagmus) (Video 18.2). Purely vertical nystagmus and purely torsional nystagmus are almost always due to a central disorder, whereas horizontal and torsional components may occur in patients with either peripheral or central disorders. Visual fixation does not affect intensity of central vestibular nystagmus whereas peripheral vestibular nystagmus attenuates with visual fixation and increases by avoiding fixation (see Figure 18.2).

Nystagmus from peripheral vestibular disorders can be categorized according to the severity of nystagmus. In the first-degree nystagmus, nystagmus may be present only during gaze away from the side of the lesion, that is only in the direction of the fast phase (seen in mild affection), in the second degree, nystagmus may be found not only during gaze away from the side of the lesion, but also when patient gazes straightforward. In the third-degree nystagmus, the nystagmus is found when the eyes are gazing center, toward and away from the side of the lesion (the most severe affection).

The characteristic features of peripheral vestibular nystagmus are given in Table 18.1.

Pathophysiology of the peripheral vestibular nystagmus

Normally, there is continuous tonic stream of impulses going from the peripheral vestibular end organs in the labyrinth to the

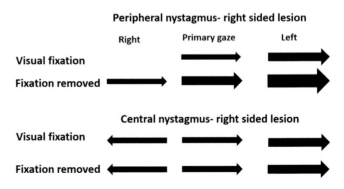

FIGURE 18.2 Direction of nystagmus in peripheral and central vestibular lesion.

TABLE 18.1: Characteristics of Peripheral Vestibular Nystagmus

- Horizontal/horizontal-rotary
- Does not change direction
- Obeys "Alexander's law"
- Accentuated by suppressing visual fixation

vestibular nuclei and these are equal on both sides. Pathological conditions affecting one side reduce its firing frequency, resulting in tonic imbalance between the two sides, which is responsible for the nystagmus and vertigo.

Normally activation of the right horizontal canal stimulates the ipsilateral medial vestibular nucleus (MVN), which gets connected to the opposite abducens nucleus complex, which stimulates the contralateral (left) lateral rectus and through the MLF stimulates the ipsilateral (right) medial rectus resulting in a tonic eye deviation to the opposite side and corrective fast phase to the same side. Thus, nystagmus due to peripheral vestibular lesion causes a unidirectional slow phase drift due to imbalance in the level of tonic neural activity in the vestibular nuclei. If the disease leads to reduced activity in the right vestibular nuclei, the left vestibular nuclei will drive the eyes in a slow phase to the right and the quick phases will be directed to the left, that is away from the side of lesion (Video 18.3).

Nystagmus in benign paroxysmal positional vertigo (BPPV)

BPPV is second most common cause of peripheral vestibulopathy. The Dix-Hallpike maneuver is a classical test for a diagnosis of BPPV involving the posterior semicircular canal (PC).[10] While seated on the examination table, the patient's head is turned 45° toward the side to be tested. The patient is then moved en bloc to a supine position, ending with the head hanging 20° below the examination table. This maneuver places the PC in the most dependent position. In posterior canal, the elicited nystagmus is a mixed up-beat and torsional with the upper pole of the eyes beating toward the lower ear. When free-floating otolithic debris is present (canalolithiasis) in the PC being tested, nystagmus usually develops with a latency of several seconds (up to 30 seconds) and resolves within 1 minute (usually within 30 seconds). The nystagmus reverses direction upon sitting and tends to habituate with repeated testing (fatiguability). The other method of diagnosing the posterior canal BPPV is the side-lying test.[11] In this test, the patient is quickly laid en bloc toward the side being tested after the head is turned 45° away from the side to be tested.

The horizontal canal variant of BPPV is elicited by the supine roll test, in which the patient's head is first flexed forward about 30° to align the horizontal canal with the earth vertical, and then turned about 90° to each side. Two types of positional nystagmus can be observed in horizontal BPPV, that is geotropic and apogeotropic. In the geotropic type, the nystagmus beats to the ground. In the supine head roll test, when head is turned to the right, the nystagmus beats to the right. When the head is turned to left, the nystagmus beats to the left. In the apogeotropic type, the nystagmus beats away from the ground. In the supine head roll test, when head is turned to the right, the nystagmus beats to the left. When the head is turned to left, the nystagmus beats to the right. The geotropic BPPV is due to canalolithiasis, whereas the apogeotropic BPPV is due to cupulolithiasis and is more persistent.

The side in which the nystagmus is stronger gives the clue to the side of affection. In the case of geotropic BPPV, the nystagmus induced by the head roll test is stronger toward the affected ear.

For example, if the head roll to right elicits more intense geotropic nystagmus than the head is rolled to the left, then the affected ear is the right. On the other hand, in the case of apogeotropic BPPV, the nystagmus induced by the head roll test is stronger toward the normal ear. For example, if head roll to right evokes more intense apogeotropic nystagmus than head roll to the left, then the affected ear is the left.[12]

Central vestibular nystagmus

A central vestibular dysfunction should be suspected when any one of the following findings is present:

1. Purely vertical or torsional spontaneous nystagmus
2. Horizontal-torsional nystagmus with the normal head-impulse test on the side contralateral to the nystagmus
3. Positional nystagmus incompatible with canalolithiasis or cupulolithiasis
4. Gaze-evoked nystagmus
5. Impaired vestibulo-ocular reflex (VOR) suppression
6. Saccadic pursuit
7. Dysmetric or slow saccades
8. Presence of skew deviation

Disturbance of central vestibular connections (the vestibular nuclei and their projections, including vestibulocerebellum) commonly causes vertical nystagmus (upbeat or downbeat) and less commonly torsional or horizontal nystagmus.

Upbeat nystagmus

Upbeat nystagmus (UBN) refers to nystagmus with fast phase upward. It most often worsens in upgaze. UBN typically increases with upgaze, usually diminishes with downgaze and is unaffected by horizontal gaze. Unlike downbeat nystagmus, upbeat nystagmus usually does not increase in lateral gaze. Convergence may enhance, suppress or reverse the direction.

UBN does not have much localizing value. UBN has been described in lesions of the midbrain, ventral pontine tegmentum, anterior cerebellar vermis, thalamus and medulla. When UBN increases in downgaze, the lesion usually involves the caudal medulla[13] (Video 18.4).

The presence of associated ocular motor abnormalities may help localize the lesion responsible for UBN.

- Saccadic ipsipulsion and skew deviation suggest a medullary lesion
- An internuclear ophthalmoplegia (INO) indicates pontine damage
- Vertical gaze palsy suggests mesencephalic dysfunction

Causes of UBN include cerebrovascular disease, multiple sclerosis, cerebellar degeneration and tumors, Wernicke's encephalopathy, encephalitis, Behçet syndrome and Leber's congenital amaurosis.

Downbeat nystagmus

Downbeat nystagmus (DBN) refers to a jerk nystagmus with the fast phase downward, seen in the primary position.

Typically, the nystagmus decreases in upgaze and worsens in downgaze. It is typically increased with convergence, with eccentric gaze, and particularly by having the patient look downward and laterally (side-pocket nystagmus) (Video 18.5). There may be a horizontal component, so the nystagmus may appear oblique on lateral gaze.[6] The nystagmus may be worsened by altering the head position, head-shaking, hyperventilation or vibration in the mastoid bone. With convergence, the nystagmus may increase, decrease or convert to UBN.

The DBN is caused by lesions of the vestibulocerebellum including the flocculus, paraflocculus, nodulus and uvula and medulla may also be the cause.[14] Typically, DBN is caused by lesions at the cervicomedullary junction, such as Arnold-Chiari malformation. Other causes include spinocerebellar degeneration, brainstem ischemia, demyelination, tumors, encephalitis, trauma, as well as hydrocephalus, Wernicke's encephalopathy. Rarely, DBN can also occur with hypomagnesemia, thiamine deficiency, B-12 deficiency and toxicity with lithium, alcohol, amiodarone, toluene, carbamazepine, phenytoin[6,15,16] or as a paraneoplastic manifestation.

Pathophysiology of upbeat and downbeat nystagmus
To understand the pathophysiology of upbeat and downbeat nystagmus, one should know the vertical VOR pathways. Normally, there is upward VOR tone from the anterior semi-circular canals (ACC) and downward VOR tone from the posterior semi-circular canals (PCC). Therefore, there is a tonic stream of impulses coming from both ACC to the upward-moving extraocular nuclei and both PCC to the downward-moving extraocular nuclei.

Impulses from the right ACC go to the ipsilateral superior vestibular nucleus, and from there fibers cross to the opposite side and ascend in the ventral tegmental tract (VTT) to reach the oculomotor complex on the contralateral side concerned with upward ocular movements, that is contralateral superior rectus subnucleus and the inferior oblique subnucleus. Since the superior rectus innervates the contralateral superior rectus muscle, stimulation of one ACC (e.g., right) results activation of ipsilateral (i.e., right) superior rectus and contralateral inferior oblique. What results is that the ipsilateral eye goes into elevation and intorsion, and the contralateral eye goes into elevation and extorsion. When the left ACC is stimulated, the ipsilateral eye goes into elevation and intorsion, and the contralateral eye (right eye) goes into elevation and extorsion (Video 18.6).

When both ACC are activated, the upward bias is added on, but the torsional action, being opposite in each case, gets canceled out by the bilateral stimulation. Hence, the net effect of bilateral ACC activation is the upward tonic activation of the extraocular muscles (Video 18.6).

When the ascending pathways are affected bilaterally as in an intra-axial pathology, the upward bias from the ACC is lost and eyes tend drift downward, resulting in corrective upward saccades with resultant upbeat nystagmus (Video 18.6). This reduction of upward VOR tone from the anterior semicircular canals can occur by lesions in the superior cerebellar peduncle (SCP), the VTT or the nucleus prepositus hypoglossi (NPH). The eyes are then deflected downward with corrective fast components upward.

The effect is the opposite in the case of stimulation of the PCC. Impulses from the each PCC go to the ipsilateral MVN, and from there fibers cross to the opposite side through the median longitudinal fasciculus (MLF) to reach the oculomotor nuclear complex on the contralateral side subserving downward ocular movement, that is the inferior rectus and superior oblique subnuclei, which innervate the ipsilateral inferior rectus and contralateral superior oblique muscles, respectively.

This results in depression and intorsion of the ipsilateral eye and depression and extorsion of the contralateral eye.

To illustrate, activation of the right PCC results in activation of the left inferior rectus/superior oblique subnucleus, resulting in activation of the left inferior rectus and right superior oblique muscles. This results in depression and intorsion of the right eye and depression and extorsion of the left eye.

When both PCCs are activated, the downward bias is added on, but the torsional action, being opposite in each case, is canceled out by the bilateral stimulation. Hence, net effect of bilateral PCC activation is the downward tonic activation of the extraocular muscle (Video 18.7).

When the ascending pathways are affected bilaterally, the downward bias from the PCC is lost and eyes tend drift upward, resulting in corrective downward saccades with resultant DBN (Video 18.7).

Superior vestibular nucleus giving rise to the VTT is normally kept inhibited by the flocculus, which is in turn inhibited by the caudal medulla (Video 18.6).

Lesions of the caudal medulla can also produce upbeat nystagmus. As mentioned earlier, a lesion in the medulla can result in disinhibition of the flocculus, which normally inhibits the superior vestibular nucleus. The disinhibited flocculus now exerts hyper-inhibition of the superior vestibular nucleus, producing a decrease in the upward bias in oculomotor system and the eyes tend drift downward with corrective upward saccade ending in upbeat nystagmus (Video 18.6).

The upward drift which is the basic pathophysiology of DBN can be caused by two mechanisms: an upward bias drift and a gaze-evoked drift.

The upward bias drift is caused by the relative predominance of the anterior SCC pathways compared with the posterior SCC projections as described above due to lesion of the bilateral MLF which carries the VOR input from the PCC. Alternatively, the superior vestibular nucleus wherein the afferent inputs from ACC end, is normally suppressed by the flocculus. Hence, a lesion of the flocculus can again result in upward bias drift due to disinhibition of the superior vestibular nucleus[17] resulting in excessive stimulation of the contralateral superior rectus and inferior oblique muscle with resultant upward bias and corrective downward saccade (Video 18.7).

DBN is a prominent manifestation of floccular and parafloccular dysfunction.

Causes of UBN and DBN are summarized in Table 18.2.[6]

Other forms of central vestibular nystagmus
Torsional nystagmus is a rarer form of central vestibular nystagmus. Purely torsional nystagmus suggests a brainstem lesion. In torsional nystagmus, the eye oscillates in a purely rotary or cyclotorsional plane. It may be present in the primary position or with either head positioning or gaze deviation. It is usually the result of central vestibular pathway lesions.

The torsional nystagmus is due to tonic imbalance in the roll plane, resulting in a tonic torsional drift of the eyes with corrective torsional fast phase beating opposite to the deviation. With pontomedullary lesions, fast phases of torsional nystagmus are contralesional (i.e., the upper pole of the eye beats to the side opposite the lesion). With medial longitudinal fasciculus (MLF) and interstitial nucleus of Cajal (INC) lesions, fast phases of torsional nystagmus are ipsilesional.

Torsional nystagmus is commonly observed in patients with a lateral medullary infarction (Wallenberg syndrome). The upper poles generally beat away from the side of the infarction, along with a contralateral hypertropia and ipsilateral saccadic

TABLE 18.2: Causes of Upbeat and Downbeat Nystagmus

Upbeat Nystagmus	Downbeat Nystagmus
Drugs	Drugs
Barbiturates	Lithium
Amitriptyline withdrawal	Amiodarone
	Metronidazole
	Antiepileptics
	Opioids
Toxins	Toxins
Nicotine	
Organoarsenic	
Organophosphates	
Infectious	Infectious
Creutzfeldt-Jakob disease	Herpes simplex encephalitis
Neurocysticercosis	West Nile encephalitis
	Legionnaire's disease
	Human T-lymphotropic virus infection
	Ciguatera toxin
	Tetanus
Inflammatory	Inflammatory
Multiple sclerosis	Multiple sclerosis
Neuromyelitis optica	Neuromyelitis optica
Paraneoplastic syndrome	Paraneoplastic syndrome
Anti-GAD antibody syndrome	Anti-GAD antibody syndrome
	Miller Fisher syndrome
Vascular	Vascular
	Stroke
	Vertebrobasilar dolichoectasia
Degenerative	Degenerative
	Spine-cerebellar atrophy
	Multi-system atrophy
Other	Other
Chiari malformation	Chiari malformation
Pseudotumor cerebri	B12 deficiency
Epileptic manifestation	Hypomagnesemia
	Heat stroke
	Gluten ataxia
	Episodic ataxias

lateropulsion. In midbrain lesions, torsional nystagmus beats toward the side of the lesion, unlike lesions lower in the brainstem, which beat away from the damaged vestibular nuclei. Lesions of the caudal vestibular nuclei or vestibular root entry zone cause torsional nystagmus with a large horizontal component.[18] Discrete lesions of the rostral part of the lateral vestibular nucleus or superior vestibular nucleus can produce torsional or mixed torsional-vertical nystagmus.

Pathophysiology of torsional nystagmus

When the inputs from both the superior and inferior semicircular canal to the brainstem extraocular nuclei are affected on one side, the torsional nystagmus results. As told before, when one superior semicircular canal input is stimulated, both the eyes go upward and makes torsional movements to the opposite side. When the posterior semicircular canal input is stimulated, both the eyes go downward and make the torsional movements to the opposite side. When both the anterior and posterior semicircular canal inputs are stimulated on one side, the vertical movements, being opposite in direction, gets canceled out, but the torsional movements are in the same direction, that is to the opposite

direction. For example, when the inputs from the right side are stimulated, the eyes make clockwise slow torsional movements when observed from the examiner's point of view. In the case of lesion of the right side, the eyes make a torsional slow phase deviation in the counterclockwise direction due to the overaction of the inputs from the left side, resulting in corrective fast component in the clockwise direction. Thus, a lateral medullary lesion on the right side results in torsional nystagmus with fast phase in the clockwise direction (Video 18.8).

Gaze-evoked nystagmus

Gaze-evoked nystagmus (GEN) refers to the nystagmus that develops when patients look into eccentric eye positions. Here, the fast component is to the point of fixation and there is no nystagmus in the primary position. When the patient looks to the right, the fast component is to the right and when the patient looks to the left, it is to the left and if the patient looks up, the fast component is upward.[6]

When the patient attempts to look in a lateral direction, the agonist activation (velocity command) is provided by abducens nuclear complex, which gets its premotor command ("pulse") from the parapontine reticular formation (PPRF). Once a saccade is completed to one side, maintaining eccentric eye position requires a tonic level of muscle innervation (*step innervation or the position command*) to oppose the elastic forces present in the orbit, which tend to restore the eye to the straight-ahead position. This step is generated by the *neural integrator*. The step is proportional to the *pulse*, which is the burst neuron activity in the PPRF. The step innervation holds the eye precisely in its new location after the saccade.

For conjugate horizontal eye movements, the neural integrator is the NPH and MVN.[19] The neural integrator for conjugate vertical gaze is in the INC.[20] The neural integrator is inherently leaky and is stabilized by the flocculus to which it is reciprocally connected.

Lesions in the neural integrator or the flocculus that stabilizes it result in a deficit in holding the gaze in the eccentric position. This defect in gaze-holding produces a slow drift of the eyes back to the primary position, resulting in a gaze-evoked nystagmus (Figure 18.3). The larger the eccentricity of the gaze, the faster

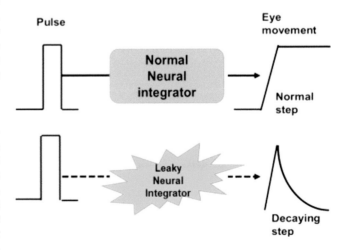

FIGURE 18.3 The perfect neural integrator (green) and leaky one (yellow) causing the centripetal drift.

the slow phase velocity. As the eye position becomes less eccentric, there is less drift. This slow drift is corrected by correcting saccades, which brings back the eye to the desired location in the orbit, resulting in nystagmus with fast phase to the point of fixation GEN.

Bilateral lesions of the neural integrator affect gaze-holding in all conjugate eye movements. Bilateral lesions of the INC result in partial failure of vertical gaze-holding.

GEN is therefore caused by lesions affecting the brainstem structures concerned with a neural integrator function or the connection with the vestibulocerebellum. With unilateral lesions of the cerebellum (flocculus), gaze-evoked nystagmus is greater on looking toward the side of lesion. The structures responsible for unidirectional GEN included the pyramid, uvula, tonsil and parts of the biventer and inferior semilunar lobules.[21]

GEN can also be caused by the side effect of various drugs, like AEDS, sedatives and alcohol. Gaze-evoked nystagmus due to medications usually occurs in both the horizontal and vertical planes.[6]

Caveat

Gaze-evoked nystagmus can sometimes be confused with end point nystagmus, which is a normal physiological phenomenon.

The following features help to differentiate end point nystagmus from gaze-evoked nystagmus.

Features of "end point nystagmus"

- It is present only in extreme lateral right and left gaze.
- It has a small amplitude.
- It is absent in upgaze.
- It is ill-sustained and fatigues over time (often just a few small beats of nystagmus are seen in each direction).

Rebound nystagmus

With persistent efforts of eccentric fixation, gaze-evoked nystagmus may quiet down and even reverse direction, so that the eye begins to drift centrifugally. If the eyes are then returned to the primary position, a short-lived nystagmus with slow drifts in the direction of the prior eccentric gaze and fast component to the opposite direction occurs (Video 18.9). This is called rebound nystagmus. This probably reflects an attempt by brainstem or cerebellar mechanisms to correct the centripetal drift of the gaze-evoked nystagmus.

Rebound nystagmus is usually seen with cerebellar disorders, but it has also been seen with lesions of the medulla in the region of the NPH and MVN. Rebound nystagmus is characteristic of flocculus-paraflocculus lesions.

Central positional nystagmus and vertigo

Paroxysmal positional vertigo and nystagmus can occur in posterior fossa lesions.[22] In central lesions, one can have downbeating nystagmus upon supine head-hanging, upbeating nystagmus upon returning from supine to the upright position, as well as apogeotropic horizontal-torsional nystagmus during the Dix-Hallpike or the supine head-roll test.[23] This is mainly seen with cerebellar strokes and tumors involving the nodulus and uvula.

Characteristics of nystagmus in distinguishing central and peripheral positional vertigo are given in Table 18.3.

TABLE 18.3: Differentiating Features between Peripheral and Central Positional Nystagmus

Nystagmus	Peripheral	Central
Appearance	Vertical and torsional	Pure vertical or upbeat
Latency	3–40 seconds	No latency
Fatigability	Yes	No
Habituation	Yes	No
Rebound	Yes	No
Reproducibility	Poor	Good
Localization	Posterior SCC or horizontal SCC	Brainstem or cerebellum

Periodic alternating nystagmus

Periodic alternating nystagmus (PAN) refers to nystagmus, which alternates direction in the primary position.[24] The nystagmus beats in one direction for about 60–90 seconds with an increasing and then decreasing intensity, followed by a brief transitional period (which may be punctuated by UBN, DBN or saccadic intrusions), and then beats in the opposite direction (Video 18.10). In order to make this diagnosis, one must observe the nystagmus for at least 3 minutes in order to see the full cycle.[25]

PAN can be congenital. Acquired PAN is usually caused by cerebellar nodular dysfunction. In rare cases, PAN may be seen with bilateral visual loss[26] and peripheral vestibulopathies, like Meniere's disease.[27] PAN arising from peripheral vestibular dysfunction is suppressed by visual fixation, has a more irregular periodicity and is associated with hearing loss but no central neurologic signs.[27]

Convergence-retraction nystagmus

There is rapid convergence with synchronous retraction of both globes caused by simultaneous contraction of all the extraocular muscles, followed by a slow divergent movement. Convergence-retraction nystagmus is not a true nystagmus, but opposing adducting saccades causing convergence of both eyes, without any slow phase. It is most often elicited by having the patient attempt to look up or by moving an optokinetic tape downward, which would normally elicit upbeating saccades. Instead of such saccades, the eyes converge and retract in the orbit. The retraction is best seen by observing the patient from the side. Convergence retraction nystagmus is one of many signs of Parinaud's dorsal midbrain syndrome. Other findings include upgaze paresis, light-near dissociation of the pupils and upper eyelid retraction.

See-saw nystagmus

See-saw nystagmus (SSN) is an unusual pattern in which one eye moves downward and extorts, while the other eye rises and intorts. The torsional component is conjugate, while the vertical is disconjugate. SSN can be of a pendular type or the jerk type, *hemi-see-saw nystagmus* (HSSN). The pendular type is usually due to a suprasellar lesion in most cases. Bitemporal hemianopsia, poor visual acuity and exodeviations are common accompaniments.

In the jerk-waveform or HSSN, half the cycle is the slow phase followed by a corrective half cycle of jerk. This type is usually seen with unilateral lesions in the region of the interstitial nucleus of Cajal in the midbrain.[28] Lesions in INC may cause either SSN or HSSN.

Congenital SSN may have no torsional component or may have a reverse torsional component so that the elevating eye extorts and the depressing eye intorts.

Dissociated jerk nystagmus

Dissociated nystagmus refers to nystagmus, which is different in both eyes. The most common cause is internuclear ophthalmoplegia.

A lesion of the MLF between the pons and midbrain causes an INO, characterized by an ipsilateral adduction deficit and a contralateral abducting nystagmus during attempted gaze away from the side of the lesion. Because the nystagmus is only observed in one eye, it is called a dissociated nystagmus. It is important to remember that myasthenia gravis may mimic INO *pseudo-internuclear ophthalmoplegia*.

INO is often bilateral, as both MLFs are near each other in the dorsal tegmentum. Vertical nystagmus is also common in INO, resulting from damage to the vestibulo-oculomotor pathways passing through the MLF.

Characteristics of unilateral INO (Video 18.11)

- Weakness of ipsilateral medial rectus for conjugate movements
- Dissociated nystagmus of contralateral abducting eye
- Skew deviation with ipsilateral hypertropia
- Asymmetrically impaired vertical VOR
- Dissociated vertical nystagmus: downbeat in ipsilateral eye, torsional in contralateral eye

Characteristics of bilateral INO

- Exotropia with bilateral adduction deficit
- Gaze-evoked vertical nystagmus
- Impaired vertical pursuit
- Impaired vertical VOR

Nystagmus and instability of gaze due to diseases affecting the visual pathways

Loss of vision due to disease of the anterior visual pathways causes instability of gaze. If the visual loss is binocular, there is nystagmus that has both horizontal and vertical components and changes direction over the course of seconds to minutes. The latter case is referred to as a "wandering null point". The waveform of the slow phase is variable, with decreasing, increasing or uniform velocity. These findings can be accounted for by an abnormal gaze-holding network (neural integrator). This abnormality is due to deprivation of visual inputs to the cerebellar or brainstem components of the neural integrator.

Monocular visual loss may lead to instability of gaze that is most obvious in the blind eye. The eye will show low frequency bidirectional drifts, which are more prominent vertically and unidirectional drifts with nystagmus occurring horizontally. Sometimes the appearance is that of a monocular vertical pendular nystagmus.

Nystagmus due to imbalance in pursuit tone

One type of nystagmus can occur when there is an asymmetry of horizontal smooth pursuit with disease of posterior cerebral hemispheres. Such patients show a constant velocity drift of the eyes toward the intact hemisphere. This is due to an imbalance in pursuit tone.

Congenital nystagmus (infantile nystagmus syndrome)

Congenital nystagmus (CN) is often noticed in the first few months of life. A family history of this disorder may be present. CN is often associated with a resting head tilt.

CN is a conjugate horizontal nystagmus and characteristically remains horizontal even in upgaze or downgaze (Video 18.12). It may be associated with a smaller torsional or vertical component. The nystagmus may change from pendular to jerk movements in different positions of gaze. The nystagmus shows a null position, in which the nystagmus is least and the visual acuity is best and patients often adopt a head turn to place the eyes in the null position to maximize visual acuity.[29]

Congenital nystagmus is increased when the child looks at a far object, whereas convergence dampens nystagmus amplitude (Video 18.12). Patients with CN do not complain of oscillopsia. Conversely, acquired nystagmus is not associated with a null position and therefore is less likely to be associated with head deviation. An additional clue suggesting infantile nystagmus is the presence of head oscillations.

CN is abolished in sleep. Two characteristic features of CN are the increasing velocity slow phase and the reversal of the normal optokinetic nystagmus such that the slow phase of eye movements moves in the direction opposite that of a rotating optokinetic stimulus. Approximately 15% of patients with CN have concomitant strabismus.

CN is not uniformly associated with poor visual acuity. However, CN may be associated with defects in the afferent visual system, such as albinism, congenital stationary night blindness or achromatopsia.

Latent nystagmus (fusional development nystagmus syndrome)

Latent nystagmus, which also appears very early in life, refers to nystagmus induced by covering one eye (Video 18.13). The nystagmus takes the form of jerk nystagmus with the fast component in the direction of the uncovered eye and the slow phase of the viewing eye beating toward the nose. Therefore, it will alternate directions depending on which eye is covered. It may be associated with congenital esotropia, dissociated vertical deviation (where the eye under the cover deviates upward), or congenital nystagmus.

Latent nystagmus that is present when both eyes are open is known as a manifest latent nystagmus. This is typically due to suppression of the vision of one eye, usually the esotropic eye.

Monocular nystagmus of childhood

Monocular nystagmus of childhood is a rare form of nystagmus manifesting in early life and is associated with anterior visual pathway lesions.

The eye movements are of small amplitude and vertical or elliptical, and the eye with nystagmus may have decreased vision, an afferent pupillary defect and optic atrophy. This pattern may be seen in benign cases such as profound amblyopia, as well as in association with glioma of the optic nerve or chiasm.

Spasmus nutans

Spasmus nutans is characterized by the triad of (1) torticollis, (2) head nodding (2–3 Hz) and (3) monocular or asymmetric nystagmus.[30] The nystagmus is the hallmark, and the other two features may or may not be present. Spasmus nutans is an intermittent, binocular, very small amplitude, high frequency (up to 15Hz), primarily horizontal, pendular nystagmus. The nystagmus may be dissociated or even monocular. It may be greater in the abducting eye, may have a vertical component, and may be more evident during convergence.

Onset of spasmus nutans is usually between the ages of 4 and 14 months and rarely up to 3 years. It typically lasts for several months but may last up to a few years. However, spasmus nutans can also occur with parasellar and hypothalamic tumors.[31,32] If there is evidence of an afferent pupillary defect or optic pallor, or endocrinologic abnormalities including poor feeding or diencephalic syndrome, spasmus nutans may be a secondary phenomenon.

Acquired pendular nystagmus

Acquired pendular nystagmus (APN) consists of involuntary, sinusoidal ocular oscillations typically ranging from 2 to 6 Hz that may be horizontal, vertical or a combination thereof including circular, elliptical or windmill-type. APN may arise from lesions affecting the dentate-rubro-olivary pathways (Guillain-Mollaret triangle), pontine tegmentum, inferior olivary nucleus (ION), cerebellum and MVN.[6,33]

There are three principal APN syndromes:

- APN associated with brainstem/cerebellar demyelinating disease (such as multiple sclerosis, adrenoleukodystrophy, toluene toxicity, Pelizaeus-Merzbacher disease, Cockayne syndrome and peroxisomal assembly disorders)[6,34]
- APN as part of the oculopalatal tremor (OPT) syndrome
- APN in Whipple disease

APN associated with a brainstem lesion is of low amplitude and high frequency (at least 4 Hz), and mainly horizontal and torsional (Video 18.14). It is usually symmetric and commonly associated with INO and ataxia.[33] The site of lesion is in the paramedian tegmental region of the brainstem,[33] for example, multiple sclerosis.

On the other hand, APN related to OPT syndrome is more irregular and oscillates at a higher amplitude and lower frequency (1–3 Hz). The oscillations can occur in the vertical and torsional planes, and sometimes disconjugate.[6,34] This tremor does not immediately after the insult, but it usually occurs months after the lesion in the Guillain-Mollaret triangle. (This triangle is formed by the red nucleus, ION and contralateral dentate nucleus.) The usual causes include pontine hemorrhage, Alexander disease, central pontine myelinolysis, etc. Moreover, it can be manifestation of the *progressive ataxia and palatal tremor syndrome*. The lesions of central tegmental tract cause hypertrophy of the ION on the same side, whereas superior cerebellar peduncle lesion causes hypertrophy of the contralateral ION. OPT may be associated with a simultaneous contraction of the branchial muscles (muscles derived from the branchial arch), the diaphragm or larynx.[6,35]

APN associated with Whipple disease is characterized by smooth, continuous, slow (1–3 Hz), pendular, convergent-divergent nystagmus. It differs from other forms of pendular nystagmus in which it is smooth and continuous with a high amplitude and slow frequency. These eye movements can persist during sleep. This nystagmus is associated simultaneous contractions of the masticatory muscles, called oculomasticatory myorhythmia. Associated neurological features include supranuclear vertical gaze palsy, and occasionally, rhythmic movements of the limbs.

Some useful clinical pearls in nystagmus

1. The chronicity of nystagmus gives a clue to the etiology of the nystagmus. Long-standing nystagmus, especially if noticed since childhood, may suggest congenital nystagmus rather than pathologically acquired nystagmus.
2. Patients with acquired nystagmus, especially types present during central visual fixation, tend to experience oscillopsia. Patients with congenital nystagmus do not complain of oscillopsia.
3. The presence of associated neurologic symptoms and signs help to identify the etiology of the nystagmus.
   a. Nystagmus accompanied by hemiparesis, dysarthria and binocular diplopia suggests a brainstem lesion.
   b. Acute-onset gaze-evoked or upbeat nystagmus with confusion and ataxia may suggest Wernicke's encephalopathy.
   c. Chronic downbeat nystagmus with slowly progressive ataxia may suggest spinocerebellar degeneration, Chiari malformation or lithium intoxication.
   d. Any acquired nystagmus type in the setting of a multifocal relapsing neurologic illness suggests multiple sclerosis.

Saccadic intrusions and oscillations

Saccadic intrusions are spontaneous eye movements that intrude steady fixation and often initiated by an attempt to produce a saccade.

Saccadic intrusions are divided into two broad categories: those with an intersaccadic interval between the saccades and those without such an interval, which is usually 200 ms.

Saccadic intrusions with an intersaccadic interval include square-wave jerks,

Macro-square-wave jerks and macrosaccadic oscillations, whereas ocular flutter and opsoclonus constitute the saccadic intrusions without an intersaccadic interval (Figure 18.4).

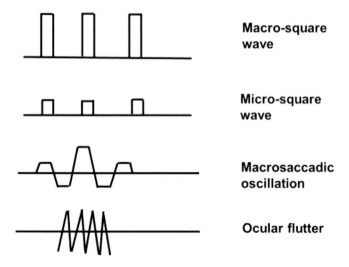

FIGURE 18.4 The various saccadic intrusions.

Saccadic intrusions with intersaccadic interval

Square wave jerks

Square wave jerks are saccades, which move the eyes from and then return them to the midline without crossing. This can be of two types depending upon the amplitude: micro- or macro-square-wave jerks. If the micro-square-wave jerks are of smaller amplitude (0.5–5°), they are called micro square waves. These micro-square-wave jerks if occur with a lower frequency (less than 20 per minute) can be seen in normal individuals and have no clinical significance. On the other hand, macro-square-wave jerks are of larger amplitude (5–15 degrees) and are almost always pathological and are seen in multiple sclerosis, progressive supranuclear palsy, multisystem atrophy, Friedreich's ataxia, etc.[36,37]

Square-wave jerks are thought to be due to lesions affecting the frontal eye fields and the superior colliculus or its inputs from the substantia nigra pars reticularis and mesencephalic reticular formation.[38] However, macro-square-wave jerks may also occur with cerebellar pathology.[39]

Macrosaccadic oscillations

Macrosaccadic oscillations are runs of repeating macro-square-wave jerks which cross the midline, and occur in a crescendo-decrescendo pattern[40] (Video 18.15). This can be thought of as an extreme and spontaneous form of cerebellar saccadic hypermetria.

This eye movement disorder is typically seen in cerebellar lesions, typically in the caudal fastigial nucleus, and may also be seen in pontine lesions.[41]

Saccadic intrusions without intersaccadic interval

Ocular flutter and opsoclonus

Ocular flutter consists of erratic bursts of very high frequency (10–25 cycles per second), back-to-back saccades that oscillate about the midline, in the horizontal plane without an intersaccadic interval between subsequent saccades (Video 18.16). When such saccades occur in multiple trajectories: horizontal, vertical and torsional, they are called as opsoclonus (Video 18.17). They occur episodically and are often provoked by shifting gaze.[42]

Flutter and opsoclonus are usually seen in pontine or cerebellar lesions.[43]

The two major causes are: paraneoplastic conditions and parainfectious brainstem encephalitis.[44] Those occurring due to parainfectious etiology are typically associated with truncal myoclonus, ataxia, and emotional lability. The infectious agents usually involved are enterovirus, West Nile virus, Lyme disease, mumps, HIV, malaria, dengue and Zika virus.[45] The antibodies seen in those with paraneoplastic etiology include anti-Hu, anti-Yo, anti-Ma, anti-amphiphysin, anti-P/Q-type calcium channel, anti-N-methyl-D-aspartate (NMDA) receptor, anti-GAD and anti-GQ1b.[46,47]

Other causes include traumatic brain injury,[48] diabetic hyperosmolar coma, etc.

Other abnormal eye movements

Ocular bobbing

This is a distinctive class of abnormal spontaneous vertical eye movements, usually seen in comatose states, which is characterized by intermittent, often conjugate, fast downward movement of the eyes followed, after a brief interval, by a slow upward movement to the primary position. It is usually seen in lesions of pons, particularly hemorrhage, tumors or infarction.[49,50]

Rarely, ocular bobbing can be seen in extra-axial posterior fossa masses,[51,52] diffuse encephalitis[53] and toxic and metabolic encephalopathies.[54] The prognosis depends upon the cause, being very poor in the more common pontine hemorrhages.

Several atypical forms of ocular bobbing have also been described. In "reverse ocular bobbing" (Video 18.18), the eyes initially move upward with a fast component, followed after a brief delay by a slow return to midposition. This type of reverse ocular bobbing is non-localizing and is seen metabolic encephalopathy.

In ocular dipping or inverse ocular bobbing (Video 18.19), there is a slow conjugate downward movement of the eyes, followed by a rapid return to midposition. This is usually seen diffuse encephalopathies like anoxic coma or after prolonged status epilepticus.[55,56]

In "reverse ocular dipping", there is a slow upward deviation of the eyes, followed by a rapid return to midposition. This is associated with metabolic encephalopathy or viral encephalitis.[57]

Roving eye movements (ping-pong gaze)

Roving eye movements are slow, conjugate, lateral and to-and-fro excursions, generally seen in normal sleep and in comatose patients with toxic, metabolic strokes[58] (Video 18.20).These movements suggest that the brainstem is intact and often indicate a toxic, metabolic conditions or alternatively bilateral hemisphere cause for coma, such as hypoxic encephalopathy.

Periodic alternating gaze deviation

Periodic alternating gaze deviation is a rare disorder of ocular motility, characterized by periods of gaze deviation lasting from 1 to 3 minutes alternating from left to right.[59] This disorder is continuous except during sleep[60] and is accompanied by a periodic gaze paresis to the side opposite the direction of the ocular deviation. This is seen in brainstem lesions.

Cyclic oculomotor paralysis with spasms

Cyclic oculomotor paralysis with spasms[61,62] is characterized by a unilateral third nerve paresis alternating with third nerve spasm lasting for 90 seconds, during which the lid elevates, the pupil constricts, the eye adducts and accommodation increases. Ten to thirty seconds later, the spasm gives way to the paretic phase, and the eye becomes abducted with ptosis and a dilated pupil and the cycle repeats itself. It is present at birth or within the first year of life. It is thought to be due to birth or childhood trauma, resulting in damage to the third nerve nucleus or its fascicles, giving rise to abnormal central as well as peripheral neuronal connections.[62]

Periodic alternating skew deviation

Periodic alternating skew deviation is characterized by a hypertropia of one eye for a period of 40–50 seconds, followed by a transition phase, during which the eyes become straight, and by a contralateral hypertropia for 40–50 seconds. Then cycle repeats itself. The site of lesion is in the midbrain at the level of the interstitial nucleus of Cajal.[63]

Pretectal pseudo-bobbing

This is characterized by arrhythmic, repetitive downward and inward eye movements at a rate ranging from one per 3 seconds to two per second and an amplitude of one-fifth to one-half of the full voluntary range[64] (Video 18.21). This form of ocular movement can be confused with ocular bobbing. However, the "V" pattern of the downward fast movement and the faster rate help to differentiate it from ocular bobbing. The site of lesion is in the pretectal region and the usual cause is obstructive hydrocephalus. This pretectal pseudo-bobbing may represent a variety of convergence nystagmus.

Conclusion

Eye fixation can be disrupted by many abnormal eye movements. Broadly these abnormal movements are classified as 'Nystagmus' and the 'Saccadic Intrusions'. Understanding the intricate network controlling the various eye movements and connecting them to various other structures like the vestibular system, the brainstem, the cerebellum and the cortex, may help in discerning the cause of abnormal eye movements in a given patient.

Multiple-Choice Questions

1. All the following features help to distinguish central vertigo from peripheral vertigo, EXCEPT:
   a. Skew deviation
   b. Direction changing nystagmus
   c. Positive head impulse test
   d. Severe imbalance while walking

   Answer:

   c. Positive head impulse test

2. All the following sites of lesion can produce upbeat nystagmus, EXCEPT:
   a. Upper midbrain
   b. Caudal medulla
   c. Flocculus
   d. Ventral tegmental tracts

   Answer:

   c. Flocculus

3. All the following statements are true regarding end point nystagmus, EXCEPT:
   a. It is present only in extreme lateral right and left gaze.
   b. It is absent in upgaze.
   c. It is ill-sustained and fatigues over time.
   d. It persists even when the patient closes one eye.

   Answer:

   d. It persists even when the patient closes one eye.

4. The pathognomonic feature of congenital nystagmus is:
   a. Nystagmus attenuates during convergence.
   b. Inverted optokinetic nystagmus.
   c. Nystagmus vector remains same when the child looks up or down.
   d. Nystagmus shows a "null" zone.

   Answer:

   b. Inverted optokinetic nystagmus.

References

1. Brandt T, Dieterich M, Strupp M. Vertigo and Dizziness: Common Complaints. New York: Springer; 2005.

2. Newman-Toker DE, Sharma P, et al. Penlight-cover test: a new bedside method to unmask nystagmus. J Neurol Neurosurg Psychiatry. 2009;80:900–903.

3. Choi KD, Oh SY, Park SH, Kim JH, Koo JW, Kim JS. Head-shaking nystagmus in lateral medullary infarction: patterns and possible mechanisms. Neurology. 2007;68:1337–1344.

4. Minagar A, Sheremata WA, Tusa RJ. Perverted head-shaking nystagmus: a possible mechanism. Neurology. 2001;57:887–889.

5. Choi KD, Kim JS, Kim HJ, Koo JW, Kim JH, Kim CY, et al. Hyperventilation-induced nystagmus in peripheral vestibulopathy and cerebellopontine angle tumor. Neurology. 2007;69:1050–1059.

6. Leigh RJ, Zee DS. The Neurology of Eye Movements. 4th ed. New York: Oxford University Press, 2006.

7. Nam J, Kim S, Huh Y, Kim JS. Ageotropic central positional nystagmus in nodular infarction. Neurology. 2009;73:1163.

8. Arai M, Terakawa I. Central paroxysmal positional vertigo. Neurology. 2005;64:1284.

9. Fernandez C, Alzate R, Lindsay JR. Experimental observations on postural nystagmus. II. Lesions of the nodulus. Ann Otol Rhinol Laryngol. 1960;69:94–114.

10. Dix MR, Hallpike CS. The pathology symptomatology and diagnosis of certain common disorders of the vestibular system. Proc R Soc Med. 1952;45:341–354.

11. Cohen HS. Side-lying as an alternative to the Dix-Hallpike test of the posterior canal. Otol Neurotol. 2004;25:130–134.

12. Bisdorff AR, Debatisse D. Localizing signs in positional vertigo due to lateral canal cupulolithiasis. Neurology. 2001;57:1085–1088.

13. Janssen JC, Larner AJ, Morris H, et al. Upbeat nystagmus: clinicoanatomical correlation. J Neurol Neurosurg Psychiatry. 1998;65:380–381.

14. Baloh RW, Yee RD. Spontaneous vertical nystagmus. Rev Neurol (Paris). 1989; 145(8–9):527–532.

15. Chrousos GA, et al. Two cases of downbeat nystagmus and oscillopsia associated with carbamazepine. Am J Ophthalmol. 1987;103(2):221–224.

16. Halmagyi GM, et al. Lithium-induced downbeat nystagmus. Am J Ophthalmol. 1989;107(6):664–670.

17. Bohmer A, Straumann D. Pathomechanism of mammalian downbeat nystagmus due to cerebellar lesion: a simple hypothesis. Neurosci Lett. 1998;250:127–130.

18. Uemura T, Cohen B. Effects of vestibular nuclei lesions on vestibulo-ocular reflexes and posture in monkeys. Acta Otolaryngol Suppl. 1973;315:1–71.

19. Lopez-Barneo J, Darlot C, Berthoz A, et al. Neuronal activity in prepositus nucleus correlated with eye movement in the alert cat. J Neurophysiol. 1982;47:329–352.

20. Fukushima K. The interstitial nucleus of Cajal and its role in the control of movements of head and eyes. Prog Neurobiol. 1987;29:107–192.

21. Baier B, Dieterich M. Incidence and anatomy of gaze-evoked nystagmus in patients with cerebellar lesions. Neurology. 2011;76:361–365.

22. Lea J. Lechner C, Halmagyi GM, Welgampola MS. Not so benign positional vertigo: paroxysmal downbeat nystagmus from a superior cerebellar peduncle neoplasm. Otol Neurotol. 2014;35(6):e204–e205.

23. Choi JY, Kim JH, Kim HJ, Glasauer S, Kim JS. Central paroxysmal positional nystagmus: characteristics and possible mechanisms. Neurology. 2015; 84(22):2238–2246.

24. Baloh RW, Honrubia V, Konrad HR. Periodic alternating nystagmus. Brain. 1976;99: 11–26.

25. Leigh RJ, Robinson DA, Zee DS. A hypothetical explanation for periodic alternating nystagmus: instability in the optokinetic-vestibular system. Ann N Y Acad Sci. 1981;374:619–635.

26. Cross SA, Smith JL, Norton EW. Periodic alternating nystagmus clearing after vitrectomy. J Clin Neuroophthalmol. 1982;2:5–11.

27. Murofushi T, Chihara Y, Ushio M, et al. Periodic alternating nystagmus in Meniere's disease: the peripheral type? Acta Otolaryngol. 2008;128:824–827.

28. Halmagyi GM, et al. Jerk-waveform see-saw nystagmus due to unilateral mesodiencephalic lesion. Brain. 1994;117:789–803.

29. Stevens DJ, Hertle RW. Relationships between visual acuity and anomalous head posture in patients with congenital nystagmus. J Pediatr Ophthalmol Strabismus. 2003;40(5): 259–264, quiz 297–298.

30. Gottlob I, Wizov SS, Reinecke RD. Spasmus nutans. A long-term follow-up. Invest Ophthalmol Vis Sci. 1995;36:2768–2771.

31. Antony JH, Ouvrier RA, Wise G: Spasmus nutans. A mistaken identity. Arch Neurol. 1980;37:373–375.

32. Lavery MA, O'Neill JF, Chu FC, et al. Acquired nystagmus in early childhood: a presenting sign of intracranial tumor. Ophthalmology. 1984;91:425–435.

33. Lopez LI, Bronstein AM, Gresty MA, et al. Clinical and MRI correlates in 27 patients with acquired pendular nystagmus. Brain. 1996;119:465–472.

34. Tilikete C, Jasse L, Pelisson D, et al. Acquired pendular nystagmus in multiple sclerosis and oculopalatal tremor. Neurology. 2011;76:1650–1657.

35. Nagaoka M, Narabayashi H. Palatal myoclonus—its remote influence. J Neurol Neurosurg Psychiatry. 1984;47:921–926.

36. Spicker S, Schulz JB, Petersen D, et al. Fixation instability and oculomotor abnormalities in Friedreich's ataxia. J Neurol. 1995;242(8):517–521.

37. Pinnock RA, McGivern RC, Forbes R, Gibson JM. An exploration of ocular fixation in Parkinson's disease, multiple system atrophy and progressive supranuclear palsy. J Neurol. 2010;257(4):533–539.

38. Gnadt JW, Noto CT, Kanwal JS. Tectal etiology for irrepressible saccades: a case study in a Rhesus monkey. F1000Res. 2013;2:85.

39. Rucker JC. Nystagmus and saccadic intrusions. Continuum (minneap minn). 2019;25(5, neuro-ophthalmology):1376–1400.

40. Selhorst JB, Stark L, Ochs AL, Hoyt WF. Disorders in cerebellar ocular motor control. II. Macrosaccadic oscillation. An oculographic, control system and clinico-anatomical analysis. Brain. 1976;99(3):509–522.

41. Kim JS, Choi KD, Oh SY, et al. Double saccadic pulses and macrosaccadic oscillations from a focal brainstem lesion. J Neurol Sci. 2007;263(1–2):118–123.

42. Digre KB. Opsoclonus in adults. Report of three cases and review of the literature. Arch Neurol. 1986;43:1165–1175.

43. Schon F, Hodgson TL, Mort D, Kennard C. Ocular flutter associated with a localized lesion in the paramedian pontine reticular formation. Ann Neurol. 2001;50(3):413–416.

44. Waisbourd M, Kesler A. Postinfectious ocular flutter. Neurology. 2009;72(11):1027.

45. Guedes BF, Vieira Filho MAA, Listik C, et al. HIV-associated opsoclonus-myoclonus-ataxia syndrome: early infection, immune reconstitution syndrome or secondary to other diseases? Case report and literature review. J Neurovirol. 2018;24(1):123–127.

46. Dubbioso R, Marcelli V, Manganelli F, et al. Anti-GAD antibody ocular flutter: expanding the spectrum of autoimmune ocular motor disorders. J Neurol. 2013;260(10):2675–2677.

47. Zaro-Weber O, Galldiks N, Dohmen C, et al. Ocular flutter, generalized myoclonus, and trunk ataxia associated with anti-GQ1b antibodies. Arch Neurol. 2008;65(5):659–661.

48. Manta A, Ugradar S, Theodorou M. Ocular flutter after mild head trauma. J Neuroophthalmol. 2018;38(4):476–478.

49. Larmande P, Limodin J, Henin D, Lapierre F. Ocular bobbing: abnormal eye movement or eye movement's abnormality? Ophthalmologica. 1983;187:161–165.

50. Zegers de Beyl D, Flament-Durand J, Borenstein S, Brunko E. Ocular bobbing and myoclonus in central pontine myelinolysis. J Neurol Neurosurg Psychiatry. 1983;46:564–565.

51. Bosch EP, Kennedy SS, Aschenbrener CA. Ocular bobbing: the myth of its localizing value. Neurology. 1975; 25:949–953.

52. Finelli PF, McEntee WJ. Ocular bobbing with extra-axial haematoma of posterior fossa. J Neurol Neurosurg Psychiatry. 1977;40:386–388.

53. Rudick R, Satran R, Eskin TA. Ocular bobbing in encephalitis. J Neurol Neurosurg Psychiatry. 1981;44:441–443.

54. Paty DW, Sherr H. Ocular bobbing in bromism: a case report. Neurology. 1972;22:526–527.

55. Newman N, Gay AJ, Heilbrun MP. Dysjugate ocular bobbing: its relation to midbrain, pontine and medullary function in a surviving patient. Neurology. 1971;21:633–637.

56. van Weerden TW, van Woerkom TCAM. Ocular dipping. Clin Neurol Neurosurg. 1982;84:221–226.

57. Mark F Mehler. The clinical spectrum of ocular bobbing and ocular dipping. Journal of Neurology, Neurosurgery, and Psychiatry. 1988;51:725–727.

58. Bateman DE. Neurological assessment of coma. J Neurol Neurosurg Psychiatr. 2001;71:i13–i17.

59. Kestenbaum A. Clinical Methods of Neuroophthalmologic Examination. New York: Grune & Stratton Inc.; 1961, pp. 381–383.

60. Goldberg RT, Gonzalez C, Breinin GM, et al. Periodic alternating gaze deviation with dissociation of head movement. Arch Ophthalmol. 1965;73:325–330.

61. Susac MJO, Smith JL. Cyclic oculomotor paresis. Neurology. 1974;24:24–27.

62. Loewenfeld IE, Thompson HS: Oculomotor paresis with cyclic spasms: a critical review of the literature and a new case. Surv Ophthalmol. 1975;20:81–124.

63. Staudenmaier C, Buncic JR. Periodic alternating gaze deviation with dissociated secondary face turn. Arch Ophthalmol. 1983;101:202–205.

64. Keane JR. Pretectal pseudobobbing. Five patients with "V"-pattern convergence nystagmus. Arch Neurol. 1985;42(6):592–594.

19A

SPECIAL CONSIDERATIONS IN GAZE
Physiology and Disorders of Saccade Velocity

Mohamed Elkasaby, Aasef G. Shaikh

Introduction

Saccades are quick simultaneous movements of both eyes and they are the fastest movements produced by the human body. The goal of saccades is to reposition the fovea on the desired object in order to enhance the visual clarity. The saccades, requiring coordination and precision, must rely on the feedback dependent complex neural network. Amongst many subtypes, the visually guided saccades are internally generated volitional eye movements. In contrast, the reflexive saccades are triggered exogenously by the appearance of a novel visual stimulus. A scanning saccade is triggered endogenously for the purpose of exploring the visual environment. The memory-guided saccades are generated internally and they are made toward the remembered location of the target. In contrast, the antisaccades are comprised of the movements that are equal in amplitude as that would have generated by the visually guided saccade but in the opposite direction. Antisaccades are also internally generated but they require inhibiting a reflexive saccade to the onset location, and voluntarily moving the eye in the other direction. Although distinct network of neurons and brain regions depend on generation of each subtype of saccade, they all share a final common pathway in the brainstem. Amplitude, timing, and velocity are the key parameters determined by the brainstem final common pathways and their influencers. Examination of kinematic changes in saccades offers critical understanding of the central pathologies, hence making saccades markers of common as well as uncommon neurological disorders and their therapies.

Anatomical substrates determining saccade velocity

Cerebral cortex

The cerebral cortex executes the visually guided saccades, and the commands are carried in two distinct pathways that converge onto the superior colliculus [1, 2]. The frontal eye field (FEF), supplementary eye field (SEF) and dorsolateral prefrontal cortex (dlPFC) comprise the first pathway. The saccade signals generated in this pathway are projected to the caudate nucleus [3–6]. The caudate directly inhibits the substantia nigra pars reticulata (SNpr) [6, 7]. Inhibition of the latter activates the superior colliculus via removal of tonic GABAergic inhibition [8–11]. The cessation of tectal inhibition initiates saccades. The parietal eye field (PEF) comprises the second pathway [1, 2]. The PEF has reciprocal connections with the FEF and it also provides input to the superior colliculus [12, 13]. The connections between the PEF and FEF participate in visual processing, while those between PEF and superior colliculus seem to affect saccade expression. The cortical lesions typically do not influence the kinematic properties of saccades, but their planning (amplitude and timing matrix) are affected [14, 15].

Superior colliculus

Layered midbrain structure called superior colliculus receives input from the frontal and parietal cortex pathways; integrates the cortical excitatory input from inhibitory basal ganglionic input; and regulates further downsteam saccade generation regions [13, 16–18]. The input from the striate, extrastriate and parietal cortex, as well as from the frontal lobes is relayed to a motor map with information about eye movement parameters occupying the ventral layers of the superior colliculus [19–22]. Non-human primate literature utilizing direct stimulation of tectal neurons demonstrated neuronal populations in the deep layers of the superior colliculus that are directly involved in saccade initiation [23, 24]. Midbrain and pontine reticular formation are projection sites of these cells; such mesencephalic regions also have premotor structures that are critical in generation of adequate saccade matrix. The superior colliculus is believed to play a part in movement initiation and determination of saccadic velocity, as well as in selecting a target to focus on [25–27].

Cerebellum

The cerebellum is not only critical as the brain's motor learning apparatus, but it also plays a crucial role in predictive mechanisms to increase the fidelity of performed movements—i.e., the "machine learning". Connected with the cortical eye fields via pontine nuclei and the superior colliculus [28–33]; the cerebellar output sends projections via its deep nuclei including the fastigial oculomotor region (FOR). The FOR output projects to the omnipause neurons (OPNs), excitatory burst neurons (EBNs) and inhibitory burst neurons (IBNs) as well as to the thalamus, superior colliculus and reticular formation [34]. FOR stimulates burst neurons during contralateral saccades and provides inhibition during ipsilateral saccades [35, 36]. This mechanism is critical for improving the saccade accuracy and calibrating for the saccade pulse-step mismatch [37–40].

OPNs

The glycine-dependent OPNs control gaze holding by inhibiting the horizontal and vertical saccade burst generators, located in the nucleus raphe interpositus of the midline pons [29, 32, 33, 41, 42]. Such inhibition is necessary for two reasons—timely cessation of the ongoing saccade and prevent intrusive saccades when steady gaze holding is desired. The task is obtained via two sources of input, one from the FOR, while the other from the tectum [29, 34–36]. The tonic activation of the OPNs results in saccade suppression, while their inactivation cause slowing of saccades; the electrical stimulation of OPNs stop saccades en route [43, 44].

Premotor burst neurons

The EBNs driving horizontal saccades are in a different mesencephalic nucleus compared to vertical EBNs [45–47]. Horizontal EBNs are in the paramedian pontine reticular formation while rostral interstitial nucleus of medial longitudinal fasciculus has vertical EBNs [48]. The EBNs are only active during saccades; their discharge rate determines saccade velocity [46–48]. The IBNs are connected with the EBNs; but in addition, IBNs project across the midline mutually inhibiting each other. Such mutually reciprocal inhibition is critical for generating post-inhibitory rebound, a mechanism critical for sufficient strength of burst ensuring rapid saccade velocity.

DOI: 10.1201/9780429020278-27

Saccade velocity in disorders affecting basal ganglia and their brainstem connections

Parkinson's disease

Parkinson's disease (PD) is one of the very common neurodegenerative condition affecting the substantia nigra pars compacta. The consequence of such degeneration is altered firing behavior of entire basal ganglia neuronal circuits (and their connections) leading to its typical deficits such as resting tremor, rigidity and bradykinesia, along with postural instability [49]. PD not only affects axial and appendicular motor system, there is prominent involvement of the eye movements such as the memory-guided saccades, convergence insufficiency and restricted gaze [50–55]. PD can substantially affect kinematics of visually guided saccades, sometimes even affecting their velocity and timing [54]. The result

of this hypometria is a "staircase" appearance of the saccade timeseries [56, 57]. While the actual velocity of the saccade may not be changed, the time it takes for the inefficient saccade to reach the target lengthens [58]. In patients with asymmetric parkinsonism, hypometria of saccades is also asymmetric and worse on the more affected side [59]. Patients with PD also appear to have increased latency in saccade initiation with verbal instruction and reduced accuracy, when compared to healthy controls [60]. However, saccades made to random visual targets are not altered [61]. PD patients show increased variability in peak saccade velocity, with decreased velocity seen only in advanced cases of the disease [62–64].

Our recent study measured visually guided saccades in 20 PD patients with high-resolution oculography. We discovered that saccades in PD are not only slow but also curved in their trajectory are interrupted. Figure 19A.1 shows an example of visually

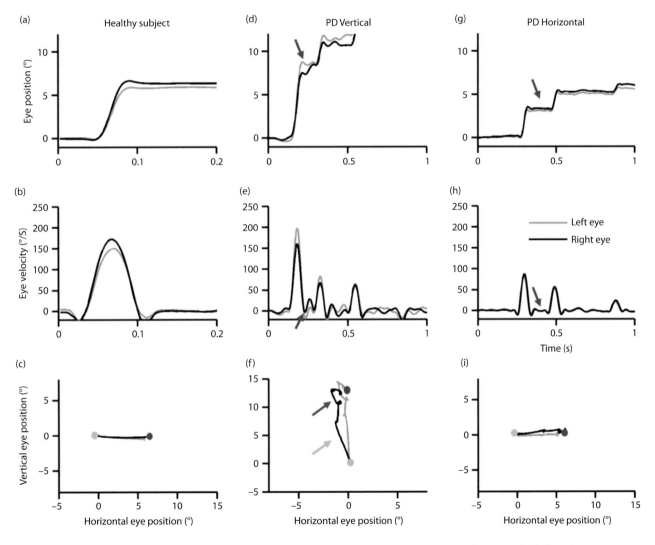

FIGURE 19A.1 Examples of visually guided saccades from healthy subject and PD patient. In first row of subplots the eye position is plotted on the y-axis, while x-axis depicts corresponding time in seconds. Black line depicts right eye, gray trace is left eye. Red arrows depict interruption in ongoing saccades. Panel A illustrates normal visually guided vertical saccade from a healthy subject. Panels (d) and (g) depict examples of visually guided vertical and horizontal saccades from the same PD subject. Middle row of subplots depicts eye velocity. Panel (b) depicts eye velocity of normal visually guided saccade recorded from a healthy subject, while panels (e) and (h) depict vertical and horizontal eye velocity respectively from a PD patient. In these subplots, the eye velocity is plotted on y-axis while x-axis illustrates corresponding time. Red arrows illustrate interruption in saccade when eye velocity was zero (panel h) or when eye moved at slower velocity in the opposite direction (panel e). The bottom row of the subplots depicts trajectories of horizontal and vertical saccades. Panel C depicts normal saccade from the healthy subject, panels (f) and (I) depict vertical and horizontal saccades in PD. Green dot is start point, red dot is stop point. Arrows in panels (f) and (i) depict curvature in saccade trajectory.

guided saccade captured from the PD patient and its comparison with the healthy subject. Figure 19A.1a and b depicts an example of a healthy subject. The y-axis in Figure 19A.1a depicts eye position, while that in Figure 19A.1b is velocity. The x-axis in both depicts corresponding time. The healthy subject has uninterrupted visually guided saccade characterized by a single peak in the velocity profile (Figure 19A.1a and b). The path of this eye movement illustrated in Figure 19A.1c has a straight trajectory. The saccades in PD patient are different compared to the healthy subject (Figure 19A.1d–i). There are three types of interruptions in the saccade trajectory. One type of "interruption" has just reduction in the saccade velocity—the eyes do not stop moving (arrows in Figure 19A.1d and e). The second type of interruption features complete cessation of the saccades, while the third type of interruption has the eyes moving in the opposite direction. The vertical saccades are not only interrupted, but they are also curved and have irregular trajectory. An example depicted in Figure 19A.1f shows upward directed initial trajectory, it then moves to the right and upward again and then to the left (green arrow Figure 19A.1f). The eyes then stop (not visible in the figure) but then make another curved movement to the target (blue arrow, Figure 19A.1f). The interruptions and irregularity in trajectories are also present in the horizontal saccades (Figure 19A.1g and h), but they are less robust (Figure 19A.1i). These deficits are consistent in all subjects. The directional disparity suggested the possibility that the abnormal saccades in PD not only reflect abnormal tectal function, but also suggest abnormal oscillatory behavior in the reciprocally innervating EBNs and IBNs that are discretely placed in the primate brain. We further speculated that impaired function of the EBNs and IBNs causes maladaptive activation of the superior colliculus. Latter may also lead to abnormal curvatures and interruption in the saccade trajectory.

Atypical Parkinsonism

Range of saccade abnormalities were described in atypical forms of parkinsonism including progressive supranuclear palsy (PSP), dementia with Lewy bodies and corticobasal degeneration (CBD). PSP, a form of tauopathy, causes supranuclear gaze and bulbar palsies, as well as postural instability with unexplained falls, cognitive dysfunction and axial rigidity [65, 66]. The hypometria and slowing of vertical saccades is more prominent in PSP, although it affects horizontal saccades as well [67]. Poor convergence ability and altered pursuit are also common. Progression of PSP results in complete loss of vertical saccade and then eventually horizontal saccade leading to complete ophthalmoplegia [68, 69]. The saccade disorders in PSP are correlated with the anatomical changes discovered in autopsy. The prominent involvement of PSP brain includes the substantia nigra pars compacta of the basal ganglia, mesencephalon, diencephalon and the brainstem reticular formation [70–72].

In 12 patients who had PSP we performed quantitative ocular motor assessment to measure kinematic properties of saccades. We discovered that both horizontal and vertical saccades were slow and had irregular trajectories and velocities. The deficits were present along both axes, but vertical saccades were prominently involved. Figure 19A.2 depicts a comparison of PSP patient with a healthy subject. An example of normal visually guided saccade from healthy subject is depicted in Figure 19A.2a–c. The normal saccade has high velocity and uninterrupted straight trajectory (Figure 19A.2a–c). The PSP patient has saccades with striking differences compared to the

healthy subject (Figure 19A.2d–i). Figure 19A.2d–i depict two examples of vertical saccades from the same PSP patient measured during the same session. One example of saccade has three types of interruptions—complete cessation (red arrow, Figure 19A.2d and e), incomplete cessation but presence of slow movement eye movement during "interruption" (blue arrow Figure 19A.2d and e) and eye movement in the opposite direction (green arrow Figure 19A.2d and e). The second example of saccade has less number of interruptions compared (Figure 19A.2g), but they are over all slow (gray arrows in Figure 19A.2e and h). In addition to interruptions, the saccades in PSP (as depicted in PD, Figure 19A.1) are also curved and irregular. For example, the first type of saccade makes upward directed trajectory first, then to the right, it halts and then crosses the midline to the left, and then finally to the target on the right (Figure 19A.2f). The trajectory shape is not only curved, but is "serpentine" (Figure 19A.2i). Interruptions and curvatures are also present in horizontal saccades (Figure 19A.2j–l), but they are less robust compared to vertical. Such interruptions and curvatures of saccades were consistently seen in all subjects.

Dementia with Lewy bodies (DLB), characterized by the presence of eosinophilic intracytoplasmic inclusions called Lewy bodies, which consist of aggregations of alpha-synuclein within neurons. The key clinical features are parkinsonism, cognitive impairment, visual hallucinations, autonomic dysfunction, a fluctuating mental state and REM sleep behavior disorder [73–75]. Hypometria as well as slowing of saccades are reported in DLB [76]. The latency of visually guided saccade initiation is increased and there are more directional errors during antisaccade tasks in patients with DLB [76, 77].

CBD is a neurodegenerative tauopathy that presents with combinations of akinesia, rigidity, dystonia, focal myoclonus, tremor, postural instability and gait changes with apraxia and alien limb phenomena [78, 79]. The slowed velocity of saccades in CBD is occasionally found, while saccade latency is always increased [53, 64, 79].

Huntington's disease

Huntington's disease (HD) is an inherited progressive neurodegenerative disorder caused by a CAG triplet repeat resulting in a defect in the protein huntingtin. This autosomal dominant disorder results in degeneration of the frontal lobe and caudate nucleus, and subsequent behavior changes, choreoathetosis and cognitive decline [80–82]. Saccade abnormalities serve as a clinical marker in Huntington's disease [83]. Early in the disease, the changes include increased latency and hypometria along with reduced velocity in either the vertical or the horizontal planes [84–88].

Saccade velocity in disorders affecting cerebellum and its brainstem connections

Spinocerebellar ataxia type 2

Spinocerebellar ataxia type 2 (SCA2) is an autosomal dominant disorder characterized by progressive ataxia, tremor, dysarthria and early neuropathy. SCA2 is caused by an unstable polyglutamine expansion within ataxin-2 [89–91]. The presence of slow saccades correlating with the size of polyglutamine expansion and inversely with ataxia severity is one of the key manifestations of SCA2 [92]. The slowing of saccades in SCA2

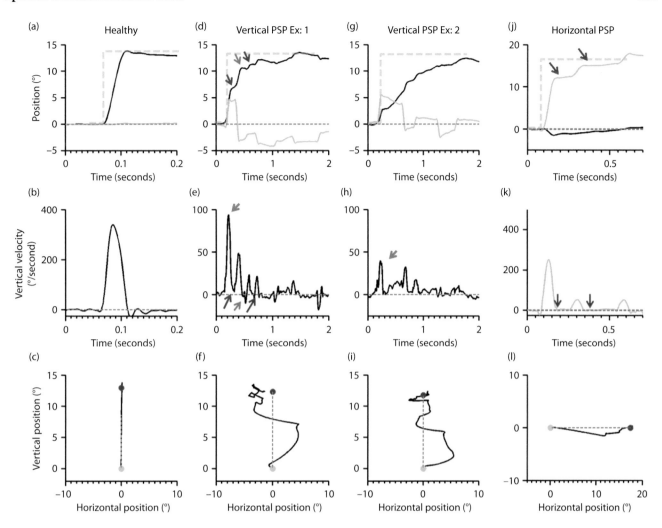

FIGURE 19A.2 Examples of visually guided saccades from healthy subject and PSP patient. In first row of subplots the eye position is plotted on the y-axis while x-axis depicts corresponding time in seconds. Black line depicts vertical eye position, while green trace illustrates horizontal eye position. Gray dashed line is a baseline depicting straight-ahead position, while blue dashed line depicts the position of the target (desired eye position). Arrows depict interruption in ongoing saccades. Blue arrow illustrates one type of interruption where the eyes continue to move at slower velocity during interruption, green arrow depicts slower eye movement in the opposite direction, while red arrow illustrates cessation of eye movement during interruption. Panel A illustrates normal visually guided vertical saccade from a healthy subject. Panels (d) and (g) depict two examples of visually guided vertical saccades from the same PSP subject is illustrated. Panel J depicts eye positions during horizontal saccade. Middle row of subplots depicts eye velocity. Panel (b) depicts eye velocity of normal visually guided saccade recorded from the healthy subject, while panels (e) and (h) depict vertical eye velocity during vertical saccade in PSP. Green line in panel (k) illustrates normal horizontal eye velocity during horizontal saccade in PSP. In these subplots, the eye velocity is plotted on y-axis while x-axis illustrates corresponding time. Red arrow illustrates interruption in saccade when eye velocity was zero, green arrow is when eye moved at slower velocity in the opposite direction, blue arrow is when eyes moved in the same direction at slower velocity. The bottom row of the subplots depicts trajectories of horizontal and vertical saccades. Panel (c) depicts normal saccade from the healthy subject, panels (f) and (i) depict vertical saccade in PSP, and panel (l) is horizontal saccade in PSP. Green dot is start point, red dot is stop point, while gray dashed line is the desired path of an eye movement. Vertical saccades have curved and serpentine path depicting the clinical phenomenon of "round the houses" sign. Similar curvature is present in horizontal saccade as well, but it is much less robust.

does not correlate with the disease duration, gender and age of onset [92]. It is noteworthy that saccade slowing can be an early manifestation of SCA2; sometimes deficits are seen even prior to other clinical manifestations [93]. Saccade velocity in SCA2 can be a sensitive and specific disease marker [94, 95]. In its most severe form, complete gaze palsy is reported in SCA2 [96]. Quantitative brain MRI has demonstrated reduced volumes in the cerebellum, pons, midbrain and frontal lobes of patients with SCA2 [97]. It is therefore suggested that the saccade slowing in SCA2 may be due to cerebellar as well as brainstem deficits involving the burst generation [97, 98]. Indeed the significant cell and synaptic density loss is often found in the parts of mesencephalon (where EBNs are located) in SCA2 suggesting impaired burst generation [99].

Spinocerebellar ataxia type 3

Spinocerebellar ataxia type 3 (SCA3) or Machado–Joseph disease is the most common autosomal dominant SCAs caused by a CAG triplet expansion in the ATXN3 gene on the long arm of chromosome 14 [100–102]. SCA3 manifests with progressive gait, stance, limb and truncal ataxia; deficits mimicking motor neuron disease such as dysarthria, poor cough, tongue fasciculations are also seen [103–105]. In addition to parkinsonism and dystonia, SCA3 also presents with abnormal eye movements—these include optokinetic or gaze-evoked nystagmus, saccadic pursuit, slow and dysmetric saccades and dysfunction of the horizontal vestibulo-ocular reflex [106–111]. Limitation of vertical gaze, most commonly in the upward direction, is also seen [112]. Abduction ophthalmoplegia with sparing of adduction is a common finding in SCA3 [112]. These patients also have an overshoot of saccades, but some have low peak velocity without dynamic overshoot [113]. MRI features diffuse atrophy of the cerebellar vermis, superior cerebellar peduncle, pontine tegmentum and frontal lobes [114, 115]. The reticulotegmental nucleus of the pons and areas where OPNs are situated also have degeneration on histopathology [116, 117]. Slowing of saccades may be due to degeneration of mesencephalic neurons responsible for the burst generation [117, 118].

Wernicke's encephalopathy

Wernicke's encephalopathy, characterized by the triad of encephalopathy, ophthalmoplegia and gait ataxia, is caused by thiamine deficiency [119]. There is a frequent association with chronic alcoholism, but it may be seen with other conditions like hyperemesis, acquired immunodeficiency syndrome, gastrointestinal surgery especially bariatric surgery and malnutrition in general [119]. Nystagmus, the most common finding, presents in form of gaze-evoked, upbeat or downbeat nystagmus; in some cases, upbeat nystagmus switches to downbeat with convergence [120, 121]. Early impairment in horizontal vestibulo-ocular reflexes are noted, but as disease progresses there is impairment in abduction, horizontal and vertical gaze palsies and inter-nuclear ophthalmoplegia that eventually becomes complete ophthalmoplegia [122–124]. Saccade slowing is rare finding in Wernicke's encephalopathy [125]. Without immediate parenteral administration thiamine, Wernicke's disease can progress to Korsakoff syndrome in which there is a striking disorder of selective anterograde and retrograde amnesia along with psychiatric symptoms. In rare cases, individuals may create imaginary events to fill in gaps in their memory (confabulation). Korsakoff syndrome may include significant abnormalities of eye movement, which include abnormal horizontal smooth pursuit eye movements, hypometria and increased saccadic durations [126, 127]. An increased number of directional errors on an antisaccade task may also be seen in these patients [128]. Wernicke's encephalopathy affects extracerebellar brainstem regions, including those responsible for burst generation, and is not predominantly cerebellar [121, 129]. Impairment of saccade burst generation is, therefore, the likely cause of the rare saccadic slowing in Wernicke's encephalopathy. In atypical cases, Wernicke's encephalopathy may also affect the substantia nigra, which could affect saccades through lack of tectal inhibition [130]. In such cases, parkinsonism is expected in addition to the slow saccades.

Syndrome of anti-GAD antibody

Glutamic acid decarboxylase (GAD) is responsible for catalyzing the conversion of glutamic acid to γ aminobutyric acid (GABA) [131]. Autoantibodies directed against this important enzyme (anti-GAD Ab) have been found in patients with insulin-dependent diabetes mellitus, epilepsy, stiff-person syndrome and late-onset cerebellar ataxia [132–135]. Patients with anti-GAD Ab may also have eye movement abnormalities that include downbeat nystagmus, loss of downward smooth pursuit, impaired ocular pursuit and cancellation of vestibulo-ocular reflex, prolonged saccade latency, saccadic dysmetria and saccadic oscillations [136–139]. There have been some reports of periodic alternating nystagmus and opsoclonus myoclonus seen in this syndrome as well [140, 141].

The saccade abnormalities seen in this syndrome could be multifactorial. Frequent hypometria, resulting in frequent interruptions of saccades with otherwise normal velocity is a classic cerebellar phenomenon [142]. We had described opsoclonus in addition to downbeat nystagmus in a patient who had increased titers of anti-GAD antibody [143]. Figure 19A.3 depicts an example of gaze holding in a patient with anti-GAD antibody, the eye movements were characterized by jerky and sinusoidal oscillations. The jerky oscillations comprised of slow ocular drift (slow-phase, black arrows, Figure 19A.3) followed by quick phase (red arrows, Figure 19A.3) suggesting downbeat nystagmus. In addition, back-to-back saccades both in horizontal vertical directions were noteworthy; in some instances they had large amplitude and low frequency (e.g., purple and green arrows, Figure 19A.3). Such oscillations suggested opsoclonus. We proposed that paucity in GABA leading to disinhibition to Purkinje target neurons at deep cerebellar and vestibular nuclei might have caused downbeat nystagmus, while increased levels of glutamate and subsequent hyperexcitability of EBNs and IBNs cause opsoclonus. Latter circuit, when hyperexcitable, lacks effects of post-inhibitory rebound, and in that case it also explains slowing of saccades in these patients. Anti-GAD antibody can also increase levels of glutamate the precursor of GABA and the substrate for the action of GAD.

Mechanistic underpinnings and computational physiology of slow saccades

Mechanistic understanding for efficient generation of saccade velocity comes from experimental and computational studies of human and non-human primate saccadic behavior. Strong correlations between the activity of premotor burst neurons, the EBNs and IBNs, with the eye velocity allowed concluding that burst generator circuits determine the robustness of saccadic drive [144–150]. OPNs were also found instrumental in generation of sufficiently strong burst facilitating high velocities of saccades. The sudden removal of OPN inhibition that is normally suppressing the burst neurons facilitate a rebound burst called post-inhibitory rebound (PIR) [148–151]. The PIR is suggested to be a key contributor for early acceleration of the saccades as it would ensure prompt increase in burst neuron discharge at the onset of saccades. Such acceleration provides adequate force to counteract viscous elastic forces hindering the rotation of the globe within in the orbit. Pharmacological inactivation of the pontine raphe interpositus, the physical location of the OPNs,

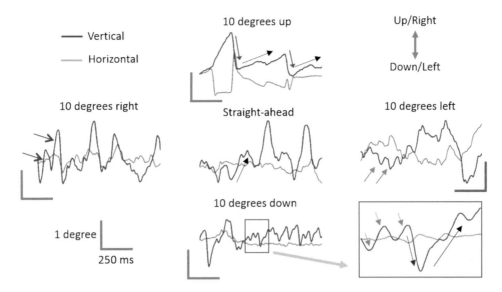

FIGURE 19A.3 Example of gaze holding in the patient with syndrome of anti-GAD antibody. Eye positions are plotted along y-axis while x-axis depicts corresponding time. One-second epochs of eye positions are illustrated in this figure. Blue traces depict vertical eye position, while gray traces are horizontal eye positions. Each panel depicts various eye-in-orbit orientations (as labeled). Red box has the trace expanded from the panel showing 10 degrees downward gaze holding. It depicts mixture of back-to-back saccades depicting opsoclonus. In addition there are superimposed upward drifts with downward quick-phase characterizing downbeat nystagmus. Green arrows point to opsoclonus, red arrows show quick phases, while black arrows show upward drifts in eye position.

in non-human primates results in slow saccades with irregular trajectories but normal latency [152–154]. Conductance-based model of saccade burst generators attributed slow saccades to reduced inhibitory neurotransmission mediated by glycine and the normal latencies to a neuronal threshold that kept burst neurons from responding to small inputs. In the model, Miura and Optican (2006) found that lower glycine levels reduced PIR by reducing low-threshold calcium currents, and also reduced NMDA currents [151]. Sustained OPNs inhibition slowed saccades but its accuracy was maintained by increasing the duration; latter might allow more time for reciprocally innervated IBN circuits time to oscillate and create high frequency ocular flutter even when saccades are slow (i.e., small, back-to-back saccades without an intersaccadic interval) [152–155]. These observations motivated the hypothesis that transient inhibition of OPNs could affect saccades in three ways: (1) via reducing peak acceleration and peak velocity secondary to the lack of an abrupt increase of the EBN firing rate in the absence of PIR; (2) via reducing deceleration, since OPNs would not turn on at the end of the saccade; and (3) via superimposing the oscillations during the saccades. We tested these predictions behaviorally in healthy human subjects by measuring the effects of sustained eye closure on saccades. It is noteworthy that sustained eye closure (or blinks) lead to inhibition of OPN activity [156].

Figure 19A.4 depicts effects of sustained eye closure on a saccade and its comparison with visually guided as well as memory guided saccade (with eyes open) in the same subject. Figure 19A.4A depicts visually guided and memory guided saccade with eyes open. A reduction in the saccade velocity to the remembered location of targets is a well-known phenomenon and it is putatively due to a reduction in premotor saccade-related activity in

the superior colliculus 15]. Consistent with the norms the peak eye velocity of saccade to remembered location was moderately reduced in our experiment when the eyes were open (Figure 19A.4c). Figure 19A.4b depicts an example of saccade to remembered location when the eyes were closed (note different time scales in left and right columns in Figure 19A.4b). The peak velocity of the saccade under closed eyelids was strikingly diminished (Figure 19A.4d). There was also a substantial reduction in peak acceleration when the saccade was made to remembered location under closed eyelids (Figure 19A.4e and f). In addition to slowing, the movement trajectory of the saccades was also irregular as clearly depicted in phase-plane plots (acceleration on ordinate and velocity on abscissa) (Figure 19A.4g and h).

The experimental results from humans and non-human primates, as well as computational simulations emphasized the hypothetical contribution of PIR to the control of saccades. These results also facilitated our understanding of the pathophysiology of slow saccades that are seen in the clinical disorders affecting the brainstem areas where OPNs, EBNs and IBNs are located [148]. The results pointed our fundamental differences between conditions that lead to injury to pontine OPNs and/or burst neurons versus those affecting the inhibitory influence of the OPNs on the burst neurons. The conditions removing inhibitory OPN control may cause saccadic oscillations as in these cases the PIR would be intact [149, 150, 155, 156]. Such scenario contrasts with condition that permanently damages OPNs where PIR would be absent. Latter manifests as slow saccades. These studies also emphasized that the lesions that affect the OPN area may also affect the burst neuron areas. Therefore, the slow saccades in these disorders may be a manifestation of a mixed deficit in OPN and burst neuron function.

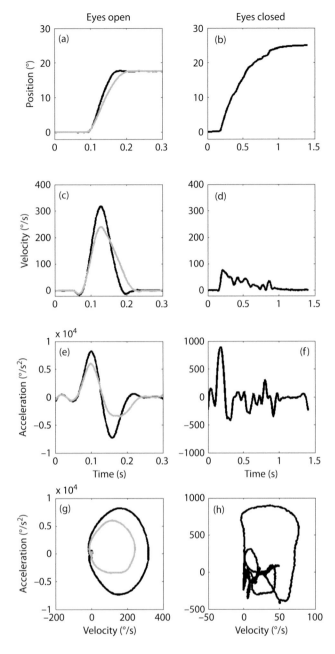

FIGURE 19A.4 Examples of a representative saccade from one subject. (a, b) Eye positions (ordinate) are plotted versus time (abscissa). (a) Black trace represents visually guided saccade and gray trace the remembered saccade. (b) Saccade made under closed eyelids. (c) Eye velocities of visually guided saccades (black) and of saccades to the remembered location (gray) are plotted versus time. (d) Eye velocity of saccade under closed eyelids is plotted versus time. (e, f) Eye acceleration (and deceleration) during a visually guided saccade, saccade to a remembered location, and saccade under closed eyelids are plotted versus time. Notice the fivefold greater time scale in panels (b), (d) and (f) as compared to (a), (c) and (e). (g) Phase plane plot comparing eye velocity with eye acceleration during visually guided (black) and memory-guided (gray) saccades. (h) Phase plane plot of the saccade made under closed eyelids.

Conclusion

Saccades are critical aspects of visual scanning behaviour executed by an elegant neural network. A detailed knowledge about the applied anatomy and physiology of the saccadic system is important to understand the central pathologies affecting them.

Acknowledgments

This work was supported by grants from Dystonia Medical Research Foundation (DMRF), American Academy of Neurology, American Parkinson's Disease Association, and Dystonia Coalition. The authors are also supported by philanthropic support to the Department of Neurology, The Allan Woll Fund.

References

1. Munoz DP. Commentary: saccadic eye movements: overview of neural circuitry. Prog Brain Res. 2002:89–96.
2. Pierrot-Deseilligny C, Milea D, Müri RM. Eye movement control by the cerebral cortex. Curr Opin Neurol. 2004;17:17–25.
3. Fox PT, Fox JM, Raichle ME, Burde RM. The role of cerebral cortex in the generation of voluntary saccades: a positron emission tomographic study. J Neurophysiol. 1985;54:348–69.
4. Pierrot-deseilligny CH, Rivaud S, Gaymard B, Agid Y. Cortical control of reflexive visually-guided saccades. Brain. 1991;114:1473–1485.
5. Berman RA, Colby CL, Genovese CR, Voyvodic JT, Luna B, Thulborn KR, et al. Cortical networks subserving pursuit and saccadic eye movements in humans: an FMRI study. Hum Brain Mapp. 1999;8:209–225.
6. Hikosaka O, Takikawa Y, Kawagoe R. Role of the basal ganglia in the control of purposive saccadic eye movements. Physiol Rev. 2000;80:953–978.
7. Nambu A, Tokuno H, Takada M. Functional significance of the cortico-subthalamo-pallidal "hyperdirect" pathway. Neurosci Res. 2002;43:111–117.
8. Fisher RS, Buchwald NA, Hull CD, Levine MS. The GABAergic striatonigral neurons of the cat: demonstration by double peroxidase labeling. Brain Res. 1986;398:148–156.
9. Francois C, Percheron G, Yelnik J. Localization of nigrostriatal, nigrothalamic and nigrotectal neurons in ventricular coordinates in macaques. Neuroscience. 1984;13:61–76.
10. Handel ARI, Glimcher PW. Quantitative analysis of substantia nigra pars reticulata activity during a visually guided saccade task. J Neurophysiol. 1999;82:3458–3475.
11. Hikosaka O, Wurtz RH. Visual and oculomotor functions of monkey substantia nigra pars reticulata. IV. Relation of substantia nigra to superior colliculus. J Neurophysiol. 1983;49:1285–1301.
12. Müri RM, Iba-Zizen MT, Derosier C, Cabanis EA, Pierrot-Deseilligny C. Location of the human posterior eye field with functional magnetic resonance imaging. J Neurol Neurosurg Psychiatry. 1996;60(4):445–448.
13. Pouget P. The cortex is in overall control of "voluntary" eye movement. Eye (London, England). 2015;29:241–245.
14. Schiller PH, True SD, Conway JL. Deficits in eye movements following frontal eye-field and superior colliculus ablations. J Neurophysiol. 1980;44(6):1175–1189.
15. Rivaud S, Müri RM, Gaymard B, Vermersch AI, Pierrot-Deseilligny C. Eye movement disorders after frontal eye field lesions in humans. Exp Brain Res. 1994;102(1):110–120.
16. Hanes DP, Wurtz RH. Interaction of the frontal eye field and superior colliculus for saccade generation. J Neurophysiol. 2001;85:804–815.
17. Baloh RW, Sills a W, Kumley WE, Honrubia V. Quantitative measurement of saccade amplitude, duration, and velocity. Neurology. 1975;25:1065–1070.
18. Leigh RJ, Kennard C. Using saccades as a research tool in the clinical neurosciences. Brain. 2004;127:460–477.
19. Illing RB, Graybiel AM. Convergence of afferents from frontal cortex and substantia nigra onto acetylcholinesterase-rich patches of the cat's superior colliculus. Neuroscience. 1985;14.
20. Sparks DL, Hartwich-Young R. The deep layers of the superior colliculus. Rev Oculomot Res. 1989;3:213–255.
21. Moschovakis AK, Scudder CA, Highstein SM. The microscopic anatomy and physiology of the mammalian saccadic system. Prog Neurobiol. 1996;50:133–254.
22. May PJ. The mammalian superior colliculus: laminar structure and connections. Prog Brain Res. 2005;151:321–378.
23. Schiller PH, Stryker M. Single-unit recording and stimulation in superior colliculus of the alert rhesus monkey. J Neurophysiol. 1972;35:915–924.
24. Sparks DL. Functional properties of neurons in the monkey superior colliculus: coupling of neuronal activity and saccade onset. Brain Res. 1978;156:1–16.
25. Krauzlis RJ. Recasting the smooth pursuit eye movement system. J Neurophysiol. 2003;91(2):591–603.
26. Bell AH. Crossmodal Integration in the Primate Superior Colliculus Underlying the Preparation and Initiation of Saccadic Eye Movements. J Neurophysiol. 2005;93(6):3659–3673.
27. Hanes DP, Smith MK, Optican LM, Wurtz RH. Recovery of saccadic dysmetria following localized lesions in monkey superior colliculus. Exp Brain Res. 2005;160(3):312–325.

28. Büttner U, Büttner-Ennever JA. Present concepts of oculomotor organization. Prog Brain Res. 2005;151:1–42.
29. Yamada J, Noda H. Afferent and efferent connections of the oculomotor cerebellar vermis in the macaque monkey. J Comp Neurol. 1987;265:224–241.
30. Thielert C -D, Thier P. Patterns of projections from the pontine nuclei and the nucleus reticularis tegmenti pontis to the posterior vermis in the rhesus monkey: A study using retrograde tracers. J Comp Neurol. 1993;337:113–126.
31. Dicke PW, Barash S, Ilg UJ, Thier P. Single-neuron evidence for a contribution of the dorsal pontine nuclei to both types of target-directed eye movements, saccades and smooth-pursuit. Eur J Neurosci. 2004;19:609–624.
32. Noda H, Sugita S, Ikeda Y. Afferent and efferent connections of the oculomotor region of the fastigial nucleus in the macaque monkey. J Comp Neurol. 1990;302:330–348.
33. Ohtsuka K, Noda H. Discharge properties of Purkinje cells in the oculomotor vermis during visually guided saccades in the macaque monkey. J Neurophysiol. 1995;74:1828–1840.
34. May PJ, Hartwich-Young R, Nelson J, Sparks DL, Porter JD. Cerebellotectal pathways in the macaque: implications for collicular generation of saccades. Neuroscience. 1990;36:305–324.
35. Fuchs AF, Robinson FR, Straube A. Role of the caudal fastigial nucleus in saccade generation. I. Neuronal discharge pattern. J Neurophysiol. 1993;70:1723–1740.
36. Kleine JF, Guan Y, Buttner U. Saccade-related neurons in the primate fastigial nucleus: what do they encode? J Neurophysiol. 2003;90:3137–3154.
37. Optican LM, Robinson DA. Cerebellar-dependent adaptive control of primate saccadic system. J Neurophysiol. 1980;44(6):1058–1076.
38. Ritchie L. Effects of cerebellar lesions on saccadic eye movements. J Neurophysiol. 1976;39(6):1246–1256.
39. Barash S, Melikyan A, Sivakov A, Zhang M, Glickstein M, Thier P. Saccadic dysmetria and adaptation after lesions of the cerebellar cortex. J Neurosci. 1999;19(24):10931–10939.
40. Straube A, Deubel H, Ditterich J, Eggert T. Cerebellar lesions impair rapid saccade amplitude adaptation. Neurology. 2001;57(11):2105–2108.
41. Selhorst JB, Stark L, Ochs AL, Hoyt WF. Disorders in cerebellar ocular motor control: II. Macrosaccadic oscillation an oculographic, control system and clinico-anatomical analysis. Brain. 1976;99(3):509–522.
42. Robinson DA. The effect of cerebellectomy on the cat's vestibulo-ocular integrator. Brain Res. 1974;71(2–3):195–207.
43. Zee DS, Yamazaki A, Butler PH, Gucer G. Effects of ablation of flocculus and paraflocculus of eye movements in primate. J Neurophysiol. 1981;46(4):878–899.
44. Ron S, Robinson DA. Eye Movements Cerebellar Evoked by in the Alert Monkey Stimulation. Vision Res. 1972;36(6):1004–1022.
45. Horn a K, Büttner-Ennever J a, Wahle P, Reichenberger I. Neurotransmitter profile of saccadic omnipause neurons in nucleus raphe interpositus. J Neurosci. 1994;14: 2032–2046.
46. Horn AKE, Büttner-Ennever JA, Büttner U. Saccadic premotor neurons in the brainstem: functional neuroanatomy and clinical implications. Neuro-Ophthalmology. 1996;16:229–240.
47. Van Gisbergen JAM, Robinson DA, Gielen S. A quantitative analysis of generation of saccadic eye movements by burst neurons. J Neurophysiol. 1981;45:417–442.
48. Scudder CA, Kaneko CR, Fuchs AF. The brainstem burst generator for saccadic eye movements: A modern synthesis. Experimental Brain Research. 2002;142(4):439–462.
49. Stewart A. Factor WJW. PARKINSON'S DISEASE Diagnosis and Clinical Management. 2004.
50. DeJong JD, Jones GM. Akinesia, hypokinesia, and bradykinesia in the oculomotor system of patients with Parkinson's disease. Exp Neurol. 1971;32(1):58–68.
51. Herishanu YO, Sharpe JA. Normal square wave jerks. Investig Ophthalmol Vis Sci. 1981;20(2):268–272.
52. Rascol O, Clanet M, Montastruc J. Abnormal ocular movements in Parkinson's disease. Brain. 1989;112 (Pt 5):1193–1214.
53. Rottach KG, Riley DE, DiScenna a O, Zivotofsky a Z, Leigh RJ. Dynamic properties of horizontal and vertical eye movements in parkinsonian syndromes. Ann Neurol. 1996;39:368–377.
54. Terao Y, Fukuda H, Yugeta A, Hikosaka O, Nomura Y, Segawa M, et al. Initiation and inhibitory control of saccades with the progression of Parkinson's disease—changes in three major drives converging on the superior colliculus. Neuropsychologia. 2011;49:1794–1806.
55. Otero-Millan J, Schneider R, Leigh RJ, Macknik SL, Martinez-Conde S. Saccades during attempted fixation in Parkinsonian disorders and recessive ataxia: from microsaccades to square-wave jerks. PLoS One. 2013;8(3):e58535.
56. Kimmig H, Haußmann K, Mergner T, Lücking CH. What is pathological with gaze shift fragmentation in Parkinson's disease? J Neurol. 2002;249:683–692.
57. Blekher T, Weaver M, Rupp J, Nichols WC, Hui SL, Gray J, et al. Multiple step pattern as a biomarker in Parkinson disease. Park Relat Disord. 2009;15:506–510.
58. Shaikh AG, Xu-Wilson M, Grill S, Zee DS. "Staircase" square-wave jerks in early Parkinson's disease. Br J Ophthalmol. 2011;95(5):705–709.
59. Choi SM, Lee SH, Choi KH, Nam TS, Kim JT, Park MS, et al. Directional asymmetries of saccadic hypometria in patients with early Parkinson's disease and unilateral symptoms. Eur Neurol. 2011;66:170–174.
60. Chambers JM, Prescott TJ. Response times for visually guided saccades in persons with Parkinson's disease: A meta-analytic review. Neuropsychologia. 2010;48(4):887–899.
61. Lueck CJ, Tanyeri S, Crawford TJ, Henderson L, Kennard C. Antisaccades and remembered saccades in Parkinson's disease. J Neurol Neurosurg Psychiatry. 1990;53(4):284–288.
62. Rottach KG, Riley DE, Discenna AO, Zivotofsky AZ, John Leigh R. Dynamic properties of horizontal and vertical eye movements in Parkinsonian syndromes. Ann Neurol. 1996;39(3):368–377.
63. White OB, Saint-cyr JA, Tomlinson RD, Sharpe JA. Ocular motor deficits in parkinson's disease: II. Control of the saccadic and smooth pursuit systems. Brain. 1983;106 (Pt 3):571–587.
64. Vidailhet M, Rivaud S, Gouider - Khouja N, Pillon B, Bonnet A - M, Gaymard B, et al. Eye movements in parkinsonian syndromes. Ann Neurol. 1994;35(4):420–426.
65. Steele J, Richardson JC, Olszewski J. Progressive Supranuclear Palsy. Ann Neurol. 1964;10:333–359.
66. Williams DR, Lees AJ, Wherrett JR, Steele JC. J. Clifford Richardson and 50 years of progressive supranuclear palsy. Neurology. 2008;70:566–573.
67. Shaikh AG, Factor SA, Juncos JL. Saccades in progressive supranuclear palsy-maladapted, irregular, curved, and slow. Mov Disord Clin Pract. 2017;4:671–681.
68. Chen AL, Riley DE, King SA, Joshi AC, Serra A, Liao K, et al. The disturbance of gaze in progressive supranuclear palsy: implications for pathogenesis. Front Neurol. 2010;1:147.
69. Bhidayasiri R, Riley DE, Somers JT, Lerner AJ, Büttner-Ennever JA, Leigh RJ. Pathophysiology of slow vertical saccades in progressive supranuclear palsy. Neurology. 2001;57:2070–2077.
70. Juncos JL, Hirsch EC, Malessa S, Duyckaerts C, Hersh LB, Agid Y. Mesencephalic cholinergic nuclei in progressive supranuclear palsy. Neurology. 1991;41(1):25–30.
71. Collins SJ, Ahlskog JE, Parisi JE, Maraganore DM. Progressive supranuclear palsy: neuropathologically based diagnostic clinical criteria. J Neurol Neurosurg Psychiatry. 1995;58(2):167–173.
72. Halliday GM, Hardman CD, Cordato NJ, Hely MA, Morris JG. A role for the substantia nigra pars reticulata in the gaze palsy of progressive supranuclear palsy. Brain. 2000;123(Pt 4):724–732.
73. Capouch SD, Farlow MR, Brosch JR. A Review of Dementia with Lewy Bodies' Impact, Diagnostic Criteria and Treatment. Neurol Ther. 2018;7(2):249–263.
74. McKeith IG, Dickson DW, Lowe J, Emre M, O'Brien JT, Feldman H, et al. Diagnosis and management of dementia with Lewy bodies: Third report of the DLB consortium. Neurology. 2005;65(12):1863–1872.
75. Walker Z, Possin KL, Boeve BF AD. Lewy body dementias. Lancet. 2015;386(10004): 1683–1697.
76. Kapoula Z, Yang Q, Vernet M, Dieudonné B, Greffard S, Verny M. Spread deficits in initiation, speed and accuracy of horizontal and vertical automatic saccades in dementia with Lewy bodies. Front Neurol. 2010;1:138.
77. Mosimann UP, Müri RM, Burn DJ, Felblinger J, O'Brien JT, McKeith IG. Saccadic eye movement changes in Parkinson's disease dementia and dementia with Lewy bodies. Brain. 2005;128(Pt 6):1267–1276.
78. Kompoliti K, Goetz CG, Boeve BF, Maraganore DM, Ahlskog JE, Marsden CD, et al. Clinical presentation and pharmacological therapy in corticobasal degeneration. Arch Neurol. 1998;55(7):957–961.
79. Mahapatra RK, Edwards MJ, Schott JM, Bhatia KP. Corticobasal degeneration. Lancet Neurology. 2004;3(12):736–743.
80. Vonsattel JP, Myers RH, Stevens TJ, Ferrante RJ, Bird ED, Richardson EP. Neuropathological classification of huntington's disease. J Neuropathol Exp Neurol. 1985;44(6):559–577.
81. Andrew SE, Goldberg YP, Kremer B, Telenius H, Theilmann J, Adam S, et al. The relationship between trinucleotide (CAG) repeat length and clinical features of Huntington's disease. Nat Genet. 1993;4(4):398–403.
82. Walker FO. Huntington's disease: the road to progress. Lancet Neurol. 2013;12(7): 624–625.
83. Lasker AG, Zee DS, Hain TC, Folstein SE, Singer HS. Saccades in Huntington's disease: initiation defects and distractibility. Neurology. 1987;37(3):364–370.
84. Kirkwood SC, Siemers E, Hodes ME, Conneally PM, Christian JC, Foroud T. Subtle changes among presymptomatic carriers of the Huntington's disease gene. J Neurol Neurosurg Psychiatry. 2000;69(6):773–779.
85. Antoniades CA, Xu Z, Mason SL, Carpenter RHS, Barker RA. Huntington's disease: Changes in saccades and hand-tapping over 3 years. J Neurol. 2010;257(11):1890–1898.
86. Leigh RJ, Newman SA, Folstein SE, Lasker AG, Jensen BA. Abnormal ocular motor control in Huntington's disease. Neurology. 1983;33:1268–1275.
87. Collewijn H, Went LN, Tamminga EP, Vegter-Van der Vlis M. Oculomotor defects in patients with Huntington's disease and their offspring. J Neurol Sci. 1988;86:307–320.
88. Lasker AG, Zee DS, Hain TC, Folstein SE, Singer HS. Saccades in Huntington's disease: slowing and dysmetria. Neurology. 1988;38:427–431.
89. Pulst S-M, Nechiporuk A, Nechiporuk T, Gispert S, Chen X-N, Lopes-Cendes I, et al. Moderate expansion of a normally biallelic trinucleotide repeat in spinocerebellar ataxia type 2. Nat Genet. 1996;14:269–276.
90. Wadia N. A clinicogenetic analysis of six Indian spinocerebellar ataxia (SCA2) pedigrees. The significance of slow saccades in diagnosis. Brain. 1998;121:2341–2355.
91. Wadia NH, Swami RK. A new form of heredo-familial spinocerebellar degeneration with slow eye movements (nine families). Brain. 1971;94:359–374.
92. Velázquez-Pérez L, Seifried C, Santos-Falcón N, Abele M, Ziemann U, Almaguer LE, et al. Saccade velocity is controlled by polyglutamine size in spinocerebellar ataxia 2. Ann Neurol. 2004;56:444–447.
93. Velázquez-Pérez L, Seifried C, Abele M, Wirjatijasa F, Rodríguez-Labrada R, Santos-Falcón N, et al. Saccade velocity is reduced in presymptomatic spinocerebellar ataxia type 2. Clin Neurophysiol. 2009;120:632–635.
94. Rodríguez-Labrada R, Velázquez-Pérez L, Auburger G, Ziemann U, Canales-Ochoa N, Medrano-Montero J, et al. Spinocerebellar ataxia type 2: Measures of saccade changes improve power for clinical trials. Mov Disord. 2016;31:570–578.
95. Seifried C, Velázquez-Pérez L, Santos-Falcón N, Abele M, Ziemann U, Almaguer LE, et al. Saccade velocity as a surrogate disease marker in spinocerebellar ataxia type 2. N Y Acad Sci. 2005;1039:524–527.
96. Klostermann W, Zühlke C, Heide W, Kömpf D, Wessel K. Slow saccades and other eye movement disorders in spinocerebellar atrophy type 1. J Neurol. 1997;244:105–111.
97. Politi LS, Bianchi Marzoli S, Godi C, Panzeri M, Ciasca P, Brugnara G, et al. MRI evidence of cerebellar and extraocular muscle atrophy differently contributing to eye movement abnormalities in SCA2 and SCA28 diseases. Investig Ophthalmol Vis Sci. 2016;57:2714–2720.

98. Rufa A, Federighi P. Fast versus slow: Different saccadic behavior in cerebellar ataxias. Ann N Y Acad Sci. 2011;1233:148–154.
99. Geiner S, Horn AKE, Wadia NH, Sakai H, Büttner-Ennever JA. The neuroanatomical basis of slow saccades in spinocerebellar ataxia type 2 (Wadia-subtype). Prog Brain Res. 2008;171:575–581.
100. Haberhausen G, Damian MS, Leweke F, Müller U. Spinocerebellar ataxia, type 3 (SCA3) is genetically identical to Machado–Joseph disease (MJD). J Neurol Sci. 1995;132:71–75.
101. Matilla T, McCall A, Subramony SH, Zoghbi HY. Molecular and clinical correlations in spinocerebellar ataxia type 3 and Machado–Joseph disease. Ann Neurol. 1995;38:68–72.
102. Ranum LP, Lundgren JK, Schut LJ, Ahrens MJ, Perlman S, Aita J, et al. Spinocerebellar ataxia type 1 and Machado–Joseph disease: incidence of CAG expansions among adult-onset ataxia patients from 311 families with dominant, recessive, or sporadic ataxia. Am J Hum Genet. 1995;57:603–608.
103. Twist EC, Casaubon LK, Ruttledge MH, Rao VS, Macleod PM, Radvany J, et al. Machado–Joseph disease maps to the same region of chromosome 14 as the spinocerebellar ataxia type 3 locus. J Med Genet. 1995;32:25–31.
104. Maruyama H, Kawakami H, Kohriyama T, Sakai T, Doyu M, Sobue G, et al. CAG repeat length and disease duration in Machado–Joseph disease: a new clinical classification. J Neurol Sci. 1997;152:166–171.
105. Riess O, Rüb U, Pastore A, Bauer P, Schöls L. SCA3: neurological features, pathogenesis and animal models. Cerebellum (London, England). 2008;7:125–137.
106. Dawson DM, Feudo P, Zubick HH, Rosenberg R, Fowler H. Electro-oculographic findings in Machado–Joseph disease 550. Neurology. 1982;32:1272–1276.
107. Hotson JR, Langston EB, Louis AA, Rosenberg RN. The search for a physiologic marker of Machado–Joseph disease 534. Neurology. 1987;37:112–116.
108. Rivaud-Pechoux S, Dürr A, Gaymard B, Cancel G, Ploner CJ, Agid Y, et al. Eye movement abnormalities correlate with genotype in autosomal dominant cerebellar ataxia type I. Ann Neurol. 1998;43:297–302.
109. Gordon CR, Joffe V, Vainstein G, Gadoth N. Vestibulo-ocular arreflexia in families with spinocerebellar ataxia type 3 (Machado–Joseph disease). J Neurol Neurosurg Psychiatry. 2003;74:1403–1406.
110. Gordon CR, Zivotofsky AZ, Caspi A. Impaired vestibulo-ocular reflex (VOR) in spinocerebellar ataxia type 3 (SCA3): bedside and search coil evaluation. J Vestib Res. 2014;24(5–6):351–355.
111. Ghasia FF, Wilmot G, Ahmed A, Shaikh AG. Strabismus and micro-opsoclonus in Machado–Joseph disease. Cerebellum. 2016;15:491–497.
112. Murofushi T, Mizuno M, Hayashida T, Yamane M, Osanai R, Ito K, et al. Neuro-otological and neuropathological findings in two cases with Machado–Joseph disease. Acta Otolaryngol. 1995;115:136–139.
113. Caspi A, Zivotofsky AZ, Gordon CR. Multiple saccadic abnormalities in spinocerebellar ataxia type 3 can be linked to a single deficiency in velocity feedback. Investig Ophthalmol Vis Sci. 2013;54:731–738.
114. Murata Y, Yamaguchi S, Kawakami H, Imon Y, Maruyama H, Sakai T, et al. Characteristic magnetic resonance imaging findings in Machado–Joseph disease. Arch Neurol. 1998;55:33–37.
115. Tokumaru AM, Kamakura K, Maki T, Murayama S, Sakata I, Kaji T, et al. Magnetic resonance imaging findings of Machado–Joseph disease: Histopathologic correlation. J Comput Assist Tomogr. 2003;27:241–248.
116. Rüb U, Bürk K, Schöls L, Brunt ER, De Vos RAI, Orozco Diaz G, et al. Damage to the reticulotegmental nucleus of the pons in spinocerebellar ataxia type 1, 2, and 3. Neurology. 2004;63:1258–1263.
117. Rüb U, Brunt ER, Gierga K, Schultz C, Paulson H, De Vos RAI, et al. The nucleus raphe interpositus in spinocerebellar ataxia type 3 (Machado–Joseph disease). J Chem Neuroanat. 2003;25:115–127.
118. Rüb U, Brunt ER, Deller T. New insights into the pathoanatomy of spinocerebellar ataxia type 3 (Machado–Joseph disease). Curr Opin Neurol. 2008;21:111–116.
119. Sechi G, Serra A. Wernicke's encephalopathy: new clinical settings and recent advances in diagnosis and management. Lancet Neurol. 2007;6:442–455.
120. Shin BS, Oh SY, Kim JS, Lee H, Kim EJ, Hwang SB. Upbeat nystagmus changes to downbeat nystagmus with upward gaze in a patient with Wernicke's encephalopathy. J Neurol Sci. 2010;298:145–147.
121. Kim K, Shin DH, Lee YB, Park KH, Park HM, Shin DJ, et al. Evolution of abnormal eye movements in Wernicke's encephalopathy: correlation with serial MRI findings. J Neurol Sci. 2012;323:77–79.
122. Cogan DG, Victor M. Ocular signs of Wernicke's disease. AMA Arch Ophthalmol. 1954;51:204–211.
123. Cox TA, Corbett JJ, Thompson HS, Lennarson L. Upbeat nystagmus changing to downbeat nystagmus with convergence. Neurology. 1981;31:891–892.
124. Delapaz MA, Chung SM, McCrary JA. Bilateral internuclear ophthalmoplegia in a patient with Wernickes encephalopathy. J Clin Neuroophthalmol. 1992;12:116–120.
125. Hamann KU. Slowed saccades in various neurological disorders. Ophthalmologica. 1979;178:357–364.
126. Kenyon RV., Becker JT, Butters N, Hermann H. Oculomotor function in Wernicke-Korsakoff's syndrome: I. Saccadic eye movements. Int J Neurosci. 1984;25:53–65.
127. Kenyon RV., Becker JT, Butters N. Oculomotor function in Wernicke-Korsakoff's syndrome: II. Smooth pursuit eye movements. Int J Neurosci. 1984;25:67–79.
128. Van Der Stigchel S, Reichenbach RCL, Wester AJ, Nijboer TCW. Antisaccade performance in Korsakoff patients reveals deficits in oculomotor inhibition. J Clin Exp Neuropsychol. 2012;34:876–886.
129. Halliday GM, Ellis J, Heard R, Caine D, Harper C. Brainstem serotonergic neurons in chronic alcoholics with and without the memory impairment of korsakoff's psychosis. J Neuropathol Exp Neurol. 1993;52:567–579.
130. Kalidass B, Sunnathkal R, Rangashamanna V, Paraswani R. Atypical Wernicke's encephalopathy showing involvement of substantia nigra. J Neuroimaging. 2012;22:204–207.
131. Watanabe M, Maemura K, Kanbara K, Tamayama T, Hayasaki H. GABA and GABA receptors in the central nervous system and other organs. Int Rev Cytol. 2002;213:1–47.
132. Solimena M, Folli F, Denis-Donini S, Comi GC, Pozza G, De Camilli P, et al. Autoantibodies to glutamic acid decarboxylase in a patient with stiff-man syndrome, epilepsy, and type I diabetes mellitus. N Engl J Med. 1988;318:1012–1020.
133. Solimena M, Folli F, Aparisi R, Pozza G, De Camilli P. Autoantibodies to GABA-ergic neurons and pancreatic beta cells in Stiff-Man syndrome. N Engl J Med. 1990;322:1555–1560.
134. Abele M, Weller M, Mescheriakov S, Burk K, Dichgans J, Klockgether T. Cerebellar ataxia with glutamic acid decarboxylase autoantibodies. Neurology. 1999;52:857–859.
135. Vianello M, Tavolato B, Giometto B. Glutamic acid decarboxylase autoantibodies and neurological disorders. Neurol Sci. 2002;23:145–151.
136. Antonini G, Nemni R, Giubilei F, Gragnani F, Ceschin V, Morino S, et al. Autoantibodies to glutamic acid decarboxylase in downbeat nystagmus. J Neurol Neurosurg Psychiatry. 2003;74:998–999.
137. Economides JR, Horton JC. Eye movement abnormalities in stiff person syndrome. Neurology. 2005;65:1462–1464.
138. Zivotofsky AZ, Siman-Tov T, Gadoth N, Gordon CR. A rare saccade velocity profile in Stiff-Person syndrome with cerebellar degeneration. Brain Res. 2006;1093:135–140.
139. Shaikh AG, Wilmot G. Opsoclonus in a patient with increased titers of anti-GAD antibody provides proof for the conductance-based model of saccadic oscillations. J Neurol Sci. 2016;362:169–173.
140. Tilikete C, Veghetto A, Trouillas P, Honnorat J. Anti-GAD antibodies and periodic alternating nystagmus. Arch Neurol. 2005;62:1300–1303.
141. Markakis I, Alexiou E, Xifaras M, Gekas G, Rombos A. Opsoclonus-myoclonus-ataxia syndrome with autoantibodies to glutamic acid decarboxylase. Clin Neurol Neurosurg. 2008;110:619–621.
142. Goffart L, Pélisson D, Guillaume A. Orienting gaze shifts during muscimol inactivation of caudal fastigial nucleus in the cat. II. Dynamics and eye-head coupling. J Neurophysiol. 1998;79:1959–1976. doi:10.1152/jn.1998.79.4.1959.
143. Shaikh AG, Wilmot G. Opsoclonus in a patient with increased titers of anti-GAD antibody provides proof for the conductance-based model of saccadic oscillations. J Neurol Sci. 2016;362:169–173.
144. Strassman A, Highstein SM, McCrea RA. Anatomy and physiology of saccadic burst neurons in the alert squirrel monkey. II. Inhibitory burst neurons. J Comp Neurol. 1986;249(3):358–380.
145. Strassman A, Highstein SM, McCrea RA. Anatomy and physiology of saccadic burst neurons in the alert squirrel monkey. I. Excitatory burst neurons. J Comp Neurol. 1986;249(3):337–357.
146. Scudder CA, Fuchs FA, Langer TP. Characteristics and functional identification of saccadic inhibitory burst neurons in the alert monkey. J Neurophysiol. 1988;59(5):1430–1454.
147. Ramat S, et al. Ocular oscillations generated by coupling of brainstem excitatory and inhibitory saccadic burst neurons. Exp Brain Res. 2005;160(1):89–106.
148. Shaikh AG, et al. A new familial disease of saccadic oscillations and limb tremor provides clues to mechanisms of common tremor disorders. Brain. 2007;130(Pt 11):3020–3031.
149. Shaikh AG, et al. Saccadic burst cell membrane dysfunction is responsible for saccadic oscillations. J Neuroophthalmol. 2008;28(4):329–336.
150. Miura K, Optican LM. Membrane channel properties of premotor excitatory burst neurons may underlie saccade slowing after lesions of omnipause neurons. J Comput Neurosci. 2006;20(1):25–41.
151. Kaneko CR. Effect of ibotenic acid lesions of the omnipause neurons on saccadic eye movements in rhesus macaques. J Neurophysiol. 1996;75(6):2229–2242.
152. Soetedjo R, Kaneko CR, Fuchs AF. Evidence against a moving hill in the superior colliculus during saccadic eye movements in the monkey. J Neurophysiol. 2002;87(6):2778–2789.
153. Soetedjo R, Kaneko CR, Fuchs AF. Evidence that the superior colliculus participates in the feedback control of saccadic eye movements. J Neurophysiol. 2002;87(2):679–695.
154. Zee DS, Robinson DA. A hypothetical explanation of saccadic oscillations. Ann Neurol. 1979;5(5):405–414.
155. Mays LE, Morrisse DW. Electrical stimulation of the pontine omnipause area inhibits eye blink. J Am Optom Assoc. 1995;66(7):419–422.
156. Edelman JA, Goldberg ME. Dependence of saccade-related activity in the primate superior colliculus on visual target presence. J Neurophysiol. 2001;86(2):676–691.

19B

SPECIAL CONSIDERATIONS IN GAZE
Disorders of Gaze Holding

Neel Fotedar, Aasef G. Shaikh

Introduction

Maintaining stable gaze on the target of interest is critical for clear vision; the brain implements a variety of mechanisms to ensure the same. When moving the head in a certain direction, the vestibulo-ocular reflex (VOR) reorients the eyes with equal amplitude and velocity in the opposite direction of head movement in order to maintain eyes on the target. When the head is not moving, there are various cerebellar and brainstem mechanisms which keep the gaze steady on the target. Such steady fixation and clear vision can be disrupted by abnormal eye movements, e.g., nystagmus. In this chapter, we will discuss the basic neurophysiological principles of gaze holding and then we will apply these principles to understand gaze-holding disorders and their pathophysiology.

The neural integrator and physiology of gaze holding

The type of eye movements that are used to scan our visual field and quickly move gaze from one target to another are called saccades. Once the gaze has been moved to the object of interest, it is important to keep it steady so that clear image is captured on the fovea. The neural integrator refers to a network of neurons in the brainstem and it is this network which is responsible for stable gaze holding. The name "integrator" refers to the fact that this network performs a mathematical integration function by which it converts the neural pulse signal for eye velocity during saccade into a steady eye position signal during gaze holding. Two different neural integrators perform this function.

When the head is steady, integration in the horizontal direction is mediated by nucleus prepositus hypoglossi (NPH) and medial vestibular nucleus (MVN), whereas the interstitial nucleus of Cajal (INC) performs the same function for vertical and torsional eye position.[1–3] Both of these are referred to as ocular motor integrators.

When the head is in motion, the vestibular integrator, which lies downstream from the ocular motor integrator, works to increase the reliability of VOR to maintain stable image on the fovea. The vestibular integrator allows for a broad range of frequencies of head oscillations over which VOR can compensate for stabilizing gaze.

David Hearly was the first to propose the concept of neural integration in 18th century, which was further described by Alexander Bain in the 1800s. Reverberation in this network of neurons leads to sustained synaptic activity, which is required to convert a neural pulse signal discharge into steady state neural firing.[4,5] This concept was further explored by David Robinson in the 1970s and 1980s.[2,6,7] The inter spike membrane potential of the network neurons changes based on gaze position and this alteration is a result of the circuit reverberations.[8–12] These reverberations, which result from auto feedback between network neurons, lead to improved efficacy of the neural integrator. For example, the schematic in Figure 19B.1 depicts an ideal neural integrator network. There are mutually excitatory connections between neurons which are part of a network and their projections to their counterparts on the contralateral side are inhibitory. The intra network mutual excitation facilitates the conversion of neuronal

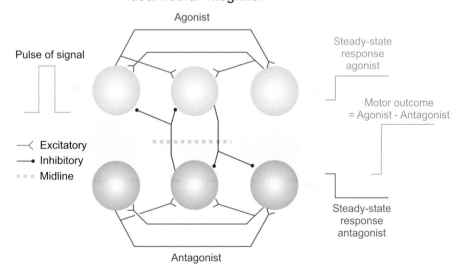

FIGURE 19B.1 Schematic diagram depicting neural network and its reciprocal connections for the function of ideal neural integrator.

DOI: 10.1201/9780429020278-28

pulse signal discharge into steady state firing; whereas the inter network mutual inhibition serves the purpose of coordinating yoked movements of agonist and antagonistic muscles. In an ideal universe, for neural integration to be perfect, the synaptic strengths within a network must be optimally tuned but this is almost impossible to achieve in real biological systems, which leads to an inherent "leaky" nature of the neural integrators. This inherent "leakiness" of the integrator leads to slow drifts, which need to be compensated by external feedback loops. Cerebellum is an important feedback source to the neural integrators.[7,13,15] The cerebellar or other deficits affecting the integrator result in various forms of nystagmus, as shown in Figure 19B.1.

Gaze-evoked nystagmus

Cerebellum becomes an important source of feedback to the ocular motor integrator, when impaired leads to unveiling of the leakiness of the integrator, which then manifests as slow drifts. The drifts are corrected by saccades to bring the eyes back to the target of interest. The farther away move from the center, higher is the drift velocity. Gaze-evoked nystagmus is defined as the slow drifts alternating with corrective saccades (depending on gaze position).[13,15]

Figure 19B.2 depicts an example of gaze-evoked nystagmus. In this figure, eye position (shown by black traces) is plotted on y-axis and corresponding time on x-axis. Each panel illustrates the eye position to aim gaze on the visual target. The eyes are relatively stable in straight-ahead position. However, when turned 30° to right, slow drifts to left deviate the eyes away from the intended target (Figure 19B.2a). These drifts are followed by rapid

corrective movement in the opposite direction, the quick phase, bringing the eyes back to the target. In contrast, right-ward drifts appear when the eyes turn 30° to the left (Figure 19B.2c). These drifts are followed by quick phases bringing the eyes back to target. The slow-phase velocity of the drifts (plotted on y-axis Figure 19B.2d) systematically changes with the eye-in-orbit position (plotted on x-axis Figure 19B.2d). The slow-phase velocity reduces as the eye in the orbit position approaches straight-ahead position. All these features are described by suboptimal neural integration of velocity commands and inability to compensate for the imperfection due to defect in the feedback system.[14,15]

Vestibular neural integrator and velocity storage mechanism

Velocity storage refers to a process which increases the bandwidth of angular VOR (aVOR), which in turn increases VOR responsivity at low frequency head rotation. The most well-known test of velocity storage is measuring pre and post rotational nystagmus kinematics during rotational testing. Normally the eyes drift in direction opposite to the direction of whole body rotation. But this angular velocity signal rapidly decays with a time constant of about 4 seconds because of the elastic properties of the cupula, thus the brain's ability to perceived ongoing rotations is limited. Because of the short time constant, the compensatory eye movements decay rather quickly; prolonging this decay is the main purpose of velocity storage. The velocity storage output decay is in turn exponential.[16] Velocity storage time constant refers to the time constant of this output decay. Inhibitory projections from parts of cerebellar cortex- nodulus and ventral uvula, via GABA affect this time constant.[16–22] Therefore, nodulus and ventral uvula lesions prolong velocity storage time constant because of disinhibition, whereas drugs with $GABA_B$ agonist activity like baclofen and 4-aminopyridine reduce it.[17,19,23]

Figure 19B.3 shows an experiment involving a healthy human subject, testing the velocity storage function and its modulation with 4-aminopyridine acting on $GABA_B$ receptors. While seated on a three-dimensional servo motor controlled rotating chair (Acutronic, Jona, Switzerland), subject's head was restrained by custom molded thermoplastic mask (Sinmed BV, Reeuwijk, The Netherlands). In Figure 19B.3a, with the subject in an upright position, results of rotations along earth vertical axis are shown. The angular vestibular response obtained in this experiment was mainly due to simulation of lateral semicircular canals (yaw-rotation, schematic inset in Figure 19B.3a). Simultaneous eye movement recordings showed a quick rise in horizontal VOR slow phase velocity, which was followed by an exponential fall with time constant of about 10 seconds (filled symbols, Figure 19B.3a). Followed by this, the subject took 10 mg 4-aminopyridine and same experiment was repeated after 30 minutes and this time, there was a much faster decay of slow phase velocity with time constant of about 6 seconds. These experiments confirm that humans have a vestibular velocity storage mechanism for horizontal VOR and that the cerebellum modulates this system via $GABA_B$ receptors.[19,24]

Similar experiments with rotations in earth vertical axis while supine (roll rotation, insert in Figure 19B.3b) or on the side with ear facing ground (pitch rotation, inset Figure 19B.3c) did not show evidence of GABAergic influence on the velocity storage. These rotations mainly involve the vertical semicircular canals and VOR was present in torsional direction for supine rotation and vertical direction for ear facing ground

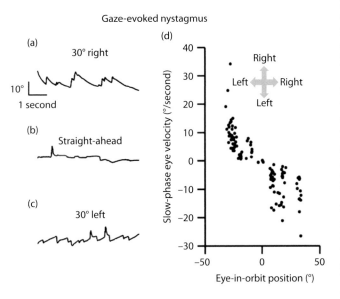

Gaze-evoked nystagmus

FIGURE 19B.2 (a–c) Example of gaze-evoked nystagmus in a patient with cerebellar atrophy. Panel (a) depicts left-drifts and right beats during rightward gaze holding, panel (b) is straight-ahead (stable) gaze holding, while panel (c) is leftward gaze holding leading to right-drifts and left beats. In panels (a–c) eye position is plotted on the y-axis while corresponding time is on the x-axis. Only horizontal eye positions are shown. (d) The summary of slow-phase velocity plotted on the y-axis while corresponding eye-in-orbit position is on the x-axis. Each dot depicts one slow-phase. Arrows in inset depict the direction. (This figure was reproduced from Shaikh et al., 2016, with permission.)

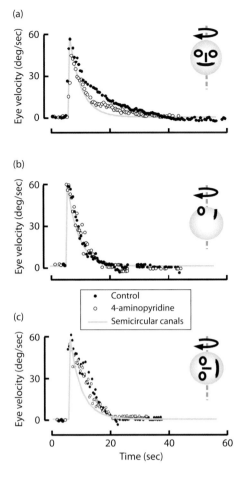

FIGURE 19B.3 Effects of constant velocity sustained rotation in yaw plane (a), roll plane (b), and pitch plane (c). Each dot depicts eye velocity (a: horizontal eye velocity; b: torsional eye velocity; c: vertical eye velocity) plotted on the y-axis while corresponding time on the x-axis. Gray line is cupular decay time constant. Filled symbols are eye velocity of rotational (and post-rotational) nystagmus before and open symbols after oral intake of 4-aminopyridine. (This figure was reproduced from Shaikh et al., 2013, with permission.)

rotation. There is no major change in torsional or vertical VOR as shown in Figures 19B.3b and c, thus depicting absence of GABAergic influence.

Gravity-dependent nystagmus

As the name refers, this type of nystagmus changes direction as head position changes with respect to direction of gravitational force. Structural lesions of the posterior vermis can cause this type of nystagmus, e.g., stroke in the posterior inferior cerebellar artery (PICA) territory.[25–30] Degenerative syndromes involving the cerebellum have also been associated with gravity-dependent nystagmus.[31–33]

It has been well described in literature that the direction and amplitude of vestibular reflexes are heavily modulated by the cerebellum[31,34,35] and any disruption of this process can lead to gravity-dependent nystagmus. Following two-step process has been proposed in literature to explain its pathophysiology.[27]

Step 1: Posterior cerebellar vermis controls the output of fastigial and vestibular nuclei; the vermis lesion causes disinhibition of these nuclei, thus leading to hyperexcitability. A similar example is gaze-evoked nystagmus, which is caused by lesion of flocculus, causing disinhibition of the neural integrators in midbrain vestibular nuclei.[14] In addition to direct flocculus lesions, any lesion of the cerebellar input fibers in inferior cerebellar peduncle (ICP) from brainstem integrators can also cause gaze-evoked nystagmus. *Step 2*: This involves the modulation of nystagmus in relation to gravity, which is related to the impaired central estimate of gravity. Experiments in monkeys have shown that they are not able to align their eye axis rotation with the gravito inertial axis during VOR when nodulus is lesioned.[28–30] Similarly, in humans, lesions of cerebellar lobule VIII and IX might impair our ability to align eye axis rotation with respect to gravity. To summarize, cerebellar cortex lesions disinhibit the deep nuclei, which produce the nystagmus and gravity-dependent modulation of nystagmus results from impairment of central estimate of gravity causing a misalignment of eye rotation axis and earth-fixed axis. Sometimes, this nystagmus can have apogeotropic features, which means that the quick phase beats away from direction of gravitation force. Figure 19B.4 shows the MRI scan of a patient with an acute infarct involving the nodulus, medial cerebellar hemisphere and lateral medulla along with ICP, and the resultant gravity-dependent nystagmus. In this patient, with left ear down, the slow phase velocity was minimum and with right ear down, it was maximum. There was no vertical nystagmus in either position. In left ear down position, the nystagmus was left beating and it changed to right beating direction with right ear down. Although the slow phase velocity in both upright and supine orientations was comparable, the patient also had upbeat and right beat nystagmus in both positions and of equal intensity (Figure 19B.4).

In some instances, the central gravity-dependent nystagmus appears very similar to the nystagmus associated with benign paroxysmal positional vertigo (BPPV) but there are some important differences between the two. Firstly, the nystagmus of BPPV follows a unique pattern in changing its direction with respect to changes in head position and secondly, the nystagmus of BPPV has a latent onset (few seconds) and is fatigable after a few seconds (has a crescendo decrescendo pattern).[36,37]

Periodic alternating nystagmus (PAN)

This type of nystagmus is defined as a central spontaneous horizontal nystagmus, which reverses its direction about every 2 minutes.[1] The velocity of the slow phase increases to a maximum level during one half cycle as evident from prominent quick phases; after reaching a maximum, the velocity starts decreasing till it reaches zero and then the direction changes. This process keeps repeating itself and the cyclic oscillation has a sinusoidal appearance (Figure 19B.5).

PAN was not well understood initially and remained a mystery but over time, study of PAN has provided significant insights into how the cerebellum modulates the temporal properties of vestibular reflexes. It has been well understood that lesions involving midline cerebellar structures produce PAN.[38] When normal subjects undergo sustained rotation at constant velocity in dark, the nystagmus is induced and it undergoes reversal because of velocity storage; this physiological observation led to initial understanding of pathogenesis of PAN.[16–18] The total duration and course of this nystagmus and its reversal are quite similar to

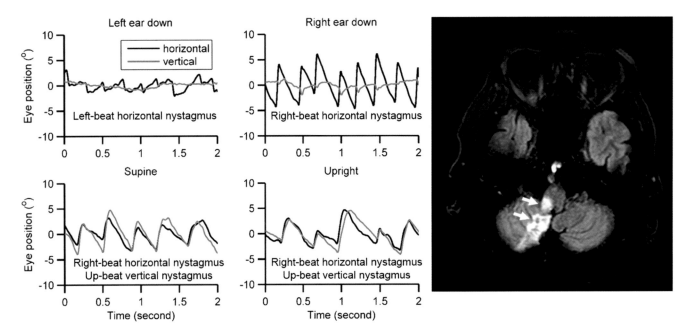

FIGURE 19B.4 Example of gravity-dependent nystagmus during various head orientations with respect to the gravity. MRI on the right side of the panel depicts infarct involving lateral medulla and posterior vermis and para-vermis hemisphere.

that of PAN. In monkeys who undergo experimental ablation of the nodulus and uvula, prolonged nystagmus is noted with rotation, suggesting that there is an excessive velocity storage (vestibular memory).[17,39] When the same monkeys are placed in a dark environment, they develop PAN but the monkeys can still suppress the nystagmus with visual fixation.[17,39] Human patients who develop PAN often have extensive cerebellar lesions, affecting not only the nodulus and ventral uvula but also other parts of vestibular cerebellum, namely flocculus and paraflocculus, which play an important role in normal visual fixation.[1] It has been suggested that the velocity storage mechanism requires inhibitory control

on vestibular commissure via metabotropic GABA$_B$ receptor, that's why baclofen which is a GABA$_B$ agonist suppresses the velocity storage mechanism in monkeys. Similarly, baclofen can abolish PAN in humans.[18,40]

PAN can have wide clinical variations. For example, in patients with ataxia-telangiectasia, cycle duration of PAN can range anywhere from 30 seconds to 4 minutes.[41] The two extreme examples are shown in Figure 19B.5. In first example, duration was 240 seconds and in second example, it was 18 seconds. Both were patients with ataxia-telangiectasia and had about similar amounts of cerebellar atrophy. This variation is believed to be due to dysfunctional recalibration via the adaptive mechanism, as has been demonstrated in the control systems model of PAN. The cycle duration of PAN seems to be affected by these alterations in adaptation gain, as shown in these models. MVN is thought to be the site of velocity storage and its neuronal intrinsic membranous properties modulate the rate of adaptation by shaping the response to sensory stimuli, hence affecting the cycle duration of PAN.

Literature combining experimental lesions, electrophysiological studies, behavioral and pharmacological studies, have offered significant insights into how the cerebellar intrinsic membrane properties control the adaptive mechanisms in normal physiological conditions and how in disease states it can manifest in a very particular fashion. It is not entirely clear why some patients manifest the disease and some don't even though they have the same structural or metabolic impairment. It is believed that genetic susceptibility may have a pivotal role in diverse presentations of the same structural deficit.

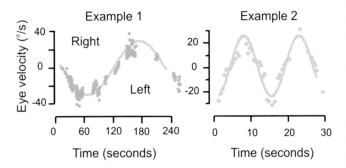

FIGURE 19B.5 An example of slow-phase velocity of periodic alternating nystagmus from two patients. Although average cycle duration of PAN is typically considered 2 minutes, the cycle duration varies among patients. Two extreme examples are illustrated here. The slow-phase velocity is plotted in colored symbols along y-axis, while corresponding time is on the x-axis. The trend of slow-phase velocity follows a sinusoidal fit function (gray line). There was a remarkable variability in the cycle duration (18 seconds and 240 seconds) in these two examples of the patients with the same diagnosis (ataxia-telangiectasia) and comparable cerebellar atrophy. (This figure was reproduced from Shaikh et al., 2009, with permission.)

Vertical nystagmus

Lesions affecting central pathways mediating vertical VOR cause vertical—downbeat (DBN) or upbeat nystagmus (UBN).[42,43] It is believed that UBN results from central imbalance of otolithic projections.[1] UBN changes direction with head position and ocular vergence also has an effect since otolith responses are modulated by the viewing distance (i.e., vergence).[44,45]

In this section, we will describe a common mechanism to explain both UBN and DBN and their gravitational modulation. The forces that influence vertical eye movements do it so through a "push-pull" mechanism; these opposing forces include the oculomotor integrator for vertical gaze holding and elastic forces of orbital soft tissue acting in both upward and downward orientation of the eyes. These forces act along a vertical axis in head fixed reference frame as represented by blue arrows in Figure 19B.6. There is one other constant vertical force that must be accounted for and that is the gravitational force (space fixed), so the "push-pull" forces need to be tuned in order to account for gravity with the help of "internal estimate of gravity". Figure 19B.6 shows the direction of internal estimate of gravity with a red arrow. In a healthy human subject who is standing upright, the two vectors (estimate of gravity and push-pull forces) are aligned and gaze is stable. In a position of nose pitched up like looking to the sky in darkness, because of no alternative cues available, a mismatch develops between the force pulling up and down by cosine of the pitching angle (because the head vertical axis is not aligned with internal estimate of gravity anymore). This causes the eyes to drift downward. On the other hand, in a nose pitched down position like looking to the ground, in darkness, the eyes drift upward. This modulation of slow phase velocity with respect to gravity is a well-known phenomenon in healthy human subjects (Figure 19B.6).[32] Patients with DBN or UBN show a similar phenomenon of gravity-dependent modulation, difference being that slow phase velocities are quite large and the sinusoidal modulation is offset in a particular direction depending on what type of nystagmus

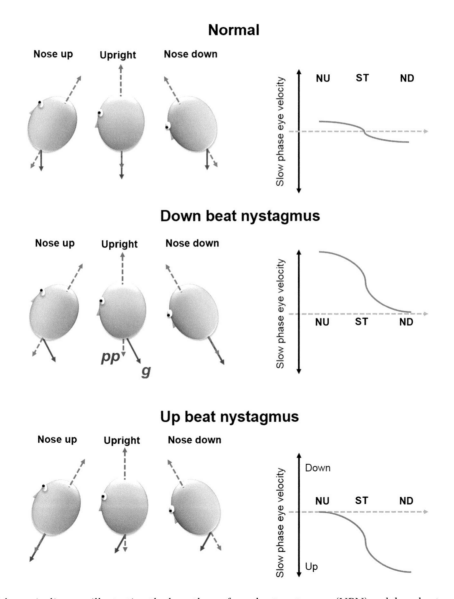

FIGURE 19B.6 Schematic diagram illustrating the hypotheses for upbeat nystagmus (UBN) and downbeat nystagmus (DBN). The caricatures on the left side of the diagrams illustrate head orientations, the blue arrows depict the direction of the head-fixed push-pull forces (**pp**), while the red arrow illustrate the internal representation of gravity (**g**). Normally, in darkness, when subjects are upright the push-pull forces align with the internal representation of gravity, but this alignment is disrupted on tilt up or down resulting in slow-phase eye velocity (as illustrated in schematic graph on the right side). Misrepresentation of the internal estimate of gravity results in UBN or DBN.

it is,[32] the offset is due to the misrepresentation of internal estimate of gravity (Figure 19B.6). For example, DBN could occur if the internal estimate of gravity is misrepresented as illustrated in Figure 19B.6. In this situation, more the subject pitches the nose up, the farther away it goes from the gravity estimate, thus making the nystagmus worse (Figure 19B.6). On the other hand, with nose pitched down, the misrepresented estimate of gravity is closer to the axis of push-pull forces, hence the nystagmus would improve. Clinically, in patients with DBN, nystagmus often gets worse in nose up position and improves in nose down position. UBN involves similar misrepresentation but in the opposite manner (Figure 19B.6). Hence, UBN is worse with nose pitched down and improves with nose pitched up.[46,47] In patients with cerebellar lesions, turning the head beyond a certain orientation can cause DBN to convert into UBN and vice versa, depending upon how severe is the misrepresentation of internal estimate of gravity.[48]

It has been well described in literature that canal otolith-convergent neurons, which lie in the vestibular nuclei in brainstem and rostral fastigial nuclei in cerebellum, represent physical laws of motion and could play a role in discriminating gravitational acceleration from otolith-coded non-gravitational acceleration, for example, inertia.[49,52,53] These neurons are also believed to be the site of vestibular velocity storage and are under inhibitory control of the nodulus.[50–53] Abnormalities in the firing rate of these neurons could be due to a variety of reasons like disinhibition due to lesions of cerebellar cortex or alterations in intrinsic membrane properties related to pharmacological or immune-related effects, thus disrupting the "calibration" of the firing rate, which alters the estimate of gravity.[31] This altered internal estimate of gravity then leads to either UBN or DBN. Focal lesions affecting flocculus frequently cause DBN; UBN is typically related to similar lesions in brainstem vestibular networks.[1]

Oculopalatal tremor

Oculopalatal tremor (OPT) is an uncommon condition, but its peculiar clinical characteristics and neuro anatomical correlate make it ideal to be studied as a "disease model" for common tremor disorders. It typically manifests in patients who have had brainstem or cerebellar stroke after few weeks to months. OPT is characterized by coarse and irregular oscillations of the eyes and palate at a frequency of about 2 Hz. These oscillations could be isolated or could develop in conjunction with similar oscillations in other muscles like pharynx, larynx, facial muscles, diaphragm and sometimes, even the extremities.

Pathologically, OPT is characterized by hypertrophic degeneration of inferior olivary (IO) nucleus along with degeneration of deep cerebellar nuclei on the contralateral side.[1] It has been theorized that OPT results from the disruption of connections between dentate nucleus and contralateral IO, the output fibers from dentate nucleus travel toward the red nucleus and then the fibers destined for IO turn caudad in central tegmental tract (CTT). The IO pseudohypertrophy is caused by disruption of CTT[54,55]. In normal physiology, there exists electrotonic coupling between dendrites of adjacent neurons in inferior olivary nucleus via connexin 36 gap junctions.[56–59] When deafferentation of IO occurs due to lesion of CTT, there is increased development of soma-somatic connexins,[55] which then leads to enhanced synchronous discharge at frequency of 1–2 Hz in independent patches of IO neurons. This synchronized signal, when transmitted to cerebellar cortex, could be responsible for maladaptive learning.

These independent patches of IO and cerebellar neurons are connected to independent sets of motorneurons producing independent pendular eye oscillations (smooth, irregular and disconjugate) in horizontal, vertical and torsional directions (Figure 19B.7c).[60] The disconjugate oscillations have different shapes (Figure 19B.7c) in all three axes and variable spectral frequency content (Figure 19B.7d). Treatment trials lend support to this hypothesis. In one of the studies where these oscillations were treated with clonazepam, evidence of decreased glucose metabolism was seen in the cerebellum but not in the inferior olive. Based on this hypothesis, it can be inferred that drugs which inhibit connexin 36, if given early in the disease course, could prevent development of maladaptive learning by inhibiting the "pacemaker" activity of inferior olive.[56] Another study has shown potential for gabapentin (alpha-2-delta calcium channel blocker) and memantine (non-competitive glutamate antagonist) in suppressing OPT in some patients,[61,62] possibly by decreasing IO synchronization via NMDA receptor blockade. NMDA receptor blockade led to decreased cerebellar cortical output, thus reducing the amplitude and frequency variability of oscillations in OPT.[61]

In the study, there was variability among the subjects in terms of effects of gabapentin and memantine; variation was also noted in the same subject among different axes of oscillations.[61,62] This is likely a result of variable expression of alpha-2-delta calcium channels and NMDA receptors among different individuals.[63] The variable expression of these receptors within the same individual between distinct IO-cerebellar oscillatory patches for all three axes could explain diversity of drug effects among different axes in the same patient.

Studying OPT has greatly enhanced our understanding of common tremor disorders. It shows how characteristics of movements can be quite different among patients who carry the same diagnosis and the variability could be described by maladaptive patterns. Essential tremor (ET) can share some analogies since it is also thought to be caused by disturbances in the inferior olivary-cerebellar circuit[64] and PET studies in such patients have shown increased activity in the olivocerebellar circuit.[65–69] A common way to study animal models of tremor is through harmaline-induced synchronized oscillations in IO,[68,70] although this mechanism of tremorogenesis is different than that in OPT but the variation in oscillation characteristics of tremor waveforms is related to cerebellar learning mechanisms, as have been described for OPT. That is why some patients with ET have regular oscillations, while others have irregular oscillations and don't show characteristics of a sinusoidal waveform.[71,72] Similarly, patients with cerebellar tremor and rubral tremor have irregular waveforms.[64] Thus, the mechanisms of pathogenesis for OPT that have been discussed in this section and the pharmacological treatment options make OPT an idea "disease model" to study and then describe the highly variable phenomenology of common tremor disorders and their therapeutic options as well.

Conclusion

An in-depth knowledge about basic neuro-physiological principles of gaze and the impact of the cerebellum and basal ganglia on these networks can help in understanding the different gaze-holding mechanisms. This may pave the way to further research aiding in developing the gaze mechanisms as clinical biomarkers of various neurological diseases.

Acknowledgments

Aasef Shaikh is supported by the Career Award from The American Academy of Neurology; George C. Cotzias Memorial Fellowship from the American Parkinson's Disease Association; Dystonia Medical Research Foundation Research Grant; and Dystonia Coalition NIH U54 TR001456.

Multiple-Choice Questions

1. Which of the following statements is true about saccade abnormalities in parkinsonism?
   a. Slowing of horizontal saccades is common initial symptom in progressive supra nuclear palsy.
   b. The latency of visually guided saccade initiation is increased and there are more directional errors during antisaccade tasks in patients with DLB.
   c. Saccade velocity is always slow in cortobasal degeneration.
   d. Patients with PD have decreased latency in saccade initiation with verbal instruction and reduced accuracy, when compared to healthy controls.

   Answer:

   b. The latency of visually guided saccade initiation is increased and there are more directional errors during antisaccade tasks in patients with DLB.

2. The eye movement abnormalities in a patient with anti-GAD Ab disease include all of the following, EXCEPT:
   a. Upbeat nystagmus
   b. Periodic alternating nystagmus
   c. Impaired ocular pursuit
   d. Prolonged saccadic latency

   Answer:

   a. Upbeat nystagmus

3. Which one of the following statements is true?
   a. Fastigial oculomotor region is critical for improving the saccade accuracy and calibrating for the saccade pulse-step mismatch.
   b. The superior colliculus is believed to play a part in movement initiation and determination of saccadic velocity.
   c. Both of the above.
   d. None of the above.

   Answer:

   d. None of the above.

4. Gravity-dependent nystagmus:
   a. Has a latent onset (few seconds) and is fatigable after a few seconds.
   b. In patients with ataxia-telangiectasia, cycle duration of PAN can range anywhere from 30 seconds to 4 minutes.
   c. UBN does not change direction with head position and ocular vergence.
   d. All are true.

   Answer:

   b. In patients with ataxia-telangiectasia, cycle duration of PAN can range anywhere from 30 seconds to 4 minutes.

5. Oculopalatal tremor:
   a. Is characterized by hypertrophic degeneration of superior olivary nucleus.
   b. Is characterized by degeneration of ipsilateral deep cerebellar nuclei.
   c. Results from the disruption of connections between dentate nucleus and contralateral inferior olivary nucleus.
   d. Results from the disruption of connections between dentate nucleus and ipsilateral inferior olivary nucleus.

   Answer:

   c. Results from the disruption of connections between dentate nucleus and contralateral inferior olivary nucleus.

References

1. Leigh RJ, Zee DS. The Neurology of Eye Movements. New York: Oxford; 2006.
2. Cannon SC, Robinson DA. Loss of the neural integrator of the oculomotor system from brainstem lesions in monkey. J Neurophysiol. 1987;57(5):1383–1409.
3. Crawford JD, Cadera W, Vilis T. Generation of torsional and vertical eye position signals by the interstitial nucleus of Cajal. Science. 1991;252(5012):1551–1553.
4. Lorente De No R. Analysis of the activity of the chains of internuncial neurons. J Neurophysiol. 1938;1:207–244.
5. Hebb DO. The Organization of Behavior. New York: Wiley; 1949.
6. Arnold DB, Robinson DA, Leigh RJ. Nystagmus induced by pharmacological inactivation of the brainstem ocular motor integrator in monkey. Vision Res. 1999;39(25):4286–4295.
7. Robinson DA. The effect of cerebellectomy on the cat's bestibulo-ocular integrator. Brain Res. 1974;71(2–3):195–207.
8. Arnold DB, Robinson DA. A learning network model of the neural integrator of the oculomotor system. Biol Cybern. 1991;64(6):447–454.
9. Cannon SC, Robinson DA. An improved neural-network model for the neural integrator of the oculomotor system: more realistic neuron behavior. Biol Cybern. 1985;53(2):93–108.
10. Aksay E, Gamkrelidze G, Seung HS, Baker R, Tank DW. In vivo intracellular recording and perturbation of persistent activity in a neural integrator. Nat Neurosci. 2001;4(2):184–193.
11. Aksay E, Olasagasti I, Mensh BD, Baker R, Goldman MS, Tank DW. Functional dissection of circuitry in a neural integrator. Nat Neurosci. 2007;10(4):494–504.
12. Miri A, Daie K, Arrenberg AB, Baier H, Aksay E, Tank DW. Spatial gradients and multidimensional dynamics in a neural integrator circuit. Nat Neurosci. 2011;14(9):1150–1159.
13. Zee DS, Yee RD, Cogan DG, Robinson DA, Engel WK. Ocular motor abnormalities in hereditary cerebellar ataxia. Brain. 1976;99(2):207–234.
14. Zee DS, Yamazaki A, Butler PH, Gucer G. Effects of ablation of flocculus and paraflocculus of eye movements in primate. J Neurophysiol. 1981;46(4):878–899.
15. Zee DS, Leigh RJ, Mathieu-Millaire F. Cerebellar control of ocular gaze stability. Ann Neurol. 1980;7(1):37–40.
16. Raphan T, Matsuo V, Cohen B. Velocity storage in the vestibulo-ocular reflex arc (VOR). Exp Brain Res. 1979;35(2):229–248.
17. Waespe W, Cohen B, Raphan T. Dynamic modification of the vestibulo-ocular reflex by the nodulus and uvula. Science. 1985;228(4696):199–202.
18. Cohen B, Helwig D, Raphan T. Baclofen and velocity storage: a model of the effects of the drug on the vestibulo-ocular reflex in the rhesus monkey. J Physiol. 1987;393:703–725.
19. Dai M, Raphan T, Cohen B. Effects of baclofen on the angular vestibulo-ocular reflex. Exp Brain Res. 2006;171(2):262–271.
20. Solomon D, Cohen B. Stimulation of the nodulus and uvula discharges velocity storage in the vestibulo-ocular reflex. Exp Brain Res. 1994;102(1):57–68.
21. Highstein SM, Rabbitt RD, Holstein GR, Boyle RD. Determinants of spatial and temporal coding by semicircular canal afferents. J Neurophysiol. 2005;93(5):2359–2370.
22. Skavenski AA, Robinson DA. Role of abducens neurons in vestibuloocular reflex. J Neurophysiol. 1973;36(4):724–738.
23. Shaikh AG, Meng H, Angelaki DE. Multiple reference frames for motion in the primate cerebellum. J Neurosci. 2004;24(19):4491–4497.
24. Shaikh AG, Marti S, Tarnutzer AA, et al. Effects of 4-aminopyridine on nystagmus and vestibulo-ocular reflex in ataxia-telangiectasia. J Neurol. 2013;260(11):2728–2735.
25. Lee H, Sohn SI, Cho YW, et al. Cerebellar infarction presenting isolated vertigo: frequency and vascular topographical patterns. Neurology. 2006;67(7):1178–1183.
26. Rubenstein RL, Norman DM, Schindler RA, Kaseff L. Cerebellar infarction—a presentation of vertigo. Laryngoscope. 1980;90(3):505–514.

27. Shaikh AG. Motion perception without nystagmus—a novel manifestation of cerebellar stroke. J Stroke Cerebrovasc Dis. 2013;23(5):1148–1156.

28. Nam J, Kim S, Huh Y, Kim JS. Ageotropic central positional nystagmus in nodular infarction. Neurology. 2009;73(14):1163.

29. Kim HA, Yi HA, Lee H. Apogeotropic central positional nystagmus as a sole sign of nodular infarction. Neurol Sci. 2012;33(5):1189–1191.

30. Johkura K. Central paroxysmal positional vertigo: isolated dizziness caused by small cerebellar hemorrhage. Stroke. 2007;38(6):e26–27.

31. Shaikh AG, Marti S, Tarnutzer AA, et al. Ataxia telangiectasia: a "disease model" to understand the cerebellar control of vestibular reflexes. J Neurophysiol. 2011;105(6):3034–3041.

32. Marti S, Palla A, Straumann D. Gravity dependence of ocular drift in patients with cerebellar downbeat nystagmus. Ann Neurol. 2002;52(6):712–721.

33. Kattah JC, Gujrati M. Familial positional downbeat nystagmus and cerebellar ataxia: clinical and pathologic findings. Ann N Y Acad Sci. 2005;1039:540–543.

34. Walker MF, Zee DS. Cerebellar disease alters the axis of the high-acceleration vestibuloocular reflex. J Neurophysiol. 2005;94(5):3417–3429.

35. Schultheis LW, Robinson DA. Directional plasticity of the vestibuloocular reflex in the cat. Ann N Y Acad Sci. 1981;374:504–512.

36. Leigh RJ, Zee DS. Neurology of Eye Movements. 4th ed. New York: Oxford; 2006.

37. Korres SG, Balatsouras DG. Diagnostic, pathophysiologic, and therapeutic aspects of benign paroxysmal positional vertigo. Otolaryngol Head Neck Surg. 2004;131(4):438–444.

38. Kornhuber HH. [Periodic alternating nystagmus (nystagmus alternans) and excitability of the vestibular system]. Archiv fur Ohren-, Nasen- und Kehlkopfheilkunde, vereinigt mit Zeitschrift fur Hals-, Nasen- und Ohrenheilkunde. 1959;174(3):182–209.

39. Waespe W, Cohen B, Raphan T. Role of the flocculus and paraflocculus in optokinetic nystagmus and visual-vestibular interactions: effects of lesions. Exp Brain Res. 1983;50(1):9–33.

40. Halmagyi GM, Rudge P, Gresty MA, Leigh RJ, Zee DS. Treatment of periodic alternating nystagmus. Ann Neurol. 1980;8(6):609–611.

41. Shaikh AG, Marti S, Tarnutzer AA, et al. Gaze fixation deficits and their implication in ataxia-telangiectasia. J Neurol Neurosurg Psychiatry. 2009;80(8):858–864.

42. Pierrot-Deseilligny C, Milea D. Vertical nystagmus: clinical facts and hypotheses. Brain. 2005;128(Pt 6):1237–1246.

43. Pierrot-Deseilligny C, Milea D, Sirmai J, Papeix C, Rivaud-Pechoux S. Upbeat nystagmus due to a small pontine lesion: evidence for the existence of a crossing ventral tegmental tract. European neurology. 2005;54(4):186–190.

44. Liao K, Walker MF, Joshi A, Reschke M, Leigh RJ. Vestibulo-ocular responses to vertical translation in normal human subjects. Exp Brain Res. 2008;185(4):553–562.

45. Liao K, Walker MF, Joshi A, Reschke M, Wang Z, Leigh RJ. A reinterpretation of the purpose of the translational vestibulo-ocular reflex in human subjects. Prog Brain Res. 2008;171:295–302.

46. Wray SH, Dalmau J, Chen A, King S, Leigh RJ. Paraneoplastic disorders of eye movements. Ann N Y Acad Sci. 2011;1233:279–284.

47. Wray SH, Martinez-Hernandez E, Dalmau J, et al. Paraneoplastic upbeat nystagmus. Neurology. 2011;77(7):691–693.

48. Helmchen C, Sprenger A, Rambold H, Sander T, Kompf D, Straumann D. Effect of 3,4-diaminopyridine on the gravity dependence of ocular drift in downbeat nystagmus. Neurology. 2004;63(4):752–753.

49. Angelaki DE, Shaikh AG, Green AM, Dickman JD. Neurons compute internal models of the physical laws of motion. Nature. 2004;430(6999):560–564.

50. Green AM, Angelaki DE. Resolution of sensory ambiguities for gaze stabilization requires a second neural integrator. J Neurosci. 2003;23(28):9265–9275.

51. Green AM, Shaikh AG, Angelaki DE. Sensory vestibular contributions to constructing internal models of self-motion. J Neural Eng. 2005;2(3):S164–179.

52. Shaikh AG, Green AM, Ghasia FF, Newlands SD, Dickman JD, Angelaki DE. Sensory convergence solves a motion ambiguity problem. Curr Biol. 2005;15(18):1657–1662.

53. Yakusheva TA, Shaikh AG, Green AM, Blazquez PM, Dickman JD, Angelaki DE. Purkinje cells in posterior cerebellar vermis encode motion in an inertial reference frame. Neuron. 2007;54(6):973–985.

54. Lapresle J, Annabi A. Olivopontocerebellar atrophy with velopharyngolaryngeal paralysis: a contribution to the somatotopy of the nucleus ambiguus. J Neuropathol Exp Neurol. 1979;38(4):401–406.

55. Ruigrok TJ, de Zeeuw CI, Voogd J. Hypertrophy of inferior olivary neurons: a degenerative, regenerative or plasticity phenomenon. Eur J Morphol. 1990;28(2–4):224–239.

56. Condorelli DF, Parenti R, Spinella F, et al. Cloning of a new gap junction gene (Cx36) highly expressed in mammalian brain neurons. Eur J Neurosci. 1998;10(3):1202–1208.

57. Devor A, Yarom Y. Coherence of subthreshold activity in coupled inferior olivary neurons. Ann N Y Acad Sci. 2002;978:508.

58. Devor A, Yarom Y. Generation and propagation of subthreshold waves in a network of inferior olivary neurons. J Neurophysiol. 2002;87(6):3059–3069.

59. Devor A, Yarom Y. Electrotonic coupling in the inferior olivary nucleus revealed by simultaneous double patch recordings. J Neurophysiol. 2002;87(6):3048–3058.

60. Shaikh AG, Hong S, Liao K, et al. Oculopalatal tremor explained by a model of inferior olivary hypertrophy and cerebellar plasticity. Brain. 2010;133(Pt 3):923–940.

61. Shaikh AG, Thurtell MJ, Optican LM, Leigh RJ. Pharmacological tests of hypotheses for acquired pendular nystagmus. Ann N Y Acad Sci. 2011;1233:320–326.

62. Thurtell MJ, Joshi AC, Leone AC, et al. Crossover trial of gabapentin and memantine as treatment for acquired nystagmus. Ann Neurol. 2010;67(5):676–680.

63. Chen LW, Tse YC, Li C, et al. Differential expression of NMDA and AMPA/KA receptor subunits in the inferior olive of postnatal rats. Brain Res. 2006;1067(1):103–114.

64. Deuschl G, Bain P, Brin M. Consensus statement of the Movement Disorder Society on Tremor. Ad Hoc Scientific Committee. Mov Disord. 1998;13 Suppl 3:2–23.

65. Hallett M, Dubinsky RM. Glucose metabolism in the brain of patients with essential tremor. J Neurol Sci. 1993;114(1):45–48.

66. Jenkins IH, Bain PG, Colebatch JG, et al. A positron emission tomography study of essential tremor: evidence for overactivity of cerebellar connections. Ann Neurol. 1993;34(1):82–90.

67. Wills AJ, Jenkins IH, Thompson PD, Findley LJ, Brooks DJ. A positron emission tomography study of cerebral activation associated with essential and writing tremor. Arch Neurol. 1995;52(3):299–305.

68. Wilms H, Sievers J, Deuschl G. Animal models of tremor. Mov. 1999;14(4):557–571.

69. Boecker H, Wills AJ, Ceballos-Baumann A, et al. The effect of ethanol on alcohol-responsive essential tremor: a positron emission tomography study. Ann Neurol. 1996;39(5):650–658.

70. Sinton CM, Krosser BI, Walton KD, Llinas RR. The effectiveness of different isomers of octanol as blockers of harmaline-induced tremor. Pflugers Arch. 1989;414(1):31–36.

71. Marshall J. Observations on essential tremor. J Neurol Neurosurg Psychiatry. 1962;25:122–125.

72. Bertrand C, Hardy J, Molina-Negro P, Martinez SN. Tremor of attitude. Confin Neurol. 1969;31(1):37–41.

20

CORTICAL VISUAL LOSS

Jason J.S. Barton

CASE STUDY

A 72-year-old male, known diabetic and hypertensive, presented 2 months prior with sudden onset of right hemiparesis and visual disturbances, due to an ischemic stroke. On examination, pupillary reflexes, visual acuity, fundus examination, and extraocular movements were normal. However, the patient was not able to perform visuospatial tasks like locating his glasses placed on table. There was difficulty in reaching out to objects shown by the examiner. The patient was able to recognize images of objects shown one at a time, but identified only one when multiple objects were visible simultaneously. What is the likely clinical syndrome based upon this patient's complaints?

Disorders that affect the brain can create a variety of visual impairments. These can be divided into two main classes. First are the impairments due to lesions of the geniculo-striate relay, up to and including striate cortex. These are typified by visual field defects that are not specific for the type of vision affected, but characterized by their retinotopy, the fact that they are spatially specific – that is, limited to certain parts of the visual field and sparing others. In this sense, they resemble lesions of any part of the neural relay that passes visual information from the retinal ganglion cells of the eye to striate cortex of the brain, of which this is the final component.

This relay ends at striate cortex, and beyond it information diverges into a large array of "extra-striate" visual regions. Lesions of these regions cause the second type of cortical visual impairment. Extra-striate deficits are not so typified by retinotopy, but instead show functional specificity, affecting certain types of visual processing but not others. Although there are many cortical regions involved in vision, they can be divided roughly into two main functional streams, a ventral and a dorsal pathway (1). The ventral pathway consists of medial occipitotemporal structures that are involved in processing color and form and in object recognition. For this reason, it is sometimes called the "What" pathway. The dorsal pathway refers to lateral occipitoparietal structures that are involved in motion processing and spatial functions such as attention, localization and targeting eye or hand movements. This is sometimes called the "Where" pathway, though some view the dorsal pathway's role more as preparing responses to the visual environment, an "Action" pathway (2). In this chapter, we follow this useful division, considering disorders of color processing or object recognition under the heading of ventral pathway disorders, and problems of motion or spatial processing as dorsal pathway disorders (3) (Figure 20.1).

Knowledge about the blood supply of the various elements of the visual pathway is another important anatomic aspect, as vascular lesions are frequent causes of cerebral visual field defects (Figure 20.2).

The geniculo-striate relay and its visual field defects

Field loss from damage to cerebral structures causes hemifield defects, meaning that the visual loss is typically located to one side of center and is present in both eyes. Patients usually complain of visual loss from hemifield defects, but not always. Lack of awareness is more likely with peripheral defects, especially those limited to the upper field. On the other hand, small central defects may masquerade as problems with reading until careful testing reveals the scotoma. Patients often confuse hemifield loss with monocular loss, for example, mistaking left hemianopia for visual loss in the left eye. Asking patients what they see with each eye covered in turn can settle this point.

Bedside or clinic testing by confrontation using finger motion and hand comparison detects about 75–90% of homonymous hemifield defects (4, 5). Good lighting and a homogenous background behind the examiner are important during testing. Each eye should be tested separately to determine how similar the defects are in the two eyes. Moving targets across the vertical meridian can be telling: a sudden change in visibility at the meridian is typical of many hemifield defects.

Hemifield defects are homonymous: they affect the same hemifield of each eye. Congruity refers to the degree of similarity of the area lost in the two eyes: congruity increases as one moves progressively from the geniculate nucleus to the striate cortex.

Hemifield defects impact patients' lives more than monocular visual loss does, because one eye cannot compensate for the other. If their field defect is large enough, patients are often not allowed to drive. How much is large enough is debatable, and the rules vary across jurisdictions. In addition to the amount of hemifield loss, how well and how frequently a hemianopic patient makes scanning eye movements to explore their blind side is an important determinant of their driving safety (6–9). However, measures of this gaze behavior have yet to be incorporated into driving evaluations.

Reading is affected when the central 5 degrees are involved, which is called hemianopic dyslexia (10–12). For languages read from left to right, a left hemianopia makes it difficult to find the start of the next line, a problem that can be helped by using a ruler with a marker. A right hemianopia slows reading speed more (11, 13, 14). Reading in these patients can be improved by using smaller type and turning the page nearly 90 degrees to skirt the field defect. Reading improves as patients with either type of hemianopia start to learn adaptive strategies (11). The free online Readright program uses leftward scrolling text to improve reading speed in right hemianopic dyslexia (15).

Other problems that some patients with hemianopia note in daily life include problems with glare, dimness, less bright colors, and depth perception. Many feel insecure in busy environments, are afraid of falling, and are unhappy with perceived limits on their ability to travel (16).

DOI: 10.1201/9780429020278-29

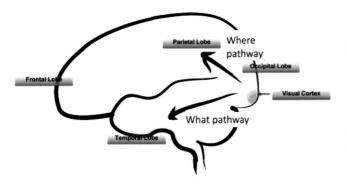

FIGURE 20.1 The occipitotemporal "what" and occipitoparietal "where" visual pathways.

There are no effective means of reversing hemifield losses. About 40% show some spontaneous improvement, usually within the first few months (17). Attempts to restore vision through training are controversial (18). Strategic compensations include training patients to scan the blind side more and putting prisms on their glasses to act much like a rear-view mirror for their blind region (19). These may help, but more evidence is needed to show that these create real-life benefits.

Lateral geniculate nucleus
The lateral geniculate nucleus is the terminus of the optic tract, whose fibers synapse in this nucleus with the neurons that give

rise to the optic radiations. This nucleus is located in the ventro-postero-lateral thalamus. It has a retinotopic organization: the macula is represented in a dorsal wedge and the far periphery is ventral, while the inferior quadrant is medial and the superior is lateral. Two arteries supply it. The lateral choroidal artery, a branch of the posterior cerebral artery, supplies the middle zone (20) while the anterior choroidal artery, a branch of the internal carotid artery, supplies its medial and lateral aspects (21, 22). This blood supply is reflected in the classic hemifield defects from partial destruction of the lateral geniculate nucleus. A lateral posterior choroidal artery stroke causes a sectoranopia (Figure 20.3a), a wedge-shaped defect emanating from the central field that straddles the horizontal meridian (20). An anterior choroidal artery stroke produces an inverse sectoranopia (Figure 20.3b), defects adjacent to the vertical meridian in the upper and lower field that spare the zone around the horizontal meridian (21–23). Ultimately, the patient will develop a subtle partial optic atrophy, but the pupil light reflexes are normal.

Optic radiations
The neurons in the lateral geniculate nucleus give rise to the optic radiations, which project to striate cortex. The radiations start as a compact bundle in the posterior internal capsule, then fan out. Because of the embryonic forward growth of the temporal horn of the lateral ventricle, the fibers for the superior quadrant project slightly anterolaterally as Meyer's loop. They then turn to project posteriorly, joining the fibers from the inferior quadrant,

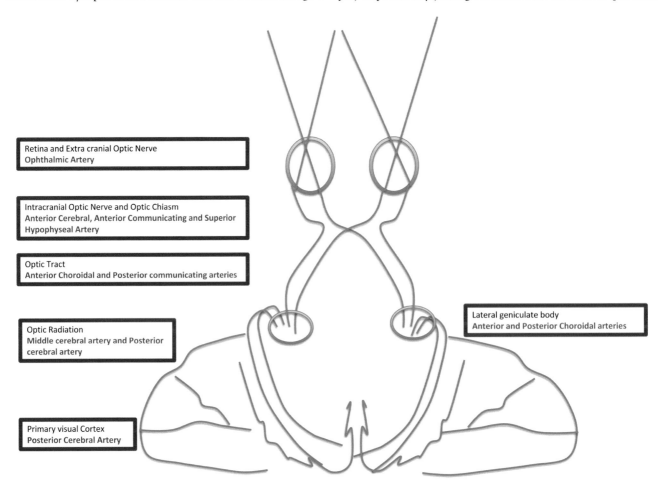

FIGURE 20.2 The blood supply of the retino-geniculo-striate visual pathway.

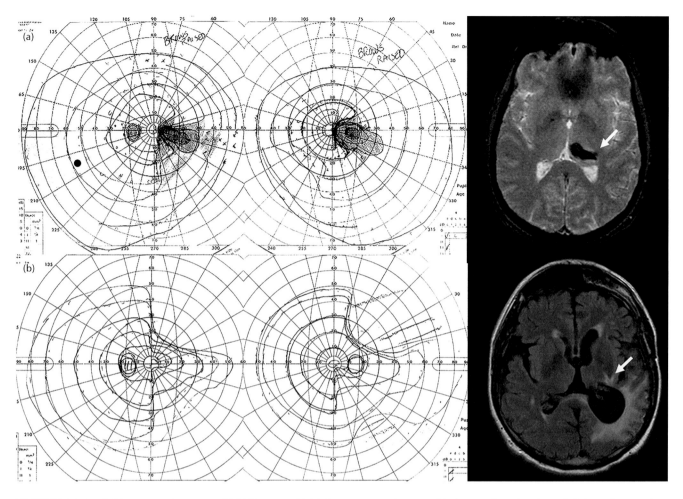

FIGURE 20.3 Goldmann perimetry and MRI images. (a) Right sectoranopia caused by hemorrhage involving left lateral geniculate nucleus (arrow). (b) Right inverse sectoranopia caused by demyelination in vicinity of left lateral geniculate nucleus and proximal optic radiations (arrow).

which have passed through inferior parietal white matter, and terminate in the calcarine fissure. Its initial portion is supplied by the anterior choroidal artery, its temporal and parietal portions by the inferior division of the middle cerebral artery and its final portion by the posterior cerebral artery. Optic radiation damage causing complete hemianopia can occur with minimal other signs if it is the initial or terminal portion that is damaged. However, in its large middle portion, complete hemianopia requires extensive damage, invariably with other signs such as hemiparesis, hemi-sensory loss, aphasia if on the left, and hemi-neglect if on the right. More common are partial hemifield defects that have a mild degree of incongruity. Superior quadrantanopia occurs with lesions of Meyer's loop (Figure 20.4a) and inferior quadrantanopia results from damage to the parietal optic radiation. These quadrantic defects usually align on the vertical meridian but seldom on the horizontal (24). Damage to the middle zone of the radiations can cause a sectoranopia like that from lateral choroidal artery infarction of the lateral geniculate nucleus (25).

Striate cortex

Striate cortex occupies the upper and lower banks of the calcarine fissure. The parieto-occipital fissure is its anterior boundary but its posterior limit is variable, extending over the first 1 or 2 centimeters

of the posterior surface of the occipital lobe. It has a systematic retinotopic map of the contralateral visual field (26–29). Central vision is located posteriorly at the occipital pole and the far periphery is anterior near the parieto-occipital fissure, while the superior field is represented in the lower bank and the inferior field in the upper bank. As is the case throughout the visual system, there is far greater representation of the central than the peripheral field: over half of striate cortex is devoted to the central 10 degrees of vision (29, 30). The striate cortex is supplied mainly by the posterior cerebral artery, with a parieto-occipital branch supplying the upper bank and a posterior temporal branch supplying the lower bank. The occipital pole is a watershed between the calcarine branch of the posterior cerebral artery and the middle cerebral artery: individual cortical and vascular variation means central vision could be supplied by either artery (31).

The hemifield defects from striate damage are highly congruent. Complete hemianopia is possible but partial defects are common. Sparing of the occipital pole causes a macula-sparing hemianopia (preservation of the central 5°) (32, 33), while sparing of the most anterior striate cortex results in sparing of the monocular temporal crescent (34, 35). A retrosplenial lesion could cause the converse, a monocular temporal crescentic scotoma only (36), but this is rare. Damage to the lower bank will cause a superior quadrantanopia and damage to the upper bank an inferior

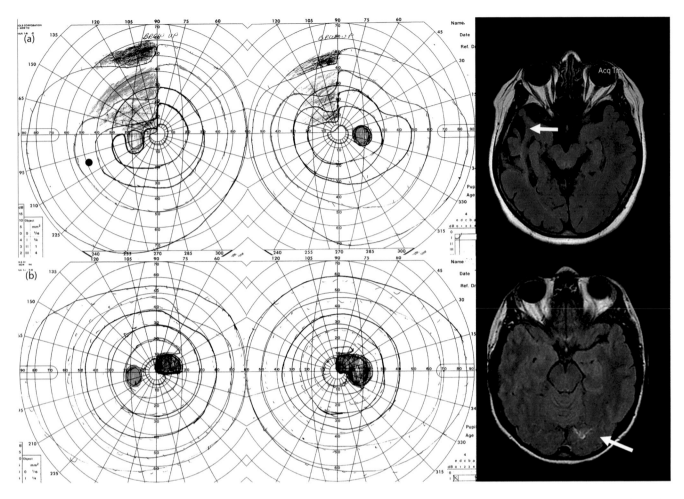

FIGURE 20.4   Goldmann perimetry and MRI images. (a) Left homonymous superior quadrantanopia caused by congenital atrophy of the right anterior temporal lobe (arrow). (b) Right homonymous hemi-macular scotoma from stroke near the left occipital pole (arrow).

quadrantanopia. Empirically, a quadrantic defect is more likely to represent striate damage than a lesion of the optic radiations (24). Striate quadrantanopia is more frequently an isolated sign or else accompanied by other visual dysfunction, such as alexia or hemi-achromatopsia, whereas a quadrantanopia from optic radiation damage usually occurs with hemiparesis, dysphasia, or amnesia (24). Small lesions that may be missed on routine MR imaging (32) can cause homonymous scotomata: small occipital pole infarcts (Figure 20.4b) can cause hemi-macular scotomata (33), and more anterior lesions cause more peripheral scotomata.

In half of patients with striate damage, the hemifield defect is an isolated finding (37). In the rest, there can be other visual deficits from ventral stream damage, such as prosopagnosia, alexia and dyschromatopsia. Amnestic syndromes can arise if the lesion extends to anterior temporal cortex and the hippocampus, as can a syndrome of agitated delirium and hemianopia (38).

Bilateral lesions
Bilateral lesions of the striate cortex or distal optic radiations are unusual but can occur. If large, the patient may have complete *cerebral blindness* (39, 40). This differs from bilateral ocular blindness by the fact that the fundi and optic discs are normal and the pupillary light reflex is intact. Incomplete bilateral hemianopia can be distinguished from bilateral ocular disease by the

congruity of the visual loss and careful search for a step defect along the vertical meridian that shows the visual loss differs between the right and left hemifields (39). Cerebral blindness is permanent in 25% (39) and permanent partial hemifield defects are the rule in those who recover. Bi-occipital lucencies on CT scans imply a poor prognosis but abnormalities on visual-evoked potentials do not correlate with severity or visual outcome (40).

Other phenomena
"Anton's syndrome" refers to the 10% of patients with cerebral blindness who deny visual problems despite lack of encephalopathy or dementia (39, 40). Denial of blindness also occurs in patients with both ocular blindness and cognitive deficits (41).

On the other hand, some studies have found that patients with unilateral hemianopia or cerebral blindness may still possess some residual visual function in their blind area, of which they may be unaware (42). This "blindsight" has been shown by many techniques, such as pointing or making saccades to a visual target in the blind field, by better-than-chance guesses about the movement, form or color of objects, or even by showing that how hemianopic patient respond to visible targets is influenced by targets in the blind hemifield (43, 44). One taxonomy groups these phenomena into three clusters (45). "Action blindsight" includes the localization of targets, "attention blindsight" refers to orienting,

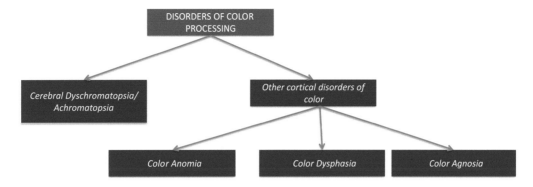

FIGURE 20.5   Overview of disorders of color processing.

inhibition of return and motion perception, and "agnosopsia" encompasses abilities to report on object properties such as form and color. These may have different anatomic explanations (45). Action blindsight may involve a subcortical pathway from the retina to superior colliculus (46, 47). Residual motion perception may involve retinotectal pathways that project via the pulvinar to extrastriate cortical regions like V5. Perception of color and form may be mediated by direct projections from surviving lateral geniculate neurons to extrastriate cortex (48). Blindsight can only be demonstrated convincingly in a laboratory, with careful control for light scatter (49, 50). While most blindsight studies have single cases or small numbers of subjects, larger samples indicate that blindsight is rare (51–53). It is not yet proven that blindsight benefits the patients who show it.

As many as half of patients with hemifield defects have "release hallucinations", also known as Charles Bonnet syndrome (54, 55). These generally occur in areas of the visual field that have absent or severely degraded input from either eye. Thus, while they understandably occur with homonymous field loss from cerebral lesions, they can also occur with bilateral ocular disease. The hallucinatory content varies from vague colors, streaks and patterns (56) to highly vivid images of people, places, and animals (57), and can change from day to day in the same person (58). This variability and their more prolonged duration distinguishes release hallucinations from visual seizures. They start days to weeks after the onset of visual loss, can be intermittent or continuous, and then stop after a few days or persist (54, 57). Release hallucinations likely originate from an inherent tendency of visual cortex to generate spontaneous patterns of neural impulses in the absence of sensory input, much like phantom limb pain. Treatment is rarely required and there is no consensus on effective medication. Most patients are aware that the hallucinations are not real and the content is seldom threatening. Patients should be reassured that these hallucinations are not a sign of mental illness but a normal physiologic response to blindness (54). Decreasing social isolation may help (59).

The ventral pathway and its disorders

The medial occipitotemporal stream stretches from the lingual and fusiform gyri posteriorly to the anterior temporal cortex. Its processing goal is to detect, recognize and identify objects in the visual environment. It includes what can be considered an intermediate level of processing, namely for color. Damage to this stream can lead to impaired color vision and disorders of object recognition. The latter can range from severe problems identifying any sort of object (the man who mistook his wife for a hat) to

more selective problems with recognizing faces (prosopagnosia), words (alexia) or places (landmark agnosia). These often but not invariably occur together as part of a ventral visual syndrome. For example, a classic conjunction is the association of apperceptive prosopagnosia, superior field defects, topographagnosia and dyschromatopsia.

Disorders of color processing (Figure 20.5)
Cerebral dyschromatopsia/achromatopsia
In cerebral achromatopsia, all sense of color is lost and the world appears in shades of gray (60–63), though sometimes with a colored tint (64, 65). In dyschromatopsia there is some residual color perception. While dyschromatopsia is more common that complete achromatopsia, both are rare. Hemi-achromatopsia is loss of color perception in the contralateral hemifield only. This is under-recognized because it is often asymptomatic (66, 67) and clinicians rarely test for it. It is usually associated with a superior quadrantanopia (66–68), in which case one can show impaired color vision only in the lower quadrant.

Most dyschromatopsic patients are aware of their color problems. They complain of trouble matching clothes, distinguishing money, and perceiving traffic lights (69). On testing, achromatopsic patients cannot name colors shown to them, while dyschromatopsic patients may be able to name broad color categories like red or yellow. They fail on finer distinctions (e.g., crimson or scarlet), but not all healthy patients have those in their verbal repertoire. One could use the pseudo-isochromatic plates designed to detect congenital red-green defects (70, 71) but with caution, as some achromatopsic patients can still see the color boundaries between the numbers and the background, particularly if the cards are held at a distance (62, 71–73). The best tests require the patient to sort color chips by either their hue (e.g., red versus green), as done with the Farnsworth-Munsell 100 Hue (Figure 20.6) or D-15 tests, or their saturation (e.g., pink versus red), as with the Sahlgren Saturation Test (74). In contrast, they can see lightness normally (63, 72, 73, 75). Cerebral achromatopsia affects all colors (63), with simply an accentuation of our normal tritan-like tendencies to struggle more with blue-yellow hues (76). In those who show recovery, color after-images may still reveal subtle anomalies (65).

To test for hemi-achromatopsia, a colored object is moved from the contralateral to the ipsilateral hemifield: the patient will note a sudden appearance of color in what had been a gray object when it crosses the vertical meridian. More detailed testing is difficult as most color tests are made for central viewing and can still be done as long as color perception is intact in one hemifield (63).

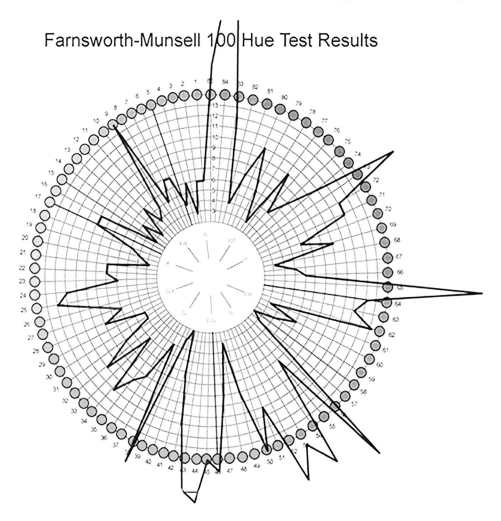

FIGURE 20.6   Results on Farnsworth-Munsell 100-hue test for a dyschromatopsic patient. Error rate is plotted against the color of the chip in a circular diagram. The further away from the central circle, the greater the errors for that region of color space. This patient shows large errors randomly distributed across all colors.

One interesting finding is that cerebral dyschromatopsia also affects "color constancy". The wavelengths sent from an object to the eye depend on both the lighting of the scene and the reflectant properties of the object's surface – that is, which wavelengths it absorbs and which it reflects (77, 78). Hence the eye receives different wavelengths from same apple under fluorescent lighting than in the midday sun, yet we perceive its "redness" as unchanging. Somehow the brain "discounts the illuminant". It does this by inferring the lighting from an average of the spectral composition from large regions of the background (77, 79). Without this calculation, our perception of the color of objects will change as the lighting changes. Although it is rare for dyschromatopsic patients to complain of unstable colors, studies have shown that they do have impaired color constancy (80–84).

On the other hand, not all color processing is lost in dyschromatopsia. The contribution of cones and retinal ganglion cells can still be seen in residual signs of trichomacy and color opponency in elegant experiments (72, 80, 85, 86). Patients can use residual color-opponent signals to see boundaries between colored areas, even though they do not know what the colors are (84). This "local chromatic contrast" can support the perception of form or motion of chromatic stimuli (87–89), and pupil responses to color (90). In contrast, striate lesions cause loss of this local chromatic contrast (91).

Achromatopsia is caused by bilateral lesions of the lingual and fusiform gyri (78, 92), as evident on neuroimaging (63, 68, 72, 73, 76, 93, 94), while hemi-achromatopsia occurs with unilateral right or left-sided lesions (95, 96) (Figure 20.7). Lesions of the middle third of the lingual gyrus are key (63, 97, 98). This region may be a

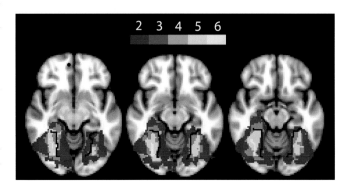

FIGURE 20.7   Overlap axial MRI diagram of lesions causing dyschromatopsia in six patients. The greatest overlap (yellow region) is in the lingual and posterior fusiform gyri, especially on the right.

human homologue of monkey area V4, which has color-selective responses (78). However, impaired color perception in monkeys occurs not with V4 lesions (99–104) but with lesions that extend to areas TE and TEO (105, 106). Human functional neuroimaging shows several color-processing regions, including V4, V8 (107, 108), and more anterior regions (109–111). Achromatopsia likely requires damage to or disconnection of several components of this color network (102, 112, 113), and the severity of the color problem reflects the extent of network damage (114).

Achromatopsia can be associated with prosopagnosia, topographagnosia and superior hemifield defects. Less frequently associated problems include general visual agnosia (72, 115), alexia (62, 94) and amnesia when damage extends to the anterior temporal lobe (62, 115).

Other cortical disorders of color

There are some unusual, often asymptomatic conditions in which patients can perceive colors but have other types of trouble with colors (Figure 20.5). *Color anomia* may be part of an interhemispheric visual-verbal disconnection when it is associated with pure alexia and right hemianopia. Loss of callosal connections prevents color information from the left hemifield (right striate cortex) from accessing the language processing of the left hemisphere (116–119). Patients with *color dysphasia* cannot state what the colors should be for line-drawn or verbally named objects (118), suggesting loss of an internal dictionary for colors. Most have lesions of the left angular gyrus that cause alexia with agraphia, Gerstmann's syndrome, and right hemifield defects. Patients with *color agnosia* cannot color line drawings correctly or state whether drawings are correctly colored (120–122). Most of these patients have left occipitotemporal lesions, some with a right hemianopia. There is even a rare developmental color agnosia that may be inherited in autosomal-dominant fashion (123).

General visual agnosia

This is a rare set of several conditions (Figure 20.8). Patients with general visual agnosia don't recognize previously familiar objects and cannot learn to recognize new objects by vision alone (124, 125). This deficit may be less dramatic with real three-dimensional objects than with line-drawn objects, which have fewer visual cues. To confirm that this is a visual disorder, the examiner should show that the patient can recognize the same objects by sound or touch. To ensure that this is agnosia rather than anomia, the patient should be asked if they know anything about the object besides its name, such as where it is found, how it is used, etc.

There are several reasons why a patient may have impaired recognition of visual objects. A traditional dichotomy distinguishes between an apperceptive variant, in which a patient's visual processing is too faulty to generate an accurate representation of the object (126), and an associative variant, in which the patient cannot link what they are seeing with what they know about objects (127). Trying to decide which variant a patient has was often decided by whether they could copy drawings accurately or match basic shapes. However, some patients make relatively correct drawings and matches through a slow laborious strategy that is not normal, suggesting that they do not see the whole object properly. Conversely, patients may draw poorly for reasons other than impaired perception (128).

More recent work has made the point that object perception involves multiple processes, such as shape coding, figure-ground segmentation, grouping and integration of features into whole objects, mapping the resulting percepts to stored structural representations, and accessing semantic information about objects (128). These processes are distinct and potentially dissociable. Correspondingly, there is now a more fractionated taxonomy of agnosia (129, 130).

Visual form (shape) agnosia

This refers to the classic failure to match simple shapes, which implies a defect in perceiving elementary properties like curvature, surface and volume (129, 131). Examples in the literature include Mr S (132) and DF (133). Shape misperception falls along a continuum, with some patients like SMK perceiving simple shapes better than complex ones (134). The residual object recognition of patients with form agnosia is fragmentary and relies on inferences from texture and color.

Some can identify shapes by tracing them with their fingers, translating visual into haptic or kinesthetic cues (135, 136). They can exploit cues processed by the dorsal stream. Thus they identify objects better when they move, and if they are allowed to move their head they can use depth cues to produce more accurate drawings of real objects (137). Even though they have trouble reporting the orientation of line segments, patients with visual agnosia can orient their grasp and reaching to the shape of an object (138, 139). Some can also recognize gestures and actions in line drawings, supporting the proposed distinction between actions and objects in perception (140).

The mechanism of visual form agnosia is debated. One possibility is a peppering of minute scotomata across their visual fields due to diffuse occipital damage (141). However, simulations in healthy subjects have not provided consistent support for this idea (142–144). A second possibility is the loss of grouping cues that define an object and therefore its shape (143, 145).

Visual form agnosia is frequently associated with diffuse occipital damage, as occurs with carbon monoxide poisoning (141, 146, 147), mercury poisoning (136), bilateral hypoxic-ischemic occipital injury or posterior cortical atrophy (Figure 20.9).

Integrative visual agnosia

Patients with this type of apperceptive agnosia can see and match simple shapes, but do not integrate such shapes into a whole object. Patient HJA is the prototype (148). Such patients match

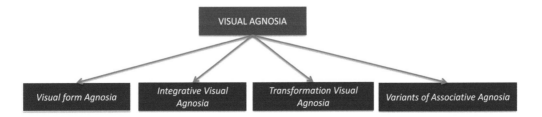

FIGURE 20.8 Overview of types of visual agnosia.

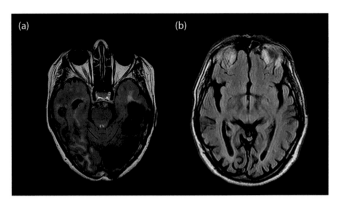

FIGURE 20.9 Axial MRI images of lesions causing apperceptive general visual agnosia. (a) Woman with severe bilateral occipitotemporal infarction. (b) Man with posterior cortical atrophy, showing gyral thinning in the occipital area.

simple forms slowly and slavishly copy drawings in a piecemeal fashion, but have trouble seeing the complex objects formed from multiple simple elements (129, 149). This creates problems with recognizing the impossibility of objects like those in Escher drawings, since these require appreciation that the local elements do not integrate into a correct global structure (150). These patients cannot tell real objects from incorrect objects that are made from parts of other objects, and have trouble seeing the objects in overlapping figures (148, 151). Causes of integrative agnosia include bilateral peri-striate occipital infarcts or a posterior variant of Alzheimer's disease (148, 151).

Transformation visual agnosia
In this rare condition, patients cannot recognize objects seen from an unusual viewpoint. The problem is attributed to failure in deriving a viewpoint-independent representation of the object's three-dimensional structure (152). These patients may not have much difficulty recognizing objects in daily life. It occurs with right occipital damage (128, 152).

Variants of associative agnosia
When perception is reasonably accurate, recognition may fail because the patient cannot understand the meaning of what they are seeing (127). This could be because their knowledge of objects has been destroyed, "semantic agnosia", or because that knowledge exists but cannot be accessed by vision, "semantic access

agnosia" (129). The distinction is made by probing verbally what patients can recall about objects. It is not clear whether semantic agnosia can ever be limited to visual information or if it is always part of a multimodal semantic problem, and therefore not really a visual agnosia (130).

There are also potential distinctions between the type of object knowledge that can't be accessed, namely stored descriptions about the object's shape versus stored knowledge about its function, location or habitat, history, etc. (153). Thus some agnosic patients can accurately describe the appearance of objects but cannot name or pantomime their use. They cannot categorize objects they see according to semantic similarity (e.g., a lion and a tiger are cats, but a bear is not) but can do so if they hear their names (153, 154).

Perhaps related is a distinction between living and non-living objects (155). More frequently, some agnosic patients have more difficulty recognizing living things (156, 157). There are many possible reasons for such a dissociation. One is that there may be separate anatomic modules in the brain for recognizing these two types of objects (158). A second reason based on function is that this dissociation may be due to the fact that living things are distinguished mainly by their shape, but non-living things by their use (159). A third argument is that non-living things are often objects that can be manipulated and therefore they can access sensorimotor representations that living things cannot (160). A fourth perceptual reason may be that animate objects involve more global processing (161) or are more similar in shape to each other than non-living things are (162).

Associative agnosia and semantic access deficits may be due to either left or bilateral damage of the parahippocampal, fusiform and lingual gyri (163, 164). In Alzheimer's disease, neurofibrillary tangles in Brodmann areas 18. 19 and 37 are linked to associative deficits in visual object recognition (165).

Disorders of face Processing
Faces are an important visual part of social interaction. They tell us who someone is, how they are feeling, whether they are looking at us, how old they are, and how trustworthy or attractive they are. Faces are perceptually complex: they have an intricate three-dimensional structure with many mobile parts, and the basic shape does not differ much between people. Nevertheless, most humans are experts in face recognition, though as with all perceptual skills people do vary in this ability (166). Failures of face recognition are considered among the best examples of impaired high-level expert processes in visual object recognition.

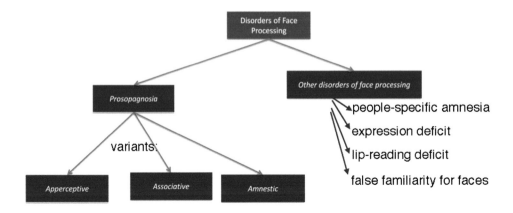

FIGURE 20.10 Overview of various types of disorders of face processing.

Prosopagnosia

Prosopagnosia refers to impaired face identity recognition. Patients with this disorder cannot recognize the faces of people they know and cannot learn to recognize the faces of new people they meet (167, 168). A rare few have an anterograde form only, in that they can recognize old acquaintances but not new people (169, 170). As with all higher-level problems of recognition, prosopagnosia needs to be distinguished from problems with face recognition due to more general problems of perception, cognition, or memory, such as macular degeneration (171), autism (172), Alzheimer's (173–175), Huntington's (176) and Parkinson's disease (177, 178).

Most patients with prosopagnosia are aware of their problem, though some cases with childhood onset or the developmental variant may not be (179–181). They report that to identify people they rely more on voices or non-facial visual cues such as a person's gait or mannerisms. They use distinctive local cues in faces such as odd glasses, hairstyles or scars, and can be misled if someone gets a new haircut. They use the context of an encounter: if they know which five people they will meet at work they can use this knowledge to improve their chances of identifying a person, though they will fail to recognize them in a random encounter on the street (179, 180, 182). These struggles can lead to social avoidance, dysphoria and occupational disability in some but not all patients (183, 184).

Faces also tell us about the direction of a person's gaze, their emotional expression, age, ethnicity and gender. Some prosopagnosic patients cannot perceive some of these aspects of faces too (179–181, 185–187), but others can (188–192). Their aesthetic sense of the attractiveness of a face is blunted (193). Given evidence that different cerebral areas encode facial identity and facial social signals like gaze and expression (194–196), such dissociations are plausible.

Diagnosing prosopagnosia requires care (197). More general problems with perception and memory need to be excluded, usually with the help of a neuropsychologist. Tests of face recognition have two formats. One uses faces already familiar to the subject. While one could use pictures of friends and family, these are usually not standardized with control subjects. One may have to resort simply to seeing if other family members can recognize the faces. There is also the possibility that the patient is recognizing an often-viewed photograph rather than the face of the person. Another possibility is to test them with famous faces from popular culture (198). The test should not ask them to name the face, but simply to indicate which faces are familiar, ideally including some anonymous faces to test their ability to tell famous and unknown faces apart (199). Although seldom done, it would also be more precise to show that they have intact familiarity for the voices or names of these famous people. The weakness of such 'famous faces' tests is that one is assuming that the person has seen those faces in the past. This has led to development of the second group of face recognition tests, which have patients learn some anonymous faces and then tests their ability to tell among a larger set of faces which ones they had seen during the learning phase and which they had not. This includes the Warrington Recognition Memory Test (200) and the Cambridge Face Memory Test (201). Some argue that the weak point of these tests is that such short-term familiarity may not truly probe the rich representations that exist for personally familiar faces.

Is prosopagnosia just about faces? This is a longstanding and still controversial issue. On one side are those who postulate that there are indeed brain regions that process only faces, and damage to these can cause a very face-selective disorder (202). On the other side are those who propose that any region of the visual brain participates in the perception of many types of objects (203): impaired face recognition may be the most dramatic and severe problem, but milder issues with object recognition can be found if testing is careful enough. Unfortunately, the literature is replete with reports of some prosopagnosic patients who cannot recognize a wide variety of objects, and others who can [for review, see (204, 205)]. There are many conceptual and technical challenges in answering this simple question. The current evidence indicates that the occasional prosopagnosic patient may have intact object recognition but the majority do not (205, 206), and any coherent explanation needs to account for both rare dissociations and frequent associations between face and object recognition problems.

As with general visual agnosia, there are functional variants of prosopagnosia (207) (Figure 20.10). Patients with apperceptive prosopagnosia cannot see the structure of faces accurately. They don't perceive the spatial arrangement of the features in a face (208, 209) and fail to show holistic effects in the way they process faces (210). They often show greater difficulty in analyzing the eye region (210–213), which is normally the most useful cue for face identification (214). In associative prosopagnosia the results of perceptual processing are disconnected from facial memories (169, 182, 207, 215, 216). In amnestic prosopagnosia there is loss of facial memories, which can be revealed by verbal tests of facial imagery (182, 217).

The apperceptive variant of prosopagnosia is frequently caused by right or bilateral damage to the lingual and fusiform gyri (Figure 20.11) located in the medial occipitotemporal cortex (182, 189, 218–223). Such lesions damage the occipital and/or fusiform face areas (208, 213, 224, 225), regions that are selectively activated by face in functional MRI studies (226–228). Damage to right or bilateral anterior temporal cortex can cause the amnestic variant (191, 217, 229). This area contains another face-responsive area, the anterior inferior temporal region (230, 231). There are rare cases from left occipitotemporal lesions, most often in patients who are left-handed (232, 233). While all these forms of acquired prosopagnosia are rare, there is also a developmental variant (234). Some claim that this may be present in as many as 2% of the general population (235), though this estimate of prevalence has been challenged (197).

Prosopagnosia from occipitotemporal lesions is often associated with achromatopsia or hemi-achromatopsia, topographagnosia and a visual hemifield defect, a left or bilateral superior quadrantanopia or a left hemianopia (182, 236–238). Prosopagnosia from anterior temporal damage can be accompanied by visual or verbal memory disturbances (220, 239) or impaired voice recognition (240). Developmental prosopagnosia and congenital amusia can occur together (241, 242).

Over the years, there have been case reports of attempts to rehabilitate prosopagnosia with various strategies and mixed results, as recently reviewed (243–245). Two perceptual training studies in larger groups have been conducted in the acquired and developmental variants, showing gains in the ability to perceive differences between faces and some modest benefits in daily life (245, 246). Coping strategies can include exploitation of face recognition technology.

Other disorders of face perception

Some patients know that a face is familiar but can't recall any information about the person. This is usually part of a multimodal problem, in that they cannot access that information from hearing the voice or the name either, and so is considered

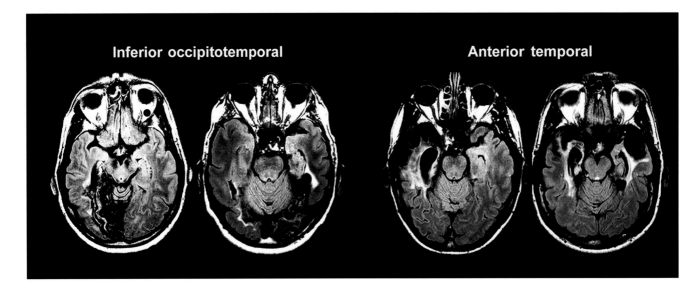

FIGURE 20.11 Axial MRI images showing lesions of four patients with prosopagnosia. Two have an apperceptive variant caused by inferior occipitotemporal lesions that affect the fusiform gyri either in the right hemisphere (left-most image) or bilaterally (second from left). Two have an amnestic variant of prosopagnosia from right or bilateral anterior temporal lesions (the two images on the right). The lesion on the left was due to a posterior cerebral arterial stroke, while the other three patients had herpes encephalitis.

a people-specific amnesia, which typically occurs with right temporal pole lesions (191, 247–249).

A less-studied aspect of face processing is the perception of dynamic social signals in faces, such as gaze, expression and even age. One older study suggested that a selective defect for facial expression occurred with left hemispheric lesions (250). However, monkey and functional imaging data suggest that impairments of these processes should be associated with damage to the right superior temporal sulcus (185, 228) and there is one report of a patient with damage to this area that affected the processing of facial expression selectively (251).

Another type of dynamic facial signal is lip-reading. Because of its relevance to language processing, one might expect this to occur with damage to face-responsive areas in the left rather than the right occipitotemporal region. Indeed, there are patients with alexia from left fusiform lesions who can still recognize the identity of faces but are impaired in lip reading (252–254).

Some patients mistakenly believe that strangers are familiar (255–257). Some of these patients with "false familiarity for faces" have impaired face recognition too but deny it (256), while others can recognize familiar people (255, 258). This false familiarity has been reported with large right middle cerebral artery strokes, most with right prefrontal damage, which may impair self-monitoring and decision-making and lead to erroneous premature judgments about faces from partial data (258).

Disorders of reading
Reading is another example of a high-level expert visual process, at least in literate humans. Like face recognition, reading is much more difficult upside down (259), indicating that we have acquired a perceptual expertise for words in a particular orientation that does not transfer readily to unusual orientations. However, reading is not just a high-level visual process. It requires low-level visual processing such as foveal resolution and intact central fields, complex pattern and form perception, attention, stable fixation and accurate saccades to shift fixation across a line, and language processing. All of these need to be considered and assessed

in a patient who complains of poor reading (Figure 20.12), even if the patient has little in the way of other complaints (260).

Reading complaints vary from slower, less efficient reading to the inability to read even single letters. The assessment of a patient with these complaints begins with visual acuity, perimetric evaluation of the central 10 degrees of vision and fundoscopic viewing of the macula. Eye movements need to be checked to exclude saccadic intrusions and nystagmus, as well as saccadic dysmetria. Acquired saccadic apraxia from bilateral frontal or parietal lesions can impair reading severely (261–264). Reading is difficult for patients with progressive supranuclear palsy because of frequent square wave jerks, hypometric and slow saccades, downgaze palsy, and dry eyes (265). Neglect and attention should be checked, perhaps with a formal neuropsychological assessment if suspected but not obvious. Finally, oral and auditory language, naming and writing should be assessed to determine if the reading problem is merely one element of a larger problem with aphasia.

The history should attempt to establish the patient's premorbid intellect and reading proficiency, to put their current reading performance in context. Reading aloud and for comprehension

Disorders of reading		
Low-level disorders:	**High-level Perceptual disorders:**	**Linguistic disorders:**
Impaired eye movements	Pure alexia	Alexia with agraphia
Hemianopic dyslexia	Hemi-alexia	Surface dyslexia
Neglect dyslexia		Phonologic dyslexia
Attentional dyslexia		Deep dyslexia

FIGURE 20.12 Overview of various types of disorders of reading.

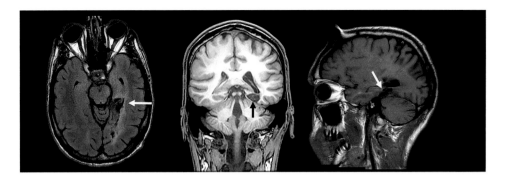

FIGURE 20.13 MRI images (axial, coronal and sagittal) of a patient with pure alexia, showing a stroke affecting the left fusiform gyrus (arrows), in the vicinity of the visual word form area.

should be tested with both single words and sentences or paragraphs. As the patient reads aloud, the examiner should listen for particular patterns and errors. Patients who complain that letters or words transiently disappear or double in the middle of the page have hemifield slide from bitemporal hemianopia (266). Mistakes or omissions of the left side of the page or the left side of individual words suggest neglect dyslexia. Patients with attentional dyslexia often read aloud normally but have trouble remembering what they have read, and complain of having to re-read lines over and over. Bizarre semantic substitutions (e.g., saying "piano" when reading the word "orchestra") point to a linguistic problem, a central dyslexia (267). The characteristic feature of pure alexia is requiring more time for longer words, the word-length effect.

Informal reading material from magazines, books or newspapers that is not too complex can be used in the clinic. If needed, there are more formal standardized assessments, such as the Wide Range Achievement and the Chapman-Cook Speed of Reading Test, which tests comprehension by having patients read paragraphs and cross out words that are incongruous with the meaning of the rest of the text.

Pure alexia (alexia without agraphia)

This is a reduction in reading proficiency that cannot be attributed to more elementary visual, ocular motor, attentional or language problems. Writing is said to be spared, but patients with pure alexia may show difficulty writing words with irregular spelling (e.g., *colonel*, *isle*), which cannot be written from their sound alone using spelling rules, and require access to an internal dictionary (268, 269). The severity of their alexia can range from an inability to read even single letters, a "global alexia" (270) that may also affect the ability to read numbers and other abstract symbols such as numbers (271), musical notation and map symbols (272, 273), to a milder version in which reading is slow and contains errors, "spelling dyslexia" or "letter-by-letter reading" (267). A key diagnostic feature is an increased word-length effect: the more letters in the word, the longer it takes for the patient to read it (274, 275). The number of letters in a word is a perceptual variable, in that it indexes the amount of perceptual work involved, as opposed to linguistic characteristics such as the frequency of a word in a language or the part of speech. While the word length effect in normal readers is only about 10–20 msec per letter, in alexic subjects it can range from a few hundred msec to a few seconds per letter (276).

The traditional explanation of pure alexia is a disconnection between visual processing and language areas in the left hemisphere (117, 277). The most common scenario is a left occipital lesion that not only causes a complete right hemianopia but also extends anteriorly to destroy callosal fibers in the splenium, forceps major, or white matter around the occipital horn (278, 279), so that information from the right occipital lobe can't access language areas in the left hemisphere. White matter lesions under the left angular gyrus may disconnect all visual input to language processors without needing a right hemianopia (280–282). More unusual cases reflect the combination of a splenial lesion and a right hemianopia from non-occipital lesions, such as left geniculate infarction (283, 284) or demyelination of the left optic radiations (285). Other cases may not be a disconnection but a selective visual agnosia from damage to the left fusiform gyrus (278, 286, 287), which contains an area activated by letters or words, the "visual word form area" (288) (Figure 20.13). Damage to this area can impair reading (289–292), but so can lesions in other regions such as the left middle temporal gyrus, which are part of a reading network (293, 294).

Just as with faces, there is debate about whether a "word-form agnosia" can only affect only words (295, 296), or if the problem with reading is only the most obvious part of a more general visual problem (297–299). Alexic patients have slower recognition and reduced perceptual span for both letters and digits (300, 301).

Pure alexia is often associated with a right hemianopia or right superior quadrantanopia, sometimes a hemi-achromatopsia or color anomia (117, 278, 302). They may have anomia for objects, whether these are seen, heard or felt, indicating some linguistic element (303). Almost all lesions causing pure alexia are in the left hemisphere, with very rare exceptions (304, 305). Most are located in the medial and inferior occipitotemporal region (270, 278, 286). The most frequent cause is left posterior cerebral artery stroke.

The prognosis for alexia depends on the cause. Global alexia can resolve into spelling dyslexia (279). Improvement may reflect reorganization of a word-processing network, with increased participation of the right fusiform region or left-sided regions around the visual word form area and the superior parietal lobule (306–308). Various approaches to rehabilitating alexia have been tried, though none have gained widespread acceptance (309, 310). These include highlighting the space between words or phrases (311, 312), oral articulation during reading (313), repetitive oral reading of text (311, 314), and finger tracing of letters (312, 315).

Other reading disorders

Disconnections of visual information from one hemifield alone have been described. In left hemi-alexia, reading is impaired in the left hemifield only because of isolated damage to the splenium or callosal fibers (289, 316). These subjects do not have right hemianopia and can read words in the right hemifield. Right hemi-alexia has been reported with a lesion of the left medial and ventral occipital lobe (317). These disorders seem rare, but reading is usually done with central vision and rarely compared between the right and left parafoveal field in either daily life or the clinic. Hence these defects are less symptomatic and their incidence probably underestimated.

In "alexia with agraphia", both reading and writing are impaired but oral and auditory language intact. It is more likely a linguistic than perceptual disorder: its characteristics suggest a deep dyslexia with deep dysgraphia – see below (269, 318, 319). It may be accompanied by other elements of Gerstmann's syndrome and some degree of anomia (320). This is associated with lesions of the left angular gyrus (277, 321) or sometimes the adjacent temporo-parietal junction (320, 322). As with pure alexia, there are occasional reports of improvement with intensive rehabilitative efforts (323).

Patients with left hemi-neglect from right parietal or frontal lesions make characteristic left-sided reading errors (324). This neglect dyslexia is the combination of a space-centered deficit, in which text on the left side of space is ignored, and an object-centered deficit, in which the left sides of words are marked by omissions (*bright* read as *right*), additions (*right* read as *bright*) or substitutions (*right* read as *light*). Vertically printed text is not affected (324). This dyslexia can rarely occur without other signs of hemi-neglect (325).

Linguistic problems can also cause some rare types of reading difficulty. These reflect the fact that there are two ways to connecting the printed word to how it sounds (267). The phonological route relies on generic pronunciation rules: this allows the reading aloud of words with regular spelling and even pseudo-words or new words the reader has never seen before. Loss of this route results in "phonological dyslexia" (326–329). The lexical route allows one to look up a word in an internal dictionary to find its pronunciation: this is the only means of knowing the pronunciation of irregularly spelled words like *yacht* and *choir*, and damage to this route causes "surface dyslexia" (330–333). "Deep dyslexia" resembles phonological dyslexia, but patients substitute words with a similar meaning for the correct one (*boat* read as *ship*) (334).

Topographagnosia
While most of us get lost occasionally in new surroundings, patients with topographagnosia get lost in familiar places such as their own neighborhood, sometimes even in their own house. A complex task like navigation draws on several cognitive skills, and topographagnosia may have a number of different causes (335).

One group gets lost because they fail to recognize familiar buildings and places. This "landmark agnosia" (336) occurs with right ventral temporo-occipital lesions (337, 338) and can accompany prosopagnosia and achromatopsia (179, 181, 189, 191, 220, 339–341). In at least some cases this disorder may be due to damage to the parahippocampal place area, a region adjacent to the fusiform face area that is activated by seeing buildings and places (342). These subjects cope by reading building signs and street names.

The hippocampus and retrosplenial cortex are involved in the formation and use of a mental map of the environment, which allows one to navigate flexibly from and between different locations (343). "Impaired cognitive map formation" is seen in congenital topographagnosia (344) and some cases of acquired topographagnosia (341). Online computerized tests are available to help diagnose failures of cognitive map formation and use, as well as landmark agnosia (www.gettinglost.ca). Use of GPS technology is a helpful way of dealing with this problem.

Right parietotemporal lesions can affect the spatial skills used to describe, follow or memorize routes (337, 345). "Egocentric disorientation" refers to the inability to represent the location of objects and buildings with respect to oneself (335). "Heading disorientation" is the failure to represent direction with respect to cues in the external environment, rather than in relation to oneself, and has been associated with posterior cingulate lesions (346).

Parahippocampal lesions have also been implicated in an "anterograde topographagnosia", in which new routes cannot be learned, though old routes are still known (347).

Dorsal occipitoparietal pathway disorders

Cerebral akinetopsia
This is a very rare disorder of motion perception. Only two cases have been well described, LM and AF (348–356). LM had no "impression" of motion in depth or of rapid motion, and fast-moving targets jumped rather than moved (349).

Tests for motion perception require computerized displays that are not available in most clinics. Smooth pursuit eye movements depend on motion perception, and LM and AF had impaired smooth pursuit (348), but one can have impaired motion perception with normal smooth pursuit and vice versa (357). Patients with akinetopsia can tell when something is moving (348) and they can see the direction of simple moving dots or patterns (349, 351, 352), but they cannot see differences in speed or discern the overall direction of flow in noisy displays that contain other elements that are stationary or moving randomly (351, 352, 358). They have trouble using motion cues in searching for objects (355) or identifying the shapes of objects defined by differences in motion between the object and the background (352, 358). They also struggle with lip-reading (354).

LM and AF had bilateral damage to the lateral occipitotemporal cortex (349, 358). Histology and functional imaging point to this as a homologue to monkey area V5 and V5a (359–362), areas in the monkey superior temporal sulcus that respond to motion specifically (363). Unilateral lateral occipitotemporal lesions are more common but at most cause only subtle complaints, such as "feeling disturbed by visually cluttered moving scenes" and trouble judging the speed and direction of cars (364, 365). Experimental tests in these subjects can show contralateral hemifield defects for various aspects of motion perception, if there is no hemianopia (366–368).

Defects that can be associated with akinetopsia include hemifield defects, problems on other visuospatial tests and poor stereopsis (352). Given the rarity of these cases, little is known about their prognosis. Some have improved over the first year (369, 370). In monkeys, recovery varies with the extent of damage (371).

Other types of motion perception can be affected by lesions elsewhere. Instead of local velocity signals, long-range integration of position data can give the impression of apparent or "high-level" motion perception, which is impaired by parietal rather than occipitotemporal lesions (372, 373). Perception of "biological motion" – for example, the walking motion seen from point sources of light attached to joints of an invisible body – is impaired by lesions of a more anterior region, the superior temporal polysensory area (374).

Bálint's Syndrome
Bálint's syndrome (375, 376) is a loosely associated triad of visuospatial dysfunctions: simultanagnosia, optic ataxia and ocular motor apraxia. These reflect disturbances in spatial attention,

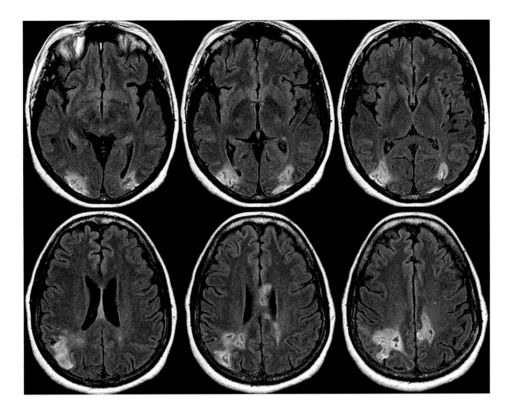

FIGURE 20.14 Axial MRI images of the bilateral strokes affecting the lateral occipital and parietal cortex in a patient with Bálint's syndrome due to primary cerebral vasculitis.

reaching guidance and saccadic initiation and targeting respectively, all spatial functions that involve distinct networks that can be affected together or in isolation. Bálint's syndrome is essentially a dorsal visual syndrome (Figure 20.14), and a counterpart to the ventral visual syndrome discussed above.

In diagnosing the various components of Bálint's syndrome, the first step is to exclude general cognitive dysfunction, hemineglect and extensive visual field defects. The latter is particularly challenging. Accurate perimetry is difficult because of the attentional problems of simultanagnosia or difficulty maintaining fixation (377–379). Nevertheless, this is critical to do: extensive peripheral scotomata leaving only "keyhole vision" can mimic all components of Bálint's syndrome (380).

Simultanagnosia
This is a deficit in attention. Classically, the term means that patients cannot pay attention to more than one object at a time. When severe, it is almost as bad as being blind or having tunnel vision, and patients may express their symptoms in those terms and behave as if blind. This underscores the fact that perception is as much about attention as it is about vision.

On bedside testing one can ask patients to describe or pick up a number of objects scattered on a table (262, 381). When describing a complex scene with multiple elements, such as the Cookie Theft Picture (382), they will miss elements or fail to realize how all the elements are related to each other in the story depicted. They will struggle with visual search tasks (383) and maintaining surveillance of large regions of space (384). Interestingly, what they perceive can depend on grouping factors. For example, they may fail at identifying multiple letters in a random string of letters, but do better if that string of letters forms a word (264). They are more likely to report

the presence of multiple objects if the objects are semantically related (383, 385).

Several phenomena point to a reduction in the capacity and flexibility of attention in simultanagnosia. Many objects have local components (e.g., wheels, door, windscreen) that together make a larger whole (e.g., car). Healthy subjects have sufficient capacity to see both the "local" components and the "global" whole, but simultanagnosic patients do not. The result is that local and global elements are placed in competition for the patient's limited attention, and the stronger percept prevails. Thus in "local capture" patients see the local elements but not the global layout (386–388). This is typified by Navon letters, large letters made from the arrangement of small letters: simultanagnosic patients may not see the large letter unless the size and density of the display is made more compelling (388, 389). On the other hand, when the global interpretation is powerful, as with Arcimboldo paintings of faces made up out of fruit, they may see the face but not the fruit, "global capture" (388).

Simultanagnosia has been linked to lesions of the dorsal occipital lobes, in Brodmann's areas 18 and 19 (384). There can also be contributions from damage to other components of a visual attention network, such as the middle frontal gyrus and white matter connections in the inferior and superior longitudinal fasciculi (390).

Optic ataxia
This refers to impaired reaching to visual targets despite normal limb strength (391) and position sense. However, the reaching problem of these patients is not always just a visual deficit. It can affect one arm more than the other (375) and impair reaching to somatosensory targets, such as the patient's own body parts (392, 393), indicating an element of dysfunctional motor programming

that can be specific to one limb in some cases or general across sensory modalities in others.

For bedside testing, the patient is simply asked to touch or grasp easily seen items at different locations around them. This is tested separately for the left and right hands and with objects to the left and right of the patient (394). They should also be asked to reach to parts of their own body with their eyes closed, to determine if the problem is limited to visual targets or also involves somatosensory ones. Pointing to the location of sounds with the eyes closed may serve a similar purpose. A more general problem suggests disturbances in multimodal parietal spatial representations (392). On the other hand, if the problem is specific to visual targets, this definitively excludes cerebellar dysmetria, which is usually also accompanied by intention tremor and dysdiadochokinesia.

Laboratory measures of manual responses sho increased latency, abnormal hand trajectories, increased variability of the end of the reach, a tendency to reach to one side as well as dissociations of distance and direction control (395–397). In optic ataxia, reaching is usually normal toward foveated objects but impaired for objects in peripheral vision, with a correlation between reaching errors and target eccentricity (398, 399). Also, reaching is characteristically worse when performed immediately to the target: a delay of a few seconds can improve both reaching accuracy (45, 400) and the ability to avoid obstacles during movement (401). This suggests that the parietal cortex may play a specific role in rapid visuomotor control, and that there are alternative routes using the ventral stream for calculating object location and guiding slow reaching movements. This is supported by observations that patients with visual agnosia have normal rapid reaching responses but are impaired if action is delayed for a few seconds (402). Additional studies in patients with unilateral optic ataxia show that the reaching errors occur in a gaze- or eye-centered map, rather than a body frame-of-reference (403–405).

Optic ataxia is associated classically with damage to the occipitoparietal lobes, at the junction between the inferior parietal lobule and the superior occipital cortex (406). However, reaching under visual guidance is mediated by recursive processes involving a sensorimotor network (407) that can be disrupted at a number of points, including parietal and frontal cortex (408, 409). Hence a variety of other lesions can cause optic ataxia, including damage to premotor cortex, cortex below the angular gyrus (397), and occipital-frontal white matter tracts (409, 410). These lesions can be unilateral (395, 409, 411), in which case the patient can have poor reaching with either the contralateral hand or to objects in the contralateral hemi-space.

Ocular motor apraxia

This term is somewhat vague in meaning, and encompasses a number of related problems with saccadic function. Patients can have trouble initiating a voluntary saccade to a visible target on command, which has also been called "psychic paralysis of gaze" (376, 412). This should be contrasted with retained reflexive saccades to suddenly appearing visual objects or sounds. They may also have "spasm of fixation" (413), a difficulty in starting saccades when a central fixation light remains visible rather than being turned off when the target appears (414, 415), which is more easily demonstrated in a laboratory. Once patients are able to make saccades, they may show "inaccurate saccadic targeting", with their eyes appearing to wander in search of the target, even though it is plainly visible (262, 391). With more complex scenes their scanning is grossly disorganized (415).

Saccadic control involves cortical regions such as the lateral intraparietal area (416) and the frontal eye field. Acquired ocular motor apraxia usually requires bilateral lesions of the frontal eye fields, inferior parietal lobes or both (262, 263, 391).

Other aspects of Bálint's syndrome

Damage to the dorsal visual system can cause other problems with spatial and temporal processing of vision, beyond the three classic elements of Bálint's syndrome. The spatial location of some stimuli can be represented in separate auditory, visual and/or somatosensory maps. Imagine looking at your hand as it taps on a table; you can see it, feel it and hear it. Some patients fail to integrate properly these separate sources of information into a coherent spatial location (417). Unreliable coarse coding of the location of object features may lead the features of one object to migrate to another object, leading to bizarre percepts (418).

Beyond these spatial problems, there can also be visuotemporal deficits, though these have been less explored than visuospatial deficits. One patient could perceive multiple stimuli presented one at a time, but could not recall the order in which they had been shown. This indicates a problem tagging objects with their occurrence in time, which was called "sequence-agnosia" (419).

Generally it is felt that the different elements of Bálint's syndrome reflect damage to separate but adjacent and somewhat overlapping networks for attention, reaching and saccades, leading to potential dissociations (262, 332, 376, 391). However, these are related functions and it has been questioned whether problems in one can contribute to the problems in another. For example, simultanagnosia used to be considered the primary defect and responsible for both optic ataxia and ocular motor apraxia (391). While this is not currently thought to be the case, deficits in peripheral attention do occur with optic ataxia (420). Impaired visuomotor control of fast movements is common to both saccades and reaching in optic ataxia (421). Therefore, even though the ocular, reaching and attentional disturbances may each have their own basis, they may also contribute to each other's manifestations.

Patients with Bálint's syndrome often have bilateral hemifield defects, usually affecting the lower quadrants more, and other visuospatial defects such as left hemineglect and astereopsis (376, 422, 423). Smooth pursuit is often impaired. Patients may complain of metamorphopsia, micropsia and macropsia, or visual perseverations such as palinopsia and monocular polyopia.

The prognosis varies with the cause: patients with infarction can recover with time, while those with posterior cortical atrophy slowly worsen. Recovery can be dissociated, with ocular motor deficits improving but not attentional abnormalities (415). Little is known about treatment: cognitive and perceptual rehabilitation may improve visual function and reaching (424).

Astereopsis

In a three-dimensional world, the distance of objects from the observer is another visuospatial perception. This has been less studied after lesions, however. In frontally eyed creatures like humans, one important clue to distance is stereovision, the disparity between the retinal images of the object in the two eyes. Patients with astereopsis may complain that the world looks flat and that they cannot tell how far away an object is, and they may misreach for objects in depth but not in direction. This occurs after bilateral occipito-parietal lesions (422, 425), sometimes in milder form with unilateral lesions. Impaired depth perception may reflect more than just astereopsis. Monocular clues to depth exist, and include relative differences in object size and color intensity (which artists exploit), and differences in the movement of near versus far objects as the observer's head moves sideways (motion parallax). It is not known if these are also dysfunctional in patients with complaints of impaired depth perception. Stereopsis can be tested with commonly available 3-D tests in eye clinics (426).

Conclusion

Visual impairment can be caused by various disorders of the brain. Cortical visual loss encompasses various disorders like visual field deficits, disorders of colour and face processing, visual agnosias, disorders of reading and stereopsis. Defects due to the impairment of the geniculostriate relay system are typified by visual field defects and the defects caused due to lesions of extrastriate visual regions show functional specificity, affecting certain types of visual processing.

Multiple-Choice Questions

1. Which of the following statements is true regarding the visual pathways?
   a. The ventral pathway consists of lateral occipitoparietal structures.
   b. The dorsal visual pathways are involved in object recognition.
   c. The dorsal pathways are involved in processing color.
   d. The dorsal visual pathways are involved in motion processing.

   Answer:

   d. The dorsal visual pathways are involved in motion processing.

2. All are true about blood supply of the visual pathway, EXCEPT:
   a. Lateral geniculate body: choroidal arteries
   b. Optic radiations: middle and posterior cerebral artery
   c. Optic tract: middle cerebral artery
   d. Retina: ophthalmic artery

   Answer:

   c. Optic tract: middle cerebral artery

3. Which of the following statements regarding cortical visual loss is NOT true?
   a. Action blindsight involves a subcortical pathway from the retina to superior colliculus.
   b. Agnosopsia encompasses abilities to report localization of targets.
   c. Charles Bonnet syndrome can arise from bilateral ocular disease.
   d. Perception of color and form may be mediated by direct projections from surviving lateral geniculate neurons to extrastriate cortex.

   Answer:

   b. Agnosopsia encompasses abilities to report localization of targets.

4. Which of the following statements regarding visual disorders is true?
   a. Visual form agnosia is frequently associated with diffuse occipital damage.
   b. Patients with apperceptive prosopagnosia can see the structure of faces accurately.

   c. Bálint's syndrome is essentially a ventral visual pathway syndrome.
   d. All are correct.

   Answer:

   a. Visual form agnosia is frequently associated with diffuse occipital damage.

References

1. Ungerleider L, Mishkin M. Two cortical visual systems. In: Ingle DJ, Mansfield RJW, Goodale MS (eds). The analysis of visual behaviour. Cambridge, MA: MIT Press; 1982. pp. 549–586.
2. Milner A, Goodale M. The visual brain in action. Oxford: Oxford University Press; 1995.
3. Martinaud O. Visual agnosia and focal brain injury. Rev Neurol (Paris). 2017; 173(7–8):451–460.
4. Johnson LN, Baloh FG. The accuracy of confrontation visual field test in comparison with automated perimetry. J Natl Med Assoc. 1991;83(10):895–898.
5. Shahinfar S, Johnson LN, Madsen RW. Confrontation visual field loss as a function of decibel sensitivity loss on automated static perimetry. Implications on the accuracy of confrontation visual field testing. Ophthalmology. 1995;102(6):872–877.
6. Hardiess G, Hansmann-Roth S, Mallot HA. Gaze movements and spatial working memory in collision avoidance: a traffic intersection task. Front Behav Neurosci. 2013;7:62.
7. Papageorgiou E, Hardiess G, Mallot HA, Schiefer U. Gaze patterns predicting successful collision avoidance in patients with homonymous visual field defects. Vision Res. 2012;65:25–37.
8. Wood JM, McGwin G, Jr., Elgin J, Vaphiades MS, Braswell RA, DeCarlo DK, et al. Hemianopic and quadrantanopic field loss, eye and head movements, and driving. Invest Ophthalmol Vis Sci. 2011;52(3):1220–1225.
9. Bahnemann M, Hamel J, De Beukelaer S, Ohl S, Kehrer S, Audebert H, et al. Compensatory eye and head movements of patients with homonymous hemianopia in the naturalistic setting of a driving simulation. J Neurol. 2015;262(2):316–325.
10. Schuett S, Heywood CA, Kentridge RW, Zihl J. The significance of visual information processing in reading: Insights from hemianopic dyslexia. Neuropsychologia. 2008;46(10):2445–2462.
11. Trauzettel-Klosinski S, Brendler K. Eye movements in reading with hemianopic field defects: the significance of clinical parameters. Graefe's Arch Clin Exp Ophthalmol. 1998;236:91–102.
12. Trauzettel-Klosinski S, Reinhard J. The vertical field border in hemianopia and its significance for fixation and reading. Invest Ophthalmol Vis Sci. 1998;39(11):2177–2186.
13. Zihl J. Eye movement patterns in hemianopic dyslexia. Brain. 1995;118:891–912.
14. de Luca M, Spinelli D, Zoccolotti P. Eye movement patterns in reading as a function of visual field defects and contrast sensitivity loss. Cortex. 1996;32:491–502.
15. Spitzyna GA, Wise RJ, McDonald SA, Plant GT, Kidd D, Crewes H, et al. Optokinetic therapy improves text reading in patients with hemianopic alexia: a controlled trial. Neurology. 2007;68(22):1922–1930.
16. de Haan GA, Heutink J, Melis-Dankers BJ, Brouwer WH, Tucha O. Difficulties in daily life reported by patients with homonymous visual field defects. J Neuroophthalmol. 2015;35(3):259–264.
17. Zhang X, Kedar S, Lynn MJ, Newman NJ, Biousse V. Natural history of homonymous hemianopia. Neurology. 2006;66(6):901–905.
18. Frolov A, Feuerstein J, Subramanian PS. Homonymous hemianopia and vision restoration therapy. Neurol Clin. 2017;35(1):29–43.
19. Rossi PW, Kheyfets S, Reding MJ. Fresnel prisms improve visual perception in stroke patients with homonymous hemianopia or unilateral visual neglect. Neurology. 1990;40(10):1597–1599.
20. Frisèn L, Holmegaard L, Rosenkrantz M. Sectoral optic atrophy and homonymous horizontal sectoranopia: a lateral choroidal artery syndrome? J Neurol Neurosurg Psychiatry. 1978;41:374–380.
21. Frisèn L. Quadruple sectoranopia and sectorial optic atrophy. A syndrome of the distal anterior choroidal artery. J Neurol Neurosurg Psychiatry. 1979;42:590–594.
22. Helgason C, Caplan L, Goodwin J, Hedges T. Anterior choroidal artery-territory infarction. Report of cases and review. Arch Neurol. 1986;43:681–686.
23. Luco C, Hoppe A, Schweitzer M, Vicuna X, Fantin A. Visual field defects in vascular lesions of the lateral geniculate body. J Neurol Neurosurg Psychiatry. 1992;55(1):12–15.
24. Jacobson D. The localizing value of a quadrantanopia. Arch Neurol. 1997;54:401–404.
25. Carter J, O'Connor P, Shacklett D, Rosenberg M. Lesions of the optic radiations mimicking lateral geniculate nucleus visual field defects. J Neurol Neurosurg Psychiatry. 1985;48:982–988.
26. Inouye T. Die Sehstorungen bei Schussverletzungen der kortikalen Sesphare. Leipzig: Engelmann; 1909.
27. Holmes G, Lister WT. Disturbances of vision from cerebral lesions with special reference to the cortical representation of the macula. Brain. 1916;39:34–73.
28. Holmes G. The organization of the visual cortex in man. Proc Royal Soc B (Biol). 1945;132:348–361.
29. Horton JC, Hoyt WF. The representation of the visual field in human striate cortex. A revision of the classic Holmes map. Arch Ophthalmol. 1991;109(6):816–824.
30. McFadzean R, Brosnahan D, Hadley D, Mutlukan E. Representation of the visual field in the occipital striate cortex. Br J Ophthalmol. 1994;78(3):185–190.
31. Smith CG, Richardson WF. The course and distribution of the arteries supplying the visual (striate) cortex. Am J Ophthalmol. 1966;61(6):1391–1396.

32. McAuley DL, Russell RW. Correlation of CAT scan and visual field defects in vascular lesions of the posterior visual pathways. J Neurol Neurosurg Psychiatry. 1979; 42(4):298–311.

33. Gray L, Galetta S, Siegal T, Schatz N. The central visual field in homonymous hemianopia. Evidence for unilateral foveal representation. Arch Neurol. 1997;54:312–317.

34. Benton S, Levy I, Swash M. Vision in the temporal crescent in occipital infarction. Brain. 1980;103:83–97.

35. Ceccaldi M, Brouchon M, Pelletier J, Poncet M. [Hemianopsia with preservation of temporal crescent and occipital infarction]. Rev Neurol (Paris). 1993;149(6–7):423–425.

36. Chavis PS, al-Hazmi A, Clunie D, Hoyt WF. Temporal crescent syndrome with magnetic resonance correlation. J Neuroophthalmol. 1997;17(3):151–155.

37. Pessin MS, Lathi ES, Cohen MB, Kwan ES, Hedges TR, 3rd, Caplan LR. Clinical features and mechanism of occipital infarction. Ann Neurol. 1987;21(3):290–299.

38. Medina J, Chokroverty S, Rubino F. Syndrome of agitated delirium and visual impairment: a manifestation of medial temporo-occipital infarction. J Neurol Neurosurg Psychiatry. 1977;40:861–864.

39. Symonds C, McKenzie I. Bilateral loss of vision from cerebral infarction. Brain. 1957;80:415–453.

40. Aldrich M, Alessi A, Beck R, Gilman S. Cortical blindness: etiology, diagnosis and prognosis. Ann Neurol. 1987;21:149–158.

41. Geschwind N. Disconnexion syndromes in animals and man. Brain. 1965;88:17–294.

42. Stoerig P, Cowey A. Blindsight in man and monkey. Brain. 1997;120:535–559.

43. Rafal R, Smith J, Krantz J, Cohen A, Brennan C. Extrageniculate vision in hemianopic humans: saccade inhibition by signals in the blind field. Science. 1990;250:118–121.

44. Intriligator JM, Xie R, Barton JJ. Blindsight modulation of motion perception. J Cogn Neurosci. 2002;14(8):1174–1183.

45. Danckert J, Rossetti Y. Blindsight in action: what can the different sub-types of blindsight tell us about the control of visually guided actions? Neurosci Biobehav Rev. 2005;29(7):1035–1046.

46. Wessinger CM, Fendrich R, Gazzaniga MS, Ptito A, Villemure J-G. Extrageniculostriate vision in humans: investigations with hemispherectomy patients. Prog Brain Res. 1996;112:405–413.

47. Pöppel E, Held R, Frost D. Residual visual function after brain wounds involving the central visual pathways in man. Nature. 1973; 243:295–296.

48. Cowey A, Stoerig P. The neurobiology of blindsight. Trends Neurosci. 1995;14:140–145.

49. Campion J, Latto R, Smith YM. Is blindsight an effect of scattered light, spared cortex, and near-threshold vision? Behavioral Brain Sci. 1983;6:423–486.

50. Barton J, Sharpe J. Smooth pursuit and saccades to moving targets in blind hemifields. A comparison of medial occipital, lateral occipital, and optic radiation lesions. Brain. 1997;120:681–699.

51. Barton JJS, Sharpe JA. Motion direction discrimination in blind hemifields. Ann Neurol. 1997;41:255–264.

52. Kasten E, Wuest S, Sabel B. Residual vision in transition zones in patients with cerebral blindness. J Clin Exp Neuropsychol. 1998;20:581–598.

53. Scharli H, Harman A, Hogben J. Blindsight in subjects with homonymous visual field defects. J Cogn Neurosci. 1999;11:52–66.

54. Teunisse RJ, Cruysberg JR, Hoefnagels WH, Verbeek AL, Zitman FG. Visual hallucinations in psychologically normal people: Charles Bonnet's syndrome. Lancet. 1996;347(9004):794–797.

55. Lepore FE. Spontaneous visual phenomena with visual loss: 104 patients with lesions of retinal and neural afferent pathways. Neurology. 1990;40(3 Pt 1):444–447.

56. Kolmel HW. Coloured patterns in hemianopic fields. Brain. 1984;107 (Pt 1):155–167.

57. Lance JW. Simple formed hallucinations confined to the area of a specific visual field defect. Brain. 1976;99(4):719–734.

58. Weinberger LM, Grant FC. Visual hallucinations and their neuro-optical correlates. Arch Ophthalmol 1940;23:166–199.

59. Cole MG. Charles Bonnet hallucinations: a case series. Can J Psychiatry. 1992; 37(4):267–270.

60. MacKay G, Dunlop JC. The cerebral lesions in a case of complete acquired colour-blindness. Scott Med Surg J. 1899;5:503.

61. Pallis CA. Impaired identification of faces and places with agnosia for colors. J Neurol Neurosurg Psychiatry. 1955;18:218.

62. Meadows JC. Disturbed perception of colors associated with localized cerebral lesions. Brain. 1974;97:615–632.

63. Rizzo M, Smith V, Pokorny J, Damasio AR. Color perception profiles in central achromatopsia. Neurology. 1993;43:995.

64. Critchley M. Acquired anomalies of colour perception of central origin. Brain. 1965;88:711.

65. Koyama S, Kezuka M, Hibino H, Tomimitsu H, Kawamura M. Evaluation of cerebral dyschromatopsia using color afterimage. Neuroreport. 2006;17(2):109–113.

66. Albert ML, Reches A, Silverberg R. Hemianopic colour blindness. J Neurol Neurosurg Psychiatry. 1975;38:546.

67. Paulson HL, Galetta SL, Grossman M, Alavi A. Hemiachromatopsia of unilateral occipitotemporal infarcts. Am J Ophthalmol. 1994;118:518.

68. Damasio A, Yamada T, Damasio H, Corbett J, McKee J. Central achromatopsia: Behavioral, anatomic and physiologic aspects. Neurology. 1980;30:1064–1071.

69. Sacks O. The case of the colour-blind painter. An Anthropologist on Mars. New York: Alfred A Knopf; 1995.

70. Hardy L, Rand G, Rittler M. AO-HRR pseudoisochromatic plates. 2nd ed: American Optical Co; 1957.

71. Ichikawa K, Hukame H, Tanabe S. Detection of acquired color vision defects by standard pseudoisochromatic plates, part 2. Doc Ophthalmol Proc. 1987;46:133.

72. Heywood CA, Cowey A, Newcombe F. Chromatic discrimination in a cortically colour blind observer. Eur J Neurosci. 1991;3:802–812.

73. Victor J, Maiese K, Shapley R, Sitdis J, Gazzaniga M. Acquired central dyschromatopsia: analysis of a case with preservation of color discrimination. Clinical Vision Sci. 1989;4:183–196.

74. Frisèn L, Kalm P. Sahlgren's saturation test for detecting and grading acquired dyschromatopsia. Am J Ophthalmol. 1981;92:252.

75. Heywood CA, Wilson B, Cowey A. A case study of cortical colour "blindness" with relatively intact achromatic discrimination. J Neurol Neurosurg Psychiatry. 1987;50:22–29.

76. Moroz D, Corrow SL, Corrow JC, Barton AR, Duchaine B, Barton JJ. Localization and patterns of cerebral dyschromatopsia: a study of subjects with prosopagnosia. Neuropsychologia. 2016;89:153–160.

77. Land E. Recent advances in retinex theory. Vision Res. 1986;26:7–21.

78. Zeki SM. A century of cerebral achromatopsia. Brain. 1990;113:1721–1777.

79. Land E, Hubel D, Livingstone M, Perry S, Burns M. Colour-generating interactions across the corpus callosum. Nature. 1983;303:616–618.

80. Kennard C, Lawden M, Morland AB, Ruddock KH. Colour identification and colour constancy are impaired in a patient with incomplete achromatopsia associated with prestriate lesions. Proc Roy Soc Lond B. 1995;260:169–175.

81. Clarke S, Walsh V, Schoppig A, Assal G, Cowey A. Colour constancy impairments in patients with lesions of the prestriate cortex. Exp Brain Res. 1998;123:154–158.

82. Hurlbert AC, Bramwell DI, Heywood C, Cowey A. Discrimination of cone contrast changes as evidence for colour constancy in cerebral achromatopsia. Exp Brain Res. 1998;123:136–144.

83. D'Zmura MD, Knoblauch K, Henaff M-A, Michel F. Dependence of color on context in a case of cortical color vision deficiency. Vision Res. 1998;38:3455–3459.

84. Kentridge RW, Heywood CA, Cowey A. Chromatic edges, surfaces and constancies in cerebral achromatopsia. Neuropsychologia. 2004;42(6):821–830.

85. Heywood CA, Nicholas JJ, Cowey A. Behavioural and electrophysiological chromatic and achromatic contrast sensitivity in an achromatopsic patient. J Neurol Neurosurg Psychiatry. 1996;61:638–643.

86. Adachi-Usami E, Tsukamoto M, Shimada Y. Color vision and color pattern evoked cortical potentials in a patient with acquired cerebral dyschromatopsia. Doc Ophthalmol. 1997;90:259–269.

87. Heywood CA, Kentridge RW, Cowey A. Form and motion from colour in cerebral achromatopsia. Exp Brain Res. 1998;123:145–153.

88. Cole G, Heywood C, Kentridge R, Fairholm I, Cowey A. Attentional capture by colour and motion in cerebral achromatopsia. Neuropsychologia. 2003;41:1837–1846.

89. Cavanagh P, Hénaff M-A, Michel F, Landis T, Troscianko T, Intriligator J. Complete sparing of high-contrast color input to motion perception in cortical color blindness. Nature Neurosci. 1998;1(3):242–247.

90. Cowey A, Alexander I, Heywood C, Kentridge R. Pupillary responses to coloured and contourless displays in total cerebral achromatopsia. Brain. 2008;131(Pt 8):2153–2160.

91. Kentridge RW, Heywood CA, Weiskrantz L. Color contrast processing in human striate cortex. Proc Natl Acad Sci U S A. 2007;104(38):15129–15131.

92. Verrey D. Hemiachromatopsie droite absolue. Arch Ophthalmol (Paris). 1888;8:289.

93. Pearlman AL, Birch J, Meadows JC. Cerebral color blindness: an acquired defect in hue discrimination. Ann Neurol. 1979;5:253.

94. Green GJ, Lessell S. Acquired cerebral dyschromatopsia. Arch Ophthalmol. 1977;95:121.

95. Freedman L, Costa L. Pure alexia and right hemiachromatopsia in posterior dementia. J Neurol Neurosurg Psychiatry. 1992;55:500–502.

96. Short RA, Graff-Radford NR. Localization of hemiachromatopsia. Neurocase. 2001;7(4):331–337.

97. Damasio H, Frank R. Three-dimensional in vivo mapping of brain lesions in humans. Arch Neurol. 1992;49:137.

98. Bouvier SE, Engel SA. Behavioral deficits and cortical damage loci in cerebral achromatopsia. Cereb Cortex. 2006;16:183–191.

99. Dean P. Visual cortex ablation and thresholds for successively presented stimuli in Rhesus monkeys: II. Hue. Exp Brain Res. 1979;35:69–83.

100. Wild HM, Butler SR, Carden D, Kulikowski JJ. Primate cortical area V4 important for colour constancy but not wavelength discrimination. Nature. 1985;313:133–135.

101. Heywood CA, Cowey A. On the role of cortical area V4 in the discrimination of hue and pattern in macaque monkeys. J Neurosci. 1987;7:2601–2617.

102. Heywood CA, Gadotti A, Cowey A. Cortical area V4 and its role in the perception of color. J Neurosci. 1992;12:4056–4065.

103. Walsh V, Kulikowski JJ, Butler SR, Carden D. The effects of lesions of area V4 on the visual abilities of macaques: colour categorization. Behav Brain Res. 1992;7:1–9.

104. Schiller P. The effects of V4 and middle temporal (MT) lesions on visual performance in the rhesus monkey. Vis Neurosci. 1993;10:717–46.

105. Cowey A, Heywood C, Irving-Bell L. The regional cortical basis of achromatopsia: a study on macaque monkeys and an achromatopsic patient. Eur J Neurosci. 2001;14: 1555–1566.

106. Heywood C, Gaffan D, Cowey A. Cerebral achromatopsia in monkeys. Eur J Neurosci. 1995;7:1064–1073.

107. Hadjikhani N, Liu A, Dale A, Cavanagh P, Tootell R. Retinotopy and color selectivity in human cortical visual area V8. Nature Neurosci. 1998;1:235–241.

108. Bartels A, Zeki S. The architecture of the colour centre in the human visual brain: new results and a review. Eur J Neurosci. 2000;12:172–193.

109. Gulyás B, Roland P. Cortical fields participating in form and colour discrimination in the human brain. Neuroreport. 1991;2:585–588.

110. Gulyás B, Heywood C, Popplewell D, Roland P, Cowey A. Visual form discrimination from color or motion cues: functional anatomy by positron emission tomography. Proc Natl Acad Sci USA. 1994;91:9965–9969.

111. Beauchamp M, Haxby J, Jennings J, DeYoe E. An fMRI version of the Farnsworth-Munsell 100-Hue test reveals multiple color-selective areas in human ventral occipito-temporal cortex. Cereb Cortex. 1999;9:257–263.

112. Merigan W. Human V4? Curr Biol. 1993;3:226–229.

113. Wandell B, Wade A. Functional imaging of the visual pathways. Neurol Clin. 2003; 21:417–444.

114. Beauchamp M, Haxby J, Rosen A, DeYoe E. A functional MRI case study of acquired cerebral dyschromatopsia. Neuropsychologia. 2000;38:1170–1179.

115. Ogden JA. Visual object agnosia, prosopagnosia, achromatopsia, loss of visual imagery, and autobiographical amnesia following recovery from cortical blindness: case M.H. Neuropsychologia. 1993;31:571.
116. Holmes G. Pure word blindness. Folia Psychiatr Neurol Neurochir Neerl. 1950;53:279.
117. Geschwind N, Fusillo M. Color-naming defects in association with alexia. Arch Neurol. 1966;15:137–146.
118. Oxbury JM, Oxbury SM, Humphrey NK. Varieties of colour anomia. Brain. 1969;92:847.
119. de Vreese LP. Two systems for color-naming defects: verbal disconnection versus colour imagery disorder. Neuropsychologia. 1991;29:1.
120. Kinsbourne M, Warrington EK. Observations on colour agnosia. J Neurol Neurosurg Psychiatry. 1964;27:296.
121. Luzzatti C, Davidoff J. Impaired retrieval of object-color knowledge with preserved color naming. Neuropsychologia. 1994;32:933–950.
122. Miceli G, Fouch E, Capasso R, Shelton J, Tomaiuolo F, Caramazza A. The dissociation of color from form and function knowledge. Nat Neurosci. 2001;4:662–667.
123. Nijboer TC, van Zandvoort MJ, de Haan EH. A familial factor in the development of colour agnosia. Neuropsychologia. 2007;45(8):1961–1965.
124. Farah M. Visual Agnosia: disorders of visual recognition and what they tell us about normal vision. Cambridge: MIT Press; 1990.
125. Riddoch M, Humphreys G. Visual agnosia. Neurol Clinics. 2003;21:501–520.
126. Lissauer H. Einfall von Seelenblindheit nebst einem Bintrag zur Theorie derselben. Arch Psychiatr Nervenkr. 1890;2:22.
127. Teuber HL. Alteration of perception and memory in man. In: Weiskrantz L (ed.), Analysis of Behavioral Change. New York: Harper & Row; 1968.
128. Humphreys GW, Riddoch MJ, Donnelly N, Freeman T, Boucart M, Müller HM. Intermediate visual processing and visual agnosia. In: Farah M, Ratcliff G (eds), The neuropsychology of high-level vision. Hillsdale, New Jersey: Lawrence Erlbaum Associates; 1994. pp. 63–101.
129. Humphreys GW, Riddoch MJ. To see but not to see: a case study of visual agnosia. London: Lawrence Erlbaum Associates; 1987.
130. Farah MJ. Visual agnosia: once more, with theory. Cogn Neuropsychol. 1988;5(3):337–346.
131. Farah MJ. Visual agnosia. 2nd ed. Cambridge: MIT Press; 2004.
132. Efron R. What is perception? Boston Studies Philosoph Sci. 1968;4:137–173.
133. Milner AD, Perrett DI, Johnston RS, Benson PJ, Jordan TR, Heeley DW, et al. Perception and action in "visual form agnosia". Brain. 1991;114 (Pt 1B):405–428.
134. Davidoff J, Warrington EK. A dissociation of shape discrimination and figure-ground perception in a patient with normal acuity. Neuropsychologia. 1993;31(1):83–93.
135. Adler A. Disintegration and restoration of optic recognition in visual agnosia: analysis of a case. Arch Neurol Psychiatr. 1944;51:243–259.
136. Landis T, Graves R, Benson DF, Hebben N. Visual recognition through kinaesthetic mediation. Psychol Med. 1982;12(3):515–531.
137. Chainey H, Humphreys GK. The real-object advantage in agnosia: evidence for a role of surface and depth information in object recognition. Cogn Neuropsychol. 2001;18:175–191.
138. Goodale MA, Milner AD, Jakobson LS, Carey DP. A neurological dissociation between perceiving objects and grasping them. Nature. 1991;349(6305):154–156.
139. James TW, Culham J, Humphrey GK, Milner AD, Goodale MA. Ventral occipital lesions impair object recognition but not object-directed grasping: an fMRI study. Brain. 2003;126(Pt 11):2463–2475.
140. Ferreira CT, Ceccaldi M, Giusiano B, Poncet M. Separate visual pathways for perception of actions and objects: evidence from a case of apperceptive agnosia. J Neurol Neurosurg Psychiatry. 1998;65(3):382–385.
141. Campion J, Latto R. Apperceptive agnosia due to carbon monoxide poisoning. An interpretation based on critical band masking from disseminated lesions. Behavioural Brain Res. 1985;15:227–240.
142. Vecera SP, Gilds KS. What is it like to be a patient with apperceptive agnosia? Conscious Cogn. 1997;6(2–3):237–266.
143. Vecera SP, Gilds KS. What processing is impaired in apperceptive agnosia? Evidence from normal subjects. J Cogn Neurosci. 1998;10(5):568–580.
144. Abrams RA, Law MB. Random visual noise impairs object-based attention. Exp Brain Res. 2002;142(3):349–353.
145. Behrmann M, Kimchi R. What does visual agnosia tell us about perceptual organization and its relationship to object perception? J Exp Psychol Hum Percept Perform. 2003;29:19–42.
146. Adler A. Course and outcome of visual agnosia. J Nervous Ment Dis. 1950;111:41–51.
147. Benson D, Greenberg J. Visual form agnosia. Arch Neurol. 1969;20:82–89.
148. Riddoch M, Humphreys G. A case of integrative visual agnosia. Brain. 1987;110:1431–1462.
149. Shelton PA, Bowers D, Duara R, Heilman KM. Apperceptive visual agnosia: a case study. Brain Cogn. 1994;25(1):1–23.
150. Delvenne JF, Seron X, Coyette F, Rossion B. Evidence for perceptual deficits in associative visual (prosop)agnosia: a single-case study. Neuropsychologia. 2004;42(5):597–612.
151. Grossman M, Galetta S, d'Esposito M. Object recognition difficulty in visual apperceptive agnosia. Brain Cogn. 1997;33:306–402.
152. Warrington EK, James M. Visual object recognition in patients with right-hemisphere lesions: axes or features? Perception. 1986;15(3):355–366.
153. Riddoch MJ, Humphreys GW. Visual object processing in optic aphasia: a case of semantic access agnosia. Cogn Neuropsychol. 1987;4:131–185.
154. Carlesimo GA, Casadio P, Sabbadini M, Caltagirone C. Associative visual agnosia resulting from a disconnection between intact visual memory and semantic systems. Cortex. 1998;34(4):563–576.
155. Caramazza A, Shelton JR. Domain-specific knowledge systems in the brain the animate-inanimate distinction. J Cogn Neurosci. 1998;10(1):1–34.
156. Farah M, McMullen P, Meyer M. can recognition of living things be selectively impaired? Neuropsychologia. 1991;29:185–193.
157. Kurbat MA. Can the recognition of living things really be selectively impaired? Neuropsychologia. 1997;35(6):813–827.
158. Kurbat MA, Farah MJ. Is the category-specific deficit for living things spurious? J Cogn Neurosci. 1998;10(3):355–361.
159. Warrington EK, Shallice T. Category specific semantic impairments. Brain. 1984;107 (Pt 3):829–854.
160. Wolk DA, Coslett HB, Glosser G. The role of sensory-motor information in object recognition: evidence from category-specific visual agnosia. Brain Lang. 2005;94(2):131–146.
161. Thomas R, Forde E. The role of local and global processing in the recognition of living and nonliving things. Neuropsychologia. 2006;44(6):982–986.
162. Humphreys GW. Cascade processes in picture identification. Cogn Neuropsychol. 1988;5:67–103.
163. Feinberg T, Schindler R, Ochoa E, Kwan P, Farah M. Associative visual agnosia and alexia without prosopagnosia. Cortex. 1994;30:395–412.
164. Capitani E, Laiacona M, Pagani R, Capasso R, Zampetti P, Miceli G. Posterior cerebral artery infarcts and semantic category dissociations: a study of 28 patients. Brain. 2009;132(Pt 4):965–981.
165. Giannakopoulos P, Gold G, Duc M, Michel JP, Hof PR, Bouras C. Neuroanatomic correlates of visual agnosia in Alzheimer's disease: a clinicopathologic study. Neurology. 1999;52(1):71–77.
166. Royer J, Blais C, Charbonneau I, Dery K, Tardif J, Duchaine B, et al. Greater reliance on the eye region predicts better face recognition ability. Cognition. 2018;181:12–20.
167. Bodamer J. Prosopagnosie. Arch Psychiatr Nervenkr. 1947;179:6–54.
168. Barton J. Disorders of face perception and recognition. Neurol Clin. 2003;21:521–548.
169. Tranel D, Damasio A. Knowledge without awareness: an autonomic index of facial recognition by prosopagnosics. Science. 1985;228:1453–1454.
170. Young A, Aggleton J, Hellawell D, Johnson M, Broks P, Hanley J. Face processing impairments after amygdalotomy. Brain. 1995;118:15–24.
171. Tejeria L, Harper RA, Artes PH, Dickinson CM. Face recognition in age related macular degeneration: perceived disability, measured disability, and performance with a bioptic device. Br J Ophthalmol. 2002;86(9):1019–1026.
172. Barton J, Cherkasova M, Hefter R, Cox T, O'Connor M, Manoach D. Are patients with social developmental disorders prosopagnosic? Perceptual heterogeneity in the Asperger and socioemotional processing disorders. Brain. 2004;127:1706–1716.
173. Mendez M, Martin R, Smyth K, Whitehouse P. Disturbances of person identification in Alzheimer's disease. A retrospective study. J Nerv Ment Dis. 1992;180:94–96.
174. Roudier M, Marcie P, Grancher A, Tzortzis C, Starkstein S, Boller F. Discrimination of facial identity and of emotions in Alzheimer's disease. J Neurol Sci. 1998;154:151–158.
175. Cronin-Coulomb A, Cronin-Coulomb M, Dunne T, Brown A, Jain K, Cipolloni P, et al. Facial frequency manipulation normalizes face discrimination in AD. Neurology. 2000;54:2316–2318.
176. Janati A. Kluver-Bucy syndrome in Huntington's chorea. J Nerv Ment Dis. 1985;173: 632–635.
177. Dewick H, Hanley J, Davies A, Playfer J, Turnbull C. Perception and memory for faces in Parkinson's disease. Neuropsychologia. 1991;29:785–802.
178. Cousins R, Hanley JR, Davies AD, Turnbull CJ, Playfer JR. Understanding memory for faces in Parkinson's disease: the role of configural processing. Neuropsychologia. 2000;38(6):837–847.
179. Young A, Ellis H. Childhood prosopagnosia. Brain Cogn. 1989;9:16–47.
180. Kracke I. Developmental prosopagnosia in Asperger syndrome: presentation and discussion of an individual case. Dev Med Child Neurol. 1994;36:873–886.
181. de Haan E, Campbell R. A fifteen year follow-up of a case of developmental prosopagnosia. Cortex. 1991;27:489–509.
182. Takahashi N, Kawamura M, Hirayama K, Shiota J, Isono O. Prosopagnosia: a clinical and anatomic study of four patients. Cortex. 1995;31:317–329.
183. Yardley L, McDermott L, Pisarski S, Duchaine B, Nakayama K. Psychosocial consequences of developmental prosopagnosia: a problem of recognition. J Psychosom Res. 2008;65(5):445–451.
184. Dalrymple KA, Fletcher K, Corrow S, das Nair R, Barton JJ, Yonas A, et al. "A room full of strangers every day": the psychosocial impact of developmental prosopagnosia on children and their families. J Psychosom Res. 2014;77(2):144–150.
185. Campbell R, Heywood C, Cowey A, Regard M, Landis T. Sensitivity to eye gaze in prosopagnosic patients and monkeys with superior temporal sulcus ablation. Neuropsychologia. 1990;28:1123–1142.
186. Humphreys K, Avidan G, Behrmann M. A detailed investigation of facial expression processing in congenital prosopagnosia as compared to acquired prosopagnosia. Exp Brain Res. 2007;176(2):356–373.
187. Stephan BC, Breen N, Caine D. The recognition of emotional expression in prosopagnosia: decoding whole and part faces. J Int Neuropsychol Soc. 2006;12(6):884–895.
188. Bruyer R, Laterre C, Seron X, Feyereisen P, Strypstein E, Pierrard E, et al. A case of prosopagnosia with some preserved covert remembrance of familiar faces. Brain Cogn. 1983;2:257–84.
189. Sergent J, Villemure J-G. Prosopagnosia in a right hemispherectomized patient. Brain. 1989;112:975–995.
190. Sergent J, Poncet M. From covert to overt recognition of faces in a prosopagnosic patient. Brain. 1990;113:989–1004.
191. Evans J, Heggs A, Antoun N, Hodges J. Progressive prosopagnosia associated with selective right temporal lobe atrophy. Brain. 1995;118:1–13.
192. Tranel D, Damasio AR, Damasio H. Intact recognition of facial expression, gender, and age in patients with impaired recognition of face identity. Neurology. 1988; 38(5):690–696.
193. Iaria G, Fox CJ, Waite C, Aharon I, Barton JJS. The contribution of the fusiform gyrus and superior temporal sulcus in processing facial attractiveness: Neuropsychological and neuroimaging evidence. Neuroscience. 2008;155:409–422.
194. Perrett D, Hietanen J, Oram M, Benson P. Organization and functions of cells responsive to faces in the temporal cortex. Phil Trans R Soc Lond B. 1992;335:23–30.
195. Gauthier I, Logothetis N. Is face recognition not so unique after all? Cogn Neuropsychol. 2000;17:125–142.

196. Haxby JV, Gobbini MI, Furey ML, Ishai A, Schouten JL, Pietrini P. Distributed and overlapping representations of faces and objects in ventral temporal cortex. Science. 2001;293(5539):2425–2430.
197. Barton JJ, Corrow SL. The problem of being bad at faces. Neuropsychologia. 2016; 89:119–124.
198. Albert M, Butters N, Levin J. Temporal gradients in retrograde amnesia of patients with alcoholic Korsakoff's disease. Arch Neurol. 1979;36:211–216.
199. Barton JJ, Cherkasova M, O'Connor M. Covert recognition in acquired and developmental prosopagnosia. Neurology. 2001;57(7):1161–1168.
200. Warrington E. Warrington recognition memory test. Los Angeles: Western Psychological Services; 1984.
201. Duchaine B, Nakayama K. Dissociations of face and object recognition in developmental prosopagnosia. J Cogn Neurosci. 2005;17:249–261.
202. Kanwisher N. Domain specificity in face perception. Nat Neurosci. 2000;3(8):759–763.
203. Behrmann M, Plaut DC. Distributed circuits, not circumscribed centers, mediate visual recognition. Trends Cogn Sci. 2013;17(5):210–219.
204. Barton JJ, Corrow SL. Selectivity in acquired prosopagnosia: the segregation of divergent and convergent operations. Neuropsychologia. 2016;83:76–87.
205. Geskin J, Behrmann M. Congenital prosopagnosia without object agnosia? A literature review. Cogn Neuropsychol. 2018;35(1–2):4–54.
206. Barton JJS, Albonico A, Susilo T, Duchaine B, Corrow SL. Object recognition in acquired and developmental prosopagnosia. Cogn Neuropsychol. 2019:1–31.
207. Damasio A, Tranel D, Damasio H. Face agnosia and the neural substrates of memory. Ann Rev Neurosci. 1990;13:89–109.
208. Barton JJ, Press DZ, Keenan JP, O'Connor M. Lesions of the fusiform face area impair perception of facial configuration in prosopagnosia. Neurology. 2002;58(1):71–78.
209. Joubert S, Felician O, Barbeau E, Sontheimer A, Barton JJ, Ceccaldi M, et al. Impaired configurational processing in a case of progressive prosopagnosia associated with predominant right temporal lobe atrophy. Brain. 2003;126(Pt 11):2537–2550.
210. Bukach CM, Bub DN, Gauthier I, Tarr MJ. Perceptual expertise effects are not all or none: spatially limited perceptual expertise for faces in a case of prosopagnosia. J Cogn Neurosci. 2006;18(1):48–63.
211. Caldara R, Schyns P, Mayer E, Smith M, Gosselin F, Rossion B. Does prosopagnosia take the eyes out of face representations? Evidence for a defect in representing diagnostic facial information following brain damage. J Cogn Neurosci. 2005;17(10):1652–1666.
212. Bukach CM, Le Grand R, Kaiser MD, Bub DN, Tanaka JW. Preservation of mouth region processing in two cases of prosopagnosia. J Neuropsychol. 2008;2(Pt 1):227–244.
213. Barton JJS. Structure and function in acquired prosospagnosia: lessons from a series of ten patients with brain damage.. J Neuropsychology. 2008;2:197–225.
214. Schyns P, Bonnar L, Gosselin F. Show me the features! Understanding recognition from the use of visual information. Psychol Sci. 2002;13:402–409.
215. de Renzi E, Faglioni P, Grossi D, Nichelli P. Apperceptive and associative forms of prosopagnosia. Cortex. 1991;27:213–221.
216. Fox CJ, Iaria G, Barton JJ. Disconnection in prosopagnosia and face processing. Cortex. 2008;44(8):996–1009.
217. Barton JJ, Cherkasova M. Face imagery and its relation to perception and covert recognition in prosopagnosia. Neurology. 2003;61(2):220–225.
218. Meadows J. The anatomical basis of prosopagnosia. J Neurol Neurosurg Psychiatry. 1974;37:489–501.
219. Damasio A, Damasio H, van Hoessen G. Prosopagnosia: anatomic basis and behavioral mechanisms. Neurology. 1982;32:331–341.
220. Landis T, Cummings J, Christen L, Bogen J, Imhof H-G. Are unilateral right posterior lesions sufficient to cause prosopagnosia? Clinical and radiological findings in six additional patients. Cortex. 1986;22:243–252.
221. de Renzi E. Prosopagnosia in two patients with CT scan evidence of damage confined to the right hemisphere. Neuropsychologia. 1986;24:385–389.
222. Michel F, Perenin M-T, Sieroff E. Prosopagnosie sans hémianopsie après lésion unilatérale occipito-temporale droite. Rev Neurol. 1986;142:545–549.
223. Schweinberger S, Klos T, Sommer W. Covert face recognition in prosopagnosia: a dissociable function? Cortex. 1995;31:517–529.
224. Rossion B, Caldara R, Seghier M, Schuller AM, Lazeyras F, Mayer E. A network of occipito-temporal face-sensitive areas besides the right middle fusiform gyrus is necessary for normal face processing. Brain. 2003;126(Pt 11):2381–2395.
225. Schiltz C, Sorger B, Caldara R, Ahmed F, Mayer E, Goebel R, et al. Impaired face discrimination in acquired prosopagnosia is associated with abnormal response to individual faces in the right middle fusiform gyrus. Cereb Cortex. 2006;16(4):574–586.
226. McCarthy G, Puce A, Gore J, Allison T. Face-specific processing in the human fusiform gyrus. J Cogn Neurosci. 1997;9:605–610.
227. Kanwisher N, McDermott J, Chun M. The fusiform face area: a module in human extrastriate cortex specialized for face perception. J Neurosci. 1997;17:4302–4311.
228. Haxby J, Hoffman E, Gobbini M. The distributed human neural system for face perception. Trends Cogn Sci. 2000;4:223–233.
229. Barton JJ, Zhao J, Keenan JP. Perception of global facial geometry in the inversion effect and prosopagnosia. Neuropsychologia. 2003;41(12):1703–1711.
230. Rajimehr R, Young JC, Tootell RB. An anterior temporal face patch in human cortex, predicted by macaque maps. Proc Natl Acad Sci U S A. 2009;106(6):1995–2000.
231. Kriegeskorte N, Formisano E, Sorger B, Goebel R. Individual faces elicit distinct response patterns in human anterior temporal cortex. Proc Natl Acad Sci U S A. 2007;104(51):20600–20605.
232. Mattson AJ, Levin HS, Grafman J. A case of prosopagnosia following moderate closed head injury with left hemisphere focal lesion. Cortex. 2000;36(1):125–137.
233. Barton JJ. Prosopagnosia associated with a left occipitotemporal lesion. Neuropsychologia. 2008;46(8):2214–2224.
234. Susilo T, Duchaine B. Advances in developmental prosopagnosia research. Curr Opin Neurobiol. 2013;23(3):423–429.
235. Bowles DC, McKone E, Dawel A, Duchaine B, Palermo R, Schmalzl L, et al. Diagnosing prosopagnosia: effects of ageing, sex, and participant-stimulus ethnic match on the Cambridge Face Memory Test and Cambridge Face Perception Test. Cogn Neuropsychol. 2009;26(5):423–455.
236. Levine D, Warach J, Farah M. Two visual systems in mental imagery: dissociation of "what" and "where" in imagery disorders due to bilateral posterior cerebral lesions. Neurology. 1985;35:1010–1018.
237. Rizzo M, Hurtig R, Damasio A. The role of scanpaths in facial recognition and learning. Ann Neurol. 1987;22:41–45.
238. Barton J, Cherkasova M, Press D, Intriligator J, O'Connor M. Perceptual function in prosopagnosia. Perception. 2004;33(8):939–956.
239. Bauer R, Verfaellie M. Electrodermal discrimination of familiar but not unfamiliar faces in prosopagnosia. Brain Cogn. 1988;8:240–252.
240. Liu RR, Pancaroglu R, Hills CS, Duchaine B, Barton JJ. Voice recognition in face-blind patients. Cereb Cortex. 2016;26(4):1473–1487.
241. Paquette S, Li HC, Corrow SL, Buss SS, Barton JJS, Schlaug G. Developmental perceptual impairments: cases when tone-deafness and prosopagnosia co-occur. Front Hum Neurosci. 2018;12:438.
242. Corrow SL, Stubbs JL, Schlaug G, Buss S, Paquette S, Duchaine B, et al. Perception of musical pitch in developmental prosopagnosia. Neuropsychologia. 2019;124:87–97.
243. DeGutis JM, Chiu C, Grosso ME, Cohan S. Face processing improvements in prosopagnosia: successes and failures over the last 50 years. Front Hum Neurosci. 2014;8:561.
244. Bate S, Bennetts RJ. The rehabilitation of face recognition impairments: a critical review and future directions. Front Hum Neurosci. 2014;8:491.
245. Davies-Thompson J, Fletcher K, Hills C, Pancaroglu R, Corrow SL, Barton JJ. Perceptual learning of faces: a rehabilitative study of acquired prosopagnosia. J Cogn Neurosci. 2017;29(3):573–591.
246. DeGutis J, Cohan S, Nakayama K. Holistic face training enhances face processing in developmental prosopagnosia. Brain. 2014;137(Pt 6):1781–1798.
247. Ellis H, Young A, Critchley E. Loss of memory for people following temporal lobe damage. Brain. 1989;1989:1469–1483.
248. Hanley J, Young A, Pearson N. Defective recognition of familiar people. Cogn Neuropsychol. 1989;6:179–210.
249. Gainotti G, Ferraccioli M, Quaranta D, Marra C. Cross-modal recognition disorders for persons and other unique entities in a patient with right fronto-temporal degeneration. Cortex. 2008;44(3):238–248.
250. Young A, Newcombe F, de Haan E, Small M, Hay D. Face perception after brain injury. Brain. 1993;116:941–959.
251. Fox CJ, Iaria G, Duchaine BC, Barton JJS. Behavioral and fMRI studies of identity and expression perception in acquired prosopagnosia. J Vision. 2008;8(6):708.
252. Campbell R, Landis T, Regard M. Face recognition and lipreading. A neurological dissociation. Brain. 1986;109:509–521.
253. Campbell R, Garwood J, Franklin S, Howard D, Landis T, Regard M. Neuropsychological studies of auditory-visual fusion illusions. Four case studies and their implications. Neuropsychologia. 1990;28(8):787–802.
254. Albonico A, Barton JJS. Face perception in pure alexia: complementary contributions of the left fusiform gyrus to facial identity and facial speech processing. Vision Sciences Society; St. Petersburg Beach; 2017.
255. Young A, Flude B, Hay D, Ellis A. Impaired discrimination of familiar from unfamiliar faces. Cortex. 1993;29:65–75.
256. Rapcsak S, Polster M, Comer J, Rubens A. False recognition and misidentification of faces following right hemisphere damage. Cortex. 1994;30:565–583.
257. Rapcsak SZ, Nielsen L, Littrell LD, Glisky EL, Kaszniak AW, Laguna JF. Face memory impairments in patients with frontal lobe damage. Neurology. 2001;57(7):1168–1175.
258. Rapcsak S, Polster M, Glisky M, Comer J. False recognition of unfamiliar faces following right hemisphere damage: neuropsychological and anatomical observations. Cortex. 1996;32:593–611.
259. Bjornstrom LE, Hills C, Hanif H, Barton JJ. Visual word expertise: a study of inversion and the word-length effect, with perceptual transforms. Perception. 2014;43(5):438–450.
260. Rodriguez AR, Barton JJ. The 20/20 patient who can't read. Can J Ophthalmol. 2015;50(4):257–264.
261. Husain M, Stein J. Rezsö Bálint and his most celebrated case. Arch Neurol. 1988;45: 89–93.
262. Holmes G. Disturbances of visual orientation. Brit J Ophthalmol. 1918;2:449–468, 506–516.
263. Pierrot-Deseilligny C, Gray F, Brunet P. Infarcts of both inferior parietal lobules with impairment of visually guided eye movements, peripheral inattention and optic ataxia. Brain. 1986;109:81–97.
264. Baylis G, Driver J, Baylis L, Rafal R. Reading of letters and words in a patient with Balint's syndrome. Neuropsychologia. 1994;32:1273–1286.
265. Friedman D, Jankovic J, McCrary J. Neuro-ophthalmic findings in progressive supranuclear palsy. J Clin Neuro-ophthalmol. 1992;12:104–109.
266. Kirkham T. The ocular symptomology of pituitary tumors. Proc Roy Soc Med. 1972;65:517–518.
267. Black S, Behrmann M. Localization in alexia. Localization and neuroimaging in neuropsychology. Academic Press; 1994. pp. 331–376.
268. Rapcsak SZ, Beeson PM. The role of left posterior inferior temporal cortex in spelling. Neurology. 2004;62(12):2221–2229.
269. Sheldon CA, Malcolm GL, Barton JJ. Alexia with and without agraphia: an assessment of two classical syndromes. Can J Neurol Sci. 2008;35(5):616–624.
270. Binder J, Mohr J. The topography of callosal reading pathways. A case control analysis. Brain. 1992;115:1807–1826.
271. Starrfelt R, Behrmann M. Number reading in pure alexia – a review. Neuropsychologia. 2011;49(9):2283–2298.
272. Horikoshi T, Asari Y, Watanabe A, Nagaseki Y, Nukui H, Sasaki H, et al. Music alexia in a patient with mild pure alexia: disturbed visual perception of non-verbal meaningful figures. Cortex. 1997;33:187–194.

273. Beversdorf D, Heilman K. Progressive ventral posterior cortical degeneration presenting as alexia for music and words. Neurology. 1998;50:657–659.
274. Bub D, Black S, Howell J. Word recognition and orthographic context effects in a letter-by-letter reader. Brain Lang. 1989;36:357–376.
275. Coslett H, Saffran E, Greenbaum S, Schwartz H. Reading in pure alexia. Brain. 1993;116:21–37.
276. Barton JJ, Hanif HM, Eklinder Bjornstrom L, Hills C. The word-length effect in reading: a review. Cogn Neuropsychol. 2014;31(5–6):378–412.
277. Dejerine J. Contributions a l'étude anatomopathologique et clinique des differentes varietes de cecite verbale. Memoires de la Societé Biologique. 1892;44:61–90.
278. Damasio A, Damasio H. The anatomic basis of pure alexia. Neurology. 1983; 33:1573–1583.
279. Lanzinger S, Weder B, Oettli R, Fretz C. Neuroimaging findings in a patient recovering from global alexia to spelling dyslexia. J Neuroimaging. 1999;9:48–51.
280. Greenblatt S. Alexia without agraphia or hemianopia. Brain. 1973;96:307–316.
281. Vincent F, Sadowsky C, Saunders R, Reeves A. Alexia without agraphia, hemianopia, or color-naming defect: a disconnection syndrome. Neurology. 1977;27:689–691.
282. Erdem S, Kansu T. Alexia without either agraphia or hemianopia in temporal lobe lesion due to herpes simplex encephalitis. J Neuro-ophthalmol. 1995;15:102–104.
283. Silver F, Chawluk J, Bosley T, Rosen M, Dann R, Sergott R, et al. Resolving metabolic abnormalities in a case of pure alexia. Neurology. 1988;38:731–735.
284. Stommel E, Friedman R, Reeves A. Alexia without agraphia associated with spleniogeniculate infarction. Neurology. 1991;41:587–588.
285. Mao-Draayer Y, Panitch H. Alexia without agraphia in multiple sclerosis: case report with magnetic resonance imaging localization. Mult Scler. 2004;10(6):705–707.
286. Kleinschmidt A, Cohen L. The neural bases of prosopagnosia and pure alexia: recent insights from functional neuroimaging. Curr Opin Neurol. 2006;19(4):386–391.
287. Leff AP, Spitsyna G, Plant GT, Wise RJ. Structural anatomy of pure and hemianopic alexia. J Neurol Neurosurg Psychiatry. 2006;77(9):1004–1007.
288. McCandliss BD, Cohen L, Dehaene S. The visual word form area: expertise for reading in the fusiform gyrus. Trends Cogn Sci 2003;7:293–299.
289. Molko N, Cohen L, Mangin J, Chochon F, Lehericy S, Le Bihan D, et al. Visualizing the neural bases of a disconnection syndrome with diffusion tensor imaging. J Cogn Neurosci. 2002;14:629–636.
290. Gaillard R, Naccache L, Pinel P, Clemenceau S, Volle E, Hasboun D, et al. Direct intracranial, FMRI, and lesion evidence for the causal role of left inferotemporal cortex in reading. Neuron. 2006;50(2):191–204.
291. Epelbaum S, Pinel P, Gaillard R, Delmaire C, Perrin M, Dupont S, et al. Pure alexia as a disconnection syndrome: new diffusion imaging evidence for an old concept. Cortex. 2008;44:962–974.
292. Martin A. Shades of Dejerine – forging a causal link between the visual word form area and reading. Neuron. 2006;50:173–175.
293. Price CJ, Devlin JT. The myth of the visual word form area. Neuroimage. 2003;19:473–481.
294. Reinke K, Fernandes M, Schwindt G, O'Craven K, Grady CL. Functional specificity of the visual word form area: general activation for words and symbols but specific network activation for words. Brain Lang. 2008;104(2):180–189.
295. Warrington E, Shallice T. Word-form dyslexia. Brain. 1980;103:99–112.
296. Cohen L, Dehaene S. Specialization within the ventral stream: the case for the visual word form area. Neuroimage. 2004;22(1):466–476.
297. Farah MJ, Wallace MA. Pure alexia as a visual impairment: a reconsideration. Cogn Neuropsychol. 1991;8:313–334.
298. Behrmann M, Nelson J, Sekuler A. Visual complexity in letter-by-letter reading: "pure" alexia is not pure. Neuropsychologia. 1998;36:1115–1132.
299. Rentschler I, Treutwein B, Landis T. Dissociation of local and global processing in visual agnosia. Vision Res. 1994;34:963–971.
300. Ingles JL, Eskes GA. A comparison of letter and digit processing in letter-by-letter reading. J Int Neuropsychol Soc. 2008;14(1):164–173.
301. Starrfelt R, Habekost T, Leff AP. Too little, too late: reduced visual span and speed characterize pure alexia. Cereb Cortex. 2009;19(12):2880–2890.
302. Lepore F. Visual deficits in alexia without agraphia. Neuro-ophthalmol. 1998;19:1–6.
303. de Renzi E, Zambolin A, Crisi G. The pattern of neuropsychological impairment associated with left posterior cerebral artery infarcts. Brain. 1987;110:1099–1016.
304. Lesniak M, Soluch P, Stepien U, Czepiel W, Seniow J. Pure alexia after damage to the right fusiform gyrus in a right-handed male. Neurol Neurochir Pol. 2014;48(5):373–377.
305. Robinson JS, Collins RL, Mukhi SV. Alexia without agraphia in a right-handed individual following right occipital stroke. Appl Neuropsychol Adult. 2016;23(1):65–69.
306. Henry C, Gaillard R, Volle E, Chiras J, Ferrieux S, Dehaene S, et al. Brain activations during letter-by-letter reading: a follow-up study. Neuropsychologia. 2005; 43(14):1983–1989.
307. Ino T, Tokumoto K, Usami K, Kimura T, Hashimoto Y, Fukuyama H. Longitudinal fMRI study of reading in a patient with letter-by-letter reading. Cortex. 2008;44(7):773–781.
308. Cohen L, Dehaene S, McCormick S, Durant S, Zanker JM. Brain mechanisms of recovery from pure alexia: a single case study with multiple longitudinal scans. Neuropsychologia. 2016;91:36–49.
309. Leff AP, Behrmann M. Treatment of reading impairment after stroke. Curr Opin Neurol. 2008;21(6):644–648.
310. Starrfelt R, Olafsdottir RR, Arendt IM. Rehabilitation of pure alexia: a review. Neuropsychol Rehabil. 2013;23(5):755–779.
311. Beeson P, Insalaco D. Acquired alexia: lessons from successful treatment. J Int Neuropsychol Soc. 1998;4:621–635.
312. Maher L, Clayton M, Barrett A, Schober-Peterson D, Rothi L. Rehabilitation of a case of pure alexia: exploiting residual reading abilities. J Int Neuropsychol Soc. 1998;4:636–647.
313. Conway T, Heilman P, Rothi L, Alexander A, Adair J, Crosson B, et al. Treatment of a case of phonological alexia with agraphia using the Auditory Discrimination in Depth (ADD) program. J Int Neuropsychol Soc. 1998;4:608–620.
314. Kim ES, Rising K, Rapcsak SZ, Beeson PM. Treatment for alexia with agraphia following left ventral occipito-temporal damage: strengthening orthographic representations common to reading and spelling. J Speech Lang Hear Res. 2015;58(5):1521–1537.
315. Nitzberg Lott S, Friedman R. can treatment for pure alexia improve letter-by-letter reading speed without sacrificing accuracy? Brain Lang. 1999;67:188–201.
316. Gazzaniga M, Freedman H. Observations on visual processes after posterior callosal section. Neurology. 1973;23:1126–1130.
317. Castro-Caldas A, Salgado V. Right hemifield alexia without hemianopia. Arch Neurol. 1984;41:84–87.
318. Cohen L, Dehaene S, Naccache L, Lehericy S, Dehaene-Lambertz G, Henaff MA, et al. The visual word form area: spatial and temporal characterization of an initial stage of reading in normal subjects and posterior split-brain patients. Brain. 2000;123 (Pt 2):291–307.
319. Glosser G, Friedman RB. The continuum of deep/phonological alexia. Cortex. 1990; 26(3):343–359.
320. Paquier PF, De Smet HJ, Marien P, Poznanski N, Van Bogaert P. Acquired alexia with agraphia syndrome in childhood. J Child Neurol. 2006;21(4):324–330.
321. Benson D. Alexia. In: Bruyn G, Klawans H, Vinken P (eds), Handbook of clinical neurology. New York: Elsevier; 1985. pp. 433–455.
322. Kawahata N, Nagata K. Alexia with agraphia due to the left posterior inferiortemporal lobe lesion – neuropsychological analysis and its pathogenetic mechanisms. Brain Lang. 1988;33:296–310.
323. Hux K, Mahrt T. Alexia and agraphia intervention following traumatic brain injury: a single case study. Am J Speech Lang Pathol. 2019:1–15.
324. Behrmann M, Moscovitch M, Black S, Mozer M. Perceptual and conceptual factors in neglect dyslexia: two contrasting case studies. Brain. 1990;113:1163–1183.
325. Patterson K, Wilson B. A rose is a nose: a deficit in initial letter identification. Cogn Neuropsychology. 1990;13:447–478.
326. Beauvois M, Dérouesné J. Phonological alexia: three dissociations. J Neurol Neurosurg Psychiatry. 1979;42:1115–1124.
327. Funnell E. Phonological processes in reading: new evidence from acquired dyslexia. Brit J Psychol. 1983;74:159–180.
328. Friedman R, Kohn S. Impaired activation of the phonological lexicon: effects upon oral reading. Brain Lang. 1990;38:278–297.
329. Friedman R. Two types of phonological alexia. Cortex. 1995;31:397–403.
330. Shallice T, Warrington E, McCarthy R. Reading without semantics. Quart J Exp Psychol. 1983;35A:111–138.
331. Patterson K, Morton J. From orthograph to phonology: an attempt at an old interpretation. In: Patterson K, Marshall J, Coltheart M (eds), Surface dyslexia. London: Erlbaum Associates; 1985. pp. 335–359.
332. Cummings J, Houlihan J, Hill M. The pattern of reading deterioration in dementia of the Alzheimer type. Brain Lang. 1986;29:315–323.
333. Friedman R, Ferguson S, Robinson S, Sunderland T. Dissociation of mechanisms of reading in Alzheimer's disease. Brain Lang. 1992;43:400–413.
334. Coltheart M. Deep dyslexia, a review of the syndrome. In: Coltheart M, Patterson K, Marshall J (eds), Deep dyslexia. London: Routledge & Kegan Paul; 1980. pp. 22–47.
335. Aguirre G, D'Esposito M. Topographical disorientation: a synthesis and taxonomy. Brain. 1999;122:1613–1628.
336. Takahashi N, Kawamura M. Pure topographical disorientation – the anatomical basis of landmark agnosia. Cortex. 2002;38(5):717–725.
337. Pai M. Topographic disorientation: two cases. J Formos Med Assoc. 1997;96:660–663.
338. McCarthy R, Evans J, Hodges J. Topographic amnesia: spatial memory disorder, perceptual dysfunction, or category specific semantic memory impairment? J Neurol Neurosurg Psychiatry. 1996;60:318–325.
339. Malone D, Morris H, Kay M, Levin H. Prosopagnosia: a double dissociation between the recognition of familiar and unfamiliar faces. J Neurol Neurosurg Psychiatry. 1982;45: 820–822.
340. Bauer R. Autonomic recognition of names and faces in prosopagnosia: a neuropsychological application of the guilty knowledge test. Neuropsychologia. 1984;22:457–469.
341. Corrow JC, Corrow SL, Lee E, Pancaroglu R, Burles F, Duchaine B, et al. Getting lost: topographic skills in acquired and developmental prosopagnosia. Cortex. 2016;76:89–103.
342. O'Craven KM, Kanwisher N. Mental imagery of faces and places activates corresponding stimulus-specific brain regions. J Cogn Neurosci. 2000;12(6):1013–1023.
343. Iaria G, Chen JK, Guariglia C, Ptito A, Petrides M. Retrosplenial and hippocampal brain regions in human navigation: complementary functional contributions to the formation and use of cognitive maps. Eur J Neurosci. 2007;25(3):890–899.
344. Iaria G, Bogod N, Fox CJ, Barton JJ. Developmental topographical disorientation: case one. Neuropsychologia. 2009;47(1):30–40.
345. de Renzi E, Faglioni P, Villa P. Topographical amnesia. J Neurol Neurosurg Psychiatry. 1977;40:498–505.
346. Takahashi N, Kawamura M, Shiota J, Kasahata N, Hirayama K. Pure topographic disorientation due to right retrosplenial lesion. Neurology. 1997;49:464–469.
347. Habib M, Sirigu A. Pure topographical disorientation: a definition and anatomical basis. Cortex. 1987;23:73–85.
348. Zihl J, von Cramon D, Mai N. Selective disturbance of movement vision after bilateral brain damage. Brain. 1983;106:313–340.
349. Zihl J, von Cramon D, Mai N, Schmid C. Disturbance of movement vision after bilateral posterior brain damage. Further evidence and follow-up observations. Brain. 1991;114:2235–2252.
350. Hess R, Baker CJ, Zihl J. The "motion-blind" patient: low-level spatial and temporal filters. J Neurosci. 1989;9:1628–1640.
351. Baker CJ, Hess R, Zihl J. Residual motion perception in a "motion-blind" patient, assessed with limited-lifetime random dot stimuli. J Neurosci. 1991;11:454–461.
352. Rizzo M, Nawrot M, Zihl J. Motion and shape perception in cerebral akinetopsia. Brain. 1995;118:1105–1127.

353. Marcar V, Zihl J, Cowey A. Comparing the visual deficits of a motion blind patient with the visual deficits of monkeys with area MT removed. Neuropsychologia. 1997;35:1459–1465.

354. Campbell R, Zihl J, Massaro D, Munhall K, Cohen M. Speechreading in the akinetopsic patient, L.M. Brain. 1997;120:1793–1803.

355. McLeod P, Heywood C, Driver J, Zihl J. Selective deficit of visual search in moving displays after extrastriate damage. Nature. 1989;339:466–467.

356. Shipp S, de Jong B, Zihl J, Frackowiak R, Zeki S. The brain activity related to residual motion vision in a patient with bilateral lesions of V5. Brain. 1994;117:1023–1038.

357. Barton J, Sharpe J, Raymond J. Directional defects in pursuit and motion perception in humans with unilateral cerebral lesions. Brain. 1996;119:1535–1550.

358. Vaina L. Functional segregation of color and motion processing in the human visual cortex: clinical evidence. Cereb Cortex. 1994;5:555–572.

359. Clarke S, Miklossy J. Occipital cortex in man: organization of callosal connections, related myelo- and cytoarchitecture, and putative boundaries of functional visual areas. J Comp Neurol. 1990;298:188–214.

360. Tootell R, Taylor J. Anatomical evidence for MT and additional cortical visual areas in humans. Cereb Cortex. 1995;5:39–55.

361. Watson J, Myers R, Frackowiak R, Hajnal J, Woods R, Mazziotta J, et al. Area V5 of the human brain: evidence from a combined study using positron emission tomography and magnetic resonance imaging. Cereb Cortex. 1993;3:79–94.

362. Barton J, Simpson T, Kiriakopoulos E, Stewart C, Guthrie B, Wood M, et al. Functional magnetic resonance imaging of lateral occipitotemporal cortex during pursuit and motion perception. Ann Neurol. 1996;40:387–398.

363. Zeki S. Cerebral akinetopsia (visual motion blindness). A review. Brain. 1991;114:811–824.

364. Vaina L, Cowey A. Impairment of the perception of second order motion but not first order motion in a patient with unilateral focal brain damage. Proc R Soc Lond B. 1996;263:1225–1232.

365. Vaina L, Makris N, Kennedy D, Cowey A. The selective impairment of the perception of first-order motion by unilateral cortical brain damage. Vis Neurosci. 1998;15:333–348.

366. Plant G, Laxer K, Barbaro N, Schiffman J, Nakayama K. Impaired visual motion perception in the contralateral hemifield following unilateral posterior cerebral lesions in humans. Brain. 1993;116:1303–1335.

367. Greenlee M, Lang H, Mergner T, Seeger W. Visual short-term memory of stimulus velocity in patients with unilateral posterior brain damage. J Neurosci. 1995;15:2287–2300.

368. Barton J, Sharpe J, Raymond J. Retinotopic and directional defects in motion discrimination in humans with cerebral lesions. Ann Neurol. 1995;37:665–675.

369. Braun D, Petersen D, Schonle P, Fahle M. Deficits and recovery of first- and second-order motion perception in patients with unilateral cortical lesions. Eur J Neurosci. 1998;10:2117–2128.

370. Barton J, Sharpe J. Ocular tracking of step-ramp targets by patients with unilateral cerebral lesions. Brain. 1998;121:1165–1183.

371. Yamasaki D, Wurtz R. Recovery of function after lesions in the superior temporal sulcus in the monkey. J Neurophysiol. 1991;66:651–673.

372. Batelli L, Cavanagh P, Intriligator J, Tramo M, Hénaff M-A, Michèl F, et al. Unilateral right parietal brain damage leads to bilateral deficit for high-level motion. Neuron. 2001;32:985–995.

373. Batelli L, Cavanagh P, Martini P, Barton J. Bilateral deficits of transient visual attention in right parietal patients. Brain. 2003;126:2164–2174.

374. Vaina LM, Gross CG. Perceptual deficits in patients with impaired recognition of biological motion after temporal lobe lesions. Proc Natl Acad Sci U S A. 2004; 101(48):16947–16951.

375. Bálint R. Seelenlahmung des "Schauens", optische Ataxie, räumliche Storung der Aufmerksamkeit. Monatschrift für Psychiatrie und Neurologie. 1909;25:51–181.

376. Hécaen H, de Ajuriaguerra J. Bálint's syndrome (psychic paralysis of visual fixation) and its minor forms. Brain. 1954;77:373–400.

377. Mackworth NH. The breakdown of vigilance during prolonged visual search. Q J Exp Psychol. 1948;1:6–121.

378. Mackworth NH, Kaplan IT, Matlay W. Eye movements during vigilance. Percept Mot Skills. 1964;18:397–402.

379. Broadbent DE. Perception and communication. New York: Pergamon Press; 1958.

380. Luria AR. Disorders of simultaneous perception in a case of bilateral occipito-parietal brain injury. Brain. 1959;82:437–449.

381. Demeyere N, Rzeskiewicz A, Humphreys KA, Humphreys GW. Automatic statistical processing of visual properties in simultanagnosia. Neuropsychologia. 2008;46(11): 2861–2864.

382. Goodglass H, Kaplan E. The assessment of aphasia and related disorders. 2nd ed. Philadelphia: Lea and Febiger; 1983.

383. Coslett H, Saffran E. Simultanagnosia. To see but not two see. Brain. 1991;114:1523–1545.

384. Rizzo M, Robin DA. Simultanagnosia: a defect of sustained attention yields insights on visual information processing. Neurology. 1990;40:447–455.

385. Coslett HB, Lie E. Simultanagnosia: effects of semantic category and repetition blindness. Neuropsychologia. 2008;46(7):1853–1863.

386. Huberle E, Karnath HO. Global shape recognition is modulated by the spatial distance of local elements – evidence from simultanagnosia. Neuropsychologia. 2006;44(6):905–911.

387. Shalev L, Mevorach C, Humphreys GW. Local capture in Balint's syndrome: effects of grouping and item familiarity. Cogn Neuropsychol. 2007;24(1):115–127.

388. Dalrymple KA, Kingstone A, Barton JJ. Seeing trees OR seeing forests in simultanagnosia: attentional capture can be local or global. Neuropsychologia. 2007;45(4):871–875.

389. Montoro PR, Luna D, Humphreys GW. Density, connectedness and attentional capture in hierarchical patterns: evidence from simultanagnosia. Cortex. 2011;47(6):706–714.

390. Chechlacz M, Rotshtein P, Hansen PC, Riddoch JM, Deb S, Humphreys GW. The neural underpinings of simultanagnosia: disconnecting the visuospatial attention network. J Cogn Neurosci. 2012;24(3):718–735.

391. Luria AR, Pravdina-Vinarskaya EN, Yarbus AL. Disturbances of ocular movement in a case of simultanagnosia. Brain. 1962;86:219–228.

392. Holmes G. Disturbances of vision caused by cerebral lesions. Brit J Ophthalmol. 1918;2:353–384.

393. Blangero A, Ota H, Delporte L, Revol P, Vindras P, Rode G, et al. Optic ataxia is not only "optic": impaired spatial integration of proprioceptive information. Neuroimage. 2007;36 (2):T61–T68.

394. Castaigne P, Rondot P, Dumas J, Tempier P. Ataxie optique localisee au cote gauche dans les deux hemichamps visuels homonymes gauches. Rev Neurol (Paris). 1975;131:23–28.

395. Perenin M, Vighetto A. Optic ataxia: a specific disruption in visuomotor mechanisms. I. Different aspects of the deficit in reaching for objects. Brain. 1988;111:643–674.

396. Jakobson L, Archibald Y, Carey D, Goodale M. A kinematic analysis of reaching and grasping movements in a patient recovering from optic ataxia. Neuropsychologia. 1991;29:803–809.

397. Rizzo M, Rotella D, Darling W. Troubled reaching after right occipito-temporal damage. Neuropsychologia. 1992;30:711–722.

398. Bonner-Jackson A, Haut K, Csernansky JG, Barch DM. The influence of encoding strategy on episodic memory and cortical activity in schizophrenia. Biol Psychiatry. 2005;58(1):47–55.

399. Himmelbach M, Karnath HO, Perenin MT, Franz VH, Stockmeier K. A general deficit of the "automatic pilot" with posterior parietal cortex lesions? Neuropsychologia. 2006;44(13):2749–2756.

400. Himmelbach M, Karnath HO. Dorsal and ventral stream interaction: contributions from optic ataxia. J Cogn Neurosci. 2005;17(4):632–40.

401. Rice NJ, Edwards MG, Schindler I, Punt TD, McIntosh RD, Humphreys GW, et al. Delay abolishes the obstacle avoidance deficit in unilateral optic ataxia. Neuropsychologia. 2008;46(5):1549–1557.

402. Goodale MA, Jakobson LS, Keillor JM. Differences in the visual control of pantomimed and natural grasping movements. Neuropsychologia. 1994;32(10):1159–1178.

403. Dijkerman HC, McIntosh RD, Anema HA, de Haan EH, Kappelle LJ, Milner AD. Reaching errors in optic ataxia are linked to eye position rather than head or body position. Neuropsychologia. 2006;44(13):2766–2773.

404. Khan AZ, Pisella L, Vighetto A, Cotton F, Luaute J, Boisson D, et al. Optic ataxia errors depend on remapped, not viewed, target location. Nat Neurosci. 2005;8(4):418–420.

405. Khan AZ, Crawford JD, Blohm G, Urquizar C, Rossetti Y, Pisella L. Influence of initial hand and target position on reach errors in optic ataxic and normal subjects. J Vis. 2007;7(5):8 1–16.

406. Karnath HO, Perenin MT. Cortical control of visually guided reaching: evidence from patients with optic ataxia. Cereb Cortex. 2005;15(10):1561–1569.

407. Battaglia Mayer A, Ferraina S, Marconi B, Bullis J, Lacquaniti F, Burnod Y, et al. Early motor influences on visuomotor transformations for reaching: a positive image of optic ataxia. Exp Brain Res. 1998;123:172–189.

408. Boller F, Cole M, Kim Y, Mack J, Patawaran C. Optic ataxia: clinical-radiological correlations with the EMIscan. J Neurol Neurosurg Psychiatry. 1975;38:954–958.

409. Nagaratnam N, Grice D, Kalouche H. Optic ataxia following unilateral stroke. J Neurol Sci. 1998;155:204–207.

410. Auerbach S, Alexander M. Pure agraphia and unilateral optic ataxia associated with a left superior parietal lobule lesion. J Neurol Neurosurg Psychiatry. 1981;44:430–432.

411. Ando S, Moritake K. Pure optic ataxia associated with a right parieto-occipital tumour. J Neurol Neurosurg Psychiatry. 1990;53:805–806.

412. Cogan DG. Congenital ocular motor apraxia. Can J Ophthalmol. 1965;1:253.

413. Holmes G. Spasm of fixation. Trans Ophthalmol Soc UK. 1930;50:253.

414. Johnston JL, Sharpe JA, Morrow MJ. Spasm of fixation: a quantitative study. J Neurol Sci. 1992;107:166.

415. Nyffeler T, Pflugshaupt T, Hofer H, Baas U, Gutbrod K, von Wartburg R, et al. Oculomotor behaviour in simultanagnosia: a longitudinal case study. Neuropsychologia. 2005;43(11):1591–1597.

416. Andersen R, Brotchie P, Mazzoni P. Evidence for the lateral intraparietal area as the parietal eye field. Curr Biol. 1992;2:840–846.

417. Valenza N, Murray MM, Ptak R, Vuilleumier P. The space of senses: impaired cross-modal interactions in a patient with Balint syndrome after bilateral parietal damage. Neuropsychologia. 2004;42(13):1737–1748.

418. McCrea SM, Buxbaum LJ, Coslett HB. Illusory conjunctions in simultanagnosia: coarse coding of visual feature location? Neuropsychologia. 2006;44(10):1724–1736.

419. Malcolm GL, Barton JJ. "Sequence Agnosia" in Balint's syndrome: defects in visuotemporal processing after bilateral parietal damage. J Cogn Neurosci. 2007;19(1):102–108.

420. Striemer C, Blangero A, Rossetti Y, Boisson D, Rode G, Vighetto A, et al. Deficits in peripheral visual attention in patients with optic ataxia. Neuroreport. 2007; 18(11):1171–1175.

421. Gaveau V, Pelisson D, Blangero A, Urquizar C, Prablanc C, Vighetto A, et al. Saccade control and eye-hand coordination in optic ataxia. Neuropsychologia. 2008;46(2): 475–486.

422. Holmes G, Horrax G. Disturbances of spatial orientation and visual attention, with loss of stereoscopic vision. Arch Neurol Psychiatry. 1919;1:385–407.

423. Rizzo M. Bálint's syndrome and associated visuospatial disorders. In: Kennard C (ed.), Bailliere's International Practice and Research. Philadelphia: W B Saunders; 1993. pp. 413–437.

424. Perez FM, Tunkel RS, Lachman EA, Nagler W. Balint's syndrome arising from bilateral posterior cortical atrophy or infarction: rehabilitation strategies and their limitation. Disabil Rehabil. 1996;18(6):300–304.

425. Rizzo M, Damasio H. Impairment of stereopsis with focal brain lesions. Ann Neurol. 1985;18:147.

426. Patterson R, Fox R. The effect of testing method in stereoanomaly. Vision Res. 1984;24:403–408.

Part V
Special Considerations in Neuro-Ophthalmology

21A

AN APPROACH TO VISUAL LOSS IN A CHILD

Muhammad Hassaan Ali, Stacy L. Pineles

CASE STUDY

A 6-month-old child presents with poor vision. The parents notice that he never makes eye contact and does not seem to track objects. He can see bright lights and they notice that when lights are turned on, and he seems to notice. They also mention that his eyes shake frequently. He has otherwise developed normally and was born full term without any complications. On examination, the patient blinks to light in each eye but does not fix or follow. His pupils are sluggish without a relative afferent pupillary defect. His intraocular pressure is normal. His anterior segment is normal and the dilated fundus examination reveals bilateral optic nerve hypoplasia with a double ring sign. Motility examination is notable for conjugate horizontal pendular nystagmus which remains horizontal in up and down gaze. The patient is orthotropic with normal ductions. The child is diagnosed with optic nerve hypoplasia. Laboratory testing for hypopituitarism is commenced and an MRI of the brain is ordered. The MRI reveals absent septum pellucidum and a thin corpus callosum. What is the diagnosis of this patient?

Introduction

Visual impairment in a generally normal child is a disturbing finding. Parents are looking ahead at a lifetime of potential visual impairment in their child and are very curious to know the cause and severity of the condition. Contingent upon the fundamental cause, the visual outcome may range from normal vision to complete visual impairment. The significance of finding an exact cause in this setting is self-evident. This section describes an approach to visual loss in a child and describes brief findings of some of the important causes of this clinical presentation.

Impaired vision in early childhood can be due to multiple causes that include congenital malformations, acquired ophthalmic disorders, or lesions of the anterior or posterior visual pathway. A careful examination of the patient can help the clinician identify some of the evident anterior segment disorders like congenital cataract, corneal opacities and refractive errors. However, some retinal pathologies like congenital stationary night blindness (CSNB), Leber's congenital amaurosis (LCA) and achromatopsia do not show any characteristic lesions on the retina in early stages and have to be diagnosed on the basis of electroretinography (ERG) (1–3). An important finding in all such cases is arteriolar narrowing and waxy disc pallor which should alert the clinician to order ERG in such cases (4). It is generally advised to wait till 1 year of life to derive conclusive findings from ERG owing to slow maturation of rod and cone maturation in the first year of life. Similarly, cerebral visual impairment may also be suspected clinically but demands detailed high-resolution neuroimaging for confirmation.

Children with mental retardation and autism represent another challenging situation for pediatric neuro-ophthalmologists since these patients may have normal visual systems despite poor visual response. Due to difficult examination of such children, the clinicians are very likely to miss occult but important ophthalmic signs and disorders in these patients. Patients with autism are increasingly reported to have congenital blindness both retinal and cortical, and vice versa. Children with autistic spectrum disorder or additional neuropsychiatric conditions like schizophrenia have disruption of magnocellular pathways in the dorsal brain which are solely responsible for motion input, and hence, these patients show delay in the development of posture and other locomotor skills (5,6).

Assessment of a visually handicapped child begins with a detailed clinical history and meticulous examination. The information gathered can then be correlated to draft a list of differential diagnoses by the treating clinician. Subsequent investigations and can then be used to reach a definitive diagnosis, and management plan can be drafted if any intervention can be done to improve the visual status of the child.

GENERAL FRAMEWORK FOR VISUAL LOSS IN A CHILD

HISTORY

Duration – Need of review of school records

- Laterality
- Diurnal variation of visual symptoms
- History of trauma or eye poking
- History of delayed development/learning disabilities
- Associated headache, photophobia
- History of trauma, family, birth, and maternal history

GENERAL PHYSICAL EXAMINATION

- Assessment of visual acuity – Notice fixation pattern, OKN, nystagmus
- Pupils
- EOM movements and strabismus examination – Movements, cover/uncover test, nystagmus
- Assessment of anterior segment
- Assessment of posterior chamber including fundus
- Cycloplegic refraction

History of an apparently blind child

Parents are the source of history in pediatric patients. It should be kept in mind that a parent or caretaker knows his or her child more than anyone else, so if they think that their baby does not have normal vision, always take it very seriously. A thorough interview of both the parents and close relatives can reveal significantly

DOI: 10.1201/9780429020278-31

useful pieces of information for underlying pathologies which can produce visual loss in the child. Interview with the parents should be utilized to build a good rapport with the parents since children with visual loss need follow-up for longer periods of time.

The following areas should be explored while taking a history of a child with vision loss:

- *Duration of vision loss*
  The parents of the child should be asked about the time elapsed since the vision loss in the child has been noted. Since children compensate their vision well with the other eye, monocular decreased vision can easily be missed for many early years of life. School or pediatrician vision screening records can be sought to explore any evidence of previous vision in the eyes in case the clinician suspects some cause of acute vision loss. Unfortunately, very few schools in developing countries have a consistent practice of pre-school vision screening, which is a common practice in developed world. For this reason, many children present very late with treatable causes of blindness in these resource-deficient countries.

- *Laterality of vision loss*
  It is always wise to assess laterality of the vision loss in children as binocular visual deficit in the absence of trauma could potentially indicate syndromic or retrochiasmal visual pathway abnormality.

- *History of trauma*
  Any child who presents with vision loss should always be evaluated for traumatic injuries to various structures of the eyes. If a positive history of head trauma is obtained, suspect occipital concussion, retinal and vitreous hemorrhages with papilloedema as potential causes of vision loss in infants and small children.

- *Headache*
  Children with vision loss secondary to migraine or due to idiopathic intracranial hypertension may present with headache.

- *Photophobia*
  The clinicians should inquire about degree of photophobia in children, if any. A positive history of photophobia should raise suspicion about congenital glaucoma, traumatic hyphema, corneal infections and iritis.

- *Birth and maternal history*
  Inquire about mode of delivery, gestational age, birth weight, any health-related events in the neonatal period, any exposure to oxygen therapy in the hospital to rule out evidence about retinopathy of prematurity (ROP). The mother should also be asked about her health during pregnancy with special emphasis on timely vaccinations and any history of fever or infection during pregnancy. Exposure to any drugs or teratogenic agents during pregnancy should also be inquired.

- *Family history*
  It is always wise to explore family of the child for any heritable diseases. The parents should be asked about history of any ocular or systemic diseases in the family.

Lastly, the parents should be inquired about any specific signs like eye poking, decreased vision at night time or in day light and child's general physical, speech and motor development. Learning abilities should also be explored and any evidence of nutritional deficiency should also be ruled out.

Having collected all the aforementioned information, the clinician now should proceed to the ophthalmic examination of the child.

Ophthalmic examination of a child with visual loss

The clinical examination of the child starts from the time the patient enters the examination room. The clinician should keenly observe the alertness and behavior of the child. A child's behavior with changing lighting in the room or if some unknown object approaches the patient should be carefully examined. Any abnormal head posture with head tilt and chin lift position should also be evaluated as these can give diagnostic clues to underlying cranial nerve palsies leading to paresis of extraocular muscles. While performing an external examination, always look for any external abnormalities like abnormal shape of the head, any craniosynostosis, heading bobbing movement, visible ptosis and nystagmus.

Vision assessment

Assessment of vision of an apparently blind child demands use of highly specialized methods or modification of the methods routinely used for evaluation of normal children. Healthy pediatric patients are usually tested by their ability to fixate and follow, steadiness of their fixation and ability to maintain fixation on an object (7). These usual techniques do not work in patients with profound visual loss as most of these patients are affixational. Therefore, it is more important to obtain an idea about the overall visual status of the child instead of trying to quantify distance or near visual acuity by using Snellen's or similar charts. Parents and closed relatives are the best possible source of information about the visual status of the children as they can inform the clinician about attentiveness, responsiveness and ability to smile while looking at close relatives which gives fair idea about gross vision of the child. Patiently playing with affected children using a variety of toys of different colors and sizes provides useful information. Can the child recognize various objects in the environment, interact with surrounding people and navigate on his own effectively? What is the response of the child to the examiner's face, objects shown to him or movement of parents nearby? What is the reaction of the child to penlight or flickering of room lights on and off? If palpebral fissures of the child widen on extinguishing the room lights, this indicates at least presence of perception of light in the affected child.

The fixation pattern of children with congenital visual defects follows a general pattern depending on the degree of vision loss: children with vision better than 20/200 follow mostly with their eyes, those with 20/200 follow with both their eyes and head and those with severe vision loss follow mostly with their head (7,8).

A preference to view objects of regard at very close range is seen occasionally in normal children, reflecting a transient behavioral pattern. Children with poor vision often do so consistently to produce linear magnification (by shortening the focal length), to damp an existing nystagmus with convergence to improve vision or, in the case of uncorrected aphakic children, to induce a miotic response to increase depth of focus and create a pinhole effect. Visual function may also be qualitatively evaluated with the optokinetic reflex. When the visual field moves with respect to the eyes, as with a rotating optokinetic drum, the eyes track the moving field to the limit of their excursion and then make a recovery saccade in the opposite direction and so on, producing optokinetic nystagmus. Cortically blind patients cannot generate optokinetic nystagmus (9).

In children with poor vision and nystagmus due to anterior visual pathway disorders, some researchers have proposed the performance of the "unequal nystagmus test" to determine which eye, if either, has better vision (10). The test is performed by noting the degree of nystagmus while the child views an attractive toy at a distance with both eyes open and then with alternate eyes covered. The nystagmus is similar in patients with similar acuity in both eyes. When the acuities are different, wider and slower excursions of nystagmus are noted in the worse eye, and faster and smaller amplitude nystagmus is noted in the better eye.

Lastly, the acuity of infants with apparently better vision may also be measured using forced choice preferential looking methods using Teller or Cardiff acuity cards and by electrophysiological tests of visual-evoked potentials (11). Both techniques are time-consuming, require special equipment and trained personnel and are costly. Until recently, these methods were generally only used in specialized pediatric ophthalmology units. In co-operative children, aged 18–24 months, it is possible to use picture optotype tests (such as Kays pictures) at very short distances. Standard optotype tests, such as the Snellen E chart, can generally only be used in children aged 3 years or above and only if the child has significant vision to see any such optotype (12). It is important that testing is carried out at the appropriate distance and, if possible, using linear optotype systems to ensure the effect of crowding is not overlooked in children with amblyopia (13). With some younger children and those unable to read, a matching test, involving matching letters on the distance chart with those on a card held at near, can be used.

Pupil examination

Assessment of pupil size and their response to a bright light can be difficult in infants but should be performed very carefully as abnormal responses can provide very useful diagnostic clues. Pupil size should be noted in dark and bright light conditions. Sometimes parents present with complaints of difference in pupil size and that finding can lead the clinician to detect an underlying retinal pathology which manifests as relative afferent pupillary defect (RAPD). Generally, presence of Marcus Gunn pupil indicates anterior visual pathway or optic nerve pathology, and a paradoxical pupillary response highlights underlying retinal pathology (14,15).

Extraocular motility and strabismus examination

The extraocular motility testing is done by having the patient look in all gaze positions. It is always recommended to quantify extraocular movements especially in cases of neurological diseases. Both pursuit movements, following any object of interest and saccadic movements, refixation on an object introduced into the field of vision should be assessed to rule out underlying neurological cause of abnormal extraocular motility. Since children are naturally interested in faces, the examiner can use her/his own face as an object of interest or some stuff toys to attract attention of the child. A common dictum for pediatric eye examination is "one toy, one look." So, the clinician can use one toy for each gaze position if the child can grossly visualize the toy.

Strabismus examination starts with corneal reflection or Hirschberg's test and by the cover-uncover test to detect manifest or hidden strabismus. The child is asked to fixate on any object of interest at far or up close and cover-uncover performed to see the pattern of strabismus. The deviation of strabismus is quantified using prism cover test. The strabismus is checked in all gaze positions both with and without glasses. If the child is unable to fixate on the target due to poor vision, the clinician can perform Krimsky's test to quantify the deviation (16). In neurological cases, care must be taken to identify primary and secondary deviation. Primary deviation is the deviation of the strabismic eye when the normal eye fixates on the target, whereas secondary deviation is the deviation of the normal eye when the paralyzed eye attempts to fixate on the target. Secondary deviation is significantly greater than primary deviation in cases of paralytic strabismus (17).

Another important aspect of extraocular motility testing is to check for presence or absence of nystagmus. Patients with cerebral visual impairment do not show infantile nystagmus whereas it is commonly seen in patients with congenital optic nerve disorders or optic tract lesions (18). Sometimes premature infants with lesions of optic radiations and periventricular leukomalacia also manifest infantile nystagmus (19). Sometimes infantile nystagmus is seen in children with grossly normal ocular anatomy but are suspected to have underlying visual sensory lesions. It is worth mentioning here that the electro-oculographic waveform of the infantile nystagmus is same irrespective of the underlying cause of nystagmus (20,21).

While examining a baby with nystagmus, care should be taken to observe any gaze direction in which the amplitude and frequency of nystagmus dampen. This is called null point or null zone and can produce abnormal head posture in the patient. Null point also implies the presence of fixation and functional vision in the affected baby. Conventional surgical procedure called Kestenbaum Anderson procedure can be performed to shift the null point to the primary gaze position which corrects abnormal head posture in these cases (22).

Examining the anterior segment

Slit lamp biomicroscope should be used to perform meticulous examination of the anterior segment of the patient. Care should be taken to examine the anatomy of the eye in layers paying attention to all the individual structures. A comprehensive examination of the adnexa, conjunctiva, sclera, cornea, anterior chamber, iris, pupil, lens and anterior vitreous phase should be performed using slit lamp. The best way to examine the child is by using a portable handheld slit lamp. If this is not available, child can be made to sit in mother's lap and asked to place his face in the chin rest of the slit lamp. If the child shows very limited cooperation, the examination can be performed using a magnifying loupe or with simple pen torch to grossly see the structures of the eyes. It is advisable to always compare structures of both the eyes.

Conjunctiva should be seen for presence of Bitot's spot which can point toward underlying vitamin A deficiency (23). Similarly, conjunctiva should be evaluated to rule out papillary or follicular conjunctivitis. Patients with papillary conjunctivitis rub their eye frequently and end up in development of keratoconus. Cornea should be evaluated to see presence of vertical Vogt striae seen in keratoconus and horizontal Haab's striae seen in congenital glaucoma and generalized opacification (24,25). Anterior chamber should be evaluated for presence of inflammatory cells to rule out pediatric uveitis. Status of the lens should be carefully examined and any evidence of congenital cataract and other congenital anomalies like Peter's anomaly or Reiger's anomaly should be evaluated paying special attention to the presence or absence of any iridocorneal or lenticulocorneal contact (26). Then, fundal glow and presence of any reaction in the anterior vitreous phase should be noted to rule out vitritis.

It is very important to document intraocular pressure (IOP) in infants. Generally, we perform portable handheld tonometers like iCare tonometer to record IOP in children (27). Non-contact air puff tonometry can also be performed in younger children who are unable to get applanation tonometry done. If the child can cooperate, applanation tonometry should be performed since it remains the gold standard IOP measurement technique (28).

Examining the posterior segment

Examination of the posterior segment of the eye should be performed after adequate pupillary dilatation. Tropicamide, phenylephrine, cyclopentolate, and atropine drops can be used to dilate the pupils depending upon the color and pigmentation of the iris. Fundus examination is essential to rule out any underlying cause of vision loss including life-threatening conditions like retinoblastoma. The examination can be made relatively easy if the parents are asked to hold and simultaneously feed the baby. Young infants can be examined by wrapping them in a sheet and getting an assistant hold the head of the baby steady. Parents should be counseled that the examination is not painful so they need not worry if the child cries during the examination. Fundus examination if usually performed using 28D or 30D lenses with indirect ophthalmoscope. If any lesion is found on the optic nerve head or macula, a magnified view can be obtained using direct ophthalmoscope. While examining the fundus always comment on the status of the optic disc, macula, periphery and retinal vasculature. Optic disc pit, foveal hypoplasia, macular scarring, abnormal macular pigmentation, bone spicule pigmentation, arteriolar attenuation and optic disc pallor can be seen in various pathologies which produce visual loss in children.

Refraction

Cycloplegic refraction should be performed in all children after instillation of cyclopentolate or atropine eye drops. Cycloplegic retinoscopy not gives us accurate refractive status of the child but also provides us diagnostic clues for final diagnosis of the patient.

Examining the family

Always consider detailed ophthalmic examination of the siblings, parents and other close family members if the child is suspected to suffer from a hereditary condition (Figure 21A.1). This examination can help not only in the early diagnosis of other siblings

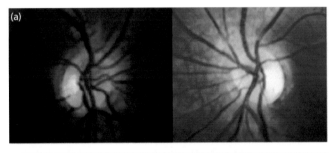
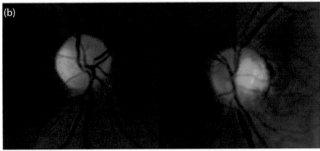

FIGURE 21A.1 A child (a) presented with moderate vision loss and decreased color vision. His examination revealed temporal optic nerve pallor. (b) Upon examining his father, similar findings were seen and a diagnosis of dominant optic atrophy was made. This was confirmed by genetic testing.

but also lead the clinician to offer genetic counseling to parents for their upcoming children.

Information for parents of apparently blind children

It is recommended to be extremely cautious about giving a final visual prognosis to the parents of apparently blind children. Care should also be taken not to attribute the condition to inheritance from either parent since that can create conflict in the family. The standard protocol is to counsel the parents for repeated ophthalmic examination and share findings of each examination in detail without giving false hopes to the parents. Lastly, it is recommended not to judge final visual outcome of the child at an early age as many children ultimately develop more than expected visual outcome later in life.

Causes of severe visual loss and blindness in children

Various studies have shown that many causes of childhood blindness are preventable or treatable if detected early. Low vision aids and visual rehabilitation should be offered to all the individuals whose pathology is unlikely to benefit from any medical or surgical treatment. Causes of childhood blindness are classified according to the anatomical site or the underlying pathology. For this chapter, we divide the causes into prenatal, perinatal and postnatal causes. Prenatal causes are the diseases which can occur from the time of conception till delivery, postnatal causes affect during or after delivery and perinatal causes affect the fetus from 28th week of gestation to 1–4 weeks after birth. Some of the major conditions that can develop during these periods are discussed below.

Prenatal onset

Congenital anomalies

Congenital anomalies in which the eyeball is either absent or abnormally small in size are called anophthalmos and microphthalmos, respectively (29). Congenital uveal coloboma is the commonest congenital anomaly which occurs when the embryonic fissure fails to fuse completely by sixth week of development (30,31). Coloboma involving the macula or the optic nerve causes severe visual loss. Many studies have shown that these anomalies are leading causes of blindness in children with congenital visual disorders in many parts of Asia (32,33). No cause of these anomalies can be detected prenatally even though detailed investigations and genetic testing have been proposed in the subsequent siblings of an affected patient. Whether there is a role of folic acid in preventing such congenital malformations remains yet to be explored. These patients are generally managed with best refractive correction and low vision aids. Some people also advocate applying laser to the margins of the coloboma to avoid any impending retinal detachment (34).

Another congenital anomaly in which the primary vitreous persists and extends from the optic disc to the vitreous base at the posterior pole of the lens is called persistent hyperplastic primary vitreous (PHPV) or more recently persistent fetal vasculature (PFV) (35). It may be unilateral or bilateral and is seldom associated with microphthalmos. Early vitrectomy can be attempted in such cases; however, the visual outcomes are suboptimal (36).

Infantile glaucoma

Any child who presents with photophobia, lacrimation and blepharospasm should be strongly suspected to have congenital glaucoma unless proved otherwise. Glaucoma in children usually occurs due to angle dysgenesis and is often associated with other congenital ocular abnormalities like Peter's and Rieger's anomaly (37,38). All children with congenital glaucoma should undergo regular testing for IOP, corneal diameter, anterior segment examination, cup to disc ratio and axial length measurement. Out of all these parameters, the corneal diameter is the most reliable indicator of severity of the glaucoma in children. A corneal diameter of greater than 14 mm indicates advanced buphthalmos and an advanced stage of the disease. Another characteristic feature of infantile glaucoma is the possibility of reversal of cup to disc ratio once pressure of the eye is controlled. Infantile glaucoma if not treated early may cause complete blindness in children. The treatment of choice is mostly surgical with goniotomy performed in eyes with clear corneas and angle filtration surgery preferred in eyes with hazy corneas (39). Complicated cases with failed filtration surgeries are usually treated with glaucoma shunt devices (40). Lastly, clinicians should always offer genetic counseling to the parents if more than one sibling gets affected.

Congenital cataract

Congenital cataract affects about 3–5/1000 infants (41). Genetics, antenatal maternal infections and metabolic disorders are considered to be the most common causes of congenital cataracts (42). Early recognition of this pathology is essential to prevent development of dense amblyopia. Pediatricians should be trained to evaluate red reflex of the newborn. If they find any abnormality in red reflex or leukocoria, they should refer the baby for evaluation by a pediatric ophthalmologist. The mother and the affected baby with congenital cataract should be screened for toxoplasmosis, rubella, cytomegalovirus and herpetic infections (TORCH infections). Similarly, pediatricians should evaluate the baby for all metabolic disorders. Rubella is still considered to be a major etiological agent in developing countries. So, the child should undergo detailed systemic evaluation to rule out any other features of congenital rubella syndrome including heart, ear and skin abnormalities.

A congenital cataract that is more than 3 mm in size or totally blocking the pupillary axis needs urgent consideration for surgical extraction (43). There is a consensus among pediatric ophthalmologists that if detected at birth, pediatric cataract surgery should be done at 6 weeks of age in cases of unilateral cataracts and at 10 weeks or later in cases of bilateral cataracts (43,44). Before 6 weeks of age, the anesthetic risk to the baby and the risk of developing aphakic glaucoma outweigh the benefits of cataract extraction. Spiculated or dot-like opacities should be observed till they cause significant visual deprivation in the child.

Timing of implantation of intraocular lens (IOL) in young patients remains a controversial issue. Many experienced surgeons advocate implanting an IOL as early as 6 months of age in cases of unilateral cataracts. But usually IOL is implanted after first year of life (45,46). Bilateral cases can be delayed up to even 2 years of age. In bilateral cases, one eye is operated in one sitting. However, if the physical condition of the baby cannot tolerate two consecutive anesthesia over a span of 1 week, bilateral surgery can be considered. In bilateral surgery in one sitting, each eye should be operated as a separate case with separate preparations and use of new instruments and drugs for each eye. In developing countries, children with bilateral cataracts are usually left aphakic with IOL implanted later in life at the age of around 8–9 years (47). The IOL power in children can be calculated using different formulas with the aim to achieve emmetropia at the age of around 7–8 years.

There is almost 100% rate of posterior capsular opacification in children after cataract surgery. In all such cases, primary posterior capsulotomy and anterior vitrectomy up to the age of 6–7 years are recommended. The anterior vitrectomy removes the solid vitreous base. The pars plana is generally avoided in children since this approach may cause suprachoroidal hemorrhage. Vitrectomy through the limbal side ports is also relatively easier for the surgeons who are trained in the anterior segment. Some surgeons prefer to perform capsulorrhexis of the posterior capsule. In such cases, anterior vitrectomy need not be performed since the vitreous phase is not disturbed. The preferable lens material for IOL in children is either hydrophobic acrylic or polymethyl methacrylate. If the children are cooperative and able to sit properly on slit amp, Nd:YAG laser capsulotomy can be done over 6 years of age after surgery (48).

Repeated refractions along with patching for treatment of amblyopia are mainstay of visual rehabilitation after pediatric cataract surgery. Glaucoma and opacification of visual axes may present as late post-operative complications (49). Detailed counseling of parents about the need for regular ophthalmic examination along with frequent refractions for correction of near and far vision are essential to help the child attain maximum visual acuity after the cataract surgery.

Retinal dystrophies

Retina dystrophies are a group of diseases which cause congenital retinal blindness. They generally present late in childhood and are common in developing countries where cousin marriages are highly prevalent. These diseases are usually managed with low vision aids that provide navigatory vision to the affected individual. LCA is a group of hereditary (mostly autosomal recessive) retinal dystrophies which produce severe visual impairment at a very early age (50). Affected children usually present with severely reduced vision, high hyperopia, sluggish or absent pupillary light reflexes and nystagmus which may be pendular to roving from very early age. The electroretinogram of these patients show markedly reduced scotopic and mesopic responses which are hallmark of this condition. The fundus may show no changes in the early stages to retinitis pigmentosa like bone spicule lesions in the late course of the disease. Oculodigital syndrome manifests with oculodigital phenomenon (constant rubbing of the eyes for retinal stimulation leading to enophthalmos), deafness, learning disabilities and epilepsy. Patients with Knobloch syndrome present with nystagmus, myopia and retinal detachment (51). Oculocutaneous albinism is usually X-linked or autosomal recessive (52). It presents with characteristic transillumination defects in iris and hypopigmented fundi and is usually associated with nystagmus. Achromatopsia is an autosomal recessive disease which produces color vision abnormalities and decreased central vision (53). Patients with achromatopsia present with photophobia and nystagmus in early childhood. The evaluation of children with retinal dystrophies is difficult as they often present early in infancy with poor vision but a relatively normal eye examination (Figure 21A.2).

Retinoblastoma

This the most common malignancy in early childhood that presents with leukocoria, esotropia or uveitis is retinoblastoma. Any patient with leukocoria should undergo dilated fundus examination with B-scan ultrasonography of the eye and subsequent orbital imaging to reach the final diagnosis. Retinoblastoma produces characteristic calcifications which are visible on

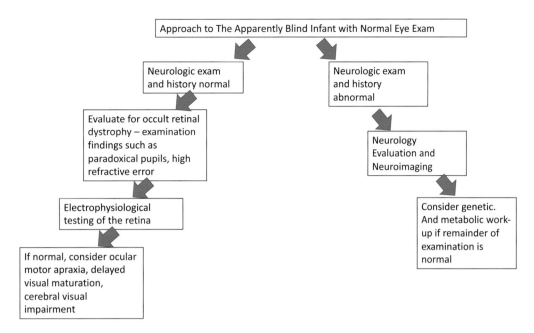

FIGURE 21A.2   Approach to the evaluation of an apparently blind infant without an obvious ophthalmic etiology.

B-scan of the eye. Early detection leads to better treatment with chemotherapy and globe preservation, whereas larger legions need enucleation after which a prosthesis is implanted in the child's eye.

Perinatal onset

Ophthalmia neonatorum

It occurs during delivery as infant passes through the birth canal. It can be prevented by antenatal screening, treatment of sexually transmitted infections (STIs) during pregnancy and proper prophylaxis. Prophylactic treatment includes topical antibiotic/antiseptic instilled immediately after birth for cleaning newborn's eyes. Treatment depends on local epidemiology of STIs and organism's sensitivity to antibiotics. If an active infection is suspected, treatment must include topical as well as systemic antibiotics to prevent extraocular infections like pneumonia.

Retinopathy of prematurity

ROP accounts for 15% of all cases of blindness in developed countries and up to 60% in developing countries (54). Many risk factors are responsible for its development. However, the most commonly implicated risk factors include degree of immaturity determined by the newborn's birth weight, gestational age and exposure to supplementary oxygen (54). Oxygen therapy is necessary to maintain adequate oxygen saturation in newborn's blood whose lungs are still immature due to premature delivery. However, it can result in permanent blindness in premature infants if given in uncontrolled fashion. Several guidelines have shown about safe upper and lower limits of O_2 saturation. Survival ratio of premature infants can be increased with improvement of neonatal care in developed as well as poor countries.

ROP is further classified according to severity (states I–V), site (zones 1–3) and extent (clock hours 1–12). Developed countries screen infants according to birth weight <1500 g, while developing countries screen individuals with even higher birth weights up to 2500 g. The recommended method of screening premature infants is by indirect ophthalmoscopy using standard 28D or 30D lens. Temporal retina is usually visualized to see the extent of development of normal retinal vasculature. Postnatal screening during the first few weeks of life helps in prompt treatment either with laser ablation of peripheral avascular retina. However, there are no successful reports that show surgery can cause marked improvement for stage IV and V ROP. Anti-vascular endothelial growth factor (anti-VEGF) drugs are beneficial for the treatment of retinal vascular disorders in adults; however, they have to be used with extreme caution in premature infants since these drugs can interfere with development of normal vasculature elsewhere in body. Alveoli and lungs are highly VEGF-sensitive and develop at the same time as does ROP, so the benefits and risks of anti-VEGF therapy should be carefully weighed before administering these agents in preterm babies. Refractive error, strabismus, amblyopia and low vision are very common in premature infants; therefore, long-term follow-up is recommended.

Optic nerve lesions and cerebral visual impairment

Optic nerve lesions and cortical visual impairment are commonly seen in developed countries as a consequence of preterm birth and birth asphyxia (Figure 21A.3). The usual clinical features are optic disc pallor and optic atrophy. These patients are usually mentally handicapped and are difficult to examine due to very limited cooperation during the examination. No medical or surgical treatment provide significant improvement in vision. Low vision aids are the mainstay of management such cases.

Postnatal onset

Common causes of corneal blindness like vitamin A deficiency, measles, trauma and trachoma are rare in infancy but are still occasionally reported from developing countries. Patients may present with corneal opacification and other associated features. If a bilateral disease is seen with keratomalacia, suspect vitamin A deficiency, which is treated with vitamin A supplementation after the age of 6 months.

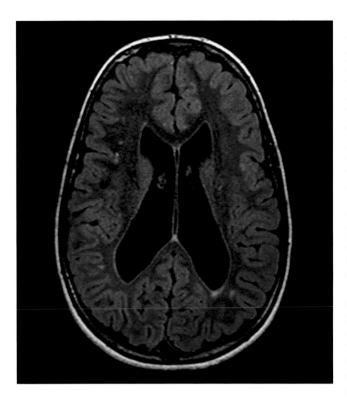

FIGURE 21A.3 An axial image from an MRI of a child who was born at 28 weeks' gestation and suffered from subsequent periventricular leukomalacia. This child presented to the ophthalmologist with unexplained vision loss and was found to have optic atrophy bilaterally which was attributed to extreme prematurity and periventricular leukomalacia.

Refractive errors are common in infants but are only treated with spectacles if they are greater than 3–4 D or are causing strabismus or asthenopic symptoms. Young patients may also present with complaints of severe itching and redness in the eyes. Consider vernal keratoconjunctivitis in such cases and check for signs of keratoconus which develops as a consequence of repeated rubbing of eyes.

Challenges in the early diagnosis and treatment of visually impaired children in developing countries

Due to shortage of specialists in developing countries, it becomes difficult to detect problem early during assessment in eye care center. In developed countries, proper referral system is maintained between health visitors, family practitioners, neonatal units, pediatric ophthalmologists and retina specialists. Since subspecialties are not well developed in resource-deficient countries, specialized eye care is not freely available. Due to financial and geographic limitations, parents are unable to avail diagnostic, curative and rehabilitative services in poor countries. Pediatric eye surgery is expensive as compared to adult surgery as it requires multidisciplinary approach including the need for general anesthetists for examination and intervention together with pediatricians and neonatologists for assessment of general health status and medical fitness of the child.

Another limitation is lack of awareness among general practitioners regarding various pediatric eye diseases. Many family practitioners advise parents to delay treatment to get child old enough to start treatment. Some physicians counsel the parents that the problem may resolve spontaneously as the child gets old or unilateral disease can be compensated with other healthy eye. These misunderstandings lead to late referrals and children present with advanced features of diseases. This is the reason that patients as old as 12–15 years are seen for the very first time with dense amblyopia. Even after timely referral, some parents delay treatment thinking that their child is too young for any ocular surgery or wear glasses.

If the child suffers from some congenital retinal disorder and there is nothing much that the ophthalmologist can do to help the patient, glasses, low vision aids and special visual rehabilitation services should be offered to the patient. Special schools for visually handicapped children can play an important role in helping to develop various cognitive and locomotor skills in such children. Parents should be counseled in detail about the visual prognosis and future career options of the child with empathy and answering all their concerns. Genetic counseling should be offered to all those parents whose more than one child gets affected with the same disease. Role of dedicated ophthalmic social workers or counselors should be emphasized here. They should be introduced to the parents at very early stages of their child's disease so that he can gradually guide parents about various aspects of the child's condition. All patients with visual impairment should undergo frequent ophthalmic visits to maintain optimal refractive correction and timely management of amblyopia.

Conclusion

Visual impairment in a child may be extremely concerning requiring a thorough neuro-ophthalmic evaluation. Detailed history and examination are required to discern the cause of visual loss in a child. Examination is the key but may often be difficult in very young children. Contingent upon the cause, the visual outcome may vary from complete recovery to severe visual loss. A systematic approach may aid in early diagnosis and treatment in these patients.

Multiple-Choice Questions

1. All of the following causes of vision loss in a child typically present with photophobia, EXCEPT:
   a. Uveitis
   b. Congenital glaucoma
   c. Optic nerve hypoplasia
   d. Cone dystrophy

   Answer:
   c. Optic nerve hypoplasia

2. Bitot spots are a sign of:
   a. Vitamin B12 deficiency
   b. Vitamin A deficiency
   c. Copper deficiency
   d. Folate deficiency

   Answer:
   b. Vitamin A deficiency

3. In a visually significant unilateral congenital cataract, the optimal time for lens extraction is:

a. 6 weeks

b. 6 months

c. 3 years

d. 2 weeks

Answer:

a. 6 weeks

References

1. Zeitz C, Robson AG, Audo I. Congenital stationary night blindness: An analysis and update of genotype–phenotype correlations and pathogenic mechanisms. Prog Retin Eye Res. 2015;45:58–110.

2. Chung DC, Traboulsi EI. Leber congenital amaurosis: Clinical correlations with genotypes, gene therapy trials update, and future directions. J Am Assoc Pediatr Ophthalmol Strabismus. 2009;13(6):587–92.

3. Kondo M, Miyake Y, Kondo N, Tanikawa A, Suzuki S, Horiguchi M, et al. Multifocal ERG findings in complete type congenital stationary night blindness. Invest Ophthalmol Vis Sci. 2001;42(6):1342–8.

4. Tsang SH, Sharma T. Congenital stationary night blindness. In: Atlas of inherited retinal diseases. Cham, Switzerland: Springer; 2018. pp. 61–4.

5. Javitt DC. When doors of perception close: Bottom-up models of disrupted cognition in schizophrenia. Annu Rev Clin Psychol. 2009;5:249–75.

6. Laycock R, Crewther SG, Crewther DP. A role for the 'magnocellular advantage' in visual impairments in neurodevelopmental and psychiatric disorders. Neurosci Biobehav Rev. 2007;31(3):363–76.

7. Pritchard C, Ellis GS. Approach to visual acuity assessment and strabismus evaluation of the pediatric patient. In: Practical management of pediatric ocular disorders and strabismus. New York, NY: Springer; 2016. pp. 3–23.

8. Hall A, Orel-Bixler D, Haegerstrom-Portnoy G. Special visual assessment techniques for multiply handicapped persons. J Vis Impair Blind. 1991;85(1):23–9.

9. Verhagen WIM, Huygen PLM, Mulleners WM. Lack of optokinetic nystagmus and visual motion perception in acquired cortical blindness. Neuro-Ophthalmol. 1997;17(4):211–8.

10. Jan JE, McCormick AQ, Hoyt CS. The unequal nystagmus test. Dev Med Child Neurol. 1988;30(4):441–3.

11. Sturm V, Cassel D, Eizenman M. Objective estimation of visual acuity with preferential looking. Invest Ophthalmol Vis Sci. 2011;52(2):708–13.

12. Rydberg A, Ericson B, Lennerstrand G, Jacobson L, Lindstedt E. Assessment of visual acuity in children aged 1½–6 years, with normal and subnormal vision. Strabismus. 1999;7(1):1–24.

13. Facchin A, Maffioletti S, Martelli M, Daini R. Different trajectories in the development of visual acuity with different levels of crowding: The Milan Eye Chart (MEC). Vision Res. 2019;156:10–6.

14. Choudhury E, Almarzouqi SJ, Morgan ML, Lee AG. Afferent Pupillary Defects, Relative (Marcus Gunn Pupil). In: Schmidt-Erfurth U, and Kohnen T. editors. Encyclopedia of ophthalmology. Berlin, Heidelberg: Springer; 2018.

15. Takizawa G, Miki A, Maeda F, Goto K, Araki S, Ieki Y, et al. Association between a relative afferent pupillary defect using pupillography and inner retinal atrophy in optic nerve disease. Clin Ophthalmol (Auckland, NZ). 2015;9:1895.

16. Agrawal S, Yadav A, Singh N. Clinical evaluation of strabismus. In: Agrawal S. editor. Strabismus. Singapore: Springer; 2019. https://doi.org/10.1007/978-981-13-1126-0_2.

17. Economides JR, Adams DL, Horton JC. Variability of ocular deviation in strabismus. JAMA Ophthalmol. 2016;134(1):63–9.

18. Papageorgiou E, McLean RJ, Gottlob I. Nystagmus in childhood. Pediatr Neonatol. 2014;55(5):341–51.

19. Jacobson L, Ygge J, Flodmark O. Nystagmus in periventricular leucomalacia. Br J Ophthalmol. 1998;82(9):1026–32.

20. Richards MD, Wong A. Infantile nystagmus syndrome: Clinical characteristics, current theories of pathogenesis, diagnosis, and management. Can J Ophthalmol Can d'Ophtalmologie. 2015;50(6):400–8.

21. Hertle RW. Nystagmus in infancy and childhood: Characteristics and evidence for treatment. Am Orthopt J. 2010;60(1):48–58.

22. Dotan G, Miller M, Strominger MB, Nelson LB. Surgical management of nystagmus. J Pediatr Ophthalmol Strabismus. 2018;55(5):280–3.

23. Mishra K, Jandial A, Sandal R, Khadwal A, Malhotra P. Night blindness, Bitot's spot and vitamin A deficiency. QJM An Int J Med. 2018;112(3):225.

24. Mocan MC, Yilmaz PT, Irkec M, Orhan M. The significance of Vogt's striae in keratoconus as evaluated by in vivo confocal microscopy. Clin Experiment Ophthalmol. 2008;36(4):329–34.

25. Mandal AK, Raghavachary C, Peguda HK. Haab's striae. Ophthalmology. 2017;124(1):11.

26. Robert M-C, Colby K. Corneal diseases in children: Congenital anomalies. In: Corneal diseases in children. Cham, Switzerland: Springer; 2017:69–85.

27. Chan WH, Lloyd IC, Symes RJ, Ashworth JL, Cosgrove E, Pilling R, et al. Accuracy of intraocular pressure measurement with the Icare tonometer in children. Asia-Pacific J Ophthalmol. 2015;4(6):357–9.

28. Moreno-Montañés J, Martínez-de-la-Casa JM, Sabater AL, Morales-Fernandez L, Sáenz C, Garcia-Feijoo J. Clinical evaluation of the new rebound tonometers Icare PRO and Icare ONE compared with the Goldmann tonometer. J Glaucoma. 2015;24(7):527–32.

29. Shah SP, Taylor AE, Sowden JC, Ragge N, Russell-Eggitt I, Rahi JS, et al. Anophthalmos, microphthalmos, and coloboma in the United Kingdom: Clinical features, results of investigations, and early management. Ophthalmology. 2012;119(2):362–8.

30. Onwochei BC, Simon JW, Bateman JB, Couture KC, Mir E. Ocular colobomata. Surv Ophthalmol. 2000;45(3):175–94.

31. Chang L, Blain D, Bertuzzi S, Brooks BP. Uveal coloboma: Clinical and basic science update. Curr Opin Ophthalmol. 2006;17(5):447–70.

32. Hornby SJ, Gilbert CE, Rahi J, Sil AK, Xiao Y, Dandona L, et al. Regional variation in blindness in children due to microphthalmos, anophthalmos and coloboma. Ophthalmic Epidemiol. 2000;7(2):127–38.

33. Muecke J, Hammerton M, Aung YY, Warrier S, Kong A, Morse A, et al. A survey of visual impairment and blindness in children attending seven schools for the blind in Myanmar. Ophthalmic Epidemiol. 2009;16(6):370–7.

34. Tripathy K, Chawla R, Sharma YR, Venkatesh P, Sagar P, Vohra R, et al. Prophylactic laser photocoagulation of fundal coloboma: Does it really help? Acta Ophthalmol. 2016;94(8):e809–10.

35. Chen C, Xiao H, Ding X. Persistent fetal vasculature. Asia-Pacific J Ophthalmol. 2019;8(1):86–95.

36. Zahavi A, Weinberger D, Snir M, Ron Y. Management of severe persistent fetal vasculature: Case series and review of the literature. Int Ophthalmol. 2019;39(3):579–87.

37. Chavarria-Soley G, Michels-Rautenstrauss K, Pasutto F, Flikier D, Flikier P, Cirak S, et al. Primary congenital glaucoma and Rieger's anomaly: Extended haplotypes reveal founder effects for eight distinct CYP1B1 mutations. Mol Vis. 2006;12:523–31.

38. Tamçelik N, Atalay E, Bolukbasi S, Çapar O, Ozkok A. Demographic features of subjects with congenital glaucoma. Indian J Ophthalmol. 2014;62(5):565.

39. Hsu C-R, Chen Y-H, Tai M-C, Lu D-W. Combined trabeculotomy-trabeculectomy using the modified Safer Surgery System augmented with MMC: Its long-term outcomes of glaucoma treatment in Asian children. Graefe's Arch Clin Exp Ophthalmol. 2018;256(6):1187–94.

40. Brandt JD, Hammel N, Fenerty C, Karaconji T. Glaucoma drainage devices. In: Surgical management of childhood glaucoma. Cham, Switzerland: Springer; 2018. pp. 99–127.

41. Yi J, Yun J, Li Z-K, Xu C-T, Pan B-R. Epidemiology and molecular genetics of congenital cataracts. Int J Ophthalmol. 2011;4(4):422.

42. Wu X, Long E, Lin H, Liu Y. Prevalence and epidemiological characteristics of congenital cataract: A systematic review and meta-analysis. Sci Rep. 2016;6:28564.

43. Lim ME, Buckley EG, Prakalapakorn SG. Update on congenital cataract surgery management. Curr Opin Ophthalmol. 2017;28(1):87–92.

44. Lambert SR. The timing of surgery for congenital cataracts: Minimizing the risk of glaucoma following cataract surgery while optimizing the visual outcome. J AAPOS Off Publ Am Assoc Pediatr Ophthalmol Strabismus/American Assoc Pediatr Ophthalmol Strabismus. 2016;20(3):191.

45. Tadros D, Trivedi RH, Wilson ME. Primary versus secondary IOL implantation following removal of infantile unilateral congenital cataract: Outcomes after at least 5 years. J Am Assoc Pediatr Ophthalmol Strabismus. 2016;20(1):25–9.

46. Yangzes S, Kaur S, Gupta PC, Sharma M, Jinagal J, Singh J, et al. Intraocular lens implantation in children with unilateral congenital cataract in the first 4 years of life. Eur J Ophthalmol. 2019;29(3):304–8.

47. Rong X, Ji Y, Fang Y, Jiang Y, Lu Y. Long-term visual outcomes of secondary intraocular lens implantation in children with congenital cataracts. PLoS One. 2015;10(7):e0134864.

48. Jacob SC, Antony CL, Govind I, Kalikivayi V. Significance of primary posterior capsulotomy using Nd: Yaglaser in pediatric cataract surgery. SM Opthalmol J. 2018;4(1):1015.

49. Chen TC, Walton DS, Bhatia LS. Aphakic glaucoma after congenital cataract surgery. Arch Ophthalmol. 2004;122(12):1819–25.

50. Miyamichi D, Nishina S, Hosono K, Yokoi T, Kurata K, Sato M, et al. Retinal structure in Leber's congenital amaurosis caused by RPGRIP1 mutations. Hum Genome Var. 2019;6(1):32.

51. Menzel O, Bekkeheien RCJ, Reymond A, Fukai N, Boye E, Kosztolanyi G, et al. Knobloch syndrome: novel mutations in COL18A1, evidence for genetic heterogeneity, and a functionally impaired polymorphism in endostatin. Hum Mutat. 2004;23(1):77–84.

52. Grønskov K, Ek J, Brondum-Nielsen K. Oculocutaneous albinism. Orphanet J Rare Dis. 2007;2(1):43.

53. Remmer MH, Rastogi N, Ranka MP, Ceisler EJ. Achromatopsia: A review. Curr Opin Ophthalmol. 2015;26(5):333–40.

54. Mantri A, Makwana M, Goyal V, Payal V, Mourya H, Sharma P, et al. A prospective study to determine the incidence of retinopathy of prematurity at a tertiary care centre in Western Rajasthan and delineate its risk factors. Int J Contemp Pediatr. 2017;4(4):1193.

21B

AN APPROACH TO OCULOMOTOR ANOMALIES IN A CHILD

Stacy L. Pineles

CASE STUDY

A 4-month-old child presents with crossed eyes since birth. The eyes were intermittently crossing for the first 6 weeks of life, and then they became constantly crossed by 2 months of age. Since then the parents have noticed that either eye can turn in and each eye turns about 50% of the time. On examination, the patient is able to fix and follow with each eye individually. His pupils are normal without a relative afferent pupillary defect. His intraocular pressure is normal. His anterior segment is normal and the dilated fundus examination is also normal with normal appearing optic nerves. Motility examination is notable for full abduction bilaterally. There is bilateral over-elevation in adduction. He has 40 prism diopters of esotropia which is comitant in all directions of gaze and an associated dissociated vertical deviation in the right eye. Lastly, mild latent nystagmus is noted on cover testing. What is the diagnosis of this patient?

OPHTHALMIC EXAMINATION OF A CHILD WITH VISUAL LOSS

- Shape of head, craniosynostosis or head bobbing movements
- Position of eyeball and eye lid
- Position of head
- Assess binocularity
- Assess visual acuity
- Assess fusion
- Assess stereoacuity
- Assess function of EOM mono-ocularly and binocularly
- Pursuits, saccades and nystagmus
- Assess ocular alignment
- Assess ocular torsion
- Fundus examination
- Cycloplegic refraction

Introduction

Oculomotor anomalies in a child can present numerous ways. An oculomotor anomaly can be long-standing and invisible to the parents or it can be acute in onset and be noticeable to the child or caretaker by the presence of diplopia or an anomalous head posture. This section describes an approach to oculomotor anomalies in a child and describes findings of some of the important causes of this clinical presentation.

Oculomotor anomalies can be neurological in nature or can be benign like due to amblyopia, refractive error or genetic predisposition. The underlying etiology can typically be determined by a careful history and physical examination. The information gathered from the history and physical examination can then be correlated to draft a list of differential diagnoses by the treating clinician. Occasionally, ancillary testing will also be required.

GENERAL FRAMEWORK – HISTORY AND EXAMINATION IN A CHILD WITH OCULOMOTOR ANOMALY

- Characterize oculo-motor palsy
- Duration and onset of the oculo-motor anomaly
- Anomalous head posture
- Associated signs and symptoms
- Associated visual loss
- Variability
- Important histories: history of trauma/family history

History of child with oculomotor anomalies

The history of a child with oculomotor anomalies is typically provided by the child's caretaker, but the child can also provide information if they are able. The following areas should be explored while taking a history of a child with an oculomotor anomaly:

- *Duration and onset of the oculomotor anomaly*
  Infantile-onset strabismus should be considered in patients with ocular misalignment that is long-standing and not associated with diplopia. Although most congenital or infantile-onset strabismus is noticeable to the parents, a congenital fourth nerve palsy may not be noticed as the child often compensates with increased fusional amplitudes or an anomalous head posture. Similarly, Duane syndrome may not be initially noticed if the patient is orthotropic in primary position. Reviewing old photographs may be beneficial for determining the onset of anomalous head postures in more subtle cases.
- *Presence of an anomalous head posture*
  An anomalous head posture can be the presenting symptom in virtually any cause of incomitant strabismus. The onset of the head posture can be a clue as to the onset of the oculomotor anomaly. Horizontal head turns can be seen in patients with cranial nerve third, fourth, and sixth palsies. They can also be seen in Duane syndrome as well as horizontal gaze palsies. A vertical head position or head tilt can be seen with cranial nerve third or fourth palsies, rare forms of Duane syndrome, "A" or "V" pattern strabismus,

DOI: 10.1201/9780429020278-32

skew deviation, monocular elevation deficiency, or congenital fibrosis of the extraocular muscles.

- *Associated signs and symptoms*
  Associated diplopia is particularly important symptom to illicit since its presence typically indicates that the strabismus is not congenital or infantile onset in nature. Furthermore, one must question the patient or their caretakers regarding the character of the strabismus including the direction of the deviation, whether it is unilateral or bilateral, variability, and whether it is associated with any other ocular or periocular findings such as pupillary abnormalities, ptosis, or symptoms of other cranial neuropathies.
- *History of trauma*
  Any child who presents with an oculomotor anomaly should always be questioned regarding trauma, specifically head trauma. Cranial nerve palsies can be traumatic or may also be due to increased intracranial pressure from an intracranial hemorrhage. Similarly, pathology in the brainstem or vestibular system (traumatic or otherwise) can result in vertical strabismus from a skew deviation or horizontal strabismus from a cranial neuropathy or internuclear ophthalmoplegia. Furthermore, an orbital fracture can cause both vertical and horizontal forms of strabismus.
- *Variability*
  Parents should be questioned with regard to variability throughout the day. If the ocular motor anomaly is worse when tired and improves upon awakening, one should consider myasthenia gravis.
- *Characterization of visual acuity*
  It is important to note whether there is any suspicion of decreased vision in one or both eyes. Sensory strabismus may appear similarly to other forms of comitant strabismus, and therefore, visual acuity in each eye is important to note. Furthermore, amblyopia can occur in the setting of most forms of early-onset ocular misalignment, thus visual acuity assessment is of utmost importance.
- *Presence of other symptoms*
  A history of headaches in association with a cranial neuropathy suggests the possibility of increased intracranial pressure, a central nervous system lesion, or migraine. Similarly, developmental delay or regression, nausea, vomiting, or other focal neurologic symptoms can suggest a neurological syndrome.
- *Family history*
  It is always wise to explore family history of the child for any heritable diseases. The parents should be asked about history of any ocular or systemic diseases in the family.

Having collected all the aforementioned information, the clinician now should proceed to the ophthalmic examination of the child.

Ophthalmic examination of a child with visual loss

The physical examination of the child starts from the time the physician enters the examination room. The clinician should observe the child's resting head posture and manifest eye position. Any abnormal head posture with head tilt and chin position should also be evaluated as these can give diagnostic clues to underlying cranial nerve palsies leading to paresis of extraocular muscles. External examination should also include an assessment of the eyelid position and evaluation for the presence of nystagmus. While performing an external examination, always look for any external abnormalities like abnormal shape of the head, any craniosynostosis, heading bobbing movement, or any other obvious physical abnormalities.

In patients with oculomotor anomalies, an assessment of binocularity is crucial to understanding the underlying disease. Furthermore, binocularity should be assessed at the beginning of the eye examination before fusion is broken down by dissociating tests. Oculomotor anomalies that disrupt fusion early in life typically are associated with permanent deficits in binocular vision; however, later-onset or intermittent oculomotor anomalies can be associated with moderate to excellent stereoacuity. Testing with the Worth-4-Dot test or Bagolini lenses can provide crude information related to gross levels of fusion. Stereoacuity testing with either a Contour Test or a Random Dot test can provide information related to higher levels of fusion.

After an assessment of binocularity, it is important to assess monocular visual acuity using age-appropriate testing. Function of the extraocular muscles should be assessed monocularly and binocularly by testing smooth pursuit, saccades, and ductions in all directions of gaze. Next ocular alignment should be tested using appropriate techniques in all cardinal directions of gaze and at near. Finally, ocular torsion can be tested objectively in patients who can cooperate with Double Maddox Rods.

A full ophthalmic examination including assessment of the pupils, anterior segment, and posterior segment is also crucial. Dilated fundus examination can also be used to evaluate for fundus torsion. Lastly, cycloplegic refraction should be performed in all children to aid in the final diagnosis and management.

Causes of oculomotor anomalies in children

Comitant strabismus
Infantile esotropia
Infantile esotropia is a comitant, constant, non-accommodative esotropia that typically begins before the age of 6 months (Figure 21B.1). The angle of esotropia is generally large and amblyopia is not common. In cases of suspected infantile esotropia, it is important to evaluate for frequently associated signs such as dissociated vertical deviation, over-elevation in adduction, latent nystagmus, and optokinetic asymmetry. In addition, one must be sure that abduction is full in each eye, and this may require testing monocularly to avoid cross-fixation. A complete eye

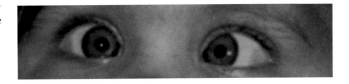

FIGURE 21B.1 A 4-month-old infant who presented with "crossing eyes" since 4 weeks of life. Her ductions were full and she also demonstrated latent nystagmus. She was diagnosed with infantile esotropia, and strabismus surgery was performed.

examination is essential to rule out other etiologies of infantile-onset esotropia such as Duane syndrome, Mobius syndrome, myasthenia gravis, early-onset accommodative esotropia, nystagmus blockage syndrome, or other neurological diseases. In addition, early-onset sensory strabismus due to poor vision in one or both eyes may present with an esotropic deviation (although sensory exotropia is more common). In cases of typical infantile esotropia, no neuroimaging is required.

Accommodative esotropia

Accommodative esotropia is an esotropia caused partially or entirely by the use of accommodation to clear vision in the presence of hyperopia. Typically, accommodative esotropia is a comitant esotropia that presents later than infantile esotropia (typically onset within ages 2–5 years) and is intermittent initially becoming more constant with time. Accommodative esotropia is typically associated with moderate-to-high hyperopia (mean +4.75D)[1] and may be associated with a high accommodative convergence to accommodation (AC/A ratio).

Acute-acquired comitant esotropia

Rarely, a child may present with a sudden-onset comitant esotropia. This syndrome is typically associated with diplopia and should be differentiated from a decompensated small-angle esotropia and accommodative esotropia. In cases of truly acute-onset acquired esotropia, neuroimaging is required to rule out central nervous system lesions such as Chiari malformation and posterior fossa lesions.[2-4] Acute esotropia is even more ominous in cases with lateral incomitance, neurological symptoms, headaches, nausea, vomiting, and increasing head circumference.

Intermittent exotropia

Intermittent exotropia is characterized by occasional outward drifting of the eyes combined with periods of binocular fusion. Intermittent exotropia may present as an intermittent unilateral eye deviation or alternating strabismus. Since intermittent exotropia is the most common form of divergent strabismus,[5] a high index of suspicion should be held for it in all cases of exotropia. The underlying cause of intermittent exotropia is not well-defined, but the characteristics are so typical that further workup is rarely indicated. Patients typically present with exotropia occurring within the first decade of life, monocular squinting in sunlight or photophobia, and normal stereopsis when in periods of fusion. In children with exotropic deviations, it is important to assess for the control of their deviation which is typically better in cases of intermittent exotropia than in other more ominous neurologic etiologies of exotropia.

Infantile exotropia

Constant exotropia in an infant is rarer than constant esotropia. When an infant presents with exotropia, a high index of suspicion should be maintained for neurologic disease. Since infantile exotropia is frequently associated with low vision, a detailed neurologic and developmental history, full assessment of visual acuity, and examination for other neurologic signs must be performed.

Incomitant strabismus

Review of cranial nerve anatomy

The three ocular motor nerves innervate the six extraocular muscles as well as the levator palpebrae superioris (LPS) and the pupillary constrictors. The oculomotor nerve innervates the LPS, superior rectus (SR), inferior rectus, medial rectus, inferior oblique, and the pupillary constrictors. The trochlear nerve innervates the superior oblique muscle, and the abducens nerve innervates the lateral rectus muscle. The pathways involved in supranuclear control of the ocular motor nerves descend from the cerebral cortex and terminate in the brainstem in the omnipause neurons (for horizontal saccades) and the rostral interstitial nucleus of the medial longitudinal fasciculus of the midbrain (vertical saccades).

The oculomotor nucleus resides in the midbrain and is divided into individual subnuclei for each extraocular muscle. Interestingly, the SR subnucleus innervates the contralateral SR muscle, while the remainder of the subnuclei innervates the ipsilateral corresponding muscles. The Edinger-Westphal nucleus, which supplies innervation to the pupillary constrictors, is shared by both sides. The oculomotor nerve fascicle exits the brainstem through the ventral midbrain in the interpeduncular fossa.

The trochlear nerve nucleus is located in the ventral pontomesencephalic junction caudal to the oculomotor nuclei. The trochlear nerve fascicles cross to innervate the contralateral superior oblique muscle and exit the brainstem dorsally beneath the inferior colliculus. The abducens nucleus resides in the dorsal pons. The abducens nerve fascicles travel ventrally and exit the brainstem at the pontomedullary junction to innervate the ipsilateral lateral rectus muscle.

All three ocular motor nerves travel through the subarachnoid space at the skull base and into the cavernous sinus. Within the cavernous sinus, they are adjacent to the first and second division of the trigeminal nerve, the internal carotid artery, and the third-order oculosympathetic fibers. In the cavernous sinus, the oculomotor nerve divides into superior and inferior divisions which innervate the (1) SR and LPS and (2) the inferior rectus, inferior oblique, medial rectus, and pupillary constrictors, respectively. The nerves then exit the cavernous sinus and traverse the orbit. The oculomotor and abducens nerves are positioned within the Annulus of Zinn, while trochlear neve lies outside of the annulus of Zinn. In-depth knowledge of the pathways of the ocular motor nerves as well as adjacent structures provides clinicians with the knowledge required to understand various clinical presentation of cranial nerve palsies with co-existent neurological syndromes.

Oculomotor nerve palsy

The presentation of an isolated oculomotor nerve palsy can vary from a complete palsy with the characteristic ptosis, mydriasis, and "down and out" appearance of the affected eye to a milder form, with any combination of affected muscles and any level of severity. When considering a third nerve palsy, a distinction is often made between a "complete" and "incomplete" palsy. A complete palsy is diagnosed when there is complete ptosis, a fixed pupil, and complete paralysis of the SR, inferior rectus, inferior oblique, and medial rectus. Historically, this distinction was thought to reflect the anatomical location of the causative lesion; however, it is now established that incomplete palsies can result from lesions anywhere along the pathway of the nerve.

When examining a patient with a suspected third nerve palsy, it is important to determine which muscles are affected in order to define whether the palsy may be divisional (superior vs. inferior). Divisional palsies are typically attributed to lesions in the pathway anterior to or within the cavernous sinus, although they have also been localized as far posteriorly as the nerve fascicle or subarachnoid space.[6–9] Evidence of aberrant regeneration should also be sought as it is considered extremely rare in ischemic etiologies and its presence in a non-congenital case should prompt practitioners to evaluate for a compressive lesion.[10]

Given the anatomy of the third nerve, there are several co-existent symptoms that should be sought on history and examination in order to localize the lesion and guide workup. Lesions of the oculomotor nucleus can result in bilateral ptosis (due to a shared LPS nucleus), contralateral or bilateral SR palsy (due to the crossing fibers of the SR nucleus), ipsilateral mydriasis and ipsilateral inferior rectus, medial rectus, and inferior oblique palsies. Although this clinical scenario is fairly classic for a nuclear lesion, there is variability in the possible presentation, and a nuclear third nerve palsy may also be mimicked by a fascicular lesion.[11] Fascicular third nerve palsies are often associated with obvious neurological symptoms due to the adjacent structures in the brainstem. In children and adults with third nerve palsies, the following symptoms should be sought to evaluate for brainstem syndromes: contralateral ataxia (Claude syndrome), contralateral hemiparesis (Weber syndrome), and contralateral tremor (Benedikt syndrome). Despite the proximal location, fascicular third nerve palsies can present with superior or inferior divisional involvement given the topographical arrangement of the nerve fibers. Rarely, nuclear and fascicular lesions can result in an isolated muscle palsy, although isolated muscle palsies should also prompt consideration of other diagnostic entities.

In the subarachnoid space, the oculomotor nerve is susceptible to compression, which may be a sign of a life-threatening condition. Uncal herniation can result in a third nerve palsy with altered mental status in a patient of any age, although compression of the third nerve by a posterior cerebral artery aneurysm is much more common in adults than pediatric patients. Due to the dorsomedial location of the pupillary fibers in the oculomotor nerve bundle, mydriasis is often the first sign of oculomotor nerve compression in the subarachnoid space. Adults and children with uncal herniation may initially present with pupillary dilation, but as the syndrome progresses, decreased consciousness, evolution of the oculomotor nerve involvement, and hemiplegia will result. Similarly, posterior communicating artery aneurysms in adults typically result in an early oculomotor nerve palsy with prominent mydriasis, but the most common accompanying symptom is pain. Within the subarachnoid space, children and adults may also develop primary tumors of

the nerves such as neuromas and schwannomas. These tumors can present at any age and typically result in a slowly progressive oculomotor nerve palsy without co-existent symptoms. Skull base tumors such as meningiomas or chordomas may also compress oculomotor nerve in this location.

In the cavernous sinus, oculomotor nerve palsies are rarely isolated. They typically occur in conjunction with trochlear or abducens nerve dysfunction, as well as evidence of trigeminal involvement or Horner syndrome. Interestingly, due to the proximity of the oculosympathetic fibers, one can find an absence of mydriasis in patients with oculomotor nerve palsy due to cavernous sinus lesions when both the parasympathetic and sympathetic fibers are equally affected. Lesions to consider in the cavernous sinus include neoplasms, cavernous sinus thrombosis, infectious etiologies, and high or low flow carotid-cavernous fistulas.

The most common cause of an oculomotor palsy in children is congenital, followed by trauma, infection and inflammation, and tumor (Table 21B.1).[12] It is estimated 18–47% of pediatric cases are of congenital origin.[13] Congenital palsies classically have pupillary involvement and aberrant regeneration. Congenital palsies have been attributed to abnormalities anywhere along the pathway of the nerve from the nucleus to the peripheral bundle. As neuroimaging techniques improve, it has become evident that some congenital palsies are in actuality secondary to neuromas or schwannoma.[14] Unlike adult patients, aneurysm is not frequently a cause of oculomotor palsy in children.[15] Ophthalmoplegic migraine should be a diagnosis of exclusion.

In patients presenting with oculomotor palsies, it is important to rule out other co-existent cranial neuropathies – the trochlear nerve can be tested by evaluating for intorsion of the eye on attempted downgaze. The movement of the conjunctival vessels can be used as a surrogate marker of the fourth nerve function in the presence of complete third nerve palsy. Common presentations of partial oculomotor palsies include divisional palsies – the superior division of the oculomotor nerve innervates the SR and LPS whereas the inferior division innervates the medial rectus, inferior rectus, inferior oblique, and pupillary constrictors. Isolated inferior rectus and inferior oblique palsies have also been reported.[16,17]

Aberrant re-innervation can arise several weeks to months after an oculomotor nerve injury or in congenital cases.[18] Aberrant re-innervation is not seen after ischemic injuries. It can present with elevation of the eyelid on attempted adduction or

TABLE 21B.1: Common Etiologies of Isolated Ocular Motor Nerve Palsy in Children

Oculomotor Nerve	Trochlear Nerve	Abducens Nerve
• Congenital	• Congenital	• Neoplasm
• Traumatic	• Traumatic	• Medulloblastoma, ependymoma, pontine glioma
• Neoplastic	• Craniofacial anomalies	• Trauma
• Midbrain astrocytoma, glioma, orbital rhabdomyosarcoma	• Neoplastic	• Meningitis
• Intrinsic nerve tumors (especially in neurofibromatosis)	• Astrocytoma, glioma	• Pneumococcus
• Meningitis	• Intrinsic nerve tumors (especially in neurofibromatosis)	• *Haemophilus influenzae*
• Pneumococcus	• Meningitis	• Tuberculosis
• *Haemophilus influenzae*	• Pneumococcus	• Lyme
• Tuberculosis	• *Haemophilus influenzae*	• Benign abducens palsy
• Lyme	• Tuberculosis	
• Migraine	• Lyme	

downgaze, adduction of the eye on attempted vertical movement, or pupillary constriction on attempted adduction.

Trochlear nerve palsy

The presentation of an isolated trochlear nerve palsy can vary depending on the severity and the age of onset. In patients with a congenital or very early onset trochlear palsy, there may be no manifest hypertropia, as these patients often develop large fusional amplitudes. In these cases, patients more typically present with torticollis or complaints of intermittent diplopia or asthenopia; a prolonged cover testing or a patch test may be required in order for the practitioner to discover the hypertropia. Conversely, acute acquired trochlear palsies more typically present with a larger manifest hypertropia, abnormal ductions, and constant cyclovertical diplopia.

When examining a patient with a suspected trochlear nerve palsy, it is important to determine whether the symptoms are acute in onset or whether they are long-standing and potentially congenital. The most common etiology of trochlear nerve palsies in children is a congenital palsy. Patients with congenital trochlear palsies frequently present with a head tilt that can be seen in childhood photographs, large fusional amplitudes, and facial asymmetry. If these historical and examination features can be proven, then further workup is not required.

The most common cause of acquired trochlear nerve palsy is trauma.[19] Trauma frequently causes trochlear palsies due to the long path of the nerves and their close proximity between the decussating nerve fibers and the tentorium, which can create contusions or pressure on the nerves. In the absence of trauma, additional diagnoses to consider vary based on the age of the patient. In young children, other etiologies of isolated trochlear palsies are extremely rare but can include vascular, increased intracranial pressure, or a central nervous system lesion.

The majority of children with congenital or acute trochlear nerve palsies present with torticollis.[20] In patients with congenital palsies, facial asymmetry may also be present. Patients with an isolated trochlear palsy typically present with an ipsilateral hypertropia, worse in contralateral gaze, and ipsilateral head tilt. This results in a contralateral face turn or tilt. In acute trochlear nerve palsies, Bielschowsky's "three-step test" may aid in localizing the lesion. The three-step test dictates that a hypertropia worse in contralateral gaze and ipsilateral head tilt is most likely related to a trochlear palsy. Of course other etiologies of strabismus may mimic a trochlear palsy and give similar results to the test; these include skew deviation (which may be differentiated by resolution in prone position), dissociated vertical deviation, myasthenia gravis, and patients with previous strabismus surgery.[21] Furthermore, long-standing trochlear palsies may not follow the rule of the three-step test due to contracture of the SR muscle and spread of comitance.

When bilateral, trochlear nerve palsies are frequently due to trauma but may also be attributed to increased intracranial pressure.[22] Bilateral trochlear palsies typically present with a V-pattern esotropia, small vertical deviation in primary position with alternating hypertopias in side gaze (right hypertropia in left gaze and left hypertropia in right gaze), and large amounts of excyclotorsion. In these cases, the three-step test is often unreliable.

In children and adults, if the history and examination are consistent with a congenital origin, then no further workup is required. In all other adults and children who do not have a congenital onset or vascular risk factors, a magnetic reference imaging (MRI) should be considered with special attention to the midbrain, cavernous sinus, and orbit. If there are any signs of meningitis, a lumbar puncture should also be considered. If neuroimaging is normal, then other diagnoses such as thyroid eye disease and myasthenia gravis should be considered and worked up if indicated.

Abducens nerve palsy

The presentation of an isolated abducens nerve palsy can vary depending on the severity of the paralysis. Patients may present with a small esotropia and face turn, or a large esotropia that precludes fusion in any direction of gaze. Due to the anatomical course of the sixth nerve, several associated symptoms must be sought in order to localize the lesion. In the sixth nerve nucleus, neurons that are destined to climb within the medial longitudinal fasciculus to innervate the contralateral medial rectus muscle for ipsilateral gaze reside. For this reason, a nuclear abducens palsy is typically associated with a gaze palsy in the ipsilateral direction. In addition, nuclear abducens palsies are also almost always associated with facial nerve palsies due to the proximity of the facial nerve nucleus and genu. As the sixth nerve traverses the petrous apex, it can be affected by intracranial pressure changes as well as by skull base tumors. In the cavernous sinus, the oculosympathetic fibers are adjacent to the abducens nerve, and therefore, a co-existent Horner syndrome must be sought.

Isolated congenital abducens nerve palsy is extremely rare because these cases typically present with Duane syndrome. True congenital abducens nerve palsy is reported though and is typically transient.[23] More commonly, sixth nerve palsy in children is due to neoplasm, trauma, post-viral inflammation, or increased intracranial pressure.[24–32] Although benign recurrent sixth nerve palsy and post-vaccination sixth nerve palsy are also relatively common in children, these should be diagnoses of exclusion, after a complete workup has been done.

In all children with an acquired sixth nerve palsy, a contrast-enhanced MRI of the brain and orbits should be obtained. Furthermore, lumbar puncture can be considered in patients with a normal brain MRI in order to evaluate for elevated intracranial pressure, meningitis, and other central nervous system infiltrative processes. Finally, an MR-venogram can also be considered in cases where elevated intracranial pressure is suspected.

Duane retraction syndrome

Duane syndrome is a common etiology of congenital abduction deficit. The disorder can present with a wide array of oculomotor anomalies, but the underlying pathogenesis is similar in all cases and involves absence of the abducens nerve and peripheral misdirection of a branch of the third nerve to the lateral rectus muscle. The misdirection of the third nerve typically leads to co-contraction of the lateral and medial rectus muscles on attempted adduction (leading to palpebral fissure narrowing) and strabismus which may be characterized by esotropia, exotropia, or hypertropia.

The most common presentation of Duane syndrome is Type I (Figure 21B.2), which is characterized by a unilateral complete lack of abduction, palpebral fissure narrowing on adduction, and esotropia. Approximately half of children with Duane syndrome are orthotropic in primary position, while the other half typically require a face turn to maintain binocular single vision.[19] Duane syndrome can be differentiated from sixth nerve palsy by the

FIGURE 21B.2   A child who presented with "crossed eyes" who was found to have complete lack of abduction coupled with a small angle esotropia and palpebral fissure narrowing on attempted adduction. The child was diagnosed with Duane syndrome, and no further workup was performed.

size of the esotropia in primary position relative to the abduction weakness. In a patient with such severe limitation to abduction, one would expect a large angle esotropia; if the esotropia is very small, then Duane syndrome should be considered.

Rarer presentations of Duane syndrome include bilateral disease, exotropic Duane syndrome, and hypertropic Duane syndrome. The exact strabismic subtype depends on the relative strength of the aberrant innervation to the lateral rectus muscle as well as co-contraction of any vertical rectus muscles on attempted adduction. Type II Duane syndrome is characterized by diminished adduction and presence of exotropia. Type III Duane syndrome presents with a reduction in both adduction and abduction.

Skew deviation
Skew deviation is a cyclovertical strabismus due to a prenuclear lesion typically within the vestibular pathway. The presentation of skew deviation is widely variable and can be horizontally comitant or incomitant and associated with either incyclo- or excyclotorsion. When it is incomitant, it may simulate a trochlear nerve palsy. However, Parulekar et al. demonstrated that skew deviations diminish in supine position, unlike trochlear nerve palsies.[33] Given that skew deviation is attributed to a central nervous system lesion, there are typically other associated neurological symptoms or signs. If a skew deviation is suspected, a full neurologic workup and neuroimaging should be sought.

Other disorders of the oculomotor system
External ophthalmoplegia
Diffuse ophthalmoplegia is rare in pediatric patients but when seen should prompt consideration of chronic progressive external ophthalmoplegia (CPEO). Other diagnoses to consider include botulism, brainstem disease, Kearns–Sayre syndrome, Miller Fisher syndrome, mitochondrial encephalopathy, and myasthenia gravis. These diagnoses can be differentiated based on history, associated symptoms, and family history.

CPEO is characterized by a slowly progressive symmetric external ophthalmoplegia typically with ptosis and diminished motility in all directions (Figure 21B.3). CPEO can be isolated and sporadically inherited or it can be syndromic and associated with autosomal dominant, recessive, or mitochondrial inheritance. Kearns–Sayre is one subtype of CPEO that is associated with pigmentary degeneration of the retina and heart block. These patients may also be affected by other neurological disorders such as cerebellar disease, mental retardation, and diabetes.[34,35] For this reason, any patient with suspected CPEO should be referred for neurologic and cardiology evaluation.

Myasthenia gravis less frequently affects children than adults but should be considered in any child with acquired strabismus or external ophthalmoplegia. It is characterized by fatigability and fluctuating muscular weakness. In most cases of pediatric myasthenia gravis, ptosis is present, and strabismus

may take any form. In juvenile myasthenia gravis, findings on the examination may include variable and fatigable ptosis, variable strabismus, diminished extraocular movements, a Cogan lid twitch, and improvement with rest or ice. In isolated ocular myasthenia gravis, ancillary testing with acetyl choline receptor antibodies is positive in only 50% of patients.[36] Therefore, the diagnosis in children is often based on clinical symptoms and improvement with rest or ice. Tensilon testing and single-fiber electromyography is very difficult in young children and is therefore not often used. In a patient in whom ocular myasthenia gravis is considered, a thorough review or systems and neurological evaluation should be performed to rule out systemic generalization. Treatment in conjunction with a neuromuscular specialist should be considered given the systemic risks of the disease.

Congenital ocular motor apraxia
Ocular motor apraxia is defined as a defect in the initiation of volitional saccades. Congenital ocular motor apraxia is typically characterized by absence of horizontal saccades but preservation of vertical eye movements and horizontal reflex movements. In order to move their eyes horizontally and achieve visual fixation, babies and children with ocular motor apraxia typically acquire a head thrust which is large in amplitude. Prior to obtaining control of their neck to perform head thrusts, these babies are often thought to be blind because of their inability to track.

Isolated ocular motor apraxia may be familial or sporadic. When sporadic, it may be isolated or in association with various developmental delays.[37–39] It also may be associated with several neurologic syndromes including Joubert syndrome, Dandy-Walker malformation, and structural brain abnormalities such as cerebellar hypoplasia, ataxia telangiectasia, or Gaucher disease type 3.[40] As children with isolated congenital ocular motor apraxia grow older, their ability to generate saccades improves. This may be attributed to a delayed maturation

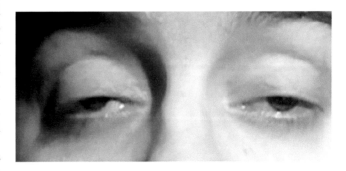

FIGURE 21B.3   A patient with chronic progressive external ophthalmoplegia who presented with progressive ptosis and severely restricted motility in all directions.

of the pathways responsible for horizontal saccades.[41] However, given the numerous association with neurologic and metabolic conditions, neuroimaging is recommended upon diagnosis in all cases.

Congenital fibrosis of the extraocular muscles (CFEOM)

CFEOM is a rare disorder characterized by fibrosis of the extra-ocular muscles, especially the inferior rectus, presenting with fixed downgaze and ptosis. The disorder may be unilateral or bilateral and may also involve the lateral rectus muscle or rarely other extraocular muscles and the LPS. Given the variable involvement of individual recuts muscles, the presentation can vary. CFEOM is attributed to an abnormality in the development of the oculomotor nerve, especially the superior branch, leading to failure of development of their target muscles. Additionally, the genetic defect leads to a co-existent orbital dysgenesis of the extraocular muscles resulting in orbital bands and adhesions.[42] CFEOM has been categorized into three subtypes: Type I is the most common subtype and is characterized by a bilateral non-progressive ophthalmoplegia with ptosis and bilateral downward fixed gaze and complete lack of supraduction bilaterally. Type II is rarer and is associated with bilateral ptosis and completely restrictive ophthalmoplegia with exotropia and poorly reactive pupils. Type III is characterized by ptosis, downward and exotropic fixed eyes, and severe restriction of the eye movements bilaterally.[43–45]

Conclusion

Oculomotor anomalies in a child can present a challenge to physicians. A good rule of thumb is to consider a workup, including neuroimaging, for all acquired anomalies. Risk stratification should include patient-specific data such as age, onset of abnormality, characteristics of the oculomotor findings, duration of symptoms, comorbid neurological signs and symptoms, and the specific type of anomaly. After risk stratification, urgency of further evaluation and treatment can be considered.

Multiple-Choice Questions

1. Duane syndrome typically presents with a:
   a. Horizontal face turn
   b. Chin-down posture
   c. Head tilt
   d. Normal head position

   Answer:
   a. Horizontal face turn

2. The most common cause of a cranial nerve three palsy in a child is:
   a. Congenital
   b. Infection
   c. Tumor
   d. Aneurysm

   Answer:
   a. Congenital

3. Which diagnosis is NOT typically associated with congenital ocular motor apraxia?
   a. Joubert syndrome
   b. Dandy-Walker malformation
   c. Muscular dystrophy
   d. Ataxia telangiectasia

   Answer:
   c. Muscular dystrophy

References

1. Dickey CF, Scott WE. The deterioration of accommodative esotropia: Frequency, characteristics, and predictive factors. J Pediatr Ophthalmol Strabismus. 1988;25(4):172–175.
2. Dikici K, Cicik E, Akman C, Kendiroglu G, Tolun H. Cerebellar astrocytoma presenting with acute esotropia in a 5 year-old girl. Case report. Int Ophthalmol. 1999;23(3):167–170.
3. Lyons C. Where the wild things are: When esotropia misbehaves. Am Orthopt J. 2012;62:61–69.
4. Musazadeh M, Hartmann K, Simon F. Late onset esotropia as first symptom of a cerebellar tumor. Strabismus. 2004;12(2):119–123.
5. Mohney BG. Common forms of childhood strabismus in an incidence cohort. Am J Ophthalmol. 2007;144(3):465–467.
6. Bhatti MT, Eisenschenk S, Roper SN, Guy JR. Superior divisional third cranial nerve paresis: Clinical and anatomical observations of 2 unique cases. Arch Neurol. 2006;63(5):771–776.
7. Guy J, Savino PJ, Schatz NJ, Cobbs WH, Day AL. Superior division paresis of the oculomotor nerve. Ophthalmology. 1985;92(6):777–784.
8. Guy JR, Day AL. Intracranial aneurysms with superior division paresis of the oculomotor nerve. Ophthalmology. 1989;96(7):1071–1076.
9. Ksiazek SM, Repka MX, Maguire A, et al. Divisional oculomotor nerve paresis caused by intrinsic brainstem disease. Ann Neurol. 1989;26(6):714–718.
10. Barr D, Kupersmith M, Turbin R, Yang S, Iezzi R. Synkinesis following diabetic third nerve palsy. Arch Ophthalmol. 2000;118(1):132–134.
11. Liu GT, Carrazana EJ, Charness ME. Unilateral oculomotor palsy and bilateral ptosis from paramedian midbrain infarction. Arch Neurol. 1991;48(9):983–986.
12. Miller NR. Solitary oculomotor nerve palsy in childhood. Am J Ophthalmol. 1977;83(1):106–111.
13. Liu GT, Volpe NJ, Galetta SL. Eye movement disorders. In: Neuro-ophthalmology: Diagnosis and management. Philadelphia, PA: Elsevier; 2010.
14. Norman AA, Farris BK, Siatkowski RM. Neuroma as a cause of oculomotor palsy in infancy and early childhood. J AAPOS. 2001;5(1):9–12.
15. Ng YS, Lyons CJ. Oculomotor nerve palsy in childhood. Can J Ophthalmol. 2005;40(5):645–653.
16. Pollard ZF. Diagnosis and treatment of inferior oblique palsy. J Pediatr Ophthalmol Strabismus. 1993;30(1):15–18.
17. Smith JL. The "nuclear third" question. J Clin Neuroophthalmol. 1982;2(1):61–63.
18. Weber ED, Newman SA. Aberrant regeneration of the oculomotor nerve: Implications for neurosurgeons. Neurosurg Focus. 2007;23(5):E14.
19. Brodsky MC. Ocular motor nerve palsies in children. In: Pediatric neuro-ophthalmology. New York, NY: Springer; 2016:325–375.
20. Kraft SP, O'Donoghue EP, Roarty JD. Improvement of compensatory head postures after strabismus surgery. Ophthalmology. 1992;99(8):1301–1308.
21. Kushner BJ. Errors in the three-step test in the diagnosis of vertical strabismus. Ophthalmology. 1989;96(1):127–132.
22. Kushner BJ. The diagnosis and treatment of bilateral masked superior oblique palsy. Am J Ophthalmol. 1988;105(2):186–194.
23. de Grauw AJ, Rotteveel JJ, Cruysberg JR. Transient sixth cranial nerve paralysis in the newborn infant. Neuropediatrics. 1983;14(3):164–165.
24. Gomez-Gosalvez F, Sala AG, Rubio A, et al. [Acquired oculomotor paralysis in the adolescent]. Rev Neurol. 2001;32(3):241–244.
25. Grewal DS, Zeid JL. Isolated abducens nerve palsy following neonatal hepatitis B vaccination. J AAPOS. 2014;18(1):75–76.
26. Afifi AK, Bell WE, Menezes AH. Etiology of lateral rectus palsy in infancy and childhood. J Child Neurol. 1992;7(3):295–299.
27. Harley RD. Paralytic strabismus in children. Etiologic incidence and management of the third, fourth, and sixth nerve palsies. Ophthalmology. 1980;87(1):24–43.
28. Kodsi SR, Younge BR. Acquired oculomotor, trochlear, and abducent cranial nerve palsies in pediatric patients. Am J Ophthalmol. 1992;114(5):568–574.
29. Moster ML, Savino PJ, Sergott RC, Bosley TM, Schatz NJ. Isolated sixth-nerve palsies in younger adults. Arch Ophthalmol. 1984;102(9):1328–1330.
30. Richards BW, Jones FR, Jr., Younge BR. Causes and prognosis in 4,278 cases of paralysis of the oculomotor, trochlear, and abducens cranial nerves. Am J Ophthalmol. 1992;113(5):489–496.
31. Robertson DM, Hines JD, Rucker CW. Acquired sixth-nerve paresis in children. Arch Ophthalmol. 1970;83(5):574–579.
32. Lee MS, Galetta SL, Volpe NJ, Liu GT. Sixth nerve palsies in children. Pediatr Neurol. 1999;20(1):49–52.

33. Parulekar MV, Dai S, Buncic JR, Wong AM. Head position-dependent changes in ocular torsion and vertical misalignment in skew deviation. Arch Ophthalmol. 2008;126(7):899–905.

34. Bau V, Zierz S. Update on chronic progressive external ophthalmoplegia. Strabismus. 2005;13(3):133–142.

35. DiMauro S, Hirano M. Mitochondrial encephalomyopathies: An update. Neuromuscul Disord. 2005;15(4):276–286.

36. Pineles SL, Avery RA, Moss HE, et al. Visual and systemic outcomes in pediatric ocular myasthenia gravis. Am J Ophthalmol. 2010;150(4):453–459 e453.

37. Jan JE, Kearney S, Groenveld M, Sargent MA, Poskitt KJ. Speech, cognition, and imaging studies in congenital ocular motor apraxia. Dev Med Child Neurol. 1998;40(2):95–99.

38. Marr JE, Green SH, Willshaw HE. Neurodevelopmental implications of ocular motor apraxia. Dev Med Child Neurol. 2005;47(12):815–819.

39. Phillips PH, Brodsky MC, Henry PM. Congenital ocular motor apraxia with autosomal dominant inheritance. Am J Ophthalmol. 2000;129(6):820–822.

40. Harris CM, Taylor DS, Vellodi A. Ocular motor abnormalities in Gaucher disease. Neuropediatrics. 1999;30(6):289–293.

41. Cogan DG, Chu FC, Reingold D. A long term follow-up of congenital ocular motor apraxia: case report. Neuroophthalmology. 1980;1:145.

42. Engle EC, Goumnerov BC, McKeown CA, et al. Oculomotor nerve and muscle abnormalities in congenital fibrosis of the extraocular muscles. Ann Neurol. 1997;41(3): 314–325.

43. Engle EC, McIntosh N, Yamada K, et al. CFEOM1, the classic familial form of congenital fibrosis of the extraocular muscles, is genetically heterogeneous but does not result from mutations in ARIX. BMC Genet. 2002;3:3.

44. Mackey DA, Chan WM, Chan C, et al. Congenital fibrosis of the vertically acting extraocular muscles maps to the FEOM3 locus. Hum Genet. 2002;110(5):510–512.

45. Traboulsi EI, Lee BA, Mousawi A, Khamis AR, Engle EC. Evidence of genetic heterogeneity in autosomal recessive congenital fibrosis of the extraocular muscles. Am J Ophthalmol. 2000;129(5):658–662.

22

RADIOLOGICAL INTERPRETATION IN NEURO-OPHTHALMOLOGY

Chirag Kamal Ahuja, Paramjeet Singh

Neuro-ophthalmology refers to a subdivision of neurology that relates to diseases of the orbit and visual pathways, as well as certain structures of the brain. It is an intriguing branch wherein, at times, it is difficult to assign its scope with respect to the pathologies that come under its ambit. For the sake of simplification, we would include all pathologies, which are related to visual pathway as well as the central/systemic ones in which the clinical manifestation of the patient relates to either visual disturbances or abnormality in ocular movements, in this chapter.

Introduction

Last three decades have seen a remarkable change in the approach to systemic diseases in general and neurological pathologies in particular, which has been secondary to the rapid evolution of imaging technology. With skull and orbital X-rays, in addition to few contrast fluoroscopic studies like ventriculography and myelography, being the only means of evaluation of neuro-orbital pathologies in previous times, evaluation of such disorders was vastly challenging and depended significantly on the clinical assessment. With the advent of ultrasound (US), computed tomography (CT) and magnetic resonance imaging (MRI), the outlook toward some of these "invincible" disorders has transformed tremendously. Though US is not as popular a modality for the detection of intracranial disorders, it was, in fact, one of the first one to be attempted to detect brain tumor by Karl Dussik, an Austrian neurologist, way back in 1942 (1). US did not catch steam in the central nervous system; however, it became hugely popular in abdominal imaging subsequently. Transcalvarial transmission of US waves was very poor. CT and MRI were subsequently introduced, which have presently become the mainstay of diagnosing neurological problems. There has been a role of catheter-related digital subtraction angiography (DSA) in vascular disorders, which not only helps in demonstration of high flow vascular disorders but also aids in the therapy in ocular disorders like obliteration of the carotico-cavernous fistula (CCF). Some salient features of these modalities are presented below, before we begin our discussion on the anatomy of the ocular nervous pathway and the imaging appearances of various diseases, which affect the same.

Ultrasonography

There is a reasonable role that US plays in the evaluation of orbital segment of neuro-ophthalmological disorders. This is due the absence of bone at this location with the eyelids and surrounding skin serving as a good transmitting media for US waves. It has added advantages in the form of its non-invasive nature, easy availability and, of-late, bedside point of care availability (portable US), if required. A relative disadvantage is the subjectivity involved in image acquisition and interpretation. Apart from the morphology of the lesions, the nature of the lesions can be assessed using the echogenicity of the various tissues.

Principle

Ultrasonography is based on the reflectivity of US waves at different acoustic interfaces within the insonating medium (1), which in the present discussion would essentially be the orbital soft tissue. The reflected US are collected by the receiver in the form of echoes and converted to electrical signals. The following are various types of US:

1. *A-mode US:* The signals received are depicted in the form of graphical spikes. The depth within the tissue is mapped on the X-axis while the echo amplitude is displayed on the Y-axis.
2. *B-mode US:* This involves generating and displaying the 2D anatomical images. The brightness (echogenicity) of the interrogated structure helps the operator in deciphering the anatomy/pathology.
3. *Doppler US:* It is based on reflection of US echoes by a moving object, in this case blood and other mobile fluids. The changes in the frequency of reflected sound waves are transformed into electrical signal in the form of images with possibility to deduce blood flow and velocity. Conventionally, red color indicates flow toward the transducer, and blue represents flow away from the transducer. It is useful for studying anatomy/pathology related to reduced/increased blood flow in the orbit, for example, CCF, central retinal artery occlusion, etc.

Eye globe being a superficial structure is best interrogated with a high-frequency transducer, 7 MHz or more. It is particularly useful in patients of cataract, vitreous hemorrhage, etc. where ophthalmoscopy is not effective to see the posteriorly placed structures due to poor "ophthalmoscope window." It is useful for follow-up of some tumors, especially in the pediatric age-group due to its non-invasive and radiation-free nature.

Computed Tomography

CT was invented by British engineer Godfrey Hounsfield of EMI Laboratories, England, and Allan Cormack of Tufts University, Massachusetts, United States, in 1972 (2). Interestingly, the first CT scan of the head took several hours to acquire and still more time to reconstruct the images. CT involves use of ionizing radiation in the form of X-rays for generating images. It is based on the principle that the X-ray beam is attenuated when it crosses a certain substance, the density of which can be measured by calculation of the attenuation coefficient of the beam. The attenuation of various tissues ranges from −1000 HU (Hounsfield units) to +1000 HU and is based on the following densities: compact bone = +1000, water = 0, fat = −100 (approximately) and air = −1000. The CT machine consists of a rotating X-ray tube in the gantry with isocenter at a mobile table where the patient is put supine. The part of the body to be imaged moves across the gantry through which X-ray beams are transmitted and received by X-ray detector rows placed diametrically opposite. The current generation multi-detector CT scanners are capable of very quick

DOI: 10.1201/9780429020278-33

acquisitions and image reconstructions both of plain CT and CT angiography/perfusion studies. CT still forms the first investigation modality of many orbito-neurological disorders.

Acquisition parameters

CT scan images can be acquired in either axial (two-dimensional [2D]) or helical (volumetric or three-dimensional [3D]) formats. Though the volume coverage of the scanned tissue is better by the helical method, it involves more radiation than its axial counterpart. The benefit of helical acquisition is the capability to reconstruct the data in any plane as well as into a true 3D image, the resolution of which depends on the thickness of original slices (the thinner the original slice, the better the resolution). Images can be acquired with or without contrast (iodine-based) administration depending on the information that is required from the scan. Data reconstructions can be either done using the maximum intensity projection (MIP), volume-rendered (VR) or surface shaded display (SSD) algorithms (Figure 22.1). Similar helical acquisition is also performed for CT angiography following rapid injection of contrast (2.5–4 mL/s) in the vein using bolus chase or fixed delay techniques.

Contraindications

CT scan is contraindicated in the following situations: iodine allergy, underlying known severe allergic disorders, renal disease with deranged creatinine, and insulin-dependent diabetes mellitus. Short interval same area multiple scans are also relatively contraindicated due to cumulative dose to the patient.

It gives better information regarding the bony walls of the orbit and skull and helps in visualizing calcifications. It is of particular significance in suspected metallic foreign body-related orbital and brain injuries where MRI is contraindicated. Due to its widespread availability, quick acquisition times and reasonably good soft tissue resolution, it is the workhorse in the initial examination of the orbito-neurological disorders.

Magnetic resonance imaging

C.J. Gorter, a Dutch physicist, is credited with the proposal of nuclear magnetic resonance (NMR) concept in 1936 which was demonstrated a year later by Isaac Rabi. Bloch and Purcell demonstrated its experimental observation in solids and liquids, independently of each other, in 1945–1946 for which they were awarded the Nobel Prize in 1952. Paul Lauterbur, Sir Peter Mansfield and Raymond Damadian were instrumental in materializing the production of the initial human MR images for which the former two received the Nobel prize in 2003 (3).

MR principles and hardware

The signal generated during MR acquisition results from magnetic interaction between nuclei of atoms (protons) of the subject/object and radiofrequency field in the presence of an external magnetic field (B0). This signal is transformed to generate images of the particular body area exposed to this process by the method of Fourier transformation. The external fixed magnetic field is generated by permanent or electro-magnets, while gradient coils generate the gradient fields. Specialized coils exist for specific body parts which snugly fit the respective area and help in generating and receiving radiofrequency signals for eventual image formation, for example, head coil. Generally, the higher the magnetic field, the better the resolution of the images.

MR acquisition sequences

Unlike CT, which involves just one type of acquisition, MR involves acquisition of multiple sequences, which collectively increase the total duration of the scan (20–40 minutes). These are useful for demonstration and characterization of various structures of the brain. Table 22.1 lists various sequences along with their characteristics.

MRI provides the best anatomical resolution and better tissue characterization of all the available imaging modalities currently. Angiography can be performed with non-contrast means using the time of flight (TOF) method. Gadolinium serves as the MR contrast, which reduces the T1 times and aids in the characterization of various lesions based on the enhancement pattern. However, MRI has its own limitations in the form of long acquisition times, higher propensity of motion artefacts and limited availability, along with contraindication for claustrophobic patients and patients with metallic implants.

Apart from structural imaging, functional imaging has also come up in the form of blood oxygen dependent (BOLD) imaging.

Digital subtraction angiography (DSA)

DSA had been and still is the gold standard of detecting cerebrovascular lesions like aneurysms, arterio-venous malformation, CCF, etc. However, due to its invasive nature, it has been replaced

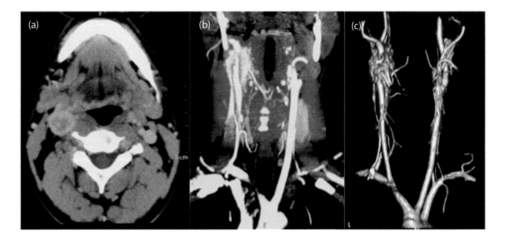

FIGURE 22.1 CT: Volumetric multidetector CT acquisition with axial base image (a) and reconstructed maximum intensity projection (MIP) (b) and volume-rendered (VR) (c) images. Hypervascular right carotid triangle lesion is appreciated consistent with paraganglioma.

TABLE 22.1: MR Pulse Sequences

S. No.	MR Pulse Sequences	Remarks
1.	T2-weighted (Figure 22.2a)	CSF appears hyperintense; gray matter is hyperintense and white matter is hypointense; most pathologies are hyperintense
2.	T1-weighted (Figure 22.2b)	CSF appears hypointense; gray matter is hypointense relative to the white matter; depicts a good gray white matter differentiation; most pathologies are hypointense
3.	FLAIR-weighted (Figure 22.2c)	T2-weighted image with suppression of CSF signal to better bring out the pathologies especially around the CSF spaces like the ventricles
4.	Diffusion-weighted (Figure 22.2d)	Better highlights cytotoxic edema, e.g., acute infarct. High signal is also seen with hypercellular tumors e.g., medulloblastoma and lesions with high-nucleocytoplasmic ratio.
5.	Susceptibility-weighted (Figure 22.2e)	Useful for demonstrating hemorrhage, calcification and mineral deposition. The calcium can be differentiated from iron by phase maps which are generated during SWI sequence.
6.	MR angiography (time of flight [TOF] and contrast enhanced [CE]) (Figure 22.2f)	Demonstrates vascular anatomy (TOF – without contrast, CE [gadolinium])
7.	MR spectroscopy	Demonstrates the biochemical milieu of the interrogated brain parenchyma, i.e., concentration of choline, creatine, N-acetyl aspartate (NAA), etc.
8.	Perfusion-weighted	Characterizes the vascularity of a lesion/cerebral parenchyma along with its blood volume and flow parameters.

Note: Due to fat content of the orbit, T1, T2 and gadolinium-enhanced T1 sequences are often done with fat saturation techniques.

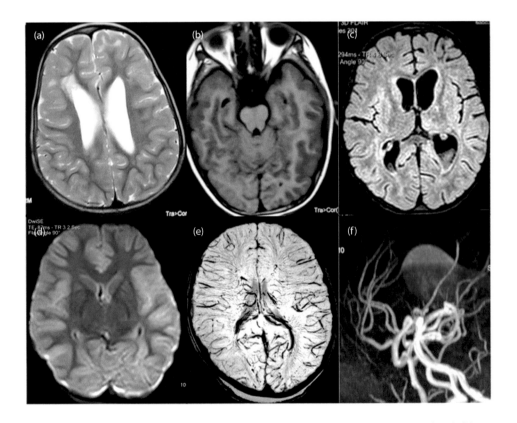

FIGURE 22.2 Magnetic resonance imaging (MRI) sequences: Axial T2-weighted (a), T1-weighted (b), FLAIR-weighted (c), diffusion-weighted (d), susceptibility-weighted (e) and time of flight (TOF) (f) MR angiography. Note that the CSF is hyperintense on T2, hypointense on T1 with suppression on FLAIR. Diffuse gyral hyperintensity is noted on diffusion sequence with prominent veins on susceptibility sequence. TOF MRA shows intracranial arterial vasculature.

by CT and MR angiography in many cases for the purpose of lesion diagnosis. It, however, holds an extremely important role in treatment of many of these lesions by endovascular route.

Principle

DSA is based on the principle of subtraction of the X-ray mask image from subsequent images, which are taken following injection of iodine-based contrast agent into the artery in which the catheter has been placed. There is complete subtraction of the bone and soft tissues, which increases the resolution of the contrast containing vascular tree tremendously (Figure 22.3).

With the advent of 3D DSA (rotational angiography) and lately four-dimensional DSA, the capability of DSA to super-resolve up to fourth- to fifth-order branches has improved. Furthermore, 3D reconstructions of the intracranial vasculature are now feasible at different time points, for example, arterial and venous phases. The relationship with surrounding structures can be depicted with 3D flat panel CT (Xper CT, dyna CT, etc.).

Indications of imaging

The indications of imaging in neuro-ophthalmological disorders can be discussed in terms of clinical perspective. The following are common requisitions for imaging by the ophthalmologist:

1. Visual loss (e.g., optic neuropathy, bitemporal hemianopia, homonymous hemianopia and amaurosis fugax)
2. Ptosis (third or multiple cranial nerve [CN] palsy, Horner's syndrome)
3. Anisocoria (pupil involving third nerve palsy)
4. Proptosis (e.g., orbital tumor/pseudotumor, thyroid eye disease, CCF, etc.)
5. Diplopia/ophthalmoparesis (multiple CN palsy, internuclear and supranuclear ophthalmoplegia, gaze palsies, and orbital lesions)
6. Nystagmus
7. Abnormalities detected on ophthalmoscopy, which may be secondary to intracranial disorders (e.g., papilledema due to intracranial hypertension, etc.).

Choosing the best imaging modality is also important in order to achieve optimal information with minimum inconvenience to the patient and the system. To optimize resources and for better targeting the imaging to particular orbital and intracranial structures, the ophthalmologist should preferably provide the localization of the presumed lesion and suspected clinical diagnosis. This would help in optimal tailoring of the MR examination. It is often said that the diagnostic yield is not only dependent on what imaging technique is being used and its interpretation but also on whether one is exploring the right place.

Anatomical considerations

This chapter will dwell on the premise that neuro-ophthalmology covers essentially all aspects of the neural components of the orbit (essentially the eyeball), the entire visual axis up till the various participating CN nuclei as well as all the supranuclear higher brain structures involved. Additionally, brain disorders having secondary manifestations in the ocular examination will also be discussed. Before embarking on this further, a brief anatomical description of the visual pathway and the nerves contributing to mobility of the eyeball is being highlighted.

Visual pathways

The visual pathway begins from the level of the retina (4, 5). The optic nerve courses through the orbit and enters the cranial compartment through the optic canal. Both the optic nerves converge in the suprasellar cistern forming the optic chiasma. The pathway continues as the optic tracts on either side and reaches the lateral geniculate body (LGN) from where the visual information is projected to the visual cortex in the respective occipital lobes through the optic radiations (geniculo-calcarine tracts).

Pathways involved in ocular movements

The ocular movements are determined by CNs III (oculomotor), IV (trochlear) and VI (abducens) through supply of the extraocular muscles, iris muscles and the adjoining region. The nuclei of the oculomotor nerve are located in the mesencephalic periaqueductal region at the level of superior quadrigeminal tubercles. The trochlear nerve nucleus also lies in the mesencephalon, inferior to

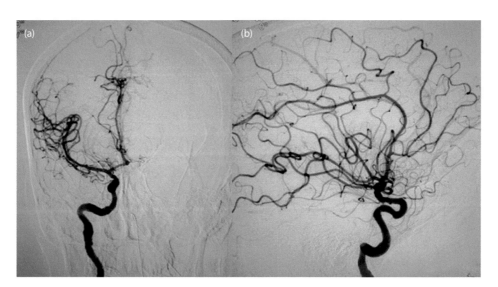

FIGURE 22.3 Digital subtraction angiography (DSA): Right internal carotid artery contrast injections with vascular depiction in the frontal (a) and lateral (b) projections.

CN III, behind the medial longitudinal fasciculus (MLF). It inner-vates the contralateral superior oblique muscles (4–7). The nucleus of the abducens nerve is located in the dorsal pons adjacent to the MLF and in front of the fourth ventricular floor (4–7). The MLF is placed along the anterior side of the mesencephalic aqueduct extending caudally up to the spinal cord. It contains association fibers, which connect the motor nuclei of ipsilateral CN III, IV, CI and XI and each CN VI with the contralateral CN III. It is essen-tial for the o-ordination of horizontal eye and vertical gaze.

Autonomic pathways

The Edinger-Westphal parasympathetic nucleus lies posterior the oculomotor nerve. It is constituted by preganglionic parasympa-thetic neurons, which join the CN III on their course toward the orbit to reach the ciliary ganglion, from which the post-ganglionic fibers emerge to innervate the pupillary constrictors and muscles of the ciliary bodies (4–7). The sympathetic pathway runs with the adventitia of the internal carotid artery (ICA), toward the cav-ernous sinus, joining the first branch of the trigeminal nerve.

Neuro-ophthalmological disorders

These disorders may be classified based on the anatomical localization into diseases of the eyeball, optic nerve and orbit, parasellar/cavernous sinus region, suprasellar region and middle cranial fossa, posterior cranial fossa along with generalized intra-cranial conditions having a bearing on vision.

Eyeball

It can be imaged by US, CT or MRI depending on the clinical input. In most cases, a good clinical history and examination often clinch the diagnosis. Sometimes ancillary investigations have to be performed depending on the supposed location of the pathology. US is the first-line investigation. However, if the window is limited or not available or an open globe is suspected which can cause extrusion of ocular contents following increased ocular pressure due to US transducer, CT should be done. CT is also the initial investigation when a foreign body injury is sus-pected (Figure 22.4).

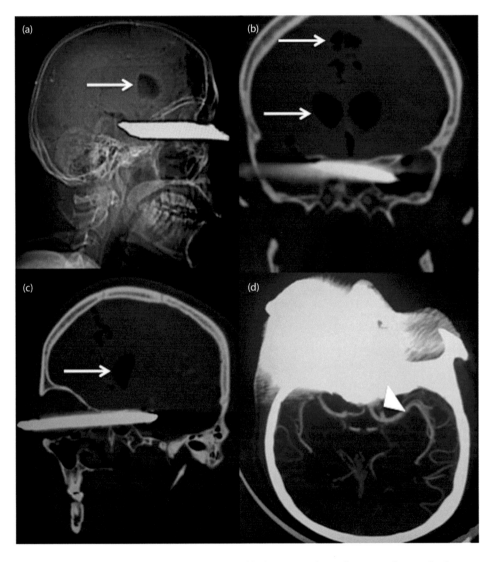

FIGURE 22.4 Metallic foreign body: Lateral skull radiograph (a) depicting the radiopaque foreign body entering the orbit with intracranial extension. Coronal (b) and oblique coronal (c) CT shows the exact projection of the foreign body extending to the contra-lateral cavernous sinus. Note the presence of pneumocephalus and pneumoventricle (arrows). CT angiography (d) shows injury to the contralateral ICA (arrowhead) but adequate distal flow through collateral route into the ACA and MCA territories.

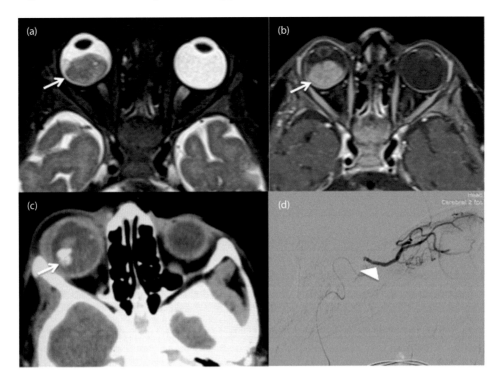

FIGURE 22.5 Retinoblastoma: Axial T2 (a), post-contrast T1-weighted (b) MRI and axial CT (c) scan demonstrate the presence of right intravitreal soft tissue having calcification (arrow) indicative of retinoblastoma. Optic nerve is not infiltrated. Ophthalmic artery (arrowhead) DSA lateral projection (d) prior to intraarterial chemotherapy shows the choroidal blush. The patient had significant regression of the lesion.

The most common intraocular tumor in the pediatric age group is retinoblastoma. The clinical manifestation is most commonly leukocoria. US and CT are sensitive modalities for the identification of the lesion with the ability to detect even small calcifications (Figure 22.5), which are seen in about 90% of these cases (8, 9). MRI adds to the information in the form of better tumor resolution, retrobulbar infiltration (Figure 22.5), CNS spread and detection of pineal/suprasellar lesions (trilateral retinoblastomas), which potentially changes the management (10). It is important to differentiate this lesion from persistent hyperplastic primary vitreous (PHPV) as the treatment of both entities is different. Apart from systemic and intravitreal injections of chemotherapeutic agents, the role of intraarterial chemotherapy has generated significant interest in a select category of patients of retinoblastoma (Figure 22.5). The posterior segment soft tissue in PHPV extends from the optic head to the posterior surface of the lens with presence of vascularity within, secondary to persistence of hyaloid vasculature (Figure 22.6). Another differentiating point is reduced axial length of the eyeball in PHPV as compared to retinoblastoma. Also, MRI is preferable to CT scan due to radiation hazards with the latter, all patients being in the childhood age. Other lesions involving

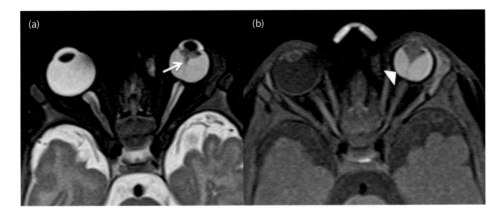

FIGURE 22.6 Persistent hyperplastic primary vitreous (PHPV): Axial T2 (a) and T1 (b) MRI shows presence of linear soft tissue extending from the optic head to the posterior surface of the lens (arrow) with small globe. Note is made of vitreous hemorrhage (arrowhead).

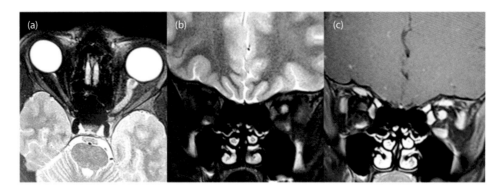

FIGURE 22.7 Optic neuritis: Axial T2 (a), coronal T2 (b) and coronal post-contrast T1 (c) MRI shows swollen left optic nerve with hyperintensity on T2 (arrow) and moderate contrast enhancement.

the posterior segment are tumors like hemangioblastomas, melanoma and metastases hemangiomas and granulomatous pathology, which have characteristic appearances on imaging. Melanoma is hypoechoic on US and may have sign of choroidal excavation indicating local invasion with increased vascularity. These lesions are typically hyperintense on T1-weighted (T1W) and hypointense on T2-weighted (TW2) MRI due to melanin content. Metastases are echogenic on US with increased vascularity and may be multiple. They are T2 hyperintense and T1 hypointense (hyperintense, if hemorrhagic) with variable (many times increased) vascularity.

Optic nerves and orbit

The optic nerve forms an important junction between the CNS and the eye globe. Apart from the immense importance it has as a sense organ/component, it forms a conduit for occurrence/spread of diseases from either side (CNS to eye globe and vice versa) and is a window to the CNS. The common inflictions of the optic nerve are inflammation (optic neuritis-isolated or as part of systemic inflammatory disorders), primary neoplasm (optic nerve glioma [ONG]), secondary involvement with lymphoproliferative syndromes and adjoining optic nerve sheath tumor (meningioma). Secondary involvement may be in the form of compression from surrounding lesions like cavernous, venolymphatic and high-flow arteriovenous malformations. Optic nerve injury can be secondary to direct (avulsion/laceration) or indirect trauma (perineural hematoma).

The clinical presentation of *optic neuritis* is unilateral vision loss, pain and afferent pupillary defect (11). The cases, which are not being explained by metabolic, hereditary, infectious, ischemic or toxic causes, warrant imaging by means of MRI. MR of the brain in most cases should also be performed as many cases of optic neuritis are the initial manifestations of demyelinating disorders namely multiple sclerosis (MS), neuromyelitis optica (NMO) and anti-MOG-associated encephalomyelitis. MRI shows the inflamed nerve to be thickened, T2 hyperintense with variable degree of patchy enhancement (Figure 22.7). The optic nerve lesions are unilateral having involvement of a short length of the nerve with preservation of the chiasma in most cases of MS, as compared to anti MOG disease which is often bilateral but also restricted to the prechiasmatic segment. The lesions involve prechiasmatic, chiasmatic and postchiasmatic segments in NMO disorder (Figure 22.8). Brain and spinal cord MRI manifestations of MS are characteristic (Figure 22.9).

Inflammatory pathologies may be in the form of sarcoidosis, inflammatory pseudotumor, thyroid ophthalmopathy, granulomatous polyangiitis, etc. Imaging shows orbital soft tissue with fat heterogeneity giving it a dirty appearance. Muscle thickening may involve single/multiple extraocular muscles with involvement of their tendinous insertions (cf, thyroid orbitopathy, which involves multiple muscle bellies sparing their tendinous insertions; Figure 22.10). Thyroid profile is also frequently deranged. Orbital cellulitis may be secondary to spread of infection from the paranasal sinuses. Although the imaging may not be different from other inflammations earlier on in the disease process, presence of sinus disease and systemic signs of fever favor it. During the latter part of the infection, there may be formation of abscess which manifests as a peripherally enhancing centrally diffusion restricting lesion (Figure 22.11). Restriction of selective ocular movements may at times be secondary to individual muscle involvement by a cysticercus cyst (Figure 22.12) or bony entrapment of its belly due to bony injury (consequence of fracture leading to muscle impingement, commonly of the inferior rectus).

The two major neoplasms related to the optic nerve are *ONG* and *optic nerve sheath meningioma (ONSM)*. Nearly all ONGs are juvenile pilocytic astrocytomas (grade I) manifesting in childhood. The former presents as a cylindrical/fusiform thickening of the nerve with no significant enhancement (Figure 22.13). It is important to determine the extent of the lesion posteriorly along the optic nerve till the chiasma for management purpose (12). MRI is the imaging modality of choice.

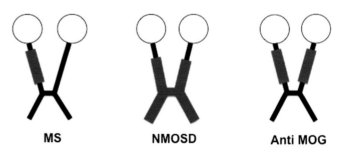

FIGURE 22.8 Diagrammatic representation of optic pathway involvement in multiple sclerosis, neuromyelitis optica spectrum disorder and anti-myelin oligodendrocyte glycoprotein-related demyelination.

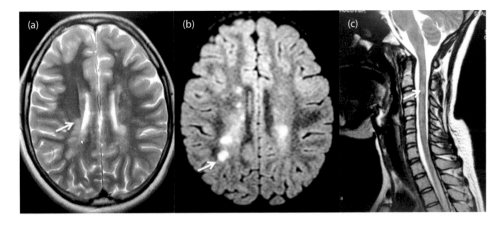

FIGURE 22.9 Multiple sclerosis (MS): Axial T2 (a), FLAIR (b) images of brain and sagittal T2 cervical spine (c) MRI depicting the characteristic oval perivenular lesions of MS involving periventricular white matter (arrows) with short segment lesions involving the cervical spinal cord.

These lesions are isointense on T1W and iso- to hyperintense on T2W sequences with variable enhancement. Calcifications are rare. Sometimes a rim of T2 hyperintensity is seen at the tumor periphery which is leptomeningeal infiltration and not expanded CSF space, as is often thought. In NF-1, the optic nerve is tortuous, kinked, buckled and diffusely enlarged. The nerve is not separately seen from the tumor unlike meningioma. ONSM usually occurs in older adults with painless, slowly progressive loss of vision and optic nerve atrophy. It may be eccentric but is usually partially circumferential causing indentation/compression of the optic nerve, many a times leading to a "tram-track" appearance (13). The enhancement is moderate to intense (Figure 22.14). The imaging differences between the two are highlighted in Table 22.2.

Lymphoproliferative disorders are actually the most common primary orbital tumors in older adult. These lesions are placed in a wide spectrum ranging from lymphoid hyperplasia to atypical lymphoid hyperplasia and lymphoma. Lymphoma is the most common of these all. It may be primary orbital or part of the systemic disease. Imaging character which differentiates these lesions from other orbital lesions is their tendency to mold to the orbital structures like the globe, optic nerve and orbital walls and roof with the tumor tending to spread around these along with bony remodeling. Due to their increased cellularity, they are

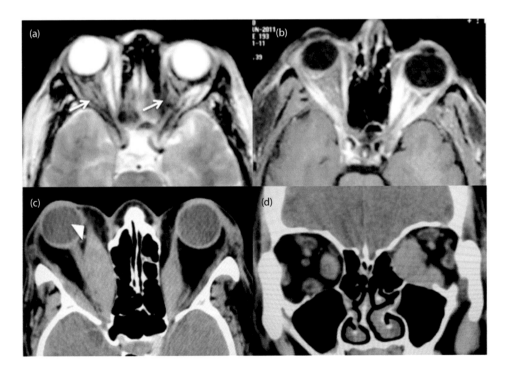

FIGURE 22.10 Inflammatory orbital pseudotumor vs thyroid orbitopathy: Axial T2-weighted (a) and post-contrast (T1)-weighted (b) MR images demonstrating T2 hypointense enhancing soft tissue along the right lateral rectus and left medial rectus (arrows). The muscle bellies also show enhancement. Compare this from diffuse fusiform enlargement of the bilateral medial and inferior recti muscles sparing their tendinous insertions (arrowhead) (c, d) in thyroid orbitopathy.

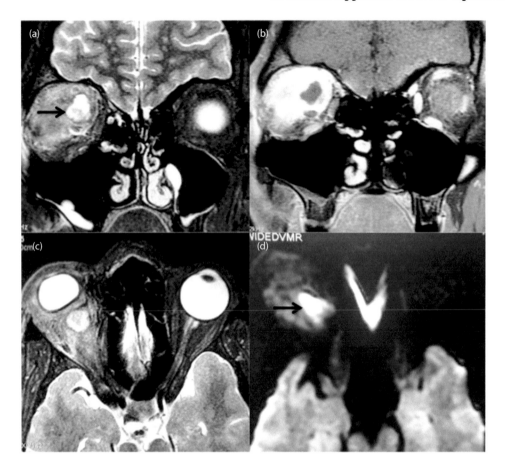

FIGURE 22.11 Orbital abscess: Coronal T2 (a), post-contrast T1 (b), axial T2 (c) and diffusion-weighted (d) MR images showing intraorbital, predominantly intraconal, inflammatory soft tissue with central breakdown (arrow) which is showing diffusion restriction suggesting abscess formation. Note the scleral indentation and compression of the eyeball from the posterior aspect.

isointense to mildly hyperintense on T2W MR sequences with moderate enhancement (Figure 22.15) and presence of moderate diffusion restriction, the latter helping in differentiating these lesions from pseudotumors (14). Differentiating these lesions on CT from other lesions is difficult. Lacrimal gland may be involved in nearly 40% of cases.

Cavernous malformation is essentially the most common vascular lesion in the orbit. They are congenital, do not spontaneously involute and show gradual growth over time. They are dilated cavernous spaces filled with blood with a surrounding fibrous pseudocapsule. On imaging, they are well circumscribed and homogenous, most commonly occurring at the lateral aspect

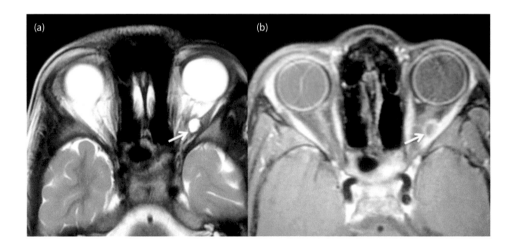

FIGURE 22.12 Orbital myocysticercus: Axial T2 (a) and post-contrast T1-weighted (b) images depicting a small cystic lesion (arrow) in relation to the left lateral rectus muscle causing lateral rectus palsy.

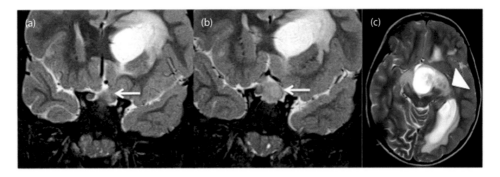

FIGURE 22.13 Hypothalamic optico-chiasmatic glioma: Coronal (a, b) and axial (c) T2-weighted MR demonstrating thickening of the left optic nerve and chiasma (arrow) with extension along the left optic tract (arrowhead).

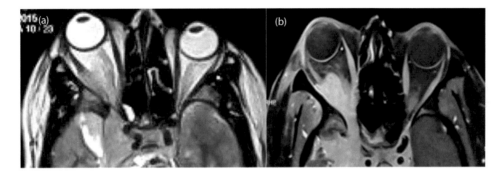

FIGURE 22.14 Cavernous sinus meningioma with orbital extension: Axial T2 (a) and post-contrast T1 (b) images showing expansile right cavernous sinus lesion having isointense (to gray matter) character on T2 and showing moderate contrast enhancement.

of the intraconal space. On MRI, they are T1 hypointense, T2 hyperintense with no discernible flow voids (15). There is progressive centripetal filling on dynamic contrast-enhanced imaging (Figure 22.16). This differentiates it from capillary hemangioma and high-flow arteriovenous malformation. Its rare malignant counterpart is hemangiopericytoma, which is derived from pericytes having spindle-shaped cells on histopathology. These are lobulated, hypervascular and aggressive with infiltrative borders.

TABLE 22.2: Comparison between Optic Nerve Glioma and Optic Nerve Sheath Meningioma

Characteristics	Optic Nerve Glioma	Optic Nerve Sheath Meningioma
Age	Children (usually <10 years)	Middle-aged (female)
Morphology	Cylindrical, fusiform, rarely eccentric	Circumferential ("tram-track appearance") or eccentric
Enhancement	Mild to moderate	Moderate to intense
Calcification	Rare (May develop following radiation)	20–50% (psammomatous)
Cystic change	May occur	Unusual
Chiasmal involvement	May occur	Unusual
Laterality	May be bilateral (in Neurofibromatosis)	Unilateral

On MRI, they are more or less isointense on T1W and T2W sequences with early moderate to intense enhancement.

Schwannomas and neurofibromas are other common neoplasms in the orbit (Figure 22.17) along with lacrimal and other mesenchymal tumors, which are however beyond the scope of this chapter. The readers are referred to dedicated articles and books on these topics.

Trauma forms a major cause of damage to the visual pathway from the level of the eyeball till the occipital lobe visual centers and the intervening pathway constituted by the optic nerve (Figure 22.18), chiasma, tracts, LGN and optic radiation. Blunt or penetrating orbital trauma may lead to open or closed globe injury. The optic nerve may receive contusion or transection resulting from bony fractures (usually at the level of optic canal). There may be entrapment of the muscle belly, commonly seen with inferior rectus resulting in restriction of superior gaze (Figure 22.19). Head injury may lead to contusions or diffuse axonal injury in the occipital lobes as a result of coup/contrecoup injury. CT is an excellent modality to delineate bony fractures. Multiplanar thin-slice reconstructions aid in the identification of even very subtle fractures. Sometimes, it is difficult to delineate soft tissue injury with CT. MRI helps in such cases with detection of signal changes in the components of visual pathways especially the optic nerves, chiasma and occipital lobes for diffuse axonal injury (DAI). High-resolution MR sequences also have a role to play in detection of subtle changes at the level of brainstem CN nuclei as well as actual visualization of the cisternal course of various nerves,

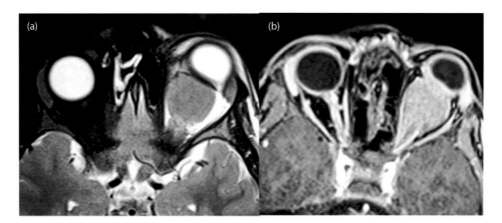

FIGURE 22.15   Orbital lymphoma: Axial T2 (a) and post-contrast T1 (b) MR images revealing a well-defined intraconal soft tissue causing indentation on the globe and deviation of the optic nerve. Note that the lesion is not infiltrating the adjoining structures.

especially CN 6, which is prone to injury due to its longest intracranial course (16–18).

Cavernous sinus and parasellar lesions

Cavernous sinus lesions present commonly in the form of either neural or vascular manifestations.

The neural is consequent to variable degree of partial/complete involvement of one/combination of CN III, IV, VI, V1 or V2 segments of the V CNs. The patients may present with

ophthalmoparesis (ptosis, diplopia), restriction of ocular movements, reduced vision and weakness or pain in trigeminal distribution. Neural involvement may also occur due to inherent nerve paresis (secondary to diabetes-related neuropathy or microvascular affliction of neural supply) or selective neural compression like PCom aneurysm causing selective third nerve compression in the supracavernous region (Figure 22.20). Vascular manifestations may be secondary to venous congestion due to cavernous sinus invasion leading to proptosis (pulsatile in CCF), chemosis,

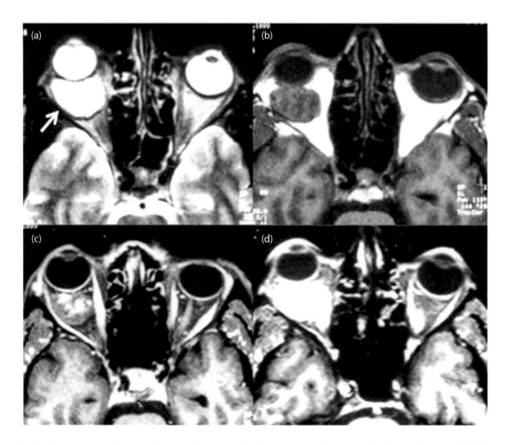

FIGURE 22.16   Orbital cavernous hemangioma: Axial T2 (a), T1 (b) and post-contrast T1 (c – late arterial, d – late venous) MR images documenting right orbital (intraconal) intensely T2 bright lesion (arrow) showing progressive enhancement in delayed phase typical of a hemangioma.

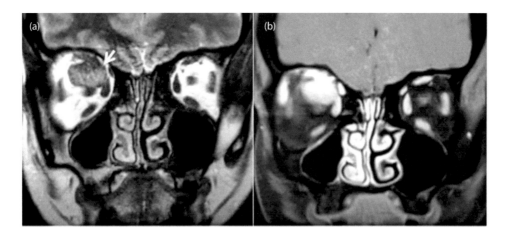

FIGURE 22.17 Orbital nerve sheath tumor: Coronal T2 (a) and post-contrast T1 (b) MR images showing right intraconal soft tissue superior to the optic nerve causing its compression leading to visual symptoms.

pain on ocular movements, etc. Orbital CT with cavernous sinus cuts is sufficient for the evaluation most of the times. Sometimes, MR has to be performed when CT is unable to detect very small lesions and characterize them.

Inflammatory pathologies involving the cavernous sinus are Tolosa–Hunt syndrome and other granulomatous lesions (pseudotumor, fungal infections).

The soft tissue in Tolosa–Hunt syndrome is localized to the orbital apex, which may extend to the cavernous sinus or along the dural attachment till the tentorium (19, 20). MRI character

of the soft tissue is T2 hypointense, T1 hypo- to isointense with moderate enhancement following gadolinium administration (Figure 22.21). There may be posterior extension of the soft tissue up to the tentorial attachment, which is better defined with MRI. The classical presentation is painful (retro-orbital pain) ophthalmoparesis. It has to be differentiated from other fungal, histiocytic soft tissue (21, 22) which may have similar character on MRI. The stark T2 hypointensity on MRI stands out, and adjoining paranasal sinus involvement is almost confirmatory for a fungal disease (Figure 22.22). Vascular invasion may occur early on during the course of the disease in aggressive fungi, for example, mucor, which may lead to arteritis with subsequent thrombosis,

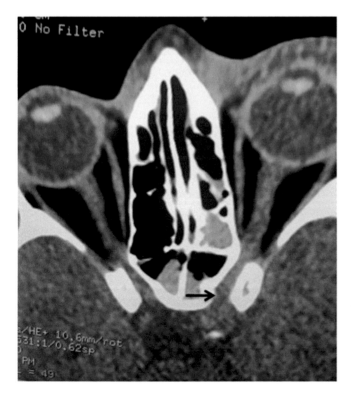

FIGURE 22.18 Traumatic optic nerve contusion: Axial CT scan demonstrating left optic nerve thickening following blunt orbital trauma. Careful observation reveals compression in the optic canal with associated soft tissue hematoma (arrow).

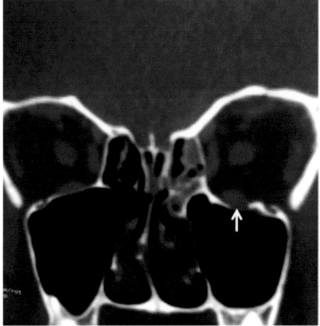

FIGURE 22.19 Traumatic inferior rectus impingement: Coronal CT image demonstrating left side inferior orbital wall fracture with impingement of the inferior rectus (arrow) muscle leading to gaze restriction.

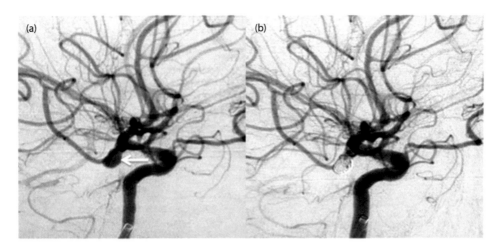

FIGURE 22.20 Oculomotor nerve palsy secondary to compression: Digital subtraction angiography (DSA) lateral view following internal carotid artery (ICA) contrast injection demonstrating aneurysm (arrow) at the communicating segment of ICA causing third cranial nerve palsy (a). Control DSA following coil embolization (b) shows complete aneurysm occlusion. The patient gradually recovered over the next few weeks.

distal embolism and infarcts. Prompt diagnosis and quick institution of therapy is of utmost importance to prevent catastrophe in these individuals.

Vascular disorders of the cavernous sinus comprise of cavernous hemangioma, CCF, large cavernous ICA aneurysms (spontaneous, dissecting or traumatic) and cavernous sinus thrombosis (spontaneous or thrombophlebitis secondary to adjoining sinus infection). Cavernous hemangioma appears as a lobulated well-circumscribed soft tissue on CT showing moderate enhancement (23). Its typical character on T2W MRI is the hyperintense nature (Figure 22.23), which helps it to differentiate it from its counterparts namely meningiomas and schwannomas. The

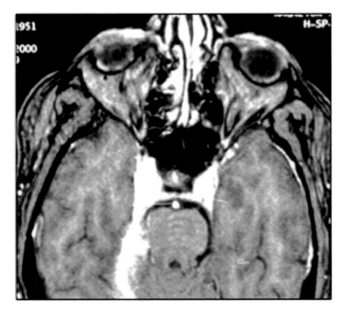

FIGURE 22.21 Tolosa–Hunt syndrome: Axial post-contrast T1-weighted MR image showing cavernous sinus soft tissue extending from the orbital apex till the tentorial attachment in a patient with retroorbital pain and ophthalmoparesis.

other typical character is progressive centripetal enhancement of the lesion on dynamic CT or MR enhancement scans. CCFs are commonly traumatic in origin presenting as pulsatile proptosis with bruit on palpation. Following head injury after a lag period of few weeks to a couple of months (sometimes immediately), they result from injury of the cavernous segment of the ICA, which subsequently ruptures into the cavernous sinus leading to a direct CCF (24). Cavernous sinus expansion is seen on CT scan with large flow voids on MRI. It is often a clinical diagnosis with imaging done mostly for the sake of completion. Endovascular embolization (with cavernous sinus packing with coils) is the safest and the most popular treatment having excellent results (Figure 22.24). Indirect CCF may be spontaneous typically occurring in middle-aged females. It is basically a dural arteriovenous fistula (AVF) with arterial feeders from branches of the external carotid artery (ECA) and venous drainage into the cavernous sinus. Mixed forms may also be seen. Treatment is again cavernous sinus coiling, which however has to be approached through the venous route due to very limited access by the arterial route. Large cavernous ICA aneurysms may cause compression of the nerves leading to symptoms. Endovascular flow diversion is the treatment of choice with reasonable occlusion rates at 1 year. Cavernous sinus thrombosis is usually secondary to spread of infection from the adjacent sphenoid sinus (Figure 22.25). Rarely, it may be secondary to hypercoagulable state or vasculitis of non-infective origin.

Neoplasms account for a vast majority of lesions of the cavernous sinus (25). The most common ones are meningiomas and nerve sheath tumors (schwannomas) with secondary involvement by pituitary adenomas and metastases contributing to the rest. A varying spectrum of lymphoproliferative disorders also present as soft tissue lesions at this location. Schwannomas are often seen to follow the course of the CN from which they arise and hence are dumble-shaped in many cases (Figure 22.26). They are T1 hypointense and T2 hyperintense with moderate heterogeneous enhancement on MRI. Intralesional microhemorrhages may be seen. Meningiomas are T1 hypo-,T2 hypo- to isointense showing moderate to intense contrast enhancement and often have a dural tail which distinguishes it from the rest of

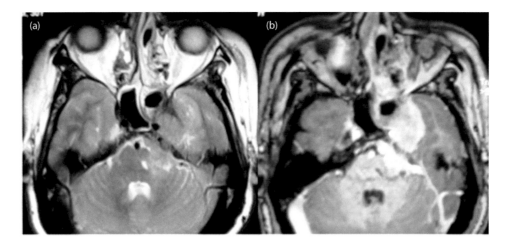

FIGURE 22.22   Fungal sinus disease with cavernous sinus invasion: Axial T2 (a) and post-contrast T1 (b) MRI showing mucosal involvement of the left sided ethmoid and sphenoid sinuses with extension to involve the cavernous sinus further extending till the cerebellopontine angle. Note the T2 hypointense nature of the soft tissue.

the lesions (Figure 22.27). Large pituitary macroadenomas have the tendency to grow and encase the cavernous sinus to varying degree (Figure 22.28). Sinus invasion may also occur which may also compromise the functioning of the CNs coursing through the sinus as well as the consequences related to venous occlusion. These tumors are heterogenous and enhance less than the pituitary parenchyma. They are epicentered in the sella turcica (26). Although they are not malignant per se, the aggressive ones can cause bony erosions and even brain parenchymal infiltration at times. Lymphoproliferative spectrum disorders can present as cavernous dural masses causing cavernous sinus syndrome. Malignant lymphomatous tissue is T1 hypointense, T2 hypo- to isointense with moderate enhancement. There are other lesions in the spectrum related to lymphocytic proliferation and sinus histiocytosis, one of which is currently referred to as Rosai–Dorfman disease (21, 27). Imaging appearance is in the form of large moderately enhancing dural-based soft tissue which may be seen at various locations in the brain related to dura, one of which is cavernous sinus dura (Figure 22.29). Treatment is surgical excision as symptoms due to compression by the large tissue are not promptly controlled by medical means. Metastases from distant primary may present as cavernous sinus masses. Such lesions show significant adjoining infiltration and bony destruction.

Suprasellar lesions

Suprasellar region is another location where an important structure of the visual pathway is situated namely the optic chiasma. The common lesions, which are centered here, are granulomatous lesions like sarcoidosis and tubercular granulomas, other meningeal inflammations like meningitis (tuberculous, cryptococcal), neoplasms like optico-chiasmatic glioma, craniopharyngioma, germ cell tumors and Langerhans cell histiocytosis (LCH).

Although not the commonest location of sarcoid granuloma, lesions in this location have to be differentiated from tubercular and fungal lesions as well as germ cell tumors. These lesions are T1 hypo- to isointense and T2 hypo- to isointense with moderate enhancement (28). The adjoining meninges may also show enhancement. Meningovasculitis is not usually a feature unlike tubercular lesions. Tubercular lesions classically appear T2 hyoto isointense with irregular enhancement, florid basal meningitis and optico-chiasmatic arachnoiditis which is the cause of visual deterioration (Figure 22.30). There may be associated parenchymal granulomas which, when interrogated with MR spectroscopy, show lipid peak.

Germ cell tumors are well circumscribed tumors sensitive to chemoradiation (29). They show T1 and T2 isointensity with

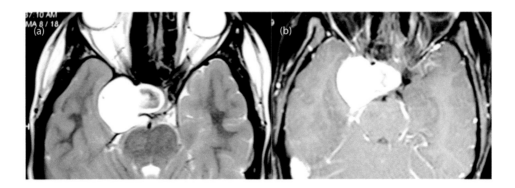

FIGURE 22.23   Cavernous sinus hemangioma: Axial T2-weighted (a) and post-contrast T1-weighted (b) images showing a well-defined intensely T2 bright cavernous sinus soft tissue showing remarkable enhancement characteristic of hemangioma.

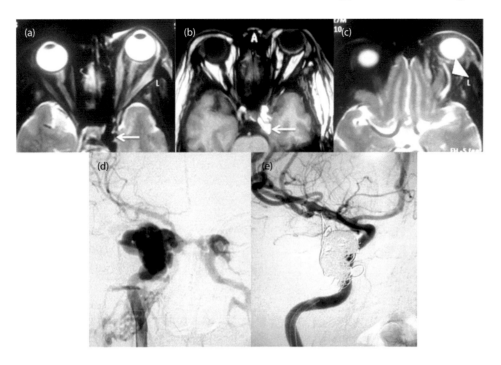

FIGURE 22.24 Traumatic carotico-cavernous fistula (CCF): Axial T2 (a, c) and T1 (b) MR images showing the exaggerated left cavernous sinus flow voids (arrows) with prominent superior ophthalmic vein (arrowhead) leading to orbital congestion and proptosis 2 weeks following trauma suggesting direct CCF. DSA (d) in another patient demonstrating contrast opacification of the cavernous sinus simultaneously with the ICA and drainage into the ipsilateral superior ophthalmic vein and contralateral cavernous sinus. Complete fistula closure following embolization (e).

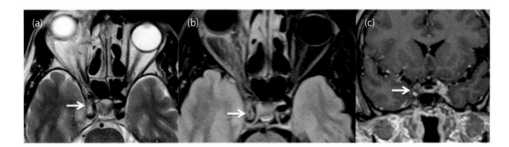

FIGURE 22.25 Cavernous sinus thrombosis (CST): Axial T2 (a), FLAIR (b) and coronal post-contrast T1 (c) MR images showing right side cavernous sinus soft tissue causing partial obliteration of ICA flow void with reduced sinus enhancement suggesting thrombosis (arrows).

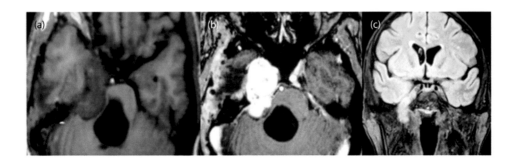

FIGURE 22.26 Cavernous sinus/Meckel's nerve sheath tumor: Axial T1 (a), post-contrast T1 (b) and coronal FLAIR (c) images demonstrating dumble-shaped tumor exiting the skull base through the neural foramen likely foramen ovale.

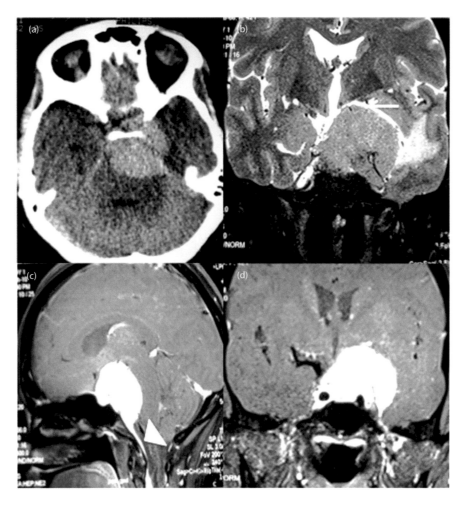

FIGURE 22.27   Cavernous sinus meningioma: Axial CT (a), T2 coronal (b) and post-contrast T1 sagittal (c) and coronal (d) MR images depicting hyperdense left cavernous sinus soft tissue with retroclival extension. The optic chiasma and left side optic tract (b) is compressed. Note the broad base and dural tail (arrowhead) in the retroclival region.

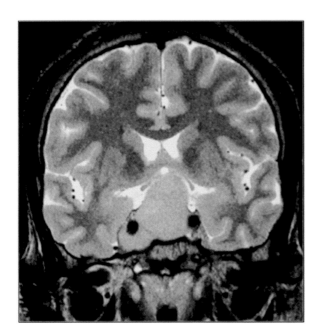

FIGURE 22.28   Pituitary macroadenoma with right cavernous sinus invasion.

moderate homogenous enhancement (Figure 22.31) and diffusion restriction on diffusion-weighted imaging. Meningeal enhancement is not seen unless there is CSF spread. There may be other lesions especially in the pineal region. Pituitary macroadenoma is the most common suprasellar neoplasm, which causes extrinsic compression on the optic chiasma leading to bitemporal campimetric field defects (cf, hypothalamic lesions, which cause inferior temporal defects due to involvement of the superior aspect of the chiasma and the fibers coursing thereof). The imaging characteristics of these tumors have been discussed elsewhere. The hypothalamic optico-chiasmatic gliomas (30), as the name suggests, arise from the elements of hypothalamus and optic chiasma. They are mostly benign WHO grade 1 tumors. They cause thickening of the optic pathway and extend along its course, many a times along the optic tracts (see fig. 22.13). They are hypointense on T1W MR images and hyperintense on T2W MR images with moderate patchy enhancement. Craniopharyngiomas have a bimodal peak. The childhood tumors may be heterogenous and show partial calcification, solid constituents and high signal intensity on T1W MRI ("motor oil" cystic component). Ninety percent of these tumors may enhance (31).

The other lesions, which affect the vision with presentation in the form of homonymous hemianopia, are lesions involving the optic radiations and occipital lobes. These form a heterogenous

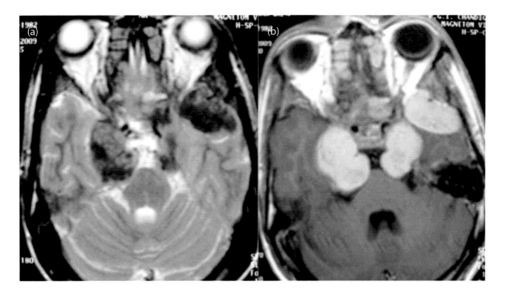

FIGURE 22.29 Rosai–Dorfman disease: Axial T2 (a) and post-contrast T1 (b)-weighted MRI showing multiple T2 hypointense dural-based intracranial lesions including bilateral cavernous sinuses with moderate enhancement. Histopathology revealed the diagnosis.

group ranging from vasogenic edema due to a host of pathologies to lesions which are strategically placed within the radiation and visual centers in the occipital lobe like granulomas (NCC, tuberculomas), neoplasms (gliomas, etc.), demyelination (MS) and vascular pathologies like posterior reversible encephalopathy syndrome (PRESS), cerebral sinovenous thrombosis (CSVT). MS is a primary demyelinating pathology classically involving periventricular white matter, corpus callosum and middle cerebellar peduncle in the brainstem. The lesions begin in the perivascular zones around the veins and thus appear oval to elongated being perpendicularly oriented to the corpus callosum (referred to as "Dawson's fingers"). There may be involvement of optic nerves (previously discussed) and spinal cord where the involvement is short segment and multifocal (cf, NMO which involves long segment central cord and has predominantly periventricular lesion distribution in the brain). The lesions are hypo- to isointense on T1W and hyperintense on T2/FLAIR-weighted MR sequences (Figure 22.9). The modified

Mc Donald criteria describe the dissemination of lesions in time and place (32) and aids in diagnosis of MS.

PRESS results from loss of cerebrovascular autoregulation, which commonly results secondary to hypertension. The lesions are classically subcortical and mainly posteriorly (parieto-occipital) placed, though they may also be in the brainstem and frontoparietal lobes. They are T2/FLAIR hyperintense, non-diffusion restricting and showing no significant enhancement (Figure 22.32). Diffusion restriction and hemorrhages may occur in atypical PRESS.

CSVT variably involves superficial and deep venous sinuses with or without cortical veins. Non-contrast CT may reveal hyperdense venous sinuses (Figure 22.33) and/or cortical veins (cord sign). There may be associated parenchymal changes in the form of congestive venous edema or venous infarcts with hemorrhage (33, 34). CECT may show filling defect in the affected sinus (empty delta sign). MRI is sensitive to the identification

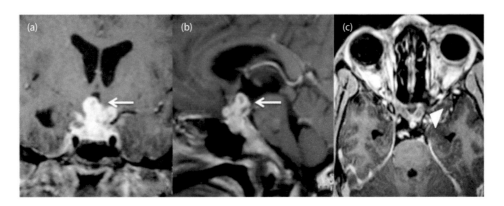

FIGURE 22.30 Tubercular meningitis with suprasellar tuberculomas (arrows) and optico-chiasmatic arachnoiditis (arrowhead) on coronal (a), sagittal (b) and axial, (c) post-contrast MRI.

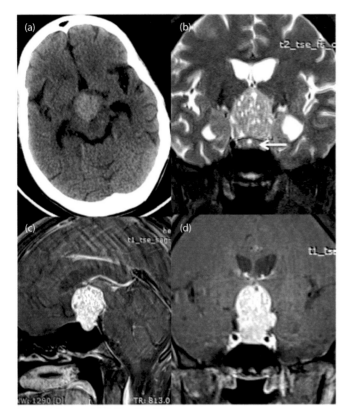

FIGURE 22.31 Suprasellar germ cell tumor: Axial CT (a) showing a well-defined suprasellar hyperdense lesion which is hyperintense on T2-weighted (b) images with moderate post-contrast enhancement (c, d) compressing on the optic chiasma. Note that the pituitary gland is seen separately on coronal T2 image (arrow).

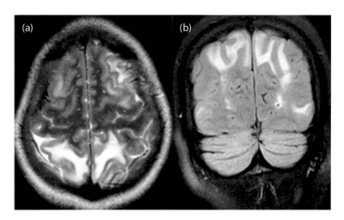

FIGURE 22.32 Posterior reversible encephalopathy syndrome (PRES)/Acute hypertensive encephalopathy: Axial T2 (a) and coronal FLAIR (b) MR images depicting the symmetrical parieto-occipital subcortical white matter involvement.

of venous thrombosis and exquisitely demonstrates the signal of thrombus according to its age. Acutely thrombosed blood appears hypointense on T2W MR imaging and becomes hyperintense with time. These thrombi are hyperintense on FLAIR-weighted sequences and hypointense (with blooming) on T2

GRE/susceptibility-weighted sequences. A filling defect is seen on CEMR. MR venography shows absent/reduced signal in thrombosed sinuses with "shaggy" appearance of the sinus wall. Contrast-enhanced MR venography may be helpful in cases where doubt still exists. Long-standing venous thrombosis leads to raised intracranial pressures (ICP) due to restriction of clearance of the venous blood from the parenchyma. There occurs a secondary equilibrium at this time, where instead of venous hemorrhages (which occur in the acute phase), dilatation of the CSF pathways (Figure 22.34a–e) happens (empty sella, prominent Meckel's caves, dilated optic nerve sheaths with papilledema) with the blood trying to find alternate routes of drainage leading occasionally to formation of dural AF fistulae. One may, at times, find segmental narrowing of the transverse sinuses, which may explain intracranial hypertension (Figure 22.34f). Whether it is the cause or result of high ICP has been debated by authors, though pressure gradient across the segment may be useful for deciding about venoplasty/stenting across the stenotic area. After excluding all other causes like brain tumors, CSF flow obstruction,

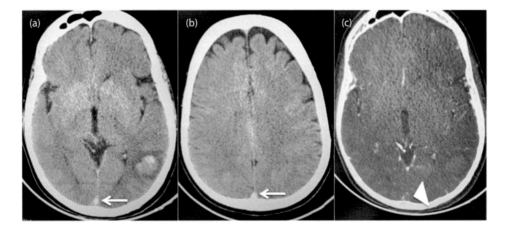

FIGURE 22.33 Cortical sinovenous thrombosis (CSVT): Non-contrast axial CT sections (a, b) revealing hyperdense superior sagittal sinus (arrow) with occipital venous hemorrhagic infarct. Contrast venography (c) shows filling defect in the corresponding sinus segment (arrowhead).

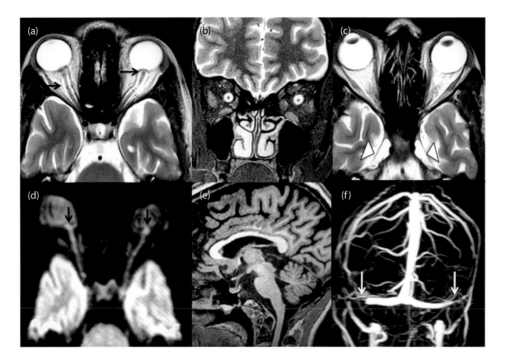

FIGURE 22.34 Intracranial hypertension: Axial T2 (a, c) coronal T2 (b), diffusion-weighted (d) and sagittal T1-weighted (e) MR images demonstrating the signs of raised intracranial pressures namely prominent perioptic CSF spaces with flattening of the optic nerve head showing diffusion restriction (black arrows), prominence of Meckel's caves (arrowheads) and partial empty sella. MR venography (f) shows bilateral transverse sinus stenosis (white arrows).

etc., these cases are classified in the category of idiopathic intracranial hypertension. The vision is affected when the pressures are transmitted to the optic nerve head leading to papilledema. Raised ICP may also lead to isolated sixth CN palsy secondary to nerve stretching, which may be bilateral owing to long cisternal course of this nerve. Identification of this false localizing sign is important in such context.

Posterior fossa/brainstem lesions

Lesions of the brainstem may involve the CN nuclei responsible for ocular movements, which lead to varying types and degrees of ophthalmoparesis causing diplopia and oscillopsia. They may be strategically located infarcts or brainstem neoplasms for

which a detailed evaluation is indicated by contrast-enhanced MRI (Figure 22.35). Demyelinating plaques (MS/NMO), tumors (brainstem gliomas) and meningovasculitis secondary to infective meningitis can all lead to compression/infiltration/infarction in the CN nuclei to varying degree, eventually resulting in ophthalmoplegia. MRI is the imaging modality of choice in these cases.

Conclusion

The advent and evolution of imaging technology has tremendously changed the diagnosis and management of various orbital and intracranial disorders. CT and MRI form the main tools for identification of neuro-ophthalmological diseases.

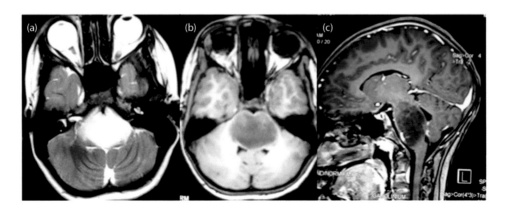

FIGURE 22.35 Diffuse pontine glioma: Axial T2 (a), T1 (b) and sagittal post-contrast T1 (c) weighted MR images showing expansile pontine lesion with minimal enhancement in a patient presenting with multiple cranial nerve palsies.

It is of utmost importance to understand the anatomy of the visual pathway prior to embarking on any diagnosis related to it. A good clinical localization by the neurologist often helps to tailor the imaging methods by the neuroradiologist, which leads to high diagnostic yield and helps in formulation of a diagnosis.

Multiple-Choice Questions

1. Which modality to image the brain and orbit uses ionizing radiation?
   a. Computed tomography
   b. Ultrasound
   c. Magnetic resonance imaging
   d. None of the above

   Answer:

   a. Computed tomography

2. "Tram-track" calcification is seen in which pathology?
   a. Optic nerve glioma
   b. Optic nerve sheath meningioma
   c. Orbital schwannoma
   d. Orbital hemangioma

   Answer:

   b. Optic nerve sheath meningioma

3. Progressive centripetal filling on dynamic contrast enhancement is seen in which cavernous sinus lesion?
   a. Schwannoma
   b. Meningioma
   c. Tolosa–Hunt syndrome
   d. Hemangioma

   Answer:

   d. Hemangioma

4. "Dawson's fingers" are described in which disease?
   a. Multiple sclerosis
   b. Neuromyelitis optica
   c. Tumefactive demyelination
   d. Primary CNS lymphoma

   Answer:

   a. Multiple sclerosis

5. Which one of the following is not a feature of intracranial hypertension?
   a. Flattening of optic nerve head
   b. Empty sella
   c. Midbrain sagging
   d. Dilated optic nerve sheath

   Answer:

   c. Midbrain sagging

References

1. https://en.wikipedia.org/wiki/Medical_ultrasound accessed on July 19, 2019.
2. https://en.wikipedia.org/wiki/CT_scan accessed on July 19, 2019.
3. https://en.wikipedia.org/wiki/History_of_magnetic_resonance_imaging accessed on July 19, 2019.
4. Balcer LJ. Anatomic review and topographic diagnosis. Ophthalmol Clin N Am. 2001;14:1–21.
5. Duong DK, Leo MM, Mitchell EL. Neuro-ophthalmology. Emerg Med Clin N Am. 2008;2:137–80.
6. Eisenkraft B, Ortiz AO. Imaging evaluation of cranial nerves 3, 4, and 6. Seminars in Ultrasound, CT and MRI. 2001;22:488–501.
7. Stalcup ST, Tuan AS, Hesselink JR. Intracranial causes of ophthalmoplegia: The visual reflex pathways. Radiographics. 2013;33:E153–69.
8. Rao AA, Naheedy JH, Chen JY, Robbins SL, Ramkumar HL. A clinical update and radiologic review of pediatric orbital and ocular tumors. J Oncol. 2013;2013:975908.
9. Galluzzi P, Hadjistilianou T, Cerase A, De Francesco S, Toti P, Venturi C. Is CT still useful in the study protocol of retinoblastoma? AJNR Am J Neuroradiol. 2009;30:1760–5.
10. de Graaf P, Göricke S, Rodjan F, Galluzzi P, Maeder P, Castelijns JA, et al. Guidelines for imaging retinoblastoma: Imaging principles and MRI standardization. Pediatr Radiol. 2012;42:2–14.
11. Margolin E. The swollen optic nerve: An approach to diagnosis and management. Pract Neurol. 2019;19(4):302–9.
12. Avery RA, Fisher MJ, Liu GT. Optic pathway gliomas. J Neuroophthalmol. 2011; 31(3):269–78.
13. Mafee MF, Goodwin J, Dorodi S. Optic nerve sheath meningiomas: Role of MR imaging. Radiol Clin North Am. 1999;37(1):37–58.
14. Sepahdari AR, Aakalu VK, Setabutr P, Shiehmorteza M, Naheedy JH, Mafee MF. Indeterminate orbital masses: Restricted diffusion at MR imaging with echo-planar diffusion-weighted imaging predicts malignancy. Radiology. 2010;256(2):554–564.
15. Ansari SA, Mafee MF. Orbital cavernous hemangioma: Role of imaging. Neuroimaging Clin N Am. 2005;15(1):137–58.
16. Thatcher J, Chang YM, Chapman MN, Hovis K, Fujita A, Sobel R, et al. Clinical-radiologic correlation of extraocular eye movement disorders: Seeing beneath the surface. Radiographics. 2016;36:2123–39.
17. Rush JA, Younge BR. Paralysis of cranial nerves III, IV, and VI. Cause and prognosis in 1000 cases. Arch Ophthalmol. 1981;99:76–9.
18. Reddy RP, Bodanapally UK, Shanmuganathan K, Van der Byl G, Dreizin D, Katzman L, et al. Traumatic optic neuropathy: Facial CT findings affecting visual acuity. Emerg Radiol. 2015;22:351–6.
19. Gordon LK. Orbital inflammatory disease: A diagnostic and therapeutic challenge. Eye (Lond). 2006;20:1196–206.
20. Tantiwongkosi B, Hesselink JR. Imaging of ocular motor pathway. Neuroimaging Clin N Am. 2015;25:425–38.
21. Rosai J, Dorfman RF. Sinus histiocytosis with massive lymphadenopathy: A newly recognized benign clinicopathological entity. Arch Pathol 1969;87:63–70.
22. Zafar MA, Waheed SS, Enam SA. Orbital aspergillus infection mimicking a tumour: A case report. Cases J. 2009;2:7860.
23. Paonessa A, Limbucci N, Gallucci M. Are bilateral cavernous hemangiomas of the orbit rare entities? The role of MRI in a retrospective study. Eur J Radiol. 2008;66:282–6.
24. Bose S. Orbital tumors. In: Levin LA, and Arnold AC, editors. Neuro ophthalmology the practical guide. New York, Stuttgart: Thieme Medical Publishers Inc; 2005. pp. 345–55.
25. Purohit BS, Vargas MI, Ailianou A, Merlini L, Poletti PA, Platon A, et al. Orbital tumours and tumour-like lesions: Exploring the armamentarium of multiparametric imaging. Insights Imaging. 2016;7:43–68.
26. Chanson P, Salenave S. Diagnosis and treatment of pituitary adenomas. Minerva Endocrinol. 2004;29(4):241–75.
27. Wang C, Kuang P, Xu F, Hu L. Intracranial Rosai–Dorfman disease with the petroclival and parasellar involvement mimicking multiple meningiomas: A case report and review of literature. Medicine (Baltimore). 2019;98(18):e15548.
28. Langrand C, Bihan H, Raverot G, Varron L, Androdias G, Borson-Chazot F, Brue T, Cathebras P, Pinede L, Muller G, Broussolle C, Cotton F, Valeyre D, Seve P. Hypothalamo-pituitary sarcoidosis: A multicenter study of 24 patients. QJM. 2012;105(10):981–95.
29. Akyüz C, Köseoğlu V, Bertan V, Söylemezoğlu F, Kutluk MT, Büyükpamukçu M. Primary intracranial germ cell tumors in children: A report of eight cases and review of the literature. Turk J Pediatr. 1999;41(2):161–72.
30. McCrea HJ, George E, Settler A, Schwartz TH, Greenfield JP. Pediatric suprasellar tumors. J Child Neurol. 2016;31(12):1367–76.
31. Rossi A, Cama A, Consales A, Gandolfo C, Garrè ML, Milanaccio C, Pavanello M, Piatelli G, Ravegnani M, Tortori-Donati P. Neuroimaging of pediatric craniopharyngiomas: A pictorial essay. J Pediatr Endocrinol Metab. 2006;19(Suppl 1):299–319.
32. Polman CH, Reingold SC, Edan G, et al. Diagnostic criteria for multiple sclerosis: 2005 revisions to the "McDonald criteria". Ann Neurol. 2005;58:840–6.
33. Thornton MJ, Ryan R, Varghese JC, et al. A three dimensional gadolinium enhanced MR venography technique for imaging central veins. Am J Roentgenol. 1999;173:999–1003.
34. Rodallec MH, Krainik A, Feydy A, et al. Cerebral venous thrombosis and multidetector CT angiography: Tips and tricks. Radiographics. 2006;26(Suppl 1):S5–18.

23

NEURO-OPHTHALMOLOGICAL FINDINGS IN PATIENTS WITH POSTERIOR CIRCULATION STROKE

Louis R. Caplan

Much of the human brain contains visually related functions. The brain territories supplied by the vertebral and basilar arteries are particularly important in perception of the visual environment and in focusing the eyes on visual objects. The symptoms and signs can be divided into those that involve afferent findings (*seeing*) and those that are efferent and oculomotor (*looking*) and pupillary abnormalities.

Seeing: Visual perception-related symptoms and signs

The most frequent region infarcted in patients with vertebrobasilar occlusive lesions and brain embolism is the temporo-occipital lobe territory supplied by the posterior cerebral arteries (PCAs).[1] Visual-related functions reside in this area. Occipito-temporal lobe hematomas present similar symptoms and signs to infarcts in the same locations.

Unilateral lesions

The most common visual field defect when one hemisphere is infarcted is a hemianopia. Patients usually report inability to see to the hemianopic side, or a void, or grayness to that side. The hemianopia is most often homonymous and congruent. The responsible lesion is usually an occipital lobe infarct (Figure 23.1). When the hemianopia is complete and splits the macula, the lesion usually involves the optic radiations subcortically or includes the calcarine cortex from the occipital pole to the anterior occipital region. In some patients, the macular, central, region of the hemianopic field adjacent to the vertical meridian is relatively spared. This central portion of the visual field is represented in the posterior portion of the striate cortex (VI) near the occipital pole. Macular sparing usually means that the occipital pole is preserved and that the lesion likely involves striate cortex rather than optic radiations. If there is macular sparing, the occipital poles are likely supplied, in addition to the PCAs, by collaterals from the middle cerebral arteries (MCAs).

Patients with occipital cortex lesions may have partial hemianopic field defects in which larger and brighter stimuli are perceived, but small dimmer stimuli are not. In contrast, lesions affecting the geniculocalcarine tracts often cause dense complete defects for all visual stimuli in the affected parts of the visual fields. Small occipital lobe infarcts can cause homonymous scotomas that are typically congruent. When the lesions are near the occipital pole, the scotomas are usually within the perimacular, central fixation area. More anterior lesions are likely to cause more peripherally placed scotomas above or below the horizontal meridian. The unpaired monocular temporal crescent of vision and the more peripheral portions of the contralateral visual fields project onto the cerebral cortex within the depth of the calcarine fissure.[2] When infarction spares the most anterior portion of the calcarine cortex, the resulting hemianopia may not be congruent and may spare the temporal crescent of vision in the eye contralateral to

the infarct. Rarely, a very far anterior, small occipital lobe infarct can involve only the temporal crescent in the contralateral eye. Homonymous sector and quadrant defects are also common. A homonymous superior quadrantanopia is caused by a lesion involving the contralateral lower bundle of the optic radiations either in Meyer's loop in the temporal lobe near the temporal horn of the lateral ventricle or in the occipital lobe affecting the striate cortex on the lower bank of the calcarine fissure (Figure 23.2). A homonymous inferior quadrantanopia is usually due to a deep parietal lobe lesion involving the upper bundle of the optic radiations or the upper bank of the calcarine cortex in the cuneus (Figure 23.3). Visual inattention and neglect of the contralateral visual field is common in patients with large unilateral infarcts.

Infarction within the lateral geniculate body (LGB) can cause a homonymous hemianopia sometimes with selective involvement or sparing of a contralateral sector of vision along the horizontal meridian. Infarction of the medial and posterior portions of the LGB in the territory of the lateral choroidal artery branch of the posterior choroidal artery usually causes a homonymous sectoranopia involving the region around the horizontal meridian. The posterior choroidal arteries are branches of the PCAs. Instead, when the infarct involves the hilum and anterolateral portions of the LGB, the territory usually supplied by the anterior choroidal artery, a branch of the internal carotid artery, the patient may have homonymous sectoranopias involving the upper and lower quadrants of the contralateral visual field but sparing the horizontal meridian.

Patients with unilateral lesions affecting the striate visual cortex often describe visual illusions and hallucinations. The illusions often occur as the visual deficit is developing or when it is clearing. The illusions are often located at the periphery of the region of visual field loss, and probably are emanating from partially damaged unstable visual cortex.

Left PCA territory infarcts

Reading, language, and memory abnormalities often are found in left PCA territory infarct patients (Table 23.1). Alexia without agraphia, also referred to as pure alexia and as pure word blindness, is a syndrome found in patients with relatively large left PCA territory infarcts. Patients with pure alexia can spell words aloud and identify words spelled to them. They are able to write correctly but later cannot read back what they had written earlier. They may retain the ability to read individual letters and usually can identify numbers. Patients who have alexia without agraphia almost invariably also have a right homonymous hemianopia or hemiachromatopsia and abnormal colornaming. Some patients also have an accompanying visual agnosia characterized by difficulty naming and identifying the nature of visual objects although the same objects are recognized when presented by sound or touch or described verbally. Another common accompanying deficit is in making new memories. The causative brain lesions invariably involve the white matter undercutting the left parastriate and peristriate regions. Infarcts

DOI: 10.1201/9780429020278-34

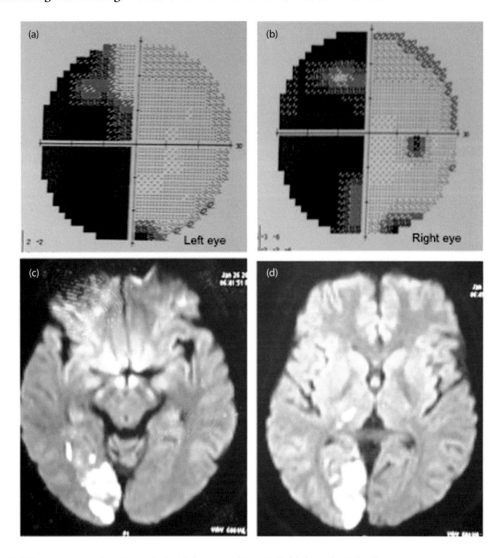

FIGURE 23.1 Left homonymous hemianopia (a, b) due to right occipital lobe infarct (c, d).

usually include the parieto-occipital and often the temporal artery branches of the left PCA. The splenium of the corpus callosum is usually directly damaged, or its exiting white matter fibers are undercut.

Right PCA territory infarcts

Visual inattention and neglect most often occurs in larger lesions involving the temporal and parietal lobe supply of the right PCA (Table 23.1). Neglect may be more common when the splenium of the corpus callosum is included in the infarct.[3] Patients with neglect usually also fail to blink to threat presented from the neglected visual field and usually have reduced optokinetic nystagmus to the neglected side. Lesions involving the deep parietal lobe and temporal lobes, undercutting area 7, the angular gyrus, and the posterior portion of the superior and middle temporal gyri cause abnormalities of ipsilateral smooth visual pursuit and optokinetic nystagmus. Lesions that cause abnormalities of smooth pursuit and optokinetic nystagmus may also involve or undercut Brodmann areas 19, 37, and 39.[4]

Patients with posteriorly located right cerebral hemisphere lesions often have defective constructional abilities and draw and copy poorly. Their drawings are characterized by: omission of some of the left side of the figures; abnormal size, angles, and proportions; and failure to improve by copying. Lesions causing constructional apraxia are usually located near the junction of the right temporal, occipital, and parietal lobes. Large right PCA territory infarcts affecting the temporal and parietal lobes, or right inferior division MCA territory infarcts involving the inferior parietal lobe are most often found. In patients with right hemispheric lesions, constructional apraxia is usually accompanied by left visual neglect and sometimes by agitation and restlessness.

Patients with right parieto-occipital lesions may have excessive difficulty finding their way about. Very severe topographical disorientation occurs in patients with bilateral upper bank, parieto-occipital lesions usually in conjunction with features of Balint's syndrome. These individuals cannot revisualize directions and describe the relationships of objects in their own rooms or houses or in a standard structure such as a baseball or football field. Otherwise alert individuals may also not identify their own location and may say that they are at very distant locales.

Bilateral lesions

Patients with bilateral (and sometimes unilateral) lesions involving the calcarine cortex or surrounding cortical zones (V2 and parastriate and peristriate cortex) show deficits in discerning motion and in detecting the nature, shape, color, and size of objects, bilaterally or within the hemianopic field (Table 23.1).

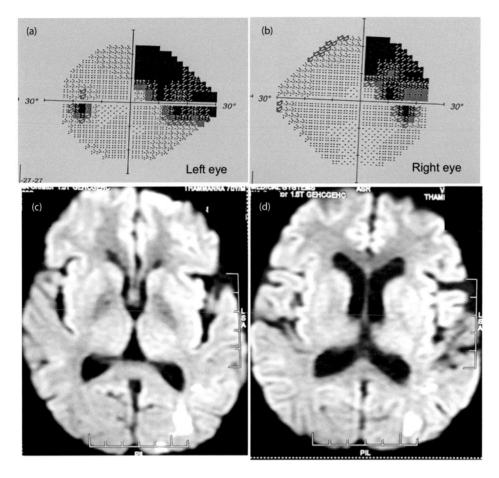

FIGURE 23.2   Right superior quadrantanopia (a, b) due to left temporal lobe infarct near temporal horn of left lateral ventricle (c, d).

One way of describing abnormalities that are located either above (upper bank) or below (lower bank) the calcarine cortex refers to aspects of visual and visual-spatial functions. The lower bank is specialized in aspects that tell *what* an object is and the upper bank relates more to the *where* aspects and visual-spatial relationships.[5,6] In area V4, including the caudal portion of the lingual and fusiform gyri (areas 18,19,37) on the lower bank of the calcarine

fissure, neurons are sensitive to color patterns. Areas within the lower bank of the calcarine cortex (fusiform and lingual gyri) are specialized for detecting the nature of objects (their color, size, shape, and name) and their movements. An example of difficulty in recognizing the nature and details of an object is prosopagnosia, defective facial recognition. Prosopagnosia is caused by lesions in the lingual and fusiform gyri, most often in the medial

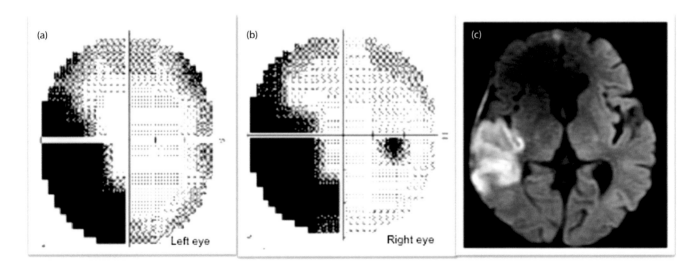

FIGURE 23.3   Left inferior quadrantanopia (a, b) due to right parieto-temporal lobe infarct (c).

TABLE 23.1: Visual Signs Present in a Patient with Posterior Cerebral Artery (PCA) Territory Infarction

Left PCA territory infarct	Right homonymous hemianopia/hemichromatopsia	
	Abnormalities in reading, language, memory	
	Alexia without agraphia	
	Visual agnosia	
Right PCA territory infarct	Left homonymous hemianopia	
	Visual inattention	
	Left visuospatial neglect	
	Abnormalities of smooth visual pursuits/OKN	
	Constructional apraxia	
	Topographical disorientation	
Bilateral PCA territory infarct	Upper bank	Defects in stereoscopy
		Asimultagnosia
		Optic ataxia
		Optic apraxia
	Lower bank	Prosopagnosia
		Defective object recognition and revisualization

portion of the fusiform gyrus, often bilaterally but occasionally unilaterally. Occasionally prosopagnosia patients have lesions in anterior temporal cortex indicating more a difficulty in remembering faces than in facial recognition. Despite severe defects in object recognition and revisualization, patients with lower bank lesions usually do not get lost, can localize objects in space, and may retain normal visual-spatial abilities. Emboli most often cause inferior calcarine bank or full PCA territory infarcts.[1]

Upper bank infarcts are much less common. The defects that result are in discerning the relationship of objects to each other and depth. Patients with bilateral inferior parietal lesions cannot revisualize where objects are located in space, for example, in picturing a map, or directions to a place. They reach for something they presume to be at a distance and hit into the object which is, in reality, very near. Stereoscopy, distance, and relationships can be tested by asking patients to look at a scene out of the window, or in the room, or even on a television screen. Three-dimensional pictures are especially useful to test for these abnormalities. The other common abnormalities are subserved under a condition termed Balint's syndrome (asimultagnosia, optic ataxia, and optic apraxia). These patients have difficulty seeing more than one object in a scene at the same time; they have difficulty coordinating hand and arm with eye movements.

Patients with bilateral occipital lobe lesions often have difficulty with depth perception.

Looking: Oculomotor and pupillary signs

Vestibulo-ocular reflex (VOR)

The vestibular nuclei in the dorsolateral medullary and pontine tegmentum and their connections with the flocculonodular lobe of the cerebellum comprise a system designed to yield information about location of the head, neck, and trunk in space. The vestibular nuclei have strong connections with the oculomotor structures that control both horizontal and vertical gaze and subserve the VOR. The VOR is a three-neuron reflex involving vestibular ganglion cells, the brainstem vestibular nuclei, and the ocular motor nuclei that allows continued visual fixation during movement in any direction. On movement of the head and/or body, the VOR generates reflex slow, conjugate eye movements in

three-dimensional space, whose direction, amplitude, and velocity adapt to head motion so that the image of an object remains stable on the retina during head or body movements.[7,8] The vestibular nuclei also project to the cerebral cortex via the thalamus to allow conscious recognition of body and head motion. The signs are most conveniently discussed in relation to anatomic regions. However, often multiple brainstem sites may be involved.

Patients with lesions that involve the vestibular system and the VOR often report vertigo, dizziness, ataxia, and dysequilibrium.[1] Sometimes objects appear to jiggle or move rhythmically (oscillopsia). Patients may describe difficulty focusing or reading while they are in motion, for example, in a moving car. Nystagmus, abnormalities of eye position, and ataxia are common abnormalities found on examination. The VOR has three different planes of activity, each subserved by different anatomical structures: the horizontal or yaw plane; the vertical, sagittal, or pitch plane; and the roll or torsional plane. The horizontal plane VOR connections are mostly in the medulla-ponto-mesencephalic regions and include structures involved in horizontal gaze. These vestibulo-ocular connections are located in the lateral and medial pontomedullary tegmentum on both sides and include: the vestibular nuclei, nuclei prepositus hypoglossi, paramedian pontine reticular formation (PPRF) lateral gaze centers, sixth nerve nuclei, medial longitudinal fasciculi (MLF), and the third nerve nuclei in the midbrain. The medial vestibular nuclei and the nuclei prepositus hypoglossi contribute to gaze holding in the horizontal plane. Lesions affecting the horizontal VOR cause rotational vertigo, postural imbalance, and horizontal nystagmus. The vertical plane VOR includes vestibular nuclei connections with structures that control vertical gaze in the rostral brainstem located in the paramedian tegmentum near the mesencephalic-diencephalic junction. Two key structures are the rostral interstitial nucleus of the MLF (riMLF) and the interstitial nucleus of Cajal (INC), a structure important in vertical gaze-holding and in eye-head coordination in the roll plane. Connections between the two sides, probably within the posterior commissure, allow coordination of the two eyes in up and down gaze. Abnormalities in this system cause up and down beat nystagmus, tilt in a pitch plane of the subjective vertical axis, and feelings of moving forward or backward or somersaulting.

Eye position and movements and pupillary signs are conveniently discussed under anatomical regions.

Thalamus

Embolism to the rostral basilar artery and medial thalamic hemorrhages are the thalamic lesions that most often are accompanied by neuro-ophthalmologic abnormalities. Lesions in the rostral midbrain tegmentum and the medial diencephalon often affect the afferent limb of the pupillary light reflex arc intercepting fibers as they pass from the optic tract to the third nerve nucleus. The pupils do not react to light. The near reflex may be preserved, the pupil reacting to convergence. Often, because unilateral or bilateral descending sympathetic fibers are also involved, the pupils are small as well as non-reactive. A magnifying glass may be needed to distinguish small, reactive "pontine pupils" from small poorly reactive "thalamic pupils." Increased intracranial pressure especially from a unilateral cerebral hemisphere mass can cause compression of the rostral brainstem and/or the third nerves. The ipsilateral pupil may first become constricted and then dilate, usually with loss of reactivity to light. The opposite pupil, contralateral to the mass, shows an initial reduction in reactivity to light followed by reduction in size and then enlargement but the pupil usually remains round.[9]

Ischemic lesions limited to the diencephalon do not affect eye position or movement. Thalamic hemorrhages cause oculomotor abnormalities because of compression of the rostral midbrain tegmentum and bleeding into and distortion of the third ventricle.

Midbrain

The structures in the most rostral portion of the midbrain tegmentum are damaged in patients with occlusions of the thalamic-subthalamic arteries, or the rostral tip of the basilar artery ("top of the basilar syndrome") or thalamic hemorrhages with postero-medial involvement or extension. Vertical plane eye motions are generated by simultaneous activation of the bilateral frontal and parieto-occipital conjugate gaze centers. Projections from these centers converge on the periaqueductal region in the brainstem tectum just beneath the collicular plate near the INC and the posterior commissure. The riMLF is also located in this region. This area is often referred to as the vertical gaze center.

There is often a disparity between vertical eye movements generated voluntarily or by following an object upward and by reflex eye movements. Vertical reflex eye movements can be generated in normal individuals by vertical oculocephalic maneuvers (vertical "doll's eyes"), by bilateral simultaneous caloric stimulation, and by inducing Bell's phenomenon. Upgaze palsy develops in patients with unilateral dorsal lesions at the mesencephalic-diencephalic junction, and stereotactically induced lesions in this region also can cause paralysis of upgaze in both eyes. In monkeys and humans, lesions that cause upgaze palsy are more often bilateral and involve the pretectal region. Fibers emerging from the riMLF probably cross in the midline within the posterior commissure so that bilateral upgaze palsy can result from lesions that involve the fibers entering or within the posterior commissure. Isolated paralysis of downgaze with preserved upgaze is rarer; the responsible lesions have been bilateral and more ventral and caudal than those that produce isolated upgaze palsy, usually located just medial to the red nuclei. In one patient with an isolated downgaze palsy, the lesions were bilateral and involved the dorsolateral periaqueductal gray including the crossing fibers of the superior colliculus. In most patients with large pretectal lesions, upgaze and downgaze are involved together and symmetrically. However, selective upgaze palsy and combined downgaze and upgaze palsy are occasionally due to a unilateral lesion of the riMLF involving the laterally spreading fibers of the posterior commissure. Some patients with pretectal lesions have both upgaze and downgaze palsy with sparing of gaze in one eye in one direction ("vertical one and a half syndrome"). In contrast to vertical gaze palsy, vertical nystagmus or isolated up or down beating nystagmus is not due to rostral brainstem lesions. Vertical nystagmus occurs with lesions of the caudal pontine and medullary tegmentum or the cerebellum.[1]

Ocular convergence is also controlled in the medial rostral midbrain tegmentum. In patients with paramedian thalamic hemorrhages or rostral basilar artery territory infarcts, one or both eyes may rest in, or down and in. This thalamic esotropia is due to an abnormality of the convergence system. Rhythmic inward beating "convergence nystagmus" can be elicited in some of these patients by asking them to look up or by watching a downward moving optokinetic stimulus. Studies of patients with convergence nystagmus show that the adducting movements are inward directed saccades and not true nystagmus. Attempted upgaze in these patients may also elicit a contraction of many extraocular muscles which causes the globes to physically jerk back into the orbit, giving rise to the term "nystagmus retractorius," a misnomer.[10,11] In some patients, upbeat or downbeat

nystagmus is also elicited by convergence. Convergence vectors may also often modify eye position and horizontal gaze. On gaze to either side, the abducting eye may also have a convergence vector that tends to pull the eye inward. This creates limitation of abduction, also called pseudo-sixth palsy. At times, spontaneous in-beating saccades can be seen in the abducting eye during attempted lateral gaze. Patients with dysconjugate gaze tend to fixate with the hyperconvergent eye so that covering this eye can lead to improved lateral excursion of the abducting eye.

Retraction of the upper eyelids, so-called Collier's sign, is also found in some patients with pretectal lesions. Eyelid retraction can be found without vertical gaze palsy. The responsible lesions that cause eyelid retraction can be unilateral and probably involve the nucleus of the posterior commissure. At times, in patients with thalamic hemorrhages that extend into the third ventricle, the eyes rest conjugately to the contralateral side. Patients with right thalamic hematomas and left hemisensory loss will have their eyes conjugately deviated to the left. This direction of deviation is opposite to that found in patients with supratentorial ischemic and hemorrhagic lesions and so has been called "wrong-way eyes" by Fisher.[12] Occasional patients with pretectal lesions will have sudden small-amplitude ocular oscillations often called "lightning-like" because of their speed and brevity. These movements are also seen in monkeys with experimentally induced pretectal vestibulo-thalamic projections in the ventrolateral thalamus. Slight vertigo and horizontal nystagmus can occur in patients with lateral thalamic infarcts.

Pons and medulla

Basilar artery occlusion most often causes infarcts that are limited to the pontine base. At times, the tegmentum is also infarcted either bilaterally or unilaterally. Pontine hemorrhages that are accompanied by neuro-ophthalmological sigs usually involve the lateral pontine tegmentum.[13]

Unilateral medial pontine lesions

These lesions often involve the MLF, abducens nucleus, or the PPRF on one side. Efferent fibers from the frontal eye fields that relate to conjugate horizontal gaze cross at the ponto-mesencephalic junction above the level of the abducens nuclei in the pons and end in the reticular gray region called the PPRF adjacent to the contralateral abducens nucleus. Lesions of the sixth nerve nucleus cause an ipsilateral conjugate gaze palsy for both voluntary and reflex-induced movements (caloric and VORs). MRI studies of patients who have a unilateral weakness of the abducting eye (sixth nerve palsy) show that the responsible lesion invariably involves the nerve fascicles of VI and not the abducens nucleus. Some patients have had an isolated sixth nerve palsy without other neurologic findings due to lesions that involved the fascicles of the abducens nerve as the nerve travels through the pontine base. Since the sixth nerve fascicles loop around the facial nuclei, involvement of the sixth nerve nucleus is usually accompanied by a peripheral type ipsilateral facial palsy. Lesions of the PPRF most likely impair voluntary conjugate horizontal gaze to the ipsilateral side with preservation of reflex-induced movements. The PPRF also mediates ipsilaterally directed saccades within the contralateral field of eye movement.

Involvement of the MLF causes an internuclear ophthalmoplegia (INO) characterized by inability to adduct the ipsilateral eye on gaze to the contralateral side accompanied usually by nystagmus of the abducting contralateral eye. At times, the eye on the side of the MLF lesion rests in the midline, but it may be deviated outward. MRI studies show that when an INO is accompanied by loss of convergence and abnormalities of abduction of the contralateral eye, the medial tegmental lesions are more extensive.[14,15] Vertical nystagmus and skew deviation often accompany an INO. The MLF contains internuclear fibers and vestibulo-oculomotor fibers important for the vertical VOR, explaining the usual presence of vertical nystagmus in patients with INOs.

Unilateral INO is often accompanied by elements of the ocular tilt reaction (OTR) in patients with lesions that involve the pons and midbrain.[16] Common findings include tilt of the subjective visual vertical, ocular torsion, and skew deviation with the eye contralateral to the INO being undermost. All components of the OTR are directed to the contralateral side.

Skew deviation is characterized by vertical misalignment of the two eyes not caused by paralysis of a single muscle or nerve. The oblique relationship is maintained through all fields of gaze. When the tegmental lesion is in the caudal pons, the ipsilateral eye usually lies below the contralateral eye, while in the rostral pons and midbrain, the ipsilateral eye usually rests above the contralateral eye. Some patients with lesions in the rostral pons involving the paramedian tegmentum in a region near the MLF have had an ipsilateral paresis of abduction accompanied at times by nystagmus of the adducting contralateral eye. Patients with lesions in the pons may have ptosis, often more severe than expected with a Horner's syndrome. The explanation for the ptosis is uncertain but it may relate to the accompanying hemiparesis or facial weakness.[17]

When the PPRF and the MLF are both involved on the same side, the resulting ophthalmoplegia is severe and patients can only move the contralateral eye in abduction to one side. This abnormality was named the "one and a half syndrome" by Fisher.[12,18] If conjugate gaze to one side is given a score of 1, normal patients with intact horizontal gaze have a score of 2. PPRF lesions abolish the conjugate gaze to one side, the ipsilateral side, and MLF lesions abolish gaze of the adducting eye to the contralateral side, removing 1/2 of gaze to that side. In total 1 and 1/2 of the total 2 points for horizontal gaze are lost. The OTR is more common in unilateral pontine tegmental lesions than in bilateral lesions.

Involvement of the unilateral medial pontine tegmentum is most common after basilar artery occlusion in which the pontine base is usually bilaterally infarcted and in patients with asymmetric pontine hematomas. Basilar branch occlusions occasionally cause infarcts extending dorsally enough to involve eye movements. More often the tegmental ischemia in patients with basilar branch occlusions is transient. In some reported patients with pontine hemorrhages extending into the tegmentum on one side but involving the midline region, patients have remained alert despite bilateral horizontal gaze paresis. The responsible lesions on MRI involved the central raphe at the midline.

Bilateral medial pontine tegmental lesions

When the medial pontine tegmentum has bilaterally lesions, patients are usually comatose and have bilateral horizontal gaze palsies. Reflex vertical gaze is preserved if the more rostral mesencephalic-diencephalic tegmental structures are spared. Often in this situation, ocular bobbing, an intermittent brisk downward movement of one or both eyes, occurs.[19,20] Bobbing can be asymmetric especially if the horizontal gaze abnormalities are asymmetric. Bobbing is more likely to affect eyes in which ocular abduction is lost. Bobbing is best understood as a form of vertical roving eye movement. Comatose patients with bilateral cerebral hemisphere lesions have free roving side-to-side movements of

their eyes. The supratentorial gaze centers have both horizontal and vertical vectors, but ordinarily horizontal gaze predominates because most of the visual action is more on an eye plane than up or down. When the left frontal eye field is stimulated ordinarily, the eyes would conjugately deviate to the right. If the right sixth nerve is paralyzed, stimulation of the left frontal eye field causes the right eye to deviate downward instead of to the right. Bilateral simultaneous stimulation of the supratentorial gaze centers results in vertical gaze because horizontal vectors are canceled. Similarly, bilateral simultaneous irrigation of both ear canals results in up or down gaze depending on whether warm or cold water is used. When horizontal gaze to one or both sides is abolished by a medial pontine lesion, then the vertical downgaze vectors predominate and bobbing occurs. At times, vergence movements are seen when patients attempt to look in the direction of a gaze palsy. In these patients, vergence movements are substituted for paretic movements.

Bilateral involvement of the MLF causes a bilateral INO in which there is no adduction of either eye but abducting nystagmus is present on gaze to either side. The eyes may rest in the midline or be deviated outward producing a bilateral exotropia (so-called "wall-eyed bilateral INO" ("WEBINO") syndrome).[1,21] This syndrome has been described in patients with tegmental pontine and midbrain lesions. Bilateral pontine tegmental lesions are usually caused by basilar artery occlusions or large pontine hemorrhages. Occasionally hydrocephalus can cause a transient WEBINO syndrome when the expanded IV ventricle compresses the junction of the pontine and midbrain tegmentum.

Lateral medullary and lateral pontine tegmental lesions

Lateral medullary infarcts sometimes extend medially enough to include the medial and superior vestibular nuclei as well as often involving the restiform body. Patients often describe sensations of turning, rotating, or pulling to the side. Oscillopsia and double vision are also commonly reported. Some patients describe the sensation as a swaying or rolling rather than true rotational spinning. Patients feel off balance and sense abnormal relation of themselves to their environment. The eyes usually lie in the midline but may drift to the contralateral side. In some patients, the eyes are strongly deviated toward the side of the lesion-lateropulsion.[22] In patients with lateral medullary infarction and lateropulsion, horizontal saccades to the side of the lesion are overshooting (hypermetric) and those to the opposite side are hypometric (undershooting).[23] When the eyes are opened, they often lie conjugately far to the ipsilateral side. Ocular torsion is also often present with the ipsilateral eye and ear located in a down position compared to the contralateral eye and ear. This ocular skew is usually maintained in all fields of gaze. Nystagmus is nearly invariable and usually has rotatory and horizontal components. The rapid component of the rotatory nystagmus usually moves the upper border of the iris toward the side of the lesion. Usually small amplitude quick nystagmus is present on gaze to the contralateral side, while slower but larger amplitude nystagmus is present on gaze to the ipsilateral side. The directional preponderance of the nystagmus and the ocular drift depend on the rostro-caudal location of the lesion and the vestibular nuclei involved.[24] Vertical nystagmus does not occur with lesions limited to the lateral medulla.

Ptosis of the ipsilateral eye is usually a part of a Horner's syndrome related to involvement of descending sympathetic nervous system fibers in the lateral tegmentum. The oculomotor abnormalities are similar in lateral pontine tegmental and lateral medullary infarcts.

Cerebellar lesions

Most descriptions of eye movement abnormalities in patients with cerebellar pathology have been found in patients with various familial and degenerative cerebellar system diseases. Eye movement abnormalities in patients with well-defined small infarcts and hemorrhages have not been studied in detail, but a few reports do describe abnormalities in some patients with localized infarcts. Cerebellar hemorrhages often compress the caudal brainstem causing oculomotor signs.

Lesions of the posterior inferior vermis in the territory of the medial branch of posterior inferior cerebellar artery (mPICA) are known to cause vertigo and vestibulo-ocular abnormalities.[25,26] Vertigo is often severe and is usually accompanied by nausea and vomiting. The entire symptom complex is dominated by vestibular symptoms and signs often leading to the erroneous diagnosis of labyrinthitis, peripheral vestibular disorder, or Meniere's disease. In patients with mPICA infarcts, the eyes may rest conjugately deviated to the side of the lesion-lateropulsion. Foveal smooth pursuit is impaired in all directions and there often is horizontal nystagmus. The nystagmus is usually in both directions of gaze but has larger amplitude when gaze is directed toward the side of the lesion. The posterior inferior vermis contains the nodulus and a major portion of the vestibulocerebellum receiving mostly projections from the vestibular nuclei. Periodic alternating nystagmus can be found in patients with an acute infarct limited to the nodulus.[27] Spontaneous horizontal nystagmus occur in the primary eye position and revers direction with cycles of about 2 minutes. The nystagmus disappear with eye fixation. Head shaking in the horizontal position elicit downbeat nystagmus. Some patients with lesions of the most posterior inferior vermis have prominent downbeat nystagmus. Most such patients have had craniocervical junction abnormalities such as Arnold Chiari syndrome with downward herniation of the cerebellar tonsils and bilateral abnormalities.

The flocculus, another component of the vestibulocerebellum, is most often supplied by anterior inferior cerebellar artery (AICA), and vertigo and nystagmus are common in patients with AICA territory infarcts. In patients with AICA territory infarcts, the brachium pontis is invariably involved, but the flocculus is the second most commonly involved structure. The AICAs also supply the eighth nerve in the cerebellopontine angle. The internal auditory artery, which supplies the eighth nerve in the internal auditory canal, and the peripheral vestibular apparatus and the cochlea, is in the vast majority of patients, a branch of AICA so that dizziness, vertigo, and nystagmus in patients with occlusion of AICA can also be due to infarction of the peripheral portion of the vestibular nerve or the labyrinth itself. Occasional patients report episodic vertigo due to peripheral labyrinthian ischemia weeks and months before developing typical AICA territory brainstem infarcts.[28] Dizziness is commonly reported in patients with superior cerebellar artery (SCA) territory infarcts, but severe vertigo and nystagmus are not common or prominent findings in SCA territory cerebellar infarcts unless the brainstem territory is also involved. Some patients with SCA territory cerebellar infarcts have an upbeating nystagmus present on gaze straight ahead probably due to involvement of the superior vermis. Hypermetria of contralaterally directed saccades and hypometria of ipsilateral saccades in patients with SCA territory cerebellar infarcts is the converse of that seen in PICA territory cerebellar infarcts. Patients with infarction limited to the lateral branch of SCA (lSCA) often have minor transient dizziness but usually do not have prominent vertigo or nystagmus.

In patients with cerebellar hemorrhages and large cerebellar infarcts, gaze palsies and sixth nerve palsies have been described. The commonest abnormality is probably weakness or delay in abduction of the eye ipsilateral to the cerebellar lesion. This often causes dysconjugate gaze and diplopia. Conjugate gaze palsy to the side of the lesion is also common. Many large cerebellar hemorrhages and infarcts are located in the cerebellar hemispheres and cause compression of structures on the floor of the fourth ventricle including the vestibular nuclei, so that some of the oculomotor findings relate to vestibular nuclei and other brainstem tegmental structure dysfunction.

Patients with cerebellar lesions of many varieties often have gaze paretic nystagmus and abnormalities of saccadic and smooth pursuit eye movements. Nystagmus is more common in patients with isolated PICA territory cerebellar infarcts than in those with cerebellar infarcts limited to the supply territory of the SCA. Especially common are inaccurate saccades which are hypermetric and overshoot the target, or hypometric, and arrive short of the target. Compensatory adjustments follow the hypometric and hypermetric saccades often with some oscillations. This abnormality of eye movements is often called ocular dysmetria and resembles the trajectory and adjustments of arm movements in patients with cerebellar lesions. Saccadic dysmetria is influenced by the initial position of the eye in the orbit, by ambient light or darkness, and by the nature of the visual target.[29] In most studies of cerebellar eye movement abnormalities, the patients have not had strokes, or the lesions were vascular but not well defined or localized.

Conclusion

Autopsy series and neuropathological studies on ocular tissues are not routinely available and hence only limited data is available in this regard. Neurologists need to be to be familiar with the pathology of neuro-ophthalmic disorders because of their implications in making diagnosis, designing treatment strategies and understanding prognosis of such disorders. Recognizing various pathological hallmarks of different infectious, inflammatory, autoimmune and neoplastic disorders involving the eye and the brain may help in making a definitive diagnosis and subsequently provide essential management clues.

Multiple-Choice Questions

1. All are midbrain stroke syndromes, EXCEPT:
   a. Benedict's
   b. Claude's
   c. Weber's
   d. Millard Gubler's

   Answer:

   d. Millard Gubler's

2. Anton's syndrome is characterized by all of the following, EXCEPT:
   a. Visual anosognosia
   b. Confabulation
   c. Visual loss
   d. Oculomotor apraxia

   Answer:

   d. Oculomotor apraxia

3. All are true regarding the infarction of lateral geniculate body, EXCEPT:
   a. Infarction of the medial and posterior portions of the LGB usually causes a homonymous sectoranopia involving the region around the horizontal meridian.
   b. The posterior choroidal arteries are branches of the PCA.
   c. Anterior choroidal artery is a branch of the middle cerebral artery.
   d. Infarction involving the hilum and anterolateral portions of the LGB may have homonymous sectoranopias involving the upper and lower quadrants of the contralateral visual field but sparing the horizontal meridian.

   Answer:

   c. Anterior choroidal artery is a branch of the middle cerebral artery.

4. In patients of posterior circulation stroke:
   a. Upper bank infarcts are commoner as compared to lower bank strokes.
   b. Emboli most often cause inferior calcarine bank or full PCA territory infarcts.
   c. Balint's syndrome occurs where patient has complete denial of blindness.
   d. The lower bank is specialized in aspects that tell *where* an object is.

   Answer:

   b. Emboli most often cause inferior calcarine bank or full PCA territory infarcts.

5. Which of the statements is NOT true with regard to "wall-eyed bilateral INO" ("WEBINO") syndrome?
   a. In patients with bilateral INO, there is no adduction of either eye but abducting nystagmus is present on gaze to either side.
   b. This syndrome has been described in patients with medullary lesions.
   c. Hydrocephalus can cause a WEBINO syndrome.
   d. Basilar artery occlusions or large pontine hemorrhages can cause WEBINO syndrome.

   Answer:

   b. This syndrome has been described in patients with medullary lesions.

References

1. Caplan LR. Vertebrobasilar ischemia and hemorrhage: Clinical findings, diagnosis, and management of posterior circulation disease, Chapter 4. In Signs and symptoms and their clinical localization. Cambridge, UK: Cambridge University Press; 2014. pp. 74–132.
2. Horton JC, Hoyt WF. The representation of the visual field in human striate cortex. A revision of the classic Holmes map. Arch Opthalmol. 1991;109:816–824.
3. Park KC, Lee BH, Kim EJ, et al. Deafferentation-disconnection neglect induced by posterior cerebral artery infarction. Neurology. 2006;66:56–61.
4. Morrow MJ, Sharpe JA. Retinotopic and directional deficits of smooth pursuit initiation after posterior cerebral hemispheric lesions. Neurology. 1993;43:595–603.
5. Mishkin M, Ungerleider LG, Macko KA. Object vision and spatial vision: Two cortical pathways. Trends Neurosci. 1983;6:414–417.
6. Ungerleider LG, Haxby JV. "What" and "where" in the human brain. Current Opinion Neurobiol. 1994;4:157–165.
7. Brandt T. Man in motion. Historical and clinical aspects of vestibular function. Brain.1991;114:2159–2174.
8. Leigh RJ, Brandt T. A reevaluation of the vestibulo-ocular reflex: New ideas of its purpose, properties, neural substrate, and disorders. Neurology. 1993;43:1288–1295.
9. Ropper AH. The opposite pupil in herniation. Neurology. 1990;40:1707–1709.
10. Sharpe JA, Hoyt WF, Rosenberg MA. Convergence evoked nystagmus: Congenital and acquired forms. Arch Neurol. 1975;32:191–194.
11. Oliva A, Rosenberg MI. Convergence evoked nystagmus. Neurology. 1990;40:161–162.
12. Fisher CM. Some neuro-ophthalmological observations. J Neurol NeurosurgPsychiatry. 1967;30:383–392.
13. Caplan, L, Goodwin, J. Lateral brainstem tegmental hemorrhage. Neurology. 1982; 32:252–260.
14. Bronstein AM, Morris J, Du Boulay G, et al. Abnormalities of horizontal gaze. Clinical, oculographic, and magnetic resonance imaging findings. I. Abducens palsy. J Neurol Neurosurg Psychiatry. 1990;53:194–199.
15. Bronstein AM, Rudge P, Gresty MA, et al. Abnormalities of horizontal gaze. Clinical, oculographic, and magnetic resonance imaging findings. II. Gaze palsy and internuclear opthalmoplegia. J Neurol Neurosurg Psychiatry. 1990;53:200–207.
16. Zwergal A, Cnyrim C, Arbusow V, Glaser M, Fesl G, Brandt T, Strupp M. Unilateral INO is associated with ocular tilt reaction in pontomesencephalic lesions. INO plus. Neurology. 2008;71:590–593.
17. Caplan LR. Ptosis. J Neurol Neurosurg Psychiatry.1974;37:1–7.
18. Pierot-Desilligny C, Chain F, Serdaru M, et al. The one and a half syndrome. Brain. 1981;104;665–699.
19. Fisher CM. Ocular bobbing. Arch Neurol 1964;11:543–546.
20. Nelson J, Johnston C. Ocular bobbing. Arch Neurol. 1970;22:348–356.
21. Pierot-Desilligny C, Caplan LR. Eye movement abnormalities. In: Caplan LR, van Gijn, editors. Stroke syndromes. 3rd ed. Cambridge: UK: Cambridge University Press;2012. pp. 67–74.
22. Meyer K, Baloh R, Krohel G, et al. Ocular lateropulsion: A sign of lateral medullary disease. Arch Optalmol. 1980;98:1614–1616.
23. Thomke F. Disorders of ocular motility. In: Urban PP, Caplan LR, editors. Brainstem disorders. Berlin: Springer; 2011. pp. 105–138.
24. Morrow MJ, Sharpe JA. Torsional nystagmus in the lateral medullary syndrome. Ann Neurol. 1988;24:396–398.
25. Amarenco P, Roullet E, Hommel M, et al. Infarction in the territory of the medial branch of the posterior inferior cerebellar artery. J Neurol Neurosurg Psychiatry. 1990;53 731–735.
26. Pierot-Desilligny C, Amarenco P, Roullet E, Marteau R. Vermal infarct with pursuit eye movement disorders. J Neurol Neurosurg Psychiatry. 1990;53:519–521.
27. Jeong H-S, Oh JY, Kim JS, et al. Periodic alternating nystagmus in isolated nodular infarction. Neurology.2007;68:956–957.
28. Oas JG, Baloh RW. Vertigo and the anterior inferior cerebellar artery syndrome.Neurol ogy.1992;42:2274–2279.
29. Gaynard B, Rivaud S, Amarenco P, Pierot-Desilligny C. Influence of visual information on cerebellar saccadic dysmetria. Ann Neurol. 1994;35:108–112.

24

TOXINS IN NEURO-OPHTHALMOLOGY

Varun K. Singh, Usha K. Misra

Introduction

Optic nerve, retina and macula are susceptible to a number of toxins which may be biological, chemicals (metals, drugs) or iatrogenic agents. With the development in medicine, science and industry, the number of toxins are increasing and toxic optic neuropathy are being recognized in greater numbers.

Toxic optic neuropathy may be associated and sometimes enhanced by comorbidities such as nutritional deficiency (B1, B6, B12, folic acid), other metabolic disorders like diabetes mellitus, renal and hepatic impairments. The associated disorders may coexist or aggravate the effect of toxin on the optic nerve.

The typical clinical features secondary to exposure to the toxic substances are bilateral vision loss, papillomacular bundle damage, central or cecocentral scotoma and reduction of color vision. The lesion can be localized to retina, chiasma, optic nerve or optic tracts. The toxic injuries are often multisystem and in the central nervous system (CNS) involve multiple fiber tracts. The systemic manifestations may include anemia, skin changes, live or kidney impairment, diarrhea, etc. Pain sensation, coordination (cerebellar and sensory ataxia) and encephalopathy may be associated in isolation or in various permutation and combination.

The clinical picture of toxic optic neuropathy and nutritional optic neuropathy are quite similar and cannot be differentiated by clinical evaluation. These are more common in developing countries because of greater exposure to toxin and prevalent malnutrition. In this chapter, common toxins affecting optic nerve will be presented, and retinal and macular toxicity will also be briefly described.

Mode of exposure

Toxic substances can enter body via different routes: inhalation, ingestion or through skin or mucus membrane absorption. The iatrogenic exposure to toxins is also possible through various routes.

Pathophysiology

The exact reason behind the susceptibility of optic nerve to various drugs is a debated topic. However, few studies have implicated mitochondrial dysfunction as the underlying mechanism. There will be incomplete oxidative phosphorylation in mitochondria and generation of reactive oxygen species (ROS), resulting in energy depletion, oxidative stress and activation of apoptosis by leakage of cytochrome c [1].

Retinal ganglion cells (RGCs) have greatest energy demands in body and higher rates of oxygen consumption [2, 3]. Even the prelaminar portion of optic nerve are metabolically more active than post-laminar portion with larger number of mitochondria, hence are more susceptible to mitochondrial dysfunction. Among the axons originating from RGCs, papillomacular bundle is more susceptible because of higher energy demands coupled with low energy production [1, 4]. Alcohol and tobacco intake are also associated with nutritional deficiency also which may contribute further to toxicity [5, 6].

Causes of toxic optic neuropathy

Heavy metals
Lead, mercury, thallium
Chemicals
Carbon mono-oxide, methanol, ethylene glycol (antifreeze)
Recreational drugs
Alcohol, tobacco, nitrous oxide

Iatrogenic

- *Antitubercular:* Isoniazid, ethambutol, streptomycin
- *Antibiotics:* Chloramphenicol, linezolid, dapsone
- *Antimalarials:* Hydroxychloroquine, chloroquine, quinine
- *Antiarrhythmic agents:* Digitalis, amiodarone
- *Anticancer agents:* Methotrexate, vincristine, cisplatin, carboplatin, raclitaxol, Lomustine (CCNU), Carmustine (BCNU)
- *Miscellaneous:* Cyclosporine, tacrolimus, αINF 2b

Clinical features

Toxic optic neuropathy present as bilateral, symmetrical painless, progressive visual loss. Change in color perception (dyschromatopsia) is often the first symptom among the many. Visual acuity disturbance may start with a blur at fixation point, i.e., relative scotoma followed by a progressive decline [7]. Examination usually shows normal light and accommodation reflex except in those who are blind. On fundoscopy, disc may appear normal, swollen or hyperemic in early stage, while in later stages, optic atrophy may ensue. Visual field testing usually reveals centrocecal scotoma.

The diagnosis of toxic optic neuropathy can be made if the following criteria are fulfilled:

- There should be a temporal relationship between toxin exposure and visual loss.
- Presence of dose–response relationship.
- Withdrawal of drug/toxin leads to improvement or halting of the progression of vision loss.
- Biological plausibility between exposure and optic nerve toxicity.
- Presence of evidence from any prior animal experiment.

Differential diagnosis

Ischemic optic neuropathy, hereditary optic neuropathy, nutritional deficiencies, inflammatory optic neuropathy and traumatic optic neuropathy are considered and are differentiated by detailed clinical evaluation and investigations. Some of the important causes of TON are briefly discussed in the following section.

Ethambutol toxicity

Ethambutol is a bacteriostatic antimicrobial agent and used as first-line anti-tuberculous therapy. It causes optic neuropathy in 1–5% of patients [8]. Its mechanism of action is chelating and disruption of one of the several metal-containing enzyme systems in the nucleic acid structures of mycobacteria. Toxic optic neuropathy involves the same mechanism.

DOI: 10.1201/9780429020278-35

The probability of optic nerve toxicity with 1 mg/kg of ethambutol is 1%, 25 mg/kg is 6% and 35 mg/kg is 18%. A dosage of 25 mg/kg is necessary for attainment of a cerebrospinal fluid (CSF) level half of that in serum. The dosage of 25 mg/kg/day for 2 months should be reduced to 15 mg/kg/day maintenance dose which is considered safe as well as effective [9]. The onset of visual symptoms starts between 2 and 8 months of initiation of drug. The recent change of guidelines suggests the prolonged usage of ethambutol up to 6 months in an alarming scenario, further predisposing an individual to ethambutol-mediated optic neuritis. Dyschromatopsia may be the earliest sign of toxicity with reduced blue-yellow color perception being the most common [8]. Visual acuity may be markedly reduced but is usually better than 20/100. There can be associated field defect like central scotomas, bitemporal field defects and peripheral field constriction [10]. Contrast sensitivity measurement has also been found effective in detecting subclinical toxicity [11]. Fundus is either normal or may show optic atrophy (Figure 24.1).

Optical coherence tomography (OCT) can detect the toxicity of ethambutol even before the changes apparent on fundus examination and has been used as an additional objective test to monitor patients on ethambutol [9]. High-risk patients are those who are older, have chronic kidney disease and taking high dose. The visual toxicity of ethambutol can be monitored by visual-evoked potentials (VEPs). In a study on 14 patients receiving ethambutol, Pattern shift visual-evoked potential (PSVEP) was abnormal in five patients; however, the symptoms were present in one patient only [12].

Discontinuation of the drug is the treatment. Recovery occurs in majority of the patients within 2 months of discontinuation of the ethambutol. Some researchers have attempted the use of high-dose vitamins including methylcobalamin and pyridoxine for patients developing ethambutol-mediated optic neuritis. Permanent loss of vision can occur if the drug is received between 6 months and 3 years. Isoniazid use has an additive effect to the ethambutol toxicity.

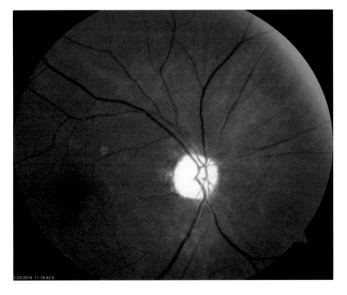

FIGURE 24.1 Fundus photograph of a 30-year-old tuberculous meningitis patient that developed optic atrophy after 6 months of ethambutol therapy.

Isoniazid toxicity

Isoniazid is one of the most important first-line antitubercular therapy. Its toxicity may be associated with bilateral optic disc swelling [13]. Bitemporal hemianopic scotomas on visual field testing is one of the peculiar feature of isoniazid toxicity. Improvement occurs with the cessation of isoniazid intake. Use of pyridoxine 25–100 mg/day may stabilize or even reverse isoniazid-induced toxic neuropathy.

Isoniazid and ethambutol are primary antitubercular drugs, and both can cause optic nerve toxicity. If stopping one does not lead to improvement in vision, then the other drug should also be stopped.

A baseline ophthalmologic examination is mandatory prior to starting ethambutol or isoniazid which includes fundus examination, color vision testing, contrast sensitivity and visual fields. A periodic ophthalmological evaluation in follow up will detect any optic nerve toxicity at its earliest.

Methanol

Methanol poisoning usually results from either accidental or suicidal ingestion of products containing methanol [14–17]. Cases are common in developing countries among poor socioeconomic classes. It is first metabolized by the enzyme alcohol dehydrogenase (ADH) in the liver, via formaldehyde to formic acid. The optic nerve toxicity develops from a combined effect of the metabolic acidosis and formate anion.

Clinical features of methanol intoxication include nausea, vomiting and abdominal pain. The CNS effects of methanol result from accumulation of formic acid within the optic nerve and leads to flashes of light. It progresses further to scotomas and scintillations. Vision loss is probably caused by interruption of mitochondrial function in the optic nerve which results in hyperemia, edema and optic nerve atrophy. Pupillary response to light is compromised and subsequently lost. Confirmation of diagnosis is by serum methanol level with gas chromatography (>20 mg/dL). Serum levels peak after 60–90 min of ingestion, but these do not correlate with the level of toxicity. Accumulation of formate leads to decrease in pH (<7.2 is a severe intoxication). Imaging findings may be suggestive with bilateral enhancing optic nerves and putaminal necrosis.

Treatment of methanol poisoning consists of supportive and specific therapy. Supportive therapy starts with airway management, correction of electrolytes and adequate hydration. Gastric lavage is beneficial within 2 h of ingestion of methanol. Metabolic acidosis needs correction with buffer like sodium bicarbonate. Hemodialysis can be done further to correct the acidosis and remove both methanol and formate. Antidote of methanol is ethanol which delays methanol metabolism to facilitate its elimination from the system by either naturally or by dialysis. Ethanol, like methanol, gets metabolized by ADH, and the enzyme has 10–20 times higher affinity for ethanol compared with methanol [18]. Fomepizole is also metabolized by the same enzyme, but it does not cause CNS depression like ethanol. But high cost and lack of availability act as limiting factor. Ethanol is commonly used and is given intravenously (IV) as a 10% solution in 5% dextrose. A loading dose of 0.6 g/kg is given followed by an IV infusion of 0.07–0.16 g/kg/h.

Linezolid

Linezolid belongs to the group of oxazolidinone antibiotics. Spectrum include activity against methicillin-resistant *Staphylococcus* species, penicillin resistant *Streptococcus* species and vancomycin-resistant enterococci. Recommended duration of therapy can be prolonged to 28 days. The probability of toxic optic neuropathy as well as peripheral neuropathy increase if treatment extends beyond a month. Mitochondrial dysfunction was postulated as the basis of toxicity. Discontinuation of drugs usually leads to vision improvement with residual deficit in central visual acuity.

Vigabatrin

It is used as antiepileptic in infantile spasm and refractory complex partial seizures. The optic neuropathy reported in 15–31% infants, 15% children and 25–30% adults [19]. Visual field defects start as bilateral nasal field defects and progress to concentric bilateral field constriction with preserved central vision. Time of onset of toxicity is age and duration-dependent. In infants, it takes 3 month, in children 11 months and in adults 9 months to appear. So visual field monitoring is recommended at baseline and at 3-month intervals in infants and 6-month intervals in adults. If the cumulative dosage is more than 3 kg, visual field needs to be checked up more frequently [20]. Treatment of vigabatrin toxicity is to stop the drug and substitute it with other antiepileptic. Vigabatrin-induced optic neuropathy was also linked to a taurine deficiency responsible for its retinal phototoxicity. It was proposed that patients taking vigabatrin could gain immediate benefit from reduced light exposures and intake of taurine-rich foods [21].

Vigabatrin produces peripheral field defect; therefore, VEP study may not be ideal for monitoring its toxicity. In one study, only 4 out of 10 patients with peripheral visual field constriction due to vigabatrin had delayed VEP [22]. The VEP prolongation is more marked if vigabatrin is combined with slow release valproate [23].

Ciprofloxacin

Ocular side effects are rare with ciprofloxacin. The incidence of blurring of vision, reduced visual acuity and color perception are reported in less than 1% cases [24]. Being aware of this uncommon side effect will be wise in the cases who receive high dose or longer course of treatment.

Deferoxamine

It is used in the treatment of hemochromatosis and also produces visual toxicity. Fundus examination is often normal; however, retinal pigment epithelium (RPE) mottling may develop later. The visual toxicity of deferoxamine can also be monitored by VEP [25].

Tropical and quinine amblyopia produce similar abnormalities [26, 27].

Dapsone

Two of the reported cases of dapsone-related optic neuropathy in literature are related to ischemic optic neuropathy in a case of dermatitis herpetiformis with type-2 diabetes mellitus and optic atrophy, respectively [28, 29].

Chloroquine

Toxicity includes keratopathy, ciliary body involvement, lens opacities and retinopathy. Retinopathy is the major concern although others are more common but benign. Risk factors of retinopathy include age, daily as well as cumulative dosage, treatment duration and coexisting retinal, renal or liver disease. Visual symptoms include decreased vision, missing central vision, glare, blurred vision, light flashes and metamorphopsia. Characteristic fundus finding is bull's-eye maculopathy. All patients have field defects including paracentral, pericentral, central and peripheral field loss. Color vision is impaired in the

advanced stage. Regular screening may be necessary to detect reversible premaculopathy. Cessation of the drug is the only effective management of the toxicity.

Amiodarone

It is a class III antiarrhythmic agent, and ocular side effects are reported in literature [30–32]. Two-thirds of cases develop reversible verticillate keratopathy. More than half patients develop blue-white anterior subcapsular cataract resulting in mild blue color vision defects. There can be slowly progressive binocular vision loss with prolonged disc swelling. Non-arteritic ischemic optic neuropathy (NAION) was also reported in patients taking amiodarone, although bilaterally [33]. Mean duration of treatment before development of vision disturbance was 9 months (1–84 months). Discontinuation of drug is the treatment after consulting cardiologist. Visual symptoms improve gradually over several months.

However, few studies failed to show an association between amiodarone therapy and vision loss [34]. Systemic cardiovascular risk factors like hypertension, diabetes mellitus, hyperlipidemia and ischemic heart disease predispose the patient to NAION rather than the amiodarone [35]. Despite all these controversies, treating physician should keep this side effect of amiodarone in his mind and ophthalmological assessment should be done at 6 monthly interval. Amiodarone results in increased latency and reduced P100 amplitude without clinical visual impairment [36].

Digitalis

Visual side effects of digitalis are less common than cardiac or other noncardiac symptoms. The spectrum of toxicity varies and includes decreased visual acuity, central scotomas or visual field reduction, photopsia most pronounced in daylight, photophobia, blurry or snowy vision, visual hallucinations, diplopia and dyschromatopsia including xanthopsia (yellow vision), cyanopsia (blue vision) and chloropsia (green vision). Dyschromatopsia can remain asymptomatic and detected only by formal testing. The mechanism of ocular toxicity postulated to be $Na^+ K^+$ ATPase inhibition [37–39]. Most appropriate test to support a diagnosis of digoxin ocular toxicity is photopic and scotopic electroretinogram (ERG) seeking for b-wave-delayed implicit time and decreased b-wave amplitude.

Phosphodiesterase type-5 (PDE-5) inhibitors

This group includes sildenafil, tadalafil and vardenafil, which are commonly used in the treatment of erectile dysfunction as well as pulmonary arterial hypertension (sildenafil). They act by increasing cyclic form of Guanosine Mono-Phosphate (cGMP) concentrations leading to systemic arterial smooth muscle relaxation and vasodilatation.

Commonly encountered visual problems were color vision defects in the blue-green to blue-purple range and increased sensitivity to light which were dose-dependent and reversible [40, 41].

Tobacco–alcohol amblyopia

It is characterized by a bilateral relative centrocecal field defect, more marked for a red or green target than white and a characteristic disturbance of color discrimination on the Farnsworth-Munsell 100 Hue Test [42]. The cause behind the vision disturbance is thought to be nutrition depletion secondary to smoking. In genetically, susceptible patients might affect sulfur metabolism, leading to chronic cyanide intoxication and deficiency of vitamin B12 [43–45].

So a diagnosis of toxic optic neuropathy should be made after exclusion of nutritional optic neuropathy, other toxic optic

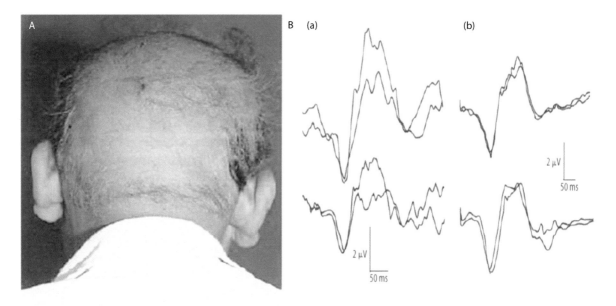

FIGURE 24.2 (A) A patient with thallium poisoning developed alopecia on Day 30. (B) VEP study of right eye showed prolonged P100 latency (126 ms) both at the 3-month (a) and 3-year follow-up (b) correlating with lack of clinical improvement in vision.

neuropathies and congenital optic neuropathies, mainly Leber Hereditary Optic Neuropathy (LHON). Treatment is tobacco abstinence and vitamin supplementation especially B1, B12 and folate. Vision may take 3–12 months for recovery.

Thallium

Thallium is highly reactive heavy metal and exists in monovalent and trivalent ionic forms. It is used in rodenticides, for optical lenses, in green colored fireworks, semiconductors, low temperature thermometers and in imitation jewelry. Soluble thallium salts such as sulfate, acetate and carbonate are highly toxic, and their fatal dose is 10–15 mg/kg. The clinical feature of thallium poisoning comprises skin manifestations, alopecia, neuropathy and other systemic manifestations (Figure 24.2A). The typical clinical picture manifests by 2–3 weeks of acute poisoning. In one study, up to 25% of patients with severe thallium poisoning have been reported to develop optic neuropathy. Early ocular involvement can be detected by visual-evoked potential testing (Figure 24.2B) [46, 47].

Chemotherapy drugs

Although advances in the field of oncology is a boon to cancer patients, the spectrum of toxicity of the chemotherapeutic agents is also worrisome. Ocular toxic effects related to the use of cytarabine include corneal epithelial toxicity and hemorrhagic conjunctivitis [48]. Methotrexate has also been noted to cause macular edema [49]. Daunorubicin inhibits proliferative vitreoretinopathy changes after surgery for retinal detachment and glaucoma filtering surgeries due to its antifibroblast action [50–52]. However, it can cause retinal toxicity with high intraocular doses. Cisplatin has been reported to cause delayed optic neuritis. Etoposide causes central retinal artery occlusion secondary to thrombosis when given intra-arterially. It exerts synergistic effect with cisplatin and causes retinal toxicities. Bleomycin causes cortical blindness with concurrent usage with cisplatin.

Nitrous oxide

Nitrous oxide is an anesthetic agent and is popular as a recreational drug due to its euphoric properties and availability as a so-called "legal high." It is usually inhaled from balloons filled from "whippits" (small, pressurized canisters of N_2O used in whipped cream dispensers). It irreversibly binds, oxidizes, inactivates and depletes vitamin B12. B12 inactivation further leads to depletion of methionine and accumulation of homocysteine as it is an essential cofactor for methionine synthase. Neurologically, B12 depletion results in demyelination leading to myelopathy, neuropathy, myeloneuropathy, cognitive changes and optic nerve toxicity. Ocular symptoms will be similar to B12 deficiency due to other causes. The visual loss is symmetric, painless and progressive. Central and centrocecal scotomas are the rule, and the optic disc will be normal in the early stages of the condition. Vision recovered usually with intramuscular injections of hydroxocobalamin unless optic atrophy becomes well established.

To understand the mechanism of vitamin B12 deficiency-associated neurological dysfunction, an animal model of cobalamin deficiency by controlled nitrous oxide exposure (1:1 N_2O and oxygen mixture) was developed. Nitrous oxide gas was administered for 90 min daily for 1 month. There was impaired motor functions (time resting, time moving, distance traveled), focal myelin loss in subcortical white matter and spinal cord and optic nerve and reduced total anti-oxidant capacity and glutathione [53]. The mechanism underlying demyelination is due to increase in tumor necrosis factor-α (TNF-α) and interleukin 6 (IL-6) and reduction of epidermal growth factor (EGF) [54]. In a study on 17 patients with vitamin B12 deficiency neurologic syndrome, P100 latency was prolonged in 17 eyes (ten patients). These patients had no visual symptom, and vision testing was normal. Six months following treatment, P100 latency improved to normal in all except four eyes. The VEP changes were related to duration of illness and antiparietal cell antibodies [52, 55].

Retinal toxicity

A variety of pharmacologic drugs can cause retinal toxicity. The toxicity can be categorized into pigmentary retinopathy, choroidal toxicity, macular edema and crystalline retinopathy. Symptoms of retinopathy includes decreased visual acuity and color vision, photopsia, field defects and metamorphopsia.

Pigmentary retinopathy
Chloroquine and hydroxychloroquine
These are antimalarial agents now used in the treatment of autoimmune diseases. It is usually noted in patient taking >3 mg/kg/day of chloroquine or >6.5 mg/kg/day of hydroxychloroquine. They bind melanin and concentrate in the iris, ciliary body and RPE altering normal physiologic function. Symptoms are blurred vision, decreased vision, scotomas and photopsias. On examination, there is blunting of the foveal reflex and pigmentary retinal changes. Classic fundus pattern is bilateral bull's-eye. Optic disc pallor and arteriovenous narrowing are late stage findings.

Thioridazine
Thioridazine is an antipsychotic agent. Use can result in decreased vision and dyschromatopsia. On clinical exam, macular pigmentary changes can develop into a "salt-and-pepper" pattern.

Choroidal toxicity

Topiramate
Topiramate, an oral anticonvulsant, is used for the treatment of seizures, prophylaxis for migraine, as well as off-label in the treatment of bipolar disorder. Ocular toxicity will lead to blurred vision, eye pain and headache. Examination shows diffuse corneal edema, shallowing of the anterior chamber and significantly raised intraocular pressure (IOP) with retinal striae. Uveal effusion or ciliary edema leads to forward displacement of the lens–iris diaphragm and thickening of the lens by relaxation of zonules. This lead to anterior chamber shallowing and induced myopia, while retinal striae are caused by vitreoretinal traction. While many of the changes are reversible with prompt cessation of the drug, cycloplegic agents are often used to reverse the anterior displacement of the lens–iris diaphragm.

Metronidazole
Metronidazole is a nitroimidazole sulfa agent used to treat anaerobic and protozoal infections. It, along with sulfa analogs such as sulfanilamide, acetazolamide and hydrochlorothiazide, causes induced bilateral myopia and anterior chamber shallowing from ciliochoroidal swelling.

Macular edema

Organophosphate
In a study on 69 spray men exposed to organophosphate and copper acetoarsenite, macular degeneration was noted in 15 out of 79 (22%) subjects (3% in controls) and was characterized by 1/6 to 1/3 disc diameter depigmented lesions in fovea, which were bilateral in 5 (Figure 24.3). Fluorescein angiography reveals focal area for pigment epithelium defect [56, 57]. These results were confirmed in an experimental study using fenthion exposure in rats [58].

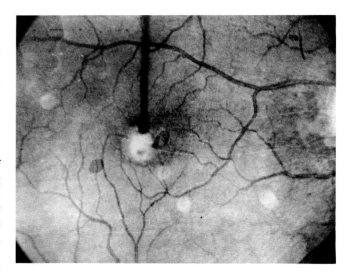

FIGURE 24.3 Fundus photograph of right eye of a pesticide worker showing macular involvement.

Latanoprost
It is a prostaglandin analog used to lower IOP by increasing uveoscleral outflow. Ocular side effects include conjunctival hyperemia, darkening of eyelashes and iris heterochromia and reversible cystoid macular edema.

Epinephrine
It acts to lower IOP by decreasing aqueous production but has been shown to induce cystoid macular edema in glaucomatous aphakic or pseudophakic patients.

Niacin
Niacin, or vitamin B3, may cause visual complaints including blurred vision, decreased vision and metamorphopsia due to development of macular edema. However, niacin-induced macular edema has the unique characteristic of being angiographically silent due to intracellular rather than extracellular fluid accumulation.

Rosiglitazone
It cause increase in retinal endothelial cell permeability and increase in vascular endothelial growth factor (VEGF) leading to intraretinal edema and blurred vision.

Crystalline retinopathy
Tamoxifen
Tamoxifen is a selective estrogen receptor modulator used in the management of breast cancer. Ocular symptoms have been noted most often with doses greater than 120 mg twice per day which is higher than therapeutic doses. Fundus evaluation demonstrates refractile intraretinal crystalline deposits concentrated primarily in the perifoveal macula.

Canthaxanthine
It is a vitamin A derivative used in the treatment of psoriasis and eczema. An oral therapy of greater than 0.5 mg/kg/day results in toxicity. On fundus exam, a doughnut-shaped ring of golden intraretinal deposits surrounds the fovea. OCT demonstrates crystalline deposition within the inner retinal layers. Fourier analysis (FA) and ERG are typically normal.

Talc

Talc retinopathy indicates a history of IV drug abuse. It deposits in the macular arterial vasculature, causing a granulomatous reaction with focal occlusion, leading to ischemia. Fundoscopy reveal refractile yellow opacities in the macula.

Conclusion

The causes of toxic optic neuropathy extend from daily use antibiotics to toxic chemicals and exposure to them are common especially in developing countries. The individual susceptibilities however vary. The potential risk of TON should be kept in the mind while treating patients with these medications. The visual functions should also be closely monitored.

Acknowledgment

We thank to Mr. Shakti Kumar for secretarial help.

Multiple-Choice Questions

1. The typical finding associated with toxic optic neuropathy is:
   a. Altitudinal field defect
   b. Unilateral visual loss
   c. Dyschromatopsia
   d. Associate chemical uveitis/conjunctivitis

   Answer:
   c. Dyschromatopsia

2. Which of the following is true about the probability of developing ethambutol-associated optic neuropathy?
   a. 10% with ethambutol 1 mg/kg/day
   b. 10% with ethambutol 15 mg/kg/day
   c. 18% with ethambutol 25 mg/kg/day
   d. 18% with ethambutol 35 mg/kg/day

   Answer:
   d. 18% with ethambutol 35 mg/kg/day

3. Dyschromatopsia is one of the early presentations with ethambutol-associated optic neuropathy. Which color perception is most affected?
   a. Red-green
   b. Blue-yellow
   c. Red-blue
   d. Blue-green

   Answer:
   b. Blue-yellow

4. Which of the following statements is TRUE about optic neuropathy due to methanol intoxication?
   a. Serum levels of methanol peak after 10–15 min of ingestion.
   b. The serum levels of methanol correlate with the level of toxicity.
   c. Gastric lavage is beneficial within 2 h of ingestion of methanol.
   d. Fomepizole used for treatment causes excessive CNS depression.

   Answer:
   c. Gastric lavage is beneficial within 2 h of ingestion of methanol.

5. Which of the following statements is NOT true about toxic optic neuropathies?
   a. Chloroquine causes keratopathy, ciliary body involvement, lens opacities, and retinopathy.
   b. Vigabatrin produces central or centrocecal field defects.
   c. Amiodarone may cause reversible verticillate keratopathy and more than half patients develop blue-white anterior subcapsular cataract resulting in mild blue color vision defects.
   d. Tobacco–alcohol amblyopia leads on to centrocecal field defect, more marked for a red or green target.

   Answer:
   b. Vigabatrin produces central or centrocecal field defects.

References

1. Wang MY, Sadun AA. Drug-related mitochondrial optic neuropathies. J Neuroophthalmol. 2013;33(2):172–8.
2. You Y, Gupta VK, Li JC, Klistorner A, Graham SL. Optic neuropathies: Characteristic features and mechanisms of retinal ganglion cell loss. Rev Neurosci. 2013;24(3):301–21.
3. Yu DY, Cringle SJ. Oxygen distribution and consumption within the retina in vascularised and avascular retinas and in animal models of retinal disease. Prog Retin Eye Res. 2001;20:175–208.
4. Pan BX, Ross-Cisneros FN, Tozer KR, Sadun AA. Mitochondrial strain index: Mathematically modeling the susceptibility of optic nerve axons in Leber's hereditary optic neuropathy. Investig. Ophthalmol. Vis. Sci. 2012;53(14):4880.
5. Danesh-Meyer H, Kubis KC, Wolf MA. Chiasmopathy? Surv Ophthalmol. 2000; 44(4):329–35.
6. Dunphy EB. Alcohol and tobacco amblyopia: A historical survey. XXXI DeSchweinitz Lecture. Am J Ophthalmol. 1969;68(4):569–78.
7. Kerrison JB. Optic neuropathies caused by toxins and adverse drug reactions. Ophthalmol Clin North Am. 2004;17(3):481–8.
8. Polak BC, Leys M, Van Lith GH. Blue-yellow colour vision changes as early symptoms of ethambutol oculotoxicity. Ophthalmologica. 1985;191(4):223–6.
9. Chai SJ, Foroozan R. Decreased retinal nerve fibre layer thickness detected by optical coherence tomography in patients with ethambutol-induced optic neuropathy. Br J Ophthalmol. 2007;91(7):895–7.
10. Phillips PH. Toxic and deficiency optic neuropathies. In: Miller NR, Newman NJ, Biousse V, et al., ediros. Walsh and Hoyt's Clinical Neuro-Ophthalmology. Baltimore: Lippincott Williams & Wilkin; 2005. pp. 447–63.
11. Salmon JF, Carmichael TR, Welsh NH. Use of contrast sensitivity measurement in the detection of subclinical ethambutol toxic optic neuropathy. Br J Ophthalmol. 1987;71(3):192–6.
12. Yiannikas C, Walsh JC. The variation of the pattern shift visual evoked response with the size of stimulus field. Electroencephalogr Clin Neurophysiol. 1983;55:424.
13. Van Stavern GP, Newman NJ. Optic neuropathies. An overview. Ophthalmol Clin North Am. 2001;14(1):61–71.
14. Bennett L Jr, Cary FH, Mitchell GL, et al. Acute methyl alcohol poisoning: A review based on experiences in an outbreak of 323 cases. Medicine. 1953;32:431–63.
15 Kane RL, Talbert W, Harlan J. A methanol poisoning outbreak in Kentucky: A clinical epidemiologic study. Arch Environ Health: An International Journal. 1968;17(1):119–29.
16. Naraqi S, Dethlefs RF, Slobodniuk RA, Sairere JS. An outbreak of acute methyl alcohol intoxication. Aust N Z J Med. 1979;9(1):65–8.
17. Swartz RD, Millman RP, Billi JE, Bondar NP, Migdal SD, Simonian SK, Monforte JR, Mcdonald FD, Harness JK, Cole KL. Epidemic methanol poisoning: Clinical and biochemical analysis of a recent episode. Medicine. 1981;60(5):373–82.
18. Beauchamp GA, Valento M, Kim J. Toxic alcohol ingestion: Prompt recognition and management in the emergency department [digest]. Emerg Med Pract. 2016;18(9):S1–S2.
19 Kedar S, Ghate D, Corbett JJ. Visual fields in neuro-ophthalmology. Indian J Ophthalmol. 2011;59(2):103.
20. Viestenz A, Mardin CY. Vigabatrin-associated bilateral simple optic nerve atrophy with visual field constriction. A case report and a survey of the literature. Der Ophthalmologe. 2003;100(5):402–5.

21. Jammoul F, Wang Q, Nabbout R, Coriat C, Duboc A, Simonutti M, Dubus E, Craft CM, Ye W, Collins SD, Dulac O. Taurine deficiency is a cause of vigabatrin-induced retinal phototoxicity. Ann Neurol. 2009;65(1):98–107.

22. Daneshvar H, Racette L, Coupland SG, Kertes PJ, Guberman A, Zackon D. Symptomatic and asymptomatic visual loss in patients taking vigabatrin. Ophthalmology. 1999;106(9):1792–8.

23. Zgorzalewicz M, Galas-Zgorzalewicz B. Visual and auditory evoked potentials during long-term vigabatrin treatment in children and adolescents with epilepsy. Clin Neurophysiol. 2000;111(12):2150–4.

24. Samarakoon N, Harrisberg B, Ell J. Ciprofloxacin-induced toxic optic neuropathy. Clin Exp Ophthalmol. 2007;35(1):102–4.

25. Taylor MJ, Keenan NK, Gallant T, Skarf B, Freedman MH, Logan WJ. Subclinical VEP abnormalities in patients on chronic deferoxamine therapy: Longitudinal studies. Electroencephalogr Clin Neurophysiol/Evoked Potentials Section. 1987;68(2):81–7.

26. Asselman P, Chadwick DW, Marsden DC. Visual evoked responses in the diagnosis and management of patients suspected of multiple sclerosis. Brain: A Journal of Neurology. 1975;98(2):261–82.

27. Gangitano JL, Keltner JL. Abnormalities of the pupil and visual-evoked potential in quinine amblyopia. Am J Ophthalmol. 1980;89(3):425–30.

28. Chalioulias K, Mayer E, Darvay A, Antcliff R. Anterior ischaemic optic neuropathy associated with Dapson. Eye (Lond). 2006;20(8):943–5.

29. Homeida M, Babikr A, Daneshmend TK. Dapsone-induced optic atrophy and motor neuropathy. Br Med J. 1980;281(6249):1180.

30. Gittinger JW, Asdourian GK. Papillopathy caused by amiodarone. Arch Ophthalmol. 1987;105(3):349–51.

31. Johnson LN, Krohel GB, Thomas ER. The clinical spectrum of amiodarone-associated optic neuropathy. J Natl Med Assoc. 2004;96(11):1477.

32. Palimar P, Cota N. Bilateral anterior ischaemic optic neuropathy following amiodarone. Eye. 1998;12(5):894–6.

33. Passman RS, Bennett CL, Purpura JM, Kapur R, Johnson LN, Raisch DW, West DP, Edwards BJ, Belknap SM, Liebling DB, Fisher MJ. Amiodarone-associated optic neuropathy: A critical review. Am J Med. 2012;125(5):447–53.

34. Mindel JS, Anderson J, Johnson G, Hellkamp A, Poole JE, Mark DB, Lee KL, Bardy GH, SCD-HeFT Investigators. Absence of bilateral vision loss from amiodarone: A randomized trial. Am Heart J. 2007;153(5):837–42.

35. Hayreh SS. Pathogenesis of some controversial non-arteritic anterior ischemic optic neuropathy clinical entities. In: Ischemic optic neuropathies. Berlin, Heidelberg: Springer; 2011. https://doi.org/10.1007/978-3-642-11852-4_15.

36. Domingues MF, Barros H, Falcão-Reis FM. Amiodarone and optic neuropathy. Acta Ophthalmologica Scandinavica. 2004;82(3p1):277–82.

37. Aronson JK. An account of foxglove and its medical uses 1785–1985. Oxford: Oxford University press; 1985. https://global.oup.com/academic/product/an-account-of-the-foxglove-and-its-medical-uses-1785-1985-9780192615015?cc=in&lang=en&#

38. Closson RG. Visual hallucinations as the earliest symptom of digoxin intoxication. Arch Neurol. 1983;40(6):386.

39. Lawrenson JG, Kelly C, Lawrenson AL, Birch J. Acquired colour vision deficiency in patients receiving digoxin maintenance therapy. Br J Ophthalmol. 2002;86(11):1259–61.

40 Kerr NM, Danesh-Meyer HV. Phosphodiesterase inhibitors and the eye. Clin Exp Ophthalmol. 2009;37(5):514–23.

41. Foulds WS, Chisholm IA, Pettigrew AR. The toxic optic neuropathies. Br J Ophthalmol. 1974;58(4):386.

42. Foulds WS, Chisholm IA, Pettigrew AR. The toxic optic neuropathies. Br J Ophthalmol. 1974;58(4):386.

43. Freeman AG. Optic neuropathy and chronic cyanide intoxication: A review. J R Soc Med. 1988;81(2):103–6.

44. Heaton JM, McCormick AJ, Freeman AG. Tobacco amblyopia: A clinical manifestation of vitamin-B12 deficiency. Lancet. 1958;2:286–90.

45. Wokes F, Moore DF. Tobacco amblyopia. The Lancet. 1958;272(7045):526–7.

46. Bohringer HR. Thallium poisoning. Toxicology. 1980;17:133–46.

47. Misra UK, Kalita J, Yadav RK, Ranjan P. Thallium poisoning: Emphasis on early diagnosis and response to haemodialysis. Postgrad Med J. 2003;79(928):103–5.

48. Schmid KE, Kornek GV, Scheithauer W, Binder S. "Update on ocular complications of systemic cancer chemotherapy. Surv Ophthalmol. 2006;51(1):19–40.

49. Millay RH, Klein ML, Shults WT, Dahlborg SA, Neuwelt EA. Maculopathy associated with combination chemotherapy and osmotic opening of the blood-brain barrier. Am J Ophthalmol. 1986;102(5):626–632. doi: 10.1016/0002-9394(86)90536-2.

50. Chhablani J, Nieto A, Hou H, Wu EC, Freeman WR, Sailor MJ, Cheng L. Oxidized porous silicon particles covalently grafted with daunorubicin as a sustained intraocular drug delivery system. Invest Ophthalmol Vis Sci. 2013;54(2):1268–79.

51. Kumar A, Nainiwal S, Choudhary I, Tewari HK, Verma LK. Role of daunorubicin in inhibiting proliferative vitreoretinopathy after retinal detachment surgery. Clin Exp Ophthalmol. 2002;30(5):348–51.

52. Varma D, Sihota R, Agarwal HC. Evaluation of efficacy and safety of daunorubicin in glaucoma filtering surgery. Eye (Lond). 2007;21(6):784–8.

53. Singh SK, Misra UK, Kalita J, Bora HK, Murthy RC. Nitrous oxide related behavioral and histopathological changes may be related to oxidative stress. Neurotoxicology. 2015;48:44–9.

54. Scalabrino G. Cobalamin (vitamin B(12)) in sub-acute combined degeneration and beyond: Traditional interpretations and novel theories. Exp Neurol. 2005;192(2):463–79.

55. Pandey S, Kalita J, Misra UK. A sequential study of visual evoked potential in patients with vitamin B12 deficiency neurological syndrome. Clin Neurophysiol 2004; 115:914–8.

56. Misra UK, Nag D, Misra NK, Krishna MC. Macular degeneration associated with chronic pesticide exposure. Lancet. 1982;1(8266):288.

57. Misra UK, Nag D, Misra NK, Mehra MK, Ray PK. Some observations on the macula of pesticide workers. Hum. Toxicol. 1985;4(2):135–45.

58. Imai H, Miyata M, Uga S, Ishikawa S. Retinal degeneration in rats exposed to an organophosphate pesticide (fenthion). Environ Res. 1983;30(2):453–65.

25

NEUROPATHOLOGY OF NEURO-OPHTHALMIC DISORDERS

Bishan Radotra

Introduction

The optic nerve and retina are extensions of the nervous system. Therefore, diseases affecting the brain may be reflected in the eyes or orbit. Conversely, some primary ophthalmic pathological conditions may initiate and produce changes in the brain; however, very limited data are available about it. The obvious reason for the lack of such data is that ocular examination is not routinely performed at autopsy. Only a few centers remove eyes as a part of central nervous system (CNS) autopsy; furthermore, in most institutions it is not practiced due to lack of awareness or even due to religious beliefs, etc. Many immune-mediated syndromes, infective diseases and tumors extend from intraocular compartment to intracranial compartment. For example, intraorbital fungal infections may extend from anterior cranial fossa. Multiple sclerosis (MS) is another example where optic chiasm/nerves are affected besides demonstrating classical periventricular white matter demyelination. The examination of ocular structures with respect to eye movements, vision and fundoscopy is part of clinical routine CNS examination. Therefore, neurologists must be familiar with neuro-ophthalmic pathology. This chapter reflects the spectrum of pathology in which a neurologist is required to understand. Any orbital pathology is likely to compress the optic nerve or the eyeball or both, and it is essential for a neurologist to appreciate these facts.

For convenience, these pathological lesions are separated into non-neoplastic and neoplastic categories.

Non-neoplastic

Giant cell arteritis

Giant cell arteritis (or temporal arteritis) is a chronic disorder, which is commonly encountered both by neurologists and ophthalmologists in their clinics. It is a disease of elderly individuals and affects large- and medium-sized arteries of the head and neck region. The superficial temporal and ophthalmic arteries are commonly affected; however, intracranial arteries are spared. The clinical manifestations of this disease are throbbing headache, jaw claudication and temporal artery tenderness besides visual symptoms which include anterior ischemic optic neuropathy, diplopia, ophthalmoplegia, retinal injury and blindness. Some patients may present with systemic symptoms such as fever, weight loss and fatigue. Biopsy is a gold standard for diagnosis; however, a negative biopsy does not rule out the disease because the disease is focal and segmental. The reasons for a negative biopsy are that either pathologist has not sampled through affected area or excised artery does not represent site of lesion. In such a scenario, serial sections must be obtained by the pathologists, and many a times some evidence of arteritis is ascertained. If serial sections are not examined by the pathologist at the time of evaluation, then the clinician should demand for it and it increased the yield for a diagnosis. Histologically, the typical granulomatous inflammation with giant cells is not commonly observed. The histology largely depends on the activity of the disease. In active stage, intimal and medial mixed inflammation consisting of lymphocytes, histiocytes and neutrophils is seen. There may be transmural inflammation associated with thickened wall and narrowed lumen (Figure 25.1). The inflamed artery will produce tenderness on palpation. The older lesions may only reveal sparse lymphocytes and intimal/medial fibrosis indicating previous episodes of inflammation. The internal elastic lamina is characteristically fragmented (Figure 25.2a and b), which can be highlighted by elastic Van Gieson's stain (Figure 25.2c). The fibrosis can be highlighted by Masson's trichrome stain. Immunohistochemistry using antibody against spinal muscular atrophy (SMA) may be used to observe loss of muscle fibers in media. Weakening of the arterial wall due to fragmentation of elastica and replacement of smooth muscle layer by fibrous tissue leads to aneurysmal dilatation of the artery. As a result of this chronic inflammatory pathology, the temporal artery becomes thickened and tortuous, which is clinically noticeable. It is worth remembering that the presence of multinucleated giant cells is not necessary for diagnosis even when the name of disease denotes it. A large segment of the artery and particularly thickened segment should be submitted for biopsy.

Progressive external ophthalmoplegia

Progressive external ophthalmoplegia (PEO) is one of the manifestations of mitochondrial disorders that affect skeletal muscle. It is also referred to as the mitochondrial myopathy. PEO is clinically characterized by external ophthalmoplegia and progressive bilateral ptosis. The other systemic symptoms are proximal muscle weakness, sensorineural hearing loss, ataxia and progressive dysphagia.[1,2]

Chronic progressive external ophthalmoplegia (CPEO) develops in mid-adulthood. When CPEO is accompanied by other symptoms of mitochondrial dysfunction, the term CPEO plus syndrome is used.[3] PEO has also been documented in about 10–15% cases of mitochondrial encephalomyopathy, lactic acidosis and stroke-like episodes (MELAS).

Clinically, ocular or generalized myasthenia gravis can resemble PEO, but the former exhibits prominent diurnal fluctuations and has acute or subacute presentation, whereas PEO manifests as progressive disease, and very rarely, it has acute presentation.[3] More than 50%cases of CPEO occur as the result of single large-scale heteroplasmic mitochondrial DNA (mtDNA) deletions, ranging in length from 1.3 to 9.1 kb.[1] The familial cases of CPEO may either be inherited maternally (mitochondrial) or these may be autosomal recessive or autosomal dominant. Nuclear genes most frequently associated with hereditary CPEO include POLG, TWNK (C10orf2), SLC25A4, RRM2B, POLG2 and SPG7.[1]

Whenever CPEO is clinically suspected, muscle biopsy is performed to confirm the diagnosis. A combination of routine hematoxylin and eosin (H&E) stain along with histochemical stains can diagnose about three-fourths of the cases, while the remaining 25% require DNA analysis.[2,3] mtDNA proliferation

DOI: 10.1201/9780429020278-36

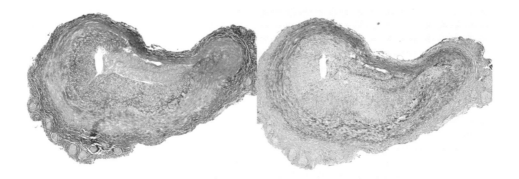

FIGURE 25.1 (a) The temporal artery shows transmural inflammation and thickening of the wall (H&E). (b) Fibrotic wall and narrowed lumen (Masson's trichrome).

occurs in response to the mtDNA point mutations which is seen as accumulation of mitochondria in subsarcolemmal location. In routine H&E stain, the accumulated subsarcolemmal mitochondria are demonstrated as basophilic material (Figure 25.3a). On modified Gomori trichrome stain, they are highlighted as red granular materials and such myofibers are typically called as ragged red fibers (RRFs) (Figure 25.3b). Succinate dehydrogenase (SDH) is encoded entirely by the nuclear DNA, and hence it is often overexpressed in mitochondrial myopathies. On SDH histochemical stain, the involved myocytes are seen as ragged blue fibers (RBFs).[3] Such myofibers often lack staining for cytochrome oxidase (COX-deficient fibers). The combined staining for COX-SDH can help in identification of COX deficient fibers, which

stand out prominently as ragged blue in appearance against the background of COX-positive yellow fibers. Therefore, combined[3] occasionally, mtDNA depletion may be observed in cases of mitochondrial myopathies, especially in those cases that result due to autosomal recessive mutations. Such cases do not show mtDNA accumulations and hence lack RRF and RBF. The identification of COX deficient fibers can help in clinching the diagnosis in such cases.[3]

It is important to remember that RRF, RBF and COX deficient fibers can occur in aging muscles and secondary to some other myopathies. Hence, cutoffs of >5% RRF at any age, >2% COX deficient fibers in <50 years and >5% COX deficient fibers in >50 years may be used to label these changes as abnormal.[3]

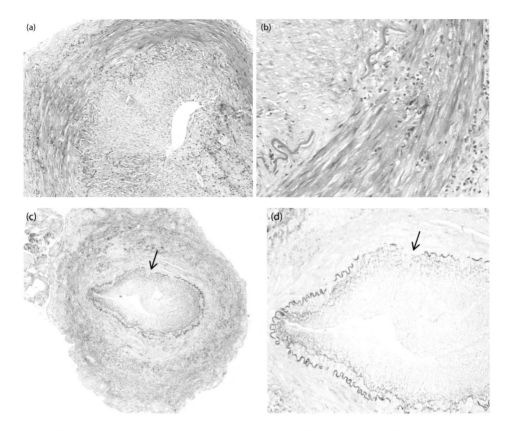

FIGURE 25.2 (a and b) The internal elastic lamina is fragmented and the arterial wall is inflamed (higher magnification). (c and d) The fragmentation of the elastic lamina is confirmed by elastic Van Gieson's stain (arrows).

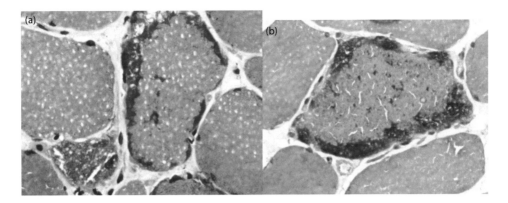

FIGURE 25.3 (a) Subsarcolemmal accumulation of basophilic material in a muscle biopsy (H&E). (b) Red-ragged fibers on modified Gomori trichrome stain (GMT).

Ultrastructural examination can show abnormal mitochondria, including variable size and shape, paracrystalline inclusions (parking lot inclusions) and abnormal swollen cristae (Figure 25.4). The findings of electron microscopy need correlation with light microscopy and clinical features, biochemical mitochondrial assays and genetic testing before a confirmed diagnosis of mitochondrial myopathy is made.[4] For mtDNA analysis, muscle biopsy serves as an appropriate sample since the amount of abnormal mtDNA is highest in muscle tissue as compared to tissue fibroblasts or white blood cells.

The treatment of visually obstructive ptosis requires surgery, especially in cases when the superior visual field is obstructed within 30 degrees of central fixation. The superior eyelid may be tethered to the frontalis muscle using a sling, in cases where considerable visual impairment is present due to severe levator palpebrae superioris involvement.[3]

IgG4-related disease

IgG4-related disease (IgG4RD) is relatively recently described immune-mediated disease of unknown cause. It is a systemic fibro-inflammatory disease, characterized by systemic as well as local increase of IgG4 positive plasma cells in affected tissues. It chiefly involves various visceral organs of body; however, cranial and spinal meninges can also be involved.[5] Therefore, IgG4RD shows wide spectrum of clinical presentations. Orbital IgG4RD is rare and manifests as lid swelling and proptosis or sometimes as apical orbital lesion. IgG4RD may involve orbit in isolation or a part of systemic involvement.[6,7] Most of the orbital IgG4RD were

previously diagnosed as orbital pseudotumor. Histologically, IgG4RD is characterized by storiform fibrosis, obliterative phlebitis and infiltration by IgG4 positive plasma cells (>40/high power field) (Figure 25.5a–c) with or without eosinophils. Serum IgG4 level is usually increased. Given the systemic implication of the disease, patients having orbital IgG4RD should be screened for the involvement of other systems, including pituitary, thyroid, salivary glands, pancreas and bile ducts.

Sarcoidosis

Sarcoidosis is a systemic granulomatous disease of unknown etiology. The organs primarily involved in this disease are lungs and hilar lymph nodes, but any organ or system may be affected. The ophthalmic involvement by sarcoidosis may occur as part of neuro-sarcoidosis,[8] although isolated orbital sarcoidosis has been rarely reported. Any structure within and around the eye can be involved independently.[9–11] The neuro-sarcoidosis mainly presents as cranial neuropathy and involvement of basal meninges, and hypothalamus may also be noted. Uncommon manifestation of neurosarcoidosis such as a combination of cranial and extracranial structures are described in some patients.[12] The optic neuropathy is seen in the form of optic nerve swelling, disc edema or optic atrophy. Additionally, posterior uveitis and periphlebitis are noticed in sarcoid optic neuropathy. Histologically, sarcoidosis shows well-formed epithelioid cell granulomas without significant lymphoid cuffing. The granulomas are discrete and devoid of caseation necrosis (Figure 25.6). The granulomas are associated with both Langhan's and foreign body type giant cells. The

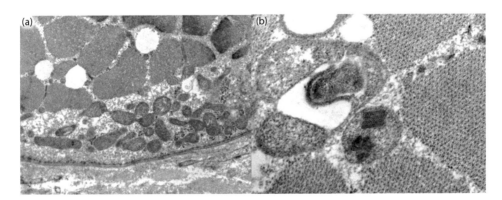

FIGURE 25.4 (a and b) Transmission electron micrograph shows subsarcolemmal accumulation of numerous abnormal mitochondria in a muscle biopsy (H&E). (b) Parking lot inclusions.

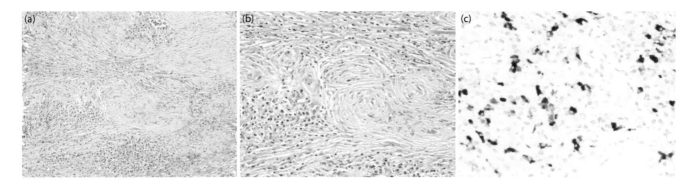

FIGURE 25.5   (a and b) The orbital tissue reveals fibrosis and extensive infiltration by inflammatory cells containing large number of plasma cells and few eosinophils. (c) IHC shows the increased number of IgG4-positive plasma cells.

asteroid and Schaumann bodies may be present in giant cells but are not characteristic for diagnosis. It is essential to exclude any infective pathology particularly tuberculous (TB)/fungal granuloma, especially in cases with isolated orbital sarcoidosis.

Optic neuritis

Optic neuritis (ON) is defined as the inflammation and swelling of the optic nerve. It is a common disease and affects individuals between 15 and 45 years of life, more so the females. It is classified according to etiology of neuritis such as autoimmunity, demyelination, infection or collagen vascular diseases.[13] It may also be classified according to the anatomical location of lesions in the optic pathway such as optic papillitis or retrobulbar neuritis. Rapid diagnosis of etiology of ON is of utmost importance because precise treatment, prevention of organ damage and prognosis depends on etiology. The accurate diagnosis requires considerable evaluation including neuroimaging and CSF examination.

The common manifestations of ON consist of acute, painful, unilateral, temporary loss of vision and flashing of lights. Bilateral, painless and severe loss of vision is uncommon. A patient with unilateral involvement typically reveals relative afferent pupillary defect which is due to difference in conduction between the affected and unaffected optic nerves.

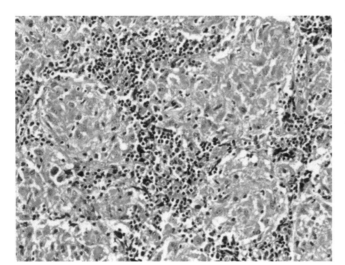

FIGURE 25.6   Naked granulomas consisting of epithelioid cells without much lymphoid cuffing in a case of sarcoidosis.

Generally, the ON is associated with MS, neuromyelitis optica (NMO) spectrum disorder and myelin oligodendrocyte glycoprotein autoantibodies (MOG-IgG) disorder. The ON is seen approximately in 70% cases of MS, and it is the presenting symptom in 25% cases.[13] Patches of chronic demyelination develop in this condition anywhere in the optic pathway. The ON in NMO may occur either alone or it may be accompanied by transverse myelitis. The myelitis may occur within 1–2 weeks to 6 months. Approximately 80% of the affected patients are seropositive for AQP4-IgG.[14] Non-whites (Asians) and women are more frequently affected by this disease compared to white population. A high risk of recurrence has been seen in this condition, and the prognosis of visual recovery is generally poor. The ON associated with MOG-IgG commonly presents as acute disseminated encephalomyelitis (ADEM) or recurrent ON. It is generally severe, painful and associated with optic disc edema, but fortunately it is steroid responsive. The differential diagnosis of retrobulbar ON may mimic compressive optic neuropathy, paraneoplastic optic neuropathy, autoimmune optic neuropathy, etc., and therefore, these need to be excluded.

The gross neuropathological findings in early stages of ON reveal a swollen and congested optic nerve. Much later, the optic nerve becomes thin, atrophic and gray-brown in color. Histologically, inflammation consists of neutrophils and perivascular T-lymphocytes which are replaced by numerous foamy macrophages within few days. The inflammation leads to demyelination, and myelin degradation products are engulfed by the macrophages. Presence of foamy macrophages in the demyelinating plaques is considered as a sign of active demyelination. Well-formed but poorly demarcated plaques are apparent in the affected optic nerve and/or optic chiasm which are highlighted by Luxol fast blue (LFB)/periodic acid Schiff (PAS) stain at this stage. The axonal component remains unaffected. With passage of time, the inflammatory process recedes, and the demyelinating plaques become sharply demarcated with no active inflammation. Such plaques are referred to as chronic plaques. The perivascular lymphocytes may still be seen in adjacent areas. The optic nerve becomes thin and atrophic. Hyaline fibrosis of the small vessels and perivascular deposition of collagen are indicative of previous episodes of inflammatory process.

A variety of viral, bacterial, parasitic and fungal infections have been reported to cause infectious ON leading to visual impairment.[15] The infection-related ON is generally a consequence of spread of infections from surrounding paranasal sinuses. The optic nerve may show necrosis and acute necrotizing inflammation (Figure 25.7a). Fungal infection such as zygomycosis involving

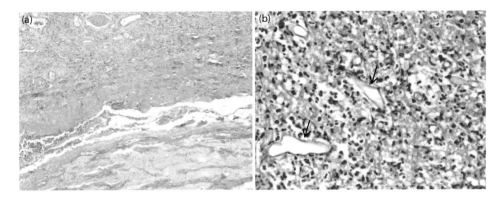

FIGURE 25.7 (a) Zygomycosis: Longitudinally cut optic surrounded by soft tissue showing inflammation and necrosis. (b) Higher power to show acute inflammation and broad fungal hyphae seen on H&E stain (arrow).

paranasal sinuses commonly in tropical countries and tends to extend into orbit where it invades optic nerve and its surrounding soft tissue. The infection spreads very rapidly and may cause bland necrosis in some cases. Broad aseptate hyphae can be seen in necrotic areas as well as inflammation even on H&E stain (Figure 25.7b).

The chronic aspergillosis of paranasal sinus is also known to spread and produce granulomatous inflammation in the orbital contents including optic nerve (Figure 25.8a and b). There is varying degree of fibrosis and ill-defined granulomatous response accompanied by numerous bizarre multinucleated giant cells containing fungal profiles. These fungi are sparse in number and may be visualized as longitudinal septate hyphae or transverse cuts which are best visualized on PAS stain. The dural covering of optic nerve must offer some protection, but in many enucleated eyeballs, optic nerve involvement has been seen (Figure 25.9a). Arteritis and vascular invasion may be seen in and around the granulomas (Figure 25.9b).

Thyroid eye disease

Thyroid eye disease (TAO), a frequent problem in neuro-ophthalmic practice, generally manifests as diplopia, proptosis and visual loss. Commonly, both eyes are affected, but unilateral and asymmetric involvement may be seen. It presents with varied manifestations such as soft tissue inflammation, eyelid retraction, proptosis, restrictive myopathy and optic neuropathy.[16] The optic neuropathy and visual loss are a result of compression by enlarged muscles on the optic nerve or pressure on the vessels

that supply it. Females are more often affected than males. The mean age is about 40 years. The severity of ocular symptoms is far more in elderly patients compared to younger patients.

Although the natural course of the disease is not fully understood, the disease occurs in two phases. In an active phase, the lids, conjunctiva and the orbit are affected by active or chronic inflammation, and it lasts for about 3–6 months. It is followed by an inactive phase, when the inflammation subsides. It is followed by proptosis and extra-ocular muscle fibrosis. About 60% patients are known to show spontaneous improvement.

The ocular manifestations in TAO result from an auto-immune inflammatory process due to antibodies to a thyroid-stimulating hormone receptor and other auto-antigens present on the orbital fibroblasts. The autoimmune process gives rise to excessive synthesis of glycosaminoglycan by fibroblasts leading to increase in orbital volume which is followed by fibrosis of eye muscles.

Leber's hereditary optic neuropathy

Leber's hereditary optic neuropathy (LHON) is a condition that is characterized by focal subacute bilateral vision loss. Young adult males are more commonly affected. It is a mitochondrial genetic disease in which point mutations in genes encoding complex 1 subunit of the respiratory chain are known to occur. LHON starts with blurring of vision in one eye, but then it involves the other eye within weeks. Pupillary reflexes are often preserved and the eye movements are painless. During the acute phase, LHON exhibits tortuous retinal vessels, telangiectatic microangiopathy and swelling of the retinal nerve fiber layer. The optic disk may

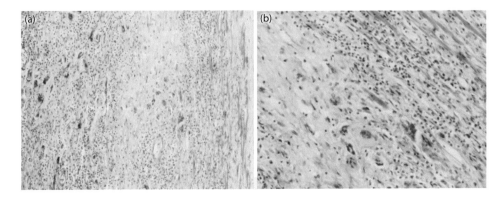

FIGURE 25.8 (a) Chronic granulomatous inflammation with multinucleate giant cells involving extraocular muscles and orbital soft tissue. (b) Higher magnification of b.

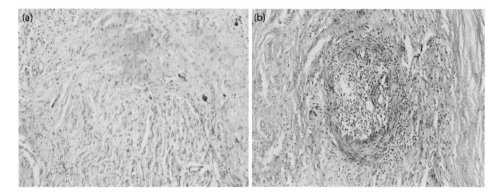

FIGURE 25.9 (a) Optic neuritis due to chronic aspergillus infection. (b) Arteritis and recanalized thrombus in a vessel around optic nerve.

look normal in about 20% cases. During the chronic phase, there is degeneration of retinal fiber layer with optic atrophy. At this point in time, it is very difficult to differentiate LHON from other causes of optic atrophy, and only genetic testing can reveal the etiology of optic atrophy.

The neuropathological findings in LHON involve retinal ganglion cell layer. There is sparing of retinal pigment layer and photoreceptor layer. A significant cell body and axonal degeneration are noticeable. These changes are accompanied by demyelination and atrophy, which may extend from the optic nerve to the lateral geniculate body. Since the point mutations in LHON are related to respiratory chain dysfunction, there is reduced ATP production, energy failure and degeneration of the retinal ganglion cells.[17]

Ocular myasthenia

Ocular myasthenia (OM) is a disorder related to the presence of antibodies to acetylcholine receptors causing dysfunction of the neuromuscular junctions. The clinical presentation in OM includes variable diplopia or ptosis or both. The symptoms worsen during late in the day. The general myasthenia gravis may develop in patients within 6 months to 2 years of manifestation of OM. About 10% patients display spontaneous remission. The disease is characterized by eye signs such as lid fatigue on prolonged upward gaze, ptosis, "peek sign," weakness of orbicularis oculi, lid flutter after blinking, etc.

The other diseases that may be associated with OM are Grave's disease, Hashimoto's thyroiditis, rheumatoid arthritis, systemic lupus erythematosus, sarcoidosis, thymoma, T-cell lymphoma, etc.

The differential diagnosis of OM gravis will include other conditions with ophthalmoplegia; for example, CPEO, cranial nerve palsies, parasellar tumors and myotonic dystrophy. Early and accurate diagnosis by multi-pronged assessment help patients avoid unnecessary treatment.[18]

Radiation-induced optic neuropathy

It is a rare but severe late-onset complication of external beam radiation therapy given for head and neck and skull-based neoplasms. Radiation-induced optic neuropathy (RION) presents as acute painless, unilateral or bilateral progressive loss of vision. The severity of vision loss may vary from mild to complete blindness. The actual pathogenesis is not fully understood, but it is thought to be due to radiation-induced ischemic necrosis of vascular endothelium by free radical damage. It is a well-known fact that mitochondria are highly sensitive to ionizing radiation. The

increased production of reactive oxygen species in radiation therapy alters mitochondrial homeostasis/function and leads to their irreversible damage. The number, morphology and distribution of mitochondria in neurons, axons and dendrites are all affected. The optic nerve gets damaged and the retinal ganglion cells are injured. The radiation dose determines the extent of damage in RION. It is suggested that anterior visual pathways is unable to tolerate more that 50Gy of cumulative radiation in fractions and less than 2Gy and the incidence of RION increases markedly at higher levels.[19] Other risk factors that are likely to increase the risk of RION are disease that affect the integrity of endothelial cells such as hypertension, hyperlipidemia, smoking and diabetes.[19] Compression of the optic nerve by a tumor and adjuvant chemotherapy may predispose the visual pathway to radiation injury.[20,21] Rong et al. have shown in their experimental work that exposure to radiation induced decline in retinal ganglion cell numbers and thinning of outer nuclear layer of retina.[22] The transmission electron microscopy revealed alterations in the mitochondrial morphology, excessive mitochondrial fragmentation and apoptosis following exposure to radiation.

Fungal infections

Invasive fungal infection of orbito-cerebral compartment is a common complication in immunocompromised patients. However, it can be encountered even in immunocompetent individuals as well.[23] The source of entry of fungus is either nasal cavity or paranasal sinuses. Invasive aspergillosis and mucormycosis are two important infections that affect orbito-cerebral compartment.

Orbital aspergillosis usually presents as a slow-growing orbital mass. Aspergillosis on histological examination shows granulomatous inflammation with numerous foreign body giant cells. There is random stromal fibrosis and variable degree of inflammation comprising of lymphocytes, plasma cells and eosinophils (Figure 25.10a). The giant cells contain fragmented fungal profiles, which are difficult to find but can be better highlighted by special stains such as PAS (Figure 25.10b) and Grocott's silver stain. The fungi are composed of septate hyphae with acute angle branching, but many a times, transverse cuts of hyphae are seen. Necrosis may be present focally unlike zygomycosis where extensive bland necrosis is present. When extension of orbital aspergillosis into intracranial compartment occurs, it may involve anterior or middle cranial fossa giving rise to basal meningitis, arteritis and necrosis of areas supplied by involved arteries

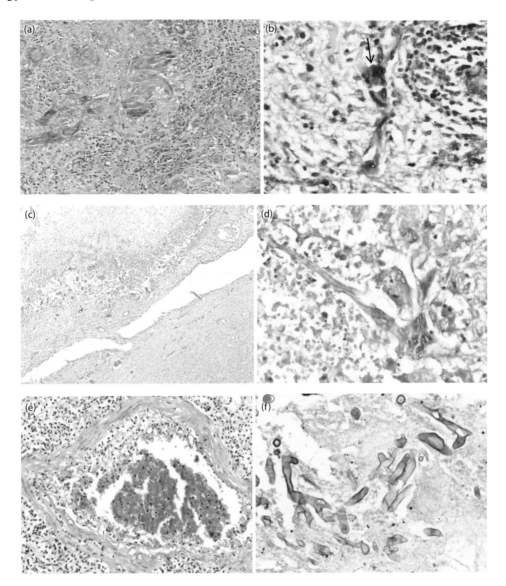

FIGURE 25.10 (a) Aspergillosis: Multiple epithelioid granulomas with multinucleate giant cells and fibrosis. (b) Higher power to show septate fungal hyphae in the giant cells on PAS stain (arrow). (c) Meninges over midbrain show granulomatous inflammation and (d) higher magnification to show giant cells and fungal hyphae in basal meningitis. (e) Orbital mucormycosis showing arteritis with invasion by fungus. (f) Numerous broad, aseptate and folded hyphae are seen on H&E stain.

(Figure 25.10c and 10d). Angio invasion and arteritic changes are the common feature of invasive aspergillosis. Aspergillus arteritis involving internal carotid artery can also present as stroke and blindness.[24]

Naso-orbital/sino-orbital mucormycosis has a fulminant clinical course. On histology, it shows extensive tissue necrosis, which can be bland or accompanied with neutrophilic infiltrate. The fungus is extremely destructive particularly in immunocompromised individuals and diabetics. It extends into the basifrontal area causing meningitis and parenchymal lesions. Compared to the aspergillus infection, granulomatous inflammation is not commonly seen in mucormycosis. Frequently, vascular necrosis, angioinvasion and thrombotic occlusion occurs which results in infarction of orbital contents (Figure 25.10e). All the orbital structures are destroyed by acute necrotizing inflammation, and

therefore, multinucleate giant cells and fibrosis are not found. Many broad, aseptate, right-angle branching fungal hyphae can be easily seen on routine H&E stain (Figure 25.10f), but these can be highlighted by PAS and silver stain. Angioinvasion is a common feature of mucormycosis, and thus mucor can invade retinal artery and vein, causing acute blindness.[25] Fungal infection from orbit is catastrophic when it spreads to brain.

Neurocysticercosis
Neurocysticercosis is a leading cause of acquired epilepsy in developing countries. The disease is worldwide but more prevalent in Southeast Asia, Africa and Brazil. It has been related to poor hygiene and sanitation, but it is largely prevalent in urban middle-class people. Although it is preventable and treatable parasitic disease, it poses a huge economic burden on health-care

system. The disease is produced by the ingestion of the eggs of Taenia solium (tapeworm), which hatch into larva in the intestine. The larva penetrates the intestinal wall, gets access into blood stream and disseminates to other body tissues such as brain, skeletal muscle, tongue, subcutaneous tissue and eyes where it gives rise to cysts. The live cyst remains protected from human immune system and does not initiate any inflammatory reaction. However, when the larva starts degenerating, the cyst wall leaks the toxins from the cyst fluid which evokes varying degree of peri-cytic inflammatory reaction including a granulomatous response. Eventually, the larva dies and disappears or gets calcified. In brain, it may produce meningeal, parenchymal, intraventricular or spinal cysts. Intraocular cysts are well described and conjunctival cysts have been seen in our surgical material. The magnetic resonance imaging (MRI) is the best technique to diagnose degree of infection, its location and evolutionary stages of the parasite. The lesions in brain are usually multiple, but sometimes solitary lesion may be demonstrated which shows contrast enhancement. In endemic countries like India, a differential diagnosis such as tuberculoma, pyogenic brain abscesses, fungal abscess, toxoplasmosis, a primary or metastatic brain tumor and infectious vasculitis all have been considered.[26] Orbital cysticercosis may involve extraocular muscle, subconjunctival space, eyelids, retro-orbital tissue and even optic nerve. Rarely, posterior segment cysticercosis such as vitreous and subretinal are also reported.[27] Depending on the location, ocular symptoms appear and may cause of blindness in endemic areas. The optic nerve per se is rarely affected. However, the involvement of other orbital tissue may compress the optic nerves which lead to disc edema and reduced vision. When the cysts are multiple or single cyst is large, ocular movements may be restricted and axial proptosis may appear. The subconjunctival cysticercosis has a thin wall, and therefore, on excision, only larva may be demonstrated on biopsy with scant accompanying inflammatory response (Figure 25.11). However, the cysts in the lid or orbital space may show chronic inflammatory reaction, or a granulomatous reaction with typical palisading histiocytes, occasional giant cells and even focal calcification.

Hemangiomas and vascular malformations

Hemangiomas and vascular malformations are commonly encountered in orbit. Such lesions may compress optic nerve and other intra-orbital structures. Various forms of vascular malformation can involve orbit, such as cavernous hemangioma, capillary hemangioma, arteriovenous malformation (AVM), lymphangioma and venous malformation. The cavernous

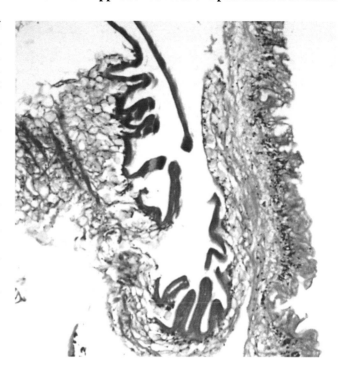

FIGURE 25.11 The histology showing only wall of the larva on excision.

hemangioma is the commonest orbital lesion seen in adults. It is a well-circumscribed tumor composed of dilated vascular channels which are lined by single layer of endothelial cells and separated by fibrous stroma (Figure 25.12a). If required endothelial cells can be highlighted by immunostaining for CD31 (Figure 25.12b). The walls may contain smooth muscle fibers.

The capillary hemangioma shows a lobulated tumor composed of capillary size vascular channels or solid clusters of proliferating endothelial cells (Figure 25.13). The stroma separating the vascular channels shows edema and myxoid changes. Few larger feeder vessels may be seen in between the lobules. The endothelial cells of hemangiomas can be outlined by immunostaining with CD31.

The lymphangioma shows dilated vascular spaces of variable thickness which are lined by single layer of lymphatic endothelium which are positive for D2-40 on immunostaining. The wall

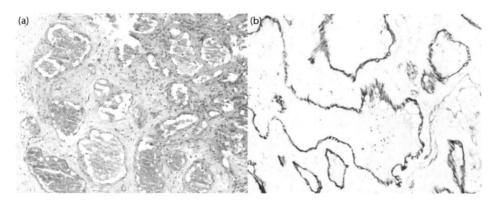

FIGURE 25.12 (a) Cavernous hemangioma consisting of dilated vascular spaces with intervening stroma (H&E). (b) IHC using anti-CD31 antibody labels endothelial cells of the cavernous spaces.

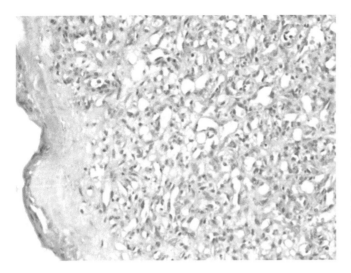

FIGURE 25.13 Capillary hemangioma showing small clusters of endothelial cells, many of which contain a lumina.

of the vascular channels in lymphangioma may show lymphoid aggregates. Venous malformation is composed of variable size vascular channels, showing variable wall thickness. The venous channels show arterialization of the wall with prominent musculature. Calcification or thrombosis of the vascular channels may be seen in AVM.[28,29]

Neoplastic

Optic pathway glioma

The optic pathway gliomas (OPG) constitutes around 66% of the primary optic pathway tumors. The optic pathway includes retina, optic nerve, optic chiasma, optic radiation and visual cortex. OPG is usually seen in children <10 years of age and these account for 3–5% of all pediatric CNS tumors. This tumor is more commonly encountered in patients with neurofibromatosis type 1. The common presenting feature depends upon the location of the tumor. The posteriorly placed tumors in the optic nerve will present either with hypothalamic symptoms or chiasmic field defects, whereas the tumor located in the anterior part of optic nerve will present with axial proptosis or visual loss. In OPG, the optic nerve gets swollen as a result of expansion of individual axonal compartments which are separated by intervening fibrous septae (Figure 25.14a).

The overlying dura, however, remain intact. In early part of disease, axons only get distorted, and therefore, visual acuity is unaffected. Later on there is visual loss because axons are destroyed. Morphologically, most of the OPGs are pilocytic astrocytoma, WHO grade 1. These are well-circumscribed tumors which typically exhibit biphasic morphology (Figure 25.14a). There are piloid areas composed of bipolar astrocytes alternating with protoplasmic areas which may show microcystic change. Rosenthal fibers and eosinophilic globular bodies (EGBs) are common finding (Figure 25.15a). The tumor shows hyalinized vessels, but necrosis and mitosis are rarely observed. Microcalcification may be seen (Figure 25.15b). Another feature in optic nerve glioma is exuberant accompanying meningothelial hyperplasia in perineural compartment. Such proliferation may mimic a meningioma and thus poses a diagnostic problem if a superficial biopsy is taken from this OPG. Rarely, grade II diffuse astrocytoma or higher histological grade gliomas are reported in optic pathway.

Retinoblastoma

Retinoblastoma is a common childhood intraocular tumor which accounts for 3% of all childhood cancers.[31] It is commonly diagnosed at an average age of 18 months but generally before the age of 5. The highest disease burden is reported from Asia and Africa, being the most populous countries with higher birth rates.[32] Retinoblastoma is caused by mutational inactivation of both alleles of the RB1 gene which maps to chromosome 13q14. The gene encodes retinoblastoma protein which acts as a tumor suppressor.[33] The retinoblastoma may occur as a bilateral tumor due to germline mutations in RB1 gene, and 15% of unilateral cases have a heritable mutation. The most common manifestation in retinoblastoma is leukocoria followed by strabismus, painful blind eye and visual loss.[32] In Southeast Asian countries, most retinoblastoma patients present late and at advanced stage of the disease. Fortunately, with current advancement in treatment protocols, the eye can be salvaged with chemotherapy particularly when the tumor is intraocular. Following chemotherapy, if there is a residual tumor, the eye is enucleated. On subsequent evaluation, when spread to extraocular compartment or to the optic nerve is demonstrated, the patient needs adjuvant radiotherapy. The pathology specimens should be evaluated in detail since all histology information is important for further treatment.[32]

The retinoblastoma arises from either the inner or outer nuclear layer of retina. It may show an endophytic or exophytic or both. The endophytic growth fills the vitreous chamber and exophytic tumor grows outwardly and lifts the retina

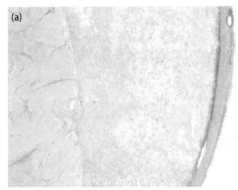
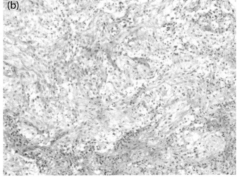

FIGURE 25.14 Optic pathway glioma: (a) The optic nerve is markedly swollen by the tumor which is restricted within dura. (b) Biphasic pattern on histology.

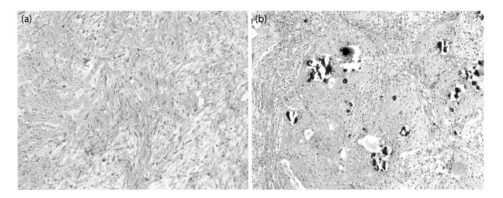

FIGURE 25.15 Optic pathway glioma: (a) Numerous Rosenthal fibers appearing as bright eosinophilic twisted structures. (b) Microcalcification is noted within tumor.[30]

(Figure 25.16a and b). The tumor looks pale necrotic mass with area of necrosis and calcification. Histological diagnosis is generally straightforward. The histology is that of a blue round cell tumor disposed in a diffuse sheet of cells (Figure 25.16c). The tumor cells contain small amount of cytoplasm and a large hyperchromatic nucleus. The cells may be polygonal in shape and exhibit variable degree of anaplasia mimicking morphology of large cell medulloblastoma. Perivascular arrangement of cells surrounding a necrotic area may be found. Cellular differentiation may either be in the form of Flexner-Wintersteiner rosettes which are composed of an "empty" lumen surrounded by columnar cells or the Homer Wright rosettes consisting of cells surrounding

a central lumen made up of their processes (Figure 25.16d).[34] The dual presence of Homer Wright and Flexner-Wintersteiner rosettes is pathognomonic for retinoblastoma. Cellular differentiation is not necessarily associated with prognosis, and therefore, it is not an important histologic parameter for evaluation. Rather the degree of anaplasia is known to be associated with outcome of the patients. Poorly differentiated tumor shows brisk mitoses. Microscopic areas of necrosis and calcification are frequently observed. Tumors with germline mutation may show multifocal tumors arising from retina. Currently, most tumors are treated with chemotherapy, and if eye is enucleated due to any indication, it may be difficult to find any residual tumor in pathology

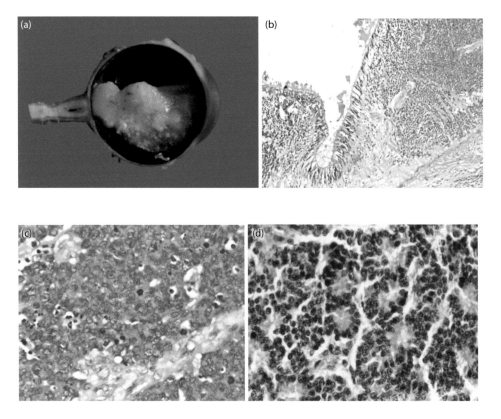

FIGURE 25.16 (a) Retinoblastoma. Pale, grayish to pink tumor occupying the entire posterior chamber. (b) The tumor lifts the retina. (c) Diffuse sheets of the anaplastic tumor cells with numerous mitoses. (d) Homer Wright rosettes consisting of cells surrounding fibrillary material.

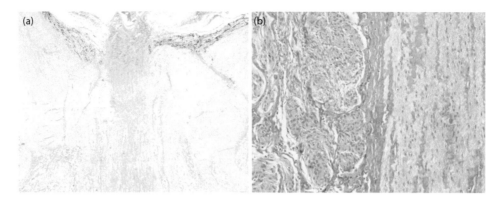

FIGURE 25.17 (a) The optic nerve is wrapped around by a meningioma. (b) Higher magnification shows meningothelial morphology, and tumor does not infiltrate the optic nerve.

specimens. In such situations, many ophthalmologists cross-check with the reporting pathologist about the presence or the absence of tumor in specific suspected locations. Further radiotherapy treatment will depend on pathologist's report. Invasion into choroid could be focal (less than 3mm in any diameter) or massive (more than 3mm in any diameter– thickness or width).[33] Some tumors may invade sclera and extend into the extraocular space. Such cases have bad prognosis. Retinoblastoma may spread along the optic nerve or through subarachnoid space to involve intracranial compartment. Optic nerve invasion should be graded as pre-laminar, post-laminar or extending up to resected margin. Massive choroid invasion, retrolaminar invasion, involvement of anterior chamber, iris, sclera and extra scleral compartment are all associated with greater chance of recurrence and metastasis. Such tumors require adjuvant radiotherapy.[33] Sudden tumor regressions are known to occur.

Meningioma

The optic pathway meningiomas constitute 1–2% of all optic pathway tumors and 1–2% of all orbital tumors. Most of the meningiomas involving optic pathway are WHO grade I, and meningothelial meningioma is the commonest among them. The optic sheath meningioma differs from adult intracranial meningiomas in two ways: (1) they occur in younger age-group, and (2) there is no female predominance. Those arising from optic nerve sheath typical grow around optic nerve meningioma and optic nerve appears to be wrapped around by the tumor (Figure 25.17a). Most of them are composed of meningothelial

cells, arranged in whorls and short fascicles and commonly display syncytial arrangement of the cells (Figure 25.17b). The individual cells are monomorphic and show intranuclear cytoplasmic pseudo inclusions. Mitosis is <4/10 high power field and necrosis is rare. Psammomatous calcification is a frequent observation. Immunohistochemically, the meningothelial cells show positivity for epithelial membrane antigen (EMA) and vimentin, but they are negative for glial fibrillary acid protein (GFAP). Optic pathway meningiomas are associated with good outcome.[35]

Schwannoma

Schwannoma is a slow-growing, benign nerve sheath tumor accounting for less than 1% of the orbital tumors and arises from branches of nerves traversing the orbit such as oculomotor, trochlear or abducens.[36–38] Due to complexity of orbital structures, it's difficult to point out the origin. Small tumors are asymptomatic, but as they grow they compress the nerve in which they arise and also the surrounding structures. Most of the patients are adult and proptosis is the commonest presentation. Lid swelling is another prominent feature. MRI is very sensitive neuro-imaging technique for diagnosis. Macroscopically, a schwannoma appears encapsulated mass with a homogeneous, grayish-white cut surface, which may contain areas of hemorrhage. Histologically, schwannoma shows hypo- and hypercellular areas (Figure 25.18a). The cells show nuclear palisading and Verocay body formation (Figure 25.18b). The individual cells show spindle-shaped nuclei with pointed ends. These cells express S-100 protein on immunostaining. Mitosis and necrosis are rarely found. Hyalinized blood vessels as well

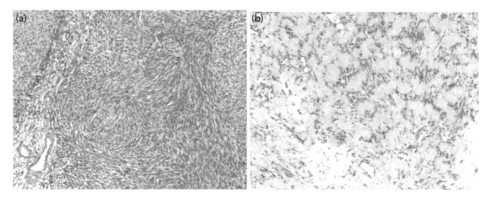

FIGURE 25.18 (a) Schwannoma consisting of fascicles of spindle cells. (b) Typical Verocay body formation.

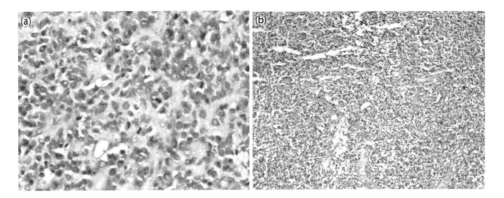

FIGURE 25.19   (a) Diffuse sheet of large lymphoid cells with numerous mitoses. (b) Diffuse positivity for CD20, a B-cell marker (IHC).

as secondary degenerative changes such as edema, variable cystic degeneration, and infiltration by foamy macrophages are common findings. Orbital schwannomas often extend into cavernous sinus. A complete surgical excision is usually curative.

Lymphomas

Lymphomas can rarely involve orbit and ocular adnexal structures. Orbital lymphomas are usually seen in older age-group. Majority of the orbital lymphomas are B-cell type (97%). Among B-cell lymphomas, almost all types of lymphoma have been reported in the orbit. The low-grade B-cell lymphomas outnumber the high-grade B-cell lymphomas. Among the low-grade B-cell lymphomas in orbit, marginal zone lymphoma (MALToma) is the commonest type, followed by follicular lymphoma and mantle cell lymphoma. Low-grade B-cell lymphomas are composed of small size lymphocytes which are 1–1.5 times the size of mature lymphocytes, and they exhibit nodular to diffuse architecture. The MALTomas show presence of lymphoepithelial lesions. Among high-grade lymphomas, diffuse large B-cell lymphoma (DLBCL) is the commonest type. It shows diffuse architecture and is composed of large lymphoid cells, 2–3 times the size of mature lymphocytes containing frequent mitoses (Figure 25.19a). Immunohistochemistry is essential for exact categorization of the lymphoma, which is essential for adequate management (Figure 25.19a). MALToma and follicular lymphoma usually carry good prognosis, while mantle cell lymphoma and DLBCL are associated with poor prognosis.[39,40]

Pseudolymphoma

Pseudolymphoma of orbit is a rare entity and pathologically shows reactive lymphoid hyperplasia. Clinically and radiologically, orbital pseudolymphoma is indistinguishable from orbital low-grade lymphoma. Histologically, pseudolymphoma shows reactive lymphoid hyperplasia with proliferation of both B and T lymphocytes (Figure 25.20). It shows different size nodules, composed of B cells, surrounded by T lymphocytes. However, it is now believed that most of the cases diagnosed as pseudolymphoma are actually low-grade B-cell lymphoma, namely MALToma. The prognosis of ocular/orbital pseudolymphoma is favorable. However, these patients should be kept in close follow-up, as certain percentage of patients may develop lymphoma.[41]

Plasmacytoma

Plasmacytoma is characterized by extramedullary clonal plasma cell proliferation. Most of the cases of plasmacytomas are associated with multiple myeloma. Pure extramedullary plasmacytoma is rare and usually involves upper aerodigestive tract. Orbital plasmacytoma is very rare.[42,43] Histology shows plasma cell proliferation, with or without amyloid deposition. The diagnosis is confirmed on IHC using anti-CD138 antibodies (Figure 25.21). The plasma cells show features of immaturity and binucleation. Orbital plasmacytomas are associated with poor prognosis.

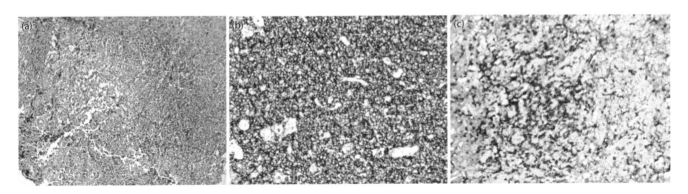

FIGURE 25.20   (a) The orbital tissue is infiltrated by reactive lymphoid cells. IHC shows positivity for both CD20 (b) and CD3 (c) markers.

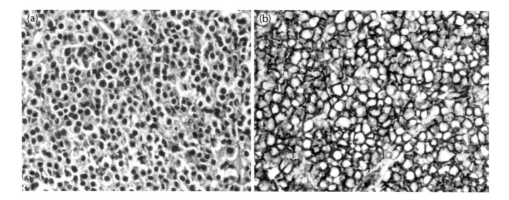

FIGURE 25.21 Orbital plasmacytoma showing sheets of atypical plasma (a) cells which are immunopositive for CD138 (b).

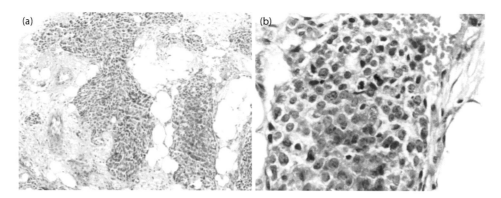

FIGURE 25.22 (a) Metastatic carcinoma from breast showing groups of malignant epithelial cells infiltrating orbital fat and fibrous tissue. (b) Higher magnification showing numerous atypical mitoses.

Metastatic carcinoma

Orbital metastasis is rare. The incidence of metastatic carcinoma varies from 1% to 13% of all orbital tumors in different studies. Orbital metastasis usually presents as proptosis in elderly patients. Rarely, orbital metastasis can be the presenting symptom of some internal malignancy. Breast is the commonest primary site of malignancy, followed by lung and prostate. Histological examination is essential to differentiate it from primary orbital pathology.[44] The histology demonstrates groups of atypical, pleomorphic epithelial cells with frequent mitoses surrounded by stromal fibroblastic reaction (Figure 25.22).

Conclusion

The brain territories supplied by the vertebral and basilar arteries are particularly important in perception of the visual environment and in focusing the eyes on visual objects. The symptoms and signs can be divided into those that involve afferent findings (seeing) and those that are efferent and oculomotor (looking), and pupillary abnormalities. Recognizing neuro-ophthalmic findings in patients with posterior circulation ischemia and haemorrhage may provide vital clues to early diagnosis aiding in prompt management of these patients.

Multiple-Choice Questions

1. Regarding giant cell arteritis, which of the following is INCORRECT?
   a. It is a chronic disease which affects elderly individuals.
   b. Presence of giant cell on histology is a must for diagnosis.
   c. Aneurysm dilatation of artery may occur due to fragmentation of elastica.
   d. A negative biopsy excludes the diagnosis.

   Answer:
   b. Presence of giant cell on histology is a must for diagnosis.

2. Chronic progressive external ophthalmoplegia is a mitochondrial disorder, which is clinically characterized by progressive bilateral ptosis, proximal muscle weakness, external ophthalmoplegia, and sensorineural hearing loss. Choose the CORRECT answer from the following:
   a. Ragged red fibers are typically seen in muscle fibers on NADH histochemical satin.
   b. COX-SDH stain is less sensitive for detection of mitochondrial myopathy than Gomori trichrome stain.
   c. Ultrastructural examination of muscle biopsy shows abnormal mitochondrial accumulation in paranuclear location.

d. The diagnosis must be confirmed by biochemical mitochondrial assays and genetic testing.

Answer:

d. The diagnosis must be confirmed by biochemical mitochondrial assays and genetic testing.

3. Orbito-cranial aspergillosis is characterized by all of the following, EXCEPT:
   a. It demonstrates chronic granulomatous inflammation of intra-orbital structures.
   b. Multinucleate giant cells are commonly encountered.
   c. Numerous fungal hyphae and extensive necrosis are frequently seen.
   d. The fungi are septate and show acute angle branching.

Answer:

c. Numerous fungal hyphae and extensive necrosis are frequently seen.

4. The optic pathway glioma (OPG) is more commonly encountered in pediatric age-group. Which of the following is INCORRECT about optic pathway gliomas?
   a. OPG manifests as an infiltrative tumor which invades overlying dura.
   b. The optic nerve is swollen and is accompanied by expansion of its individual compartments.
   c. Typically, biphasic pattern on histology may be seen.
   d. The presence of Rosenthal fibers is a diagnostic feature on histology.

Answer:

a. OPG manifests as an infiltrative tumor which invades overlying dura.

References

1. Heighton JN, Brady LI, Sadikovic B, Bulman DE, Tarnopolsky MA. Genotypes of chronic progressive external ophthalmoplegia in a large adult-onset cohort. Mitochondrion. 2019;49:227–31.
2. Chen T, Pu C, Shi Q, et al. Chronic progressive external ophthalmoplegia with inflammatory myopathy. Int J Clin Exp Pathol. 2014;7(12):8887–92.
3. McClelland C, Manousakis G, Lee MS. Progressive external ophthalmoplegia. Curr Neurol Neurosci Rep. 2016;16(6):53.
4. Lucas C-H G and Margeta M. Educational case–Mitochondrial myopathy. Acad Pathol.2019;6:1–6.
5. Radotra BD, Aggarwal A, Kapoor A, Singla N, Chaterjee D. An orphan disease: IgG4-related pachymeningitis: Report of two cases. J Neurosurg Spine. 2016;2:790–4.
6. Andron A, Hostovsky A, Nair AG, Sagiv O, Schiby G, Simon GB. The impact ofIgG-4-ROD on the diagnosis of orbital tumors: A retrospective analysis. Orbit. 2017;36(6):359–64.
7. Andrew NH, Sladden N, Kearney DJ, Selva D. An analysis of IgG4-related disease (IgG4-RD) among idiopathic orbital inflammations and benign lymphoid hyperplasias using two consensus-based diagnostic criteria for IgG4-RD. Br J Ophthalmol. 2015;99(3):376–81.
8. Mavrikakis I, Rootman J. Diverse clinical presentations of orbital sarcoid. Am J Ophthalmol. 2007;144(5):769–75.
9. Demirci H, Christianson MD. Orbital and adnexal involvement in sarcoidosis: Analysis of clinical features and systemic disease in 30 cases. Am J Ophthalmol. 2011;151(6):1074–80.
10. Lacomis D. Neurosarcoidosis. Curr Neuropharmacol. 2011;9:429–36.
11. Pasadhika S and Rosenbaum JT. Ocular sarcoidosis. Clin Chest Med. 2015;36:669–83.
12. Modi M, Bhatia R, Jain R, Lal V, Radotra BD, Aggarwal A. Uncommon manifestations of neurosarcoidosis. Neurol India. 2004;52:280–1.
13. Bennett JL. Optic neuritis. Continuum (Minneap Minn) Author manuscript; available in PMC 2020 Aug 1. Published in final edited form as: Continuum (Minneap Minn). 2019;25(5):1236–64.
14. Jarius S, Whildemann B, Paul F. Neuromyelitis optica: Clinical features, immunopathogenesis and treatment. Clin Exp Immunol. 2014;176:149–64.
15. Kahloun R, Abroug N, Ksiaa I, Mahmoud A, Zeghidi H, Zaouali S, Khairallah M. Infectious optic neuropathies: A clinical update. Eye Brain. 2015;7:59–81.
16. Sahli E, Gunduz K. Thyroid-associated ophthalmopathy. Turk J Ophthalmol. 2017;47:94–105.
17. Man PYW, Turnbull DM, Chinnery PF. Leber hereditary optic neuropathy. J Med genet. 2002;39:162–9.
18. MacVie OP, Majid MA, Husssin HM, Ung T, Manners RM, Ormerod I, Pawade J, Harrad RA. Idiopathic isolated orbicularis weakness. Eye (Lond). 2012;26:746–8.
19. Ferguson I, Huecker J, Huang J, McClelland C, Stavern GV. Risk factors for radiation-induced optic neuropathy: A case-control study. Clin Exp Ophthalmol. 2017;45(6):592–7.
20. Deng X, Yang Z, Liu R, et al. The maximum tolerated dose of gamma radiation to the optic nerve during gamma knife radiosurgery in an animal study. Stereotact Funct Neurosurg. 2013;91(2):79–91.
21. Guy J, Mancuso A, Beck R, et al. Radiation-induced optic neuropathy: Amagnetic resonance imaging study. J Neurosurg. 1991;74(3):426–32.
22. Rong R, Xia X, Peng H, Li H, You M, Liang Z, Yao F, Yao X, Xiong K, Huang J, Zhou R, Ji D. Cdk5-mediated Drp1 phosphorylation drives mitochondrial defects and neuronal apoptosis in radiation-induced optic neuropathy. Cell Death Dis.2020;11(9):720.
23. Adulkar NG, Radhakrishnan S, Vidhya N, Kim U. Invasive sino-orbital fungal infections in immunocompetent patients: A clinico-pathological study. Eye (Lond). 2019;33(6):988–94.
24. Chatterjee D, Radotra BD, Mukherjee KK. Aspergillus arteritis of the right internal carotid artery resulting in massive stroke. Neurol India. 2016;64(5):1089–91.
25. Bawankar P, Lahane S, Pathak P, Gonde P, Singh A. Central retinal artery occlusion as the presenting manifestation of invasive rhino-orbital-cerebral mucormycosis. Taiwan J Ophthalmol. 2020;10(1):62–5.
26. Sinha S and Sharma BS. Neurocysticercosis: A review of current status and management. J Clin Neurosci. 2009;16:867–76.
27. Dhiman R, Devi S, Duraipandi K, Chandra P, Vanathi M, Tandon R, Sen S. Cysticercosis of the eye. Int J Ophthalmol. 2017;10:1319–24.
28. Colletti G, Biglioli F, Poli T, Dessy M, Cucurullo M, Petrillo M, Tombris S, Waner M, Sesenna E. Vascular malformations of the orbit (lymphatic, venous, arteriovenous): Diagnosis, management and results. J Craniomaxillofac Surg. 2019;47(5):726–40.
29. Calandriello L, Grimaldi G, Petrone G, Rigante M, Petroni S, Riso M, Savino G. Cavernous venous malformation (cavernous hemangioma) of the orbit: Current concepts and a review of the literature. Surv Ophthalmol. 2017;62(4):393–403.
30. Fried I, Tabori U, Tihan T, Reginald A, Bouffet E. Optic pathway gliomas: A review. CNS Oncol. 2013;2(2):143–59.
31. Rao R and Honavar SG. Retinoblastoma. Ind J Pediatr. 2017;84:937–944.
32. Dimaras H, Kimani K, Dimba EA, Gonsdahl P, White A, Chan HSL, Gallie BL. Retinoblastoma. Lancet. 2012;379:1436–46.
33. Singh L and Kashyap S. Update on pathology of retinoblastoma. Int J Ophthalmol. 2018;11:2011–16.
34. Dimaras H and Corson TW. Retinoblastoma, the visible CNS tumor: A review. J Neurosci Res. 2019;97:29–44.
35. Furdová A, Babál P, Kobzová D. Optic nerve orbital meningioma. Cesk Slov Oftalmol. Spring 2018;74(1):23–30.
36. Yong KL, Beckman TJ, Cranstoun M, Sullivan TJ. Orbital schwannoma-management and clinical outcomes. Ophthalmic Plast Reconstr Surg. 2020;36:590–5.
37. Pointdujour-Lim R, Lally SE, Shields JA, Eagle RC Jr, Shields CL. Orbital schwannoma: Radiographic and histopathologic correlation in 15 cases. Ophthalmic Plast Reconstr Surg. 2018;34(2):162–7.
38. Kim KS, Jung JW, Yoon KC, Kwon YJ, Hwang JH, Lee SY. Schwannoma of the orbit. Arch Craniofac Surg. 2015;16:67–72.
39. Olsen TG, Heegaard S. Orbital lymphoma. Surv Ophthalmol. 2019;64(1):45–66.
40. Ahmed OM, Ma AK, Ahmed TM, Pointdujour-Lim R. Epidemiology, outcomes, and prognostic factors of orbital lymphoma in the United States. Orbit. 2020;2:1–6.
41. Andrew NH, Coupland SE, Pirbhai A, Selva D. Lymphoid hyperplasia of the orbit and ocular adnexa: A clinical pathologic review. Surv Ophthalmol. 2016;61:778–90.
42. Wang SSY, Lee MB, George A, Wang SB, Blackwell J, Moran S, Francis IC. Five cases of orbital extramedullary plasmacytoma: Diagnosis and management of an aggressive malignancy. Orbit. 2019;38(3):218–25.
43. Adkins JW, Shields JA, Shields CL, Eagle RC Jr, Flanagan JC, Campanella PC. Plasmacytoma of the eye and orbit. Int Ophthalmol. 1996–1997;20(6):339–43.
44. Allen RC. Orbital metastases: When to suspect? When to biopsy? Middle East Afr J Ophthalmol. 2018;25(2):60–64.

ANSWERS TO CASE STUDIES

Page 67:

Retrobulbar optic neuritis secondary to primary demyelinating diseases should be considered in view of typical history and normal optic disc examination. Presence of multiple T2 hyperintense lesions involving juxtacortical and subcortical white matter was a giveaway in this patient suggesting optic neuritis due to Multiple sclerosis. This chapter discusses about the differentials of optic neuritis and their characteristic features.

Page 81:

Presence of bilateral disc oedema, preserved visual acuity with constricted visual fields in the background of obesity, chronic headache and transient visual obscuration suggest increased intracranial pressure. Detailed evaluation should be done in such scenario to rule out secondary causes. Idiopathic intracranial hypertension/Pseudotumor cerebri syndrome should be considered after ruling out other causes.

Page 90:

Involvement of both the optic nerve and orbital structures suggests an orbital inflammatory syndrome. In this case prominent involvement of lacrimal glands should raise suspicion of granulomatous inflammation like sarcoidosis.

Page 99:

Presence of thick exudates and opto-chiasmatic arachnoiditis suggests infectious granulomatous inflammatory causes like tuberculosis in this clinical scenario. This chapter discusses the differentials of infectious causes of optic nerve involvement.

Page 108:

History of acute/subacute visual loss in a patient with vascular risk factors should alert a physician towards possibility of ischemic optic neuropathy. Other clues in this patient were presence of inferior hemifield deficit and prior history of similar illness in the other eye.

Page 120:

Presence of peripapillary hemorrhages and creamy white exudates with severe, bilateral and rapid diminution of vision suggests an atypical optic neuritis. In addition, imaging finding of enlarged optic nerves and chiasma with the above clinical findings suggest an infiltrative pathology.

Page 129:

Long standing malabsorption can lead on to nutritional deficiencies of various vitamins like Vitamin B12. In addition, tobacco is itself a risk factor for the development of nutritional optic neuropathy. Imaging can be normal in such cases or may show optic atrophy in long standing cases.

Page 138:

Hereditary optic neuropathy is an important differential in patients presenting with subacute, painless, central visual loss. Often the involvement is either sequential or bilateral. Overall visual prognosis in these conditions is guarded.

Page

Normal ophthalmic examination with inconsistent visual symptoms should raise suspicion of non-organic visual loss. These cases must be evaluated very carefully in order to not to miss a subtle underlying treatable cause.

Page 158:

Dilated pupil with a slow, attenuated or absent light reflex is suggestive of damage to the postganglionic parasympathetic fibers. The pupils may show a preserved or even exaggerated accommodation reflex (light near dissociation) because of the important anatomical factors as described in this chapter.

Page 163:

Ocular motor cranial neuropathies may occur in a host of clinical conditions. While local, structural and vascular causes are common culprits, a detailed knowledge about the anatomical localization of these nerves often provide vital clues to diagnosis.

Page 170:

Fluctuating ptosis with fatigability and diurnal variation are hallmarks of a postganglionic neuromuscular junction defect. Other causes of impaired neuromuscular transmission should be borne into mind in suggestive clinical scenarios.

Page 178:

Combination of optic nerve involvement with other orbital structures like extraocular muscles and characteristic imaging findings in right cavernous sinus and orbital apex suggest ongoing inflammatory process. A physician should rule out secondary causes of orbital inflammatory syndrome before considering benign/idiopathic aetiologies.

Page 185:

Congenital cranial dysinnervation syndromes should be considered when encountered with congenital, nonprogressive or familial cranial musculature deficits. The disorders are broadly classified into ones with predominantly horizontal ocular motility restriction, with predominantly vertical ocular motility restriction and those affecting facial muscles. This chapter deals with how to approach such a patient with brief description of these disorders.

Page 193:

Rhino-orbital-cerebral mucormycosis are angio-invasive fungal infections common in individuals with risk factors like immunosuppression, uncontrolled diabetes, organ transplant, underlying malignancy, trauma etc. Infection associated ocular cranial nerve palsies should be considered in clinically suggestive scenarios specially in the background of predisposing factors.

Page 210:

Parinaud's syndrome is a neuro-ophthalmic syndrome characterized by up-gaze palsy, convergence retraction nystagmus and light near dissociation which results from the affection of dorsal midbrain region. Damage to the vertical gaze center, its supranuclear connections and decussating fibers of the pretectal nucleus in the posterior commissure leads on to this constellation of symptoms.

Page 221:

Multidirectional, rapid, chaotic, conjugate, arrhythmic saccadic intrusions without intersaccadic interval are termed as opsoclonus. Neuroblastoma, paraneoplastic brain involvement and infectious/para infectious aetiologies are some of the common causes.

Page 249:
Balint's syndrome is a triad of visuo-spatial dysfunctions-simultagnosia, optic ataxia and oculomotor apraxia. It is an essentially a dorsal visual syndrome.

Page 270:
The child is likely to be having optic nerve hypoplasia.

Page 278:
The chid is having infantile esotropia.

INDEX

Note: Locators in *italics* represent figures and **bold** indicate tables in the text.